STEP-UP TO USMLE Step 1

2013

STEP-UP

TO

USMLE Step 1

2013

Brian Jenkins, MD
Family Medicine
President, and Chief Educator
Doctors in Training.com, LLC
Fort Worth, Texas

Samir Mehta, MD
Assistant Professor
Department of Orthopaedic Surgery
Chief, Orthopaedic Trauma Service
The Hospital of the University of Pennsylvania
Philadelphia, Pennsylvania

Michael McInnis, MD
Internal Medicine
Chief Educator
Doctors in Training.com, LLC
Fort Worth, Texas

Chris Lewis, MD
Family Medicine
Chief Educator
Doctors in Training.com, LLC
Austin, Texas

Sonia Mehta, MD
Resident Physician
Department of Ophthalmology
Scheie Eye Institute
University of Pennsylvania
Philadelphia, Pennsylvania

LCDR Edmund A. Milder, MC USNR
Department of Pediatrics
Naval Medical Center
San Diego, California

Sonul Mehta, MD
Resident Physician
Department of Ophthalmology
Georgetown University/Washington Hospital Center
Washington, District of Columbia

Adam J. Mirarchi, MD
Assistant Professor
Department of Orthopaedic Surgery
Oregon Health & Science University
Portland, Oregon

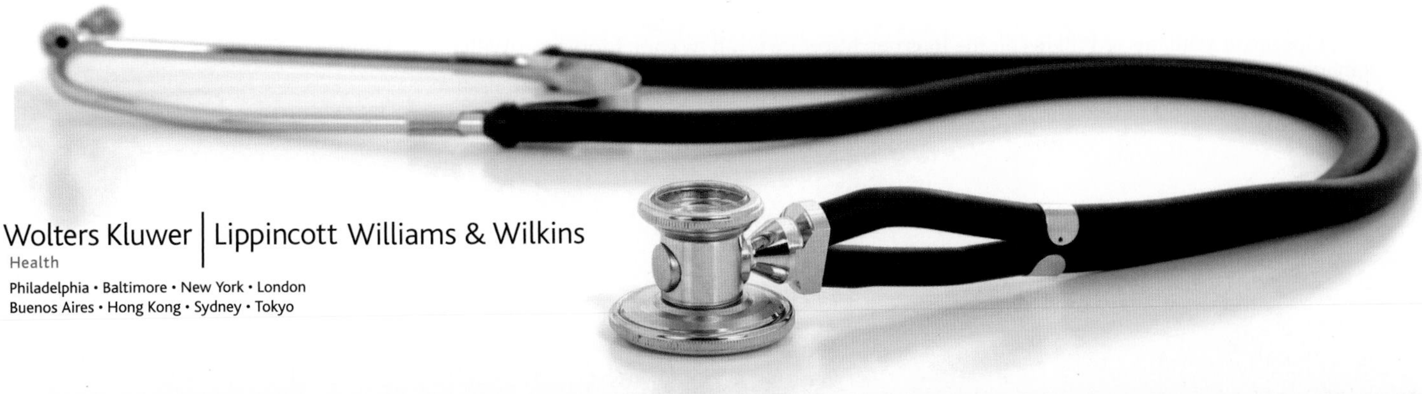

Wolters Kluwer Health | Lippincott Williams & Wilkins
Philadelphia • Baltimore • New York • London
Buenos Aires • Hong Kong • Sydney • Tokyo

Publisher: Michael Tully
Acquisitions Editor: Susan Rhyner
Product Manager: Stacey Sebring
Marketing Manager: Joy Fisher-Williams
Designer: Doug Smock
Compositor: Absolute Service, Inc.

351 West Camden Street
Baltimore, MD 21201

Two Commerce Square
2001 Market Street
Philadelphia, PA 19103

Printed in China

9 8 7 6 5 4 3 2 1

Library of Congress Cataloging-in-Publication Data

Step-up to USMLE step 1 : 2013 / Samir Mehta ... [et al.].
p. ; cm.
Includes bibliographical references and index.
ISBN 978-1-4511-7694-0
I. Mehta, Samir.
[DNLM: 1. Clinical Medicine--United States--Outlines. WB 18.2]

616.0076--dc23

2012041521

DISCLAIMER

Care has been taken to confirm the accuracy of the information present and to describe generally accepted practices. However, the authors, editors, and publisher are not responsible for errors or omissions or for any consequences from application of the information in this book and make no warranty, expressed or implied, with respect to the currency, completeness, or accuracy of the contents of the publication. Application of this information in a particular situation remains the professional responsibility of the practitioner; the clinical treatments described and recommended may not be considered absolute and universal recommendations.

The authors, editors, and publisher have exerted every effort to ensure that drug selection and dosage set forth in this text are in accordance with the current recommendations and practice at the time of publication. However, in view of ongoing research, changes in government regulations, and the constant flow of information relating to drug therapy and drug reactions, the reader is urged to check the package insert for each drug for any change in indications and dosage and for added warnings and precautions. This is particularly important when the recommended agent is a new or infrequently employed drug.

Some drugs and medical devices presented in this publication have Food and Drug Administration (FDA) clearance for limited use in restricted research settings. It is the responsibility of the health care provider to ascertain the FDA status of each drug or device planned for use in their clinical practice.

To purchase additional copies of this book, call our customer service department at **(800) 638-3030** or fax orders to **(301) 223-2320**. International customers should call **(301) 223-2300**.

Visit Lippincott Williams & Wilkins on the Internet: http://www.lww.com. Lippincott Williams & Wilkins customer service representatives are available from 8:30 am to 6:00 pm, EST.

RRS1211

Contributors

We would like to extend our thanks to all the reviewers and contributors to previous editions and extend special thanks to the contributors to this edition who have helped review and update this text to reflect the most current knowledge in their respective fields.

JENNIFER SHUFORD, MD
Infectious Disease
Austin, Texas

HAMPTON RICHARDS, MD
Obstetrics and Gynecology
Dallas, Texas

How to Contribute

Interested in medical publishing? Contribute to Step-Up!

Student suggestions and feedback are always welcomed and appreciated by the Step-Up team. Please send feedback and suggestions for new study material and test-taking strategies by writing to the authors at the website provided. Students can also directly submit new mnemonics, quick hits, tables, and figures. For each original entry incorporated into the text, students' names will be listed and personally acknowledged in the next edition. If duplicate entries are received, the first to submit will be acknowledged.

To make an entry or provide feedback and suggestions, simply visit http://www.lww.com and click Contact LWW.

Disclaimer:
Please note: submissions become the property of LWW.

Contents

Chapter 6. The Renal System

Chapter 7. The Endocrine System

Chapter 8. The Reproductive System

Where do I find...?

Strategies for Success: A Guide to Effective Preparation for the USMLE Step 1

As the first national licensure exam encountered during a medical career, the USMLE Step 1 is often a source of anxiety for the medical student.

As with most things in life, having a systematic plan can be helpful in approaching what at first seems like an enormous task—preparing for the boards. The authors of *Step-Up to the USMLE Step 1* have created this guide below to direct you in effectively preparing for and excelling on the boards.

The first section of the guide will introduce you to the exam and the test makers. It will also familiarize you with the exam structure, content, testing environment, and interface. Finally, it will review how the test is scored and how to register for the exam.

The second section of the guide details successful preparation strategies. In this section, you will learn tips for creating study schedules and gathering study materials as well as strategies for effective studying. At the end of this section, you will find a blank study schedule you can use as a basis for creating your personalized study schedule.

THE EXAM: THE USMLE STEP 1

The National Board of Medical Examiners

The USMLE is a joint endeavor by the National Board of Medical Examiners (NBME) and Federation of State Medical Boards (FSMB). Step 1 is the first of three exams medical students and graduates need to pass in order to become licensed physicians in the United States. The NBME was founded in 1915 in Philadelphia, Pennsylvania, and administered its first exam in 1916. The first exams were largely essay-based and were organized around testing the basic science subjects of anatomy, physiology, biochemistry, pathology, pharmacology, microbiology, and behavioral science. The exam has evolved over the years. In the early 1990s, after years of culminated efforts, the USMLE was introduced. This test embraced the systems-based practice of medicine and adopted a clinically oriented question format. In 1992, Step 1 replaced the Federation Licensing Examination (FLEX) and now serves as the single exam for international medical graduates seeking U.S. medical licensure. In 1999, the test became computer based and in 2005, the FRED software was adopted.

> **QUICK HIT**
>
> The USMLE Step 1 is designed to test basic science points in clinical vignettes. Know the test and you will prepare for it better!

Test Structure

The exam consists of 322 questions administered in seven blocks of 46 questions each with 60 minutes per block (Table 1). The eighth block is a survey consisting of 11 questions. Students are allotted 45 minutes of authorized break time that can be taken anytime between blocks. At the beginning of the exam, you will be presented with a 15-minute tutorial. This tutorial is also available on the NBME website: http://www.usmle.org/practice-materials/index.html. If the tutorial is taken prior to the exam date, it can be skipped on exam day—allowing you an extra 15 minutes for break time. You can also gain extra break time by finishing blocks earlier.

> **QUICK HIT**
>
> After the seventh block, a screen appears to move on to the eighth block. The eighth block is not a question block. It is a survey of your testing experience consisting of 11 questions. Don't be fooled!

TABLE 1 Time Breakdown of the USMLE Step 1 Exam

Tutorial	15 minutes (added to break time if skipped)
Question blocks	7 hours (60 minutes per block)
Break time	45 minutes (includes time for lunch)

Breaks can be taken between blocks when you wish. Figure 1 shows two suggested test day schedules. The first schedule is the traditional one-break schedule made for the student who likes one large midday break (Figure 1). The second schedule is for those students who prefer multiple breaks in order to stay fresh and to prevent testing fatigue. Both schedules may be modified to individual preferences.

Test Content

The exam consists of multiple-choice questions; each question contains a question stem followed by five or more answer choices. Nearly 75% of questions begin with a clinical vignette or patient scenario. Students may also be asked direct questions. What kinds of

QUICK HIT

Prior to test day, take the exam tutorial offered on the NBME website. On exam day, skip the tutorial and gain an extra 15 minutes of break time.

FIGURE 1 Structure of the USMLE Step 1 Exam

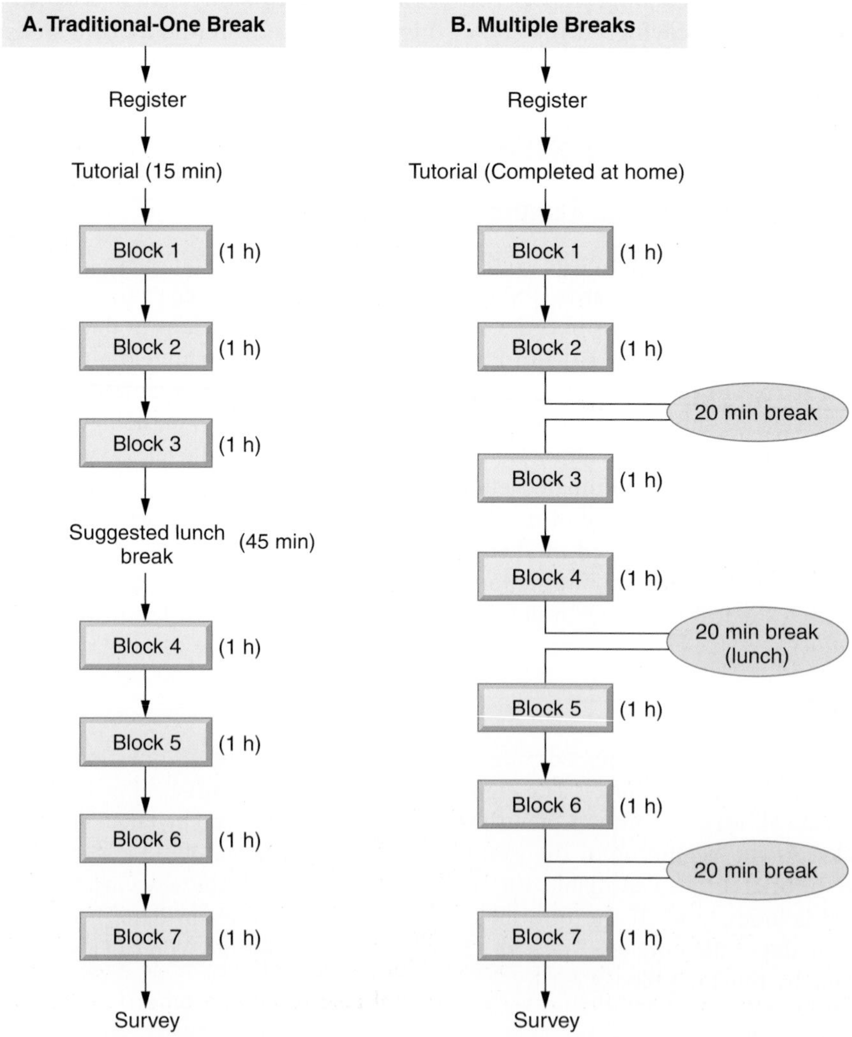
A. Traditional-One Break
Register
Tutorial (15 min)
Block 1 (1 h)
Block 2 (1 h)
Block 3 (1 h)
Suggested lunch break (45 min)
Block 4 (1 h)
Block 5 (1 h)
Block 6 (1 h)
Block 7 (1 h)
Survey
B. Multiple Breaks
Register
Tutorial (Completed at home)
Block 1 (1 h)
Block 2 (1 h)
20 min break
Block 3 (1 h)
Block 4 (1 h)
20 min break (lunch)
Block 5 (1 h)
Block 6 (1 h)
20 min break
Block 7 (1 h)
Survey

questions are not seen on the test? Question stems including "all of the following except," "not," and matching-style questions are never included in Step 1 exams.

Often, examinees will be presented with answer choices that are partially correct. In these instances, it is important to pick the option that best answers the statement in the question stem and move on.

Questions may range in difficulty from medium to hard. Although the questions vary from test to test and year to year, the proportion of question difficulty does not.

Something important for you to remember: Anywhere from 10% to 20% of questions seen on exam day are experimental questions that are not scored. Therefore, when presented with a difficult question with options that seem partially correct, it is important to select an answer that best fits and move on.

Test Environment

In general, Prometric centers share a generic design. There is the reception area where you will register on the morning of the exam, place your belongings in a locker, and return to take breaks. Beyond this is the examination area where only certain items are allowed: a government-issued identification card (typically a driver's license or passport) and a locker key. Everything else, including cell phones, pagers, digital watches, PDAs, books, notes, wallets, food, and beverages, goes into the locker. The examination area consists of a series of cubicles with computers. Test-takers are given noise reducer muffs, a dry-erase board, markers, and a dry eraser to use as needed during the exam. Proctors walk through the rooms periodically to make sure test rules are obeyed. When taking an authorized break after a block is completed, you will need to leave the examination area, present an identification card, and sign a book. The process is repeated when you return to the testing area after the break. When you return to the cubicle, the computer will ask for your candidate identification number, which is written at the top of the dry erase board. As soon as you enter the candidate identification number into the computer, the next testing block begins.

QUICK HIT

Not everyone will be taking the Step 1. All types of testing take place at the Prometric center and tests are started at different times of the day. Don't be surprised when other test-takers come and go at different times than you do.

QUICK HIT

The testing interface allows you to annotate text in the question stem. These can be helpful tools, but be wary of the clock; they can also cause you to waste valuable testing time.

Test Interface

The NBME offers an online tutorial that reviews exam procedures and the testing interface. Briefly, the testing interface for each block consists mainly of a single question and answer choices below it (Figure 2). Above this is a panel with several icons. Clicking on the appropriate icons allows you to perform that specific function. Clicking on the "mark" button will mark the question for that block, allowing you to return to the question at the end of the set. Next to the mark button are navigation buttons including a "previous" button and "next" button. These move you back one question or forward one question. Clicking on the "labs" button displays the normal lab values screen. Four options are offered: blood, hematologic, cerebrospinal, and sweat/urine/BMI. You can also write a note next to the text by clicking on the "notes" button. Finally, clicking the "calculator" button brings up a calculator to use for basic math functions.

On the left part of the screen is a panel with a running list of 46 questions. The question that is currently being viewed is highlighted in blue. Incomplete questions have a dot next to the item number and completed questions have no dot. When you mark questions with the mark function, a red flag appears next to that question. You can directly click on that question to return to it at any time before the block ends.

QUICK HIT

There is no penalty for guessing or benefit in leaving a question blank on the USMLE Step 1. Select answer choices as you move through and complete the block. If you are unsure of your answer, mark the question. If you have time at the end of the block, you can easily return to it and reconsider your initial response.

Test Scoring

Examinees receive their score via an electronic score report 3 to 6 weeks after taking the exam. The score report consists of three key pieces of information. First, it states whether the examinee has passed or failed. Second, it displays a score in a three-digit scale and two-digit scale that reflects how well the examinee performed on the content of the exam. The mean score on the exam is 225 with a standard deviation of 21. Passing on the three-digit scale is 188, which corresponds to 75 on the two-digit scale. The minimum passing score is subject to change by the NBME, although it is not expected to change for a few years. Finally, there is a table depicting the examinee's performance profile by basic science subject and organ system. The examinee's medical school also receives a report containing

QUICK HIT

If you have concerns about or fear of taking computer-based tests, consider visiting a Prometric center ahead of time to take a practice exam with the testing interface.

FIGURE 2 Testing interface

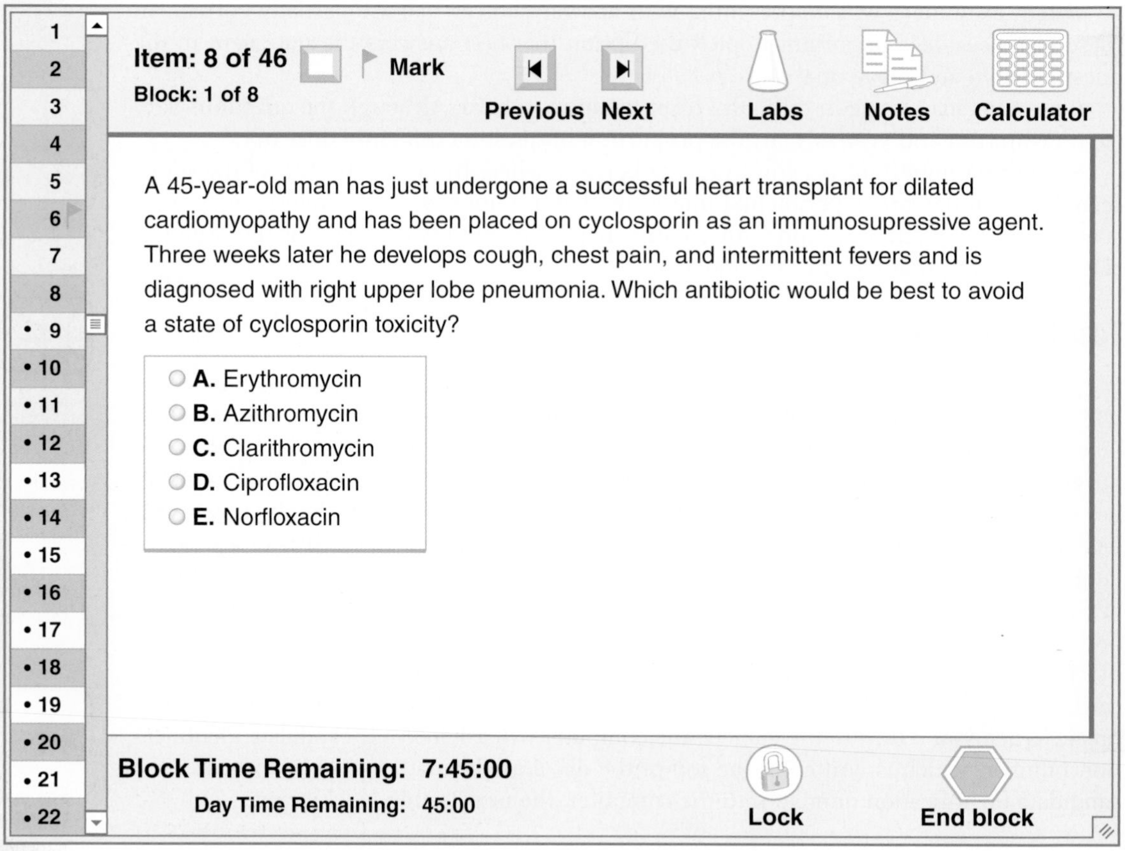
1
2
3
4
5
6
7
8
• 9
• 10
• 11
• 12
• 13
• 14
• 15
• 16
• 17
• 18
• 19
• 20
• 21
• 22
Item: 8 of 46
Block: 1 of 8
Mark
Previous
Next
Labs
Notes
Calculator
A 45-year-old man has just undergone a successful heart transplant for dilated cardiomyopathy and has been placed on cyclosporin as an immunosupressive agent. Three weeks later he develops cough, chest pain, and intermittent fevers and is diagnosed with right upper lobe pneumonia. Which antibiotic would be best to avoid a state of cyclosporin toxicity?
A. Erythromycin
B. Azithromycin
C. Clarithromycin
D. Ciprofloxacin
E. Norfloxacin
Block Time Remaining: 7:45:00
Day Time Remaining: 45:00
Lock
End block

(Adapted from http://www.usmle.org/Orientation/2009/menu.html.)

QUICK HIT

The minimum passing score on the USMLE Step 1 is 188. This number generally corresponds to getting 60% to 70% of exam questions right.

pass/fail status, digit score, and group performance profile. During the residency application process, residency programs receive a transcript containing pass/fail status and the digit score without the performance profile (Figure 3).

When preparing for the exam, the goal is two-tiered. Your first objective should be to pass the exam so that you can be on your way to becoming a licensed physician in the United States. Also, passing the exam is often linked to proceeding to the third year of medical school and getting your medical degree. The second objective is doing the best

QUICK HIT

88% to 93% of the United States and Canadian medical students pass the exam on their first attempt. Compare this to the U.S. bar exam, which has a passing rate of 67%.

FIGURE 3 **Mean scores for matched U.S. seniors by specialty.** The numbers displayed are mean values for USMLE Step 1 Score for matched U.S. seniors by specialty.

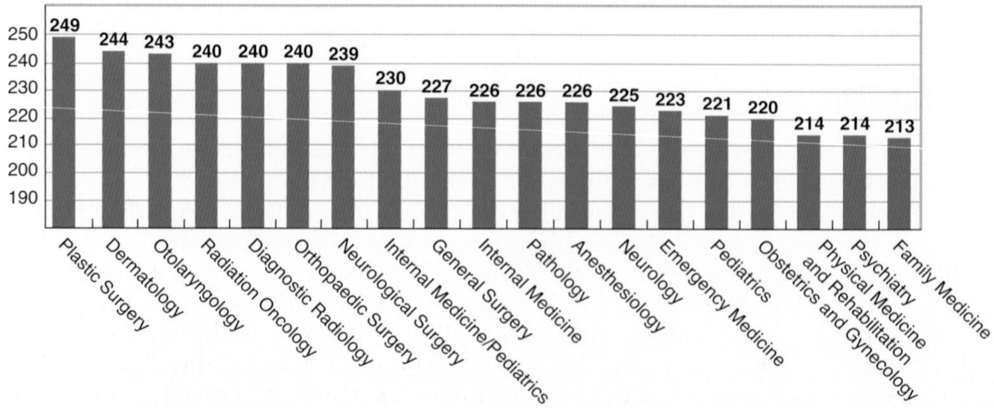
250
240
230
220
210
200
190
249
244
243
240
240
240
239
230
227
226
226
226
225
223
221
220
214
214
213
Plastic Surgery
Dermatology
Otolaryngology
Radiation Oncology
Diagnostic Radiology
Orthopaedic Surgery
Neurological Surgery
Internal Medicine/Pediatrics
General Surgery
Internal Medicine
Pathology
Anesthesiology
Neurology
Emergency Medicine
Pediatrics
Obstetrics and Gynecology
Physical Medicine and Rehabilitation
Psychiatry
Family Medicine

(Adapted from http://www.nrmp.org/data/chartingoutcomes2011.pdf.)

you can so that you can make yourself a competitive applicant for the residency of your choice. Certain highly competitive residency programs such as orthopaedic surgery and ophthalmology use Step 1 scores in the selection process.

It is important to note that the Step 1 score is only one of many factors that weigh in on the residency selection process. Programs make use of other applicant characteristics such as clinical rotation grades, research, publications, and reference letters. Having insight into your academic portfolio and defining your personal goals may be helpful in guiding your studies for Step 1.

QUICK HIT

You should register for the exam 6 to 8 months prior to your anticipated exam date.

Registering to Take the Exam

Six to eight months prior to the anticipated exam date, you will likely be prompted by your school to begin the registration process for taking the exam. The Step 1 application packet can be downloaded from the USMLE web site: http://www.usmle.org. Applicants must select a 3-month time period to take the exam (e.g., April–May–June, June–July–August). The application includes a form requiring a passport-sized photo that must be certified by the school registrar. The NBME processes the submitted application and sends out a scheduling permit.

QUICK HIT

Schedule your test as soon as possible after receiving the scheduling permit in order to receive the location and time of your choice.

The scheduling permit contains a unique candidate identification number, which is necessary in order to schedule the exam and take the exam. After receiving the scheduling permit, you should attempt to schedule your exam as soon as possible in order to receive the location and time of your choice. Scheduling occurs on a first-come, first-served basis, and testing centers fill up quickly during popular testing times of the year. Specific instructions on scheduling the test are delineated on the scheduling permit and require calling Prometric 1-800-633-3926 or logging into the Prometric site at http://www.prometric.com. A list of Prometric testing centers nearest you can be found on the Prometric website. Of note, testing centers are closed the for first 2 weeks of January, during major holidays, and generally on Sundays. Also, the exam can be started at different times of the day for those preferring the early or late hours of the day. Generally, Step 1 is taken by second-year medical students finishing their second year of medical school. Some relevant information to consider when scheduling your exam is your second year end date and third year start date. Because most curricula end in May, and students allow themselves a study time of 1 month, most students take the exam in June.

QUICK HIT

The scheduling permit needs to be presented on the day of the exam. Put it in a safe place. Copies will not be accepted.

If for some reason you need to reschedule your exam, you will need to call or visit the Prometric website. The rescheduled date must fall within the 3-month eligibility period selected earlier during the registration process (also found on your scheduling permit). Also, to avoid a rescheduling fee, Prometric should be contacted before noon EST 5 business days prior to the testing date.

QUICK HIT

To avoid a rescheduling fee, contact Prometric before noon EST 5 business days before the scheduled testing date.

PREPARING FOR THE EXAM: STUDY STRATEGIES

Study Materials

The first step to preparing for the exam is collecting and familiarizing yourself with study materials. You can start this step years before you actually take the exam. When starting medical school, consider purchasing a comprehensive review text such as *Step-Up to the USMLE Step 1*. The purpose of this is to begin reading, annotating, and familiarizing yourself with the test and content of the book. You might also consider investing early in subject-based reviews as you study those subjects in medical school. Finally, consider purchasing one or a series of question banks. Question banks allow you the opportunity to practice and apply learned concepts, solidifying the exam preparation process.

You should also take advantage of USMLE resources officially provided by the NBME. The NBME offers a free sample test consisting of 143 questions: http://www.usmle.org/practice-materials/index.html. For those examinees who would like to practice taking the exam with the testing interface, a mock testing situation can be set up at a Prometric center. This additional service costs $42. Students are provided with a score report at the end, although no explanations are offered online or at the testing center. The Comprehensive Basic Science Self-Assessment (CBSSA) is a 200-question test offered by the NBME, presented in four blocks of 50 questions each. Students must register to take the exam online and are charged $50 for this service. The website to create an account is https://nsasnbme.org/nsasweb/servlet/mesa_main. After taking the test, students are provided with a performance profile outlining the student's strengths and weaknesses.

FIGURE 4 Suggested study schedule: organ systems-based

Sunday	Monday	Tuesday	Wednesday	Thursday	Friday	Saturday
1	2 NERVOUS	3	4	5 CARDIO	6	7
8 RESPIR	9	10 GASTRO	11	12 RENAL	13	14
15 ENDO	16	17 REPRO	18	19 MUSCULO	20	21 HEME
22 LYMPH	23 BASIC CONCEPTS	24	25 WRAP UP DAYS	26	27	28
29	30					

Study Schedule

After collecting study materials, the next step is creating a study schedule. Preparation for the USMLE Step 1 can start years before actually taking the exam. As mentioned earlier, as you prepare for your medical school classes, read and annotate review texts along with studying syllabi and textbooks for classes. The purpose of this is to familiarize yourself with the text.

In the months prior to the exam, you should register for the exam, schedule the exam, and collect study materials including a question bank. Familiarize yourself with your study materials and attend campus review sessions.

The month before the exam, create and follow a study schedule. The purpose of the study schedule is to cover each of the disciplines tested on the exam. Typically, most medical students are provided 1 month to study for the exam. When students are creating a study schedule, oftentimes, the most challenging feat is determining how many days to allocate toward one discipline. Figures 4 and 5 are suggested study schedules that have been successful for students in the past. The first study schedule is organized by organ

FIGURE 5 Suggested study schedule: basic science-based

Sunday	Monday	Tuesday	Wednesday	Thursday	Friday	Saturday
1	2 PATHOLOGY	3	4	5 PHYSIOLOGY	6	7
8	9	10 PHARMACOLOGY	11	12	13 MICRO/	14
15 IMMUNO	16	17 BIOCHEM	18	19	20 BEHAV SCI	21
22 ANATOMY (including embryology, histology)	23 NEURO	24	25 WRAP UP DAYS	26	27	28
29	30					

TABLE 2 **Order for Organ System and Basic Science Schedule**

Order for Organ System Schedule	Order for Basic Science Schedule
Basic concepts/general	Physiology
Endocrine	Pathology
Nervous	Behavioral science
Cardiovascular	Microbiology/immunology
Respiratory	Pharmacology
Renal	Biochemistry
Gastrointestinal	Neuroanatomy
Musculoskeletal	Gross anatomy/embryology/histology
Reproductive	
Heme/lymph	

system and the second by basic science discipline. These schedules are only suggested schedules. Individual schedules should be tailored to your needs, keeping in mind your individual strengths and weaknesses, high-yield topics for the exam, and available time to study.

The suggested study schedules in Figures 4 and 5 assume 28 days available for study, including the day before the USMLE. If you have more or fewer days, adjust the schedule accordingly. For example, if you have 31 days, add ½ day to Behavioral Science, ½ day to Gross Anatomy/Embryology, 1 day off, and 1 day to wrap-up. In these suggested schedules, 2 to 3 days are allocated for wrap-up before the exam, 1 to 2 days are scheduled as days off as rewards for doing your work, and 24 days are full study days. In general, when determining the order of subjects to study, the general strategy should be longer-term memory subjects early and shorter-term memory subjects late (Table 2). Also, when determining how many days to allocate certain subjects or organ systems, provide more days for heavily tested subjects like pathology and physiology (Table 3).

TABLE 3 **Allocation of Days**

Allocation of Days by Organ System		Allocation of Days by Basic Science	
Organ System	**Days**	**Basic Science**	**Days**
Nervous	3.5	Pathology	4
Cardiovascular	3	Physiology	4
Respiratory	2.5	Pharmacology	4
Gastrointestinal	2	Microbiology/immunology	4
Renal	2.5	Biochemistry	3
Endocrine	2.5	Behavioral science	1.5
Reproductive	2	Gross anatomy/embryology/histology	1.5
Musculoskeletal	2	Neuroanatomy	2
Heme/lymph	2		
Basic concepts/general	2		

TABLE 4 **Suggested Daily Study Schedule**

Time	Activity
8:00 a.m.–12:00 p.m.	Study
12:00 p.m.–1:00 p.m.	Lunch
1:00 p.m.–5:00 p.m.	Study
5:00 p.m.–8:00 p.m.	Exercise, dinner, errands, phone calls
8:00 p.m.–10:00 p.m. (or 11:00 p.m.)	Questions

In the month prior to the exam, you should also create and follow a daily schedule. Table 4 contains a sample daily study schedule. The daily schedule should allot time for studying review texts, reading cases/clinical vignettes, and doing questions. While studying texts, you should not only read but also spend time understanding concepts and memorizing key facts. Tools that help with understanding and memorizing information include organizing information into tables, charts, and figures; using mnemonics; and applying information in daily practice, such as in clinics and caring for patients. Books with clinical cases and vignettes are based on this premise and provide an opportunity to integrate studied information. Doing questions is another excellent method of reinforcing and remembering learned information. An online question bank of more than 450 USMLE format questions based on commonly tested facts has been included with this text and can be accessed via this website: www.thePoint.lww.com/StepUp4e. Moreover, clinical vignettes and questions simulate the test day experience. Make sure you also include in your schedule time to relax and do other things that are important to you (work out, spend time with friends and family, etc.).

The night before the exam, relax and gather your required materials (orange permit slip, government-issued photo ID). Make sure you know how to get to the testing center and have confirmed with the testing center your test time and date. Get a good night's rest!

Study Strategies

Studying is a two-stage process. First, learn the basic definitions and concepts. The best method of accomplishing this is reading. Second, recognize and remember key facts. This is the hardest stage and one that most students neglect. Helpful strategies include:

1. Memorization—Use study aids like mnemonics, flashcards, tables, and figures.
2. Active learning—Engage in active learning by applying the concepts to scenarios, clinical settings, and mini-case presentations.
3. Questions—Apply learned concepts by doing questions.
4. Study groups—Discuss studied material and quiz each other; these activities are helpful in retaining information.

ONLINE RESOURCES

Table 5 summarizes important NBME websites and online resources available to you as you prepare for the USMLE.

PERSONALIZED STUDY SCHEDULE

Use the blank study schedule (Figure 6) on the following page to build your own based on the tips included in this chapter and your own areas of strength and weakness.

TABLE 5 Important Websites for Preparing for the USMLE Step 1

	Website	Description	Cost
NBME	http://www.nbme.org	Find general information and updates on the USMLE Step 1	N/A
Application materials	http://www.usmle.org	Apply to take the USMLE Step 1	$560
Scheduling the exam	http://www.prometric.com	Schedule your exam	N/A
FRED software tutorial and practice questions	http://www.usmle.org/practice-materials/index.html	Select option "Tutorial and Practice Test Items For Multiple Choice Questions." This contains a tutorial on the FRED software, familiarizes you with the testing interface, and contains over 140 sample questions. After taking this tutorial, you may skip the tutorial on test day, providing yourself with an extra 15 minutes in break time	Free
CBSSA	http://www.nbme.org/Students/sas/overview.html	The CBSSA contains USMLE Step 1 format questions designed by the NBME. There are 200 questions in four blocks of 50 questions each. Register to create an account and then follow instructions for CBSSA	$50
Step-Up to the USMLE Step 1 Question Bank	www.thePoint.lww.com/StepUp4e	Includes more than 350 questions in USMLE format with explanations preparing you for the most commonly tested facts on the USMLE	Free
Step-Up to the USMLE Step 1 website	http://www.lww.com/Step-Up	Ask the authors questions, become a student contributor for the next edition, provide feedback on this text	N/A

FIGURE 6 Blank study schedule

PERSONALIZED STEP 1 STUDY SCHEDULE

Use this blank calendar to create your own personalized Step 1 study schedule. Determine your preference for systems-based review or subject-based review, identify your strong areas and weak areas, and create your study schedule.

______ SYSTEMS-BASED ______ SUBJECT-BASED

Strong areas: ________________________________

Weak areas: ________________________________

Sunday	Monday	Tuesday	Wednesday	Thursday	Friday	Saturday
1	2	3	4	5	6	7
8	9	10	11	12	13	14
15	16	17	18	19	20	21
22	23	24	25	26	27	28
29	30					

TEST DAY TIPS

- Bring a cooler with ice, water, juice, or a sports drink. Pack a lunch. Bring some fruits and snacks. (You may not be able to predict what you're going to want to eat, so it's better to bring too much than too little.) Eat light, not heavy.
- Consider getting out in the sun and/or stretching during your breaks.
- Bring a light sweater or sweatshirt in case the testing center is cold.
- Don't forget your ID and USMLE pass.
- Take your breaks when you need them. (Example: 2 sections → break → 2 sections → break → 1 section → break → 2 sections) Some breaks may need to be longer than others. Don't be afraid to take a small 5-minute bathroom break.
- Expect 5 to 10 questions in each section that you have never seen before. If you expect this, then you won't become anxious when it happens (and it *will* happen).
- Bring your own watch to keep track of your break time!
- Consider answering 10 practice questions prior to going into the test center for "warm-up" (but don't look at the answers, in case you are incorrect).

What should I put on my markerboard prior to the start of the test?

- Don't write on your markerboard for more than 5 minutes before you start your test.
- Put whatever you want, but you may want to consider the following:
  - Developmental milestones
  - Important pharmacokinetic equations
  - Error square
  - Sensitivity, specificity, PPV, NPV, OR, RR, equations, and square
  - Lung volume diagram

Basic Concepts

1

DNA, RNA, AND PROTEIN

I. Chemical components of DNA and RNA

A. DNA and RNA are made up of nucleotides, which contain:
   1. A **nitrogenous base**—either a purine or pyrimidine (Figure 1-1)
      a. **Purines** are formed from
         - Aspartate
         - Carbon dioxide (CO_2)
         - Glutamate
         - Glycine
         - N10-formyltetrahydrofolate
      b. **Pyrimidines** are formed from
         - Aspartate
         - CO_2
         - Glutamate
   2. A **pentose sugar**—either a **ribose** for RNA or a **2-deoxyribose** for DNA
   3. One, two, or three phosphate groups forming a -monophosphate, -diphosphate, or -triphosphate, respectively (Figure 1-2)

B. Nucleoside triphosphates (NTP) are linked together by a 3′-5′ phosphodiester bond to form single-stranded RNA or DNA.

C. **Adenine** (A) binds to **thymine** (T), whereas **guanine** (G) binds to **cytosine** (C) in DNA. **Uracil** (U) replaces thymine (T) in RNA.

> **QUICK HIT**
> DNA synthesis can be prevented by nucleoside analogs such as cytosine arabinoside, zidovudine, and acyclovir. These types of drugs are useful in antiviral and anticancer therapy.

II. DNA replication

A. It is **semiconservative**—when two DNA molecules are created from the original helix, one strand of parental DNA is incorporated with each new daughter strand.

B. It takes place in the S phase of the cell cycle (Figure 1-3).

C. DNA strand separation requires several proteins.
   1. **DnaA**—20 to 50 of these proteins aggregate at the origin of replication and begin to separate the DNA strands.
   2. **Single-strand binding** (SSB) proteins bind cooperatively to further separate the two strands of DNA.
   3. **DNA helicase** unwinds the DNA.

D. Supercoiling is prevented by DNA **topoisomerase** types I and II.

E. Replication process in prokaryotic cells (Figure 1-4)
   1. An RNA primer is placed on the separated DNA strands by RNA polymerase (also called **primase**) before replication can begin.
   2. Only one RNA primer is needed on the leading strand; on the lagging strand, however, a new primer is required as the replication fork opens.
      a. Leading strand
         - The leading strand produces a continuously elongating strand of new DNA.

> **QUICK HIT**
> In eukaryotic cells, replication is accomplished by POL enzymes similar to those in prokaryotic cells. POL α performs primase activity like prokaryotic primase; POL δ synthesizes the leading DNA strand; POL ϵ synthesizes the lagging strand; and POL β repairs and excises primers, similar to DNA polymerase I.

FIGURE 1-1 Bases

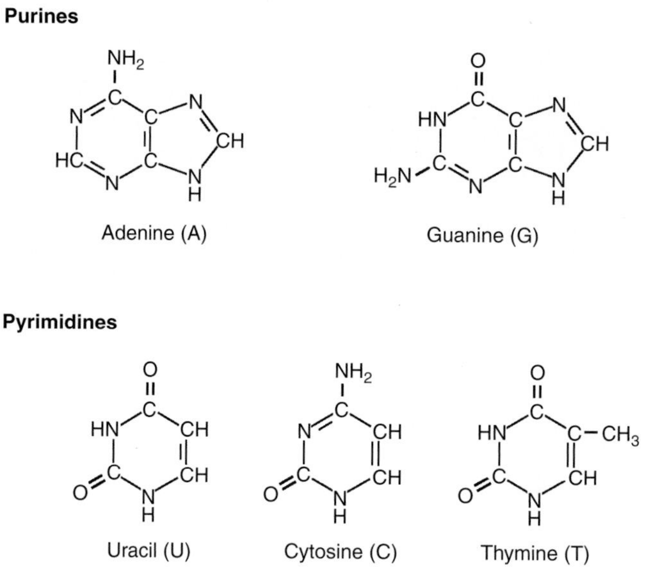
Purines
Adenine (A)
Guanine (G)
Pyrimidines
Uracil (U)
Cytosine (C)
Thymine (T)

C, carbon; H, hydrogen; N, nitrogen; O, oxygen.

FIGURE 1-2 Nucleotide structure

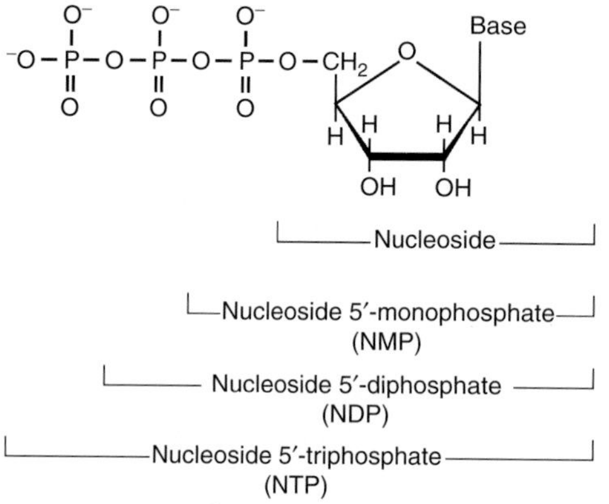
Base
Nucleoside
Nucleoside 5′-monophosphate
(NMP)
Nucleoside 5′-diphosphate
(NDP)
Nucleoside 5′-triphosphate
(NTP)

C, carbon; H, hydrogen; O, oxygen; P, phosphate.

FIGURE 1-3 The cell cycle

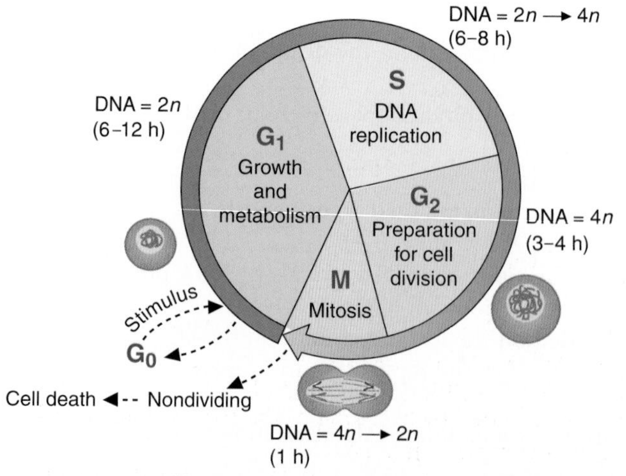
DNA = 2n → 4n
(6–8 h)
S
DNA replication
DNA = 2n
(6–12 h)
G1
Growth and metabolism
G2
Preparation for cell division
DNA = 4n
(3–4 h)
M
Mitosis
Stimulus
G0
Cell death
Nondividing
DNA = 4n → 2n
(1 h)

(Reprinted with permission from Lieberman M, Marks AD. *Marks' Basic Medical Biochemistry: A Clinical Approach.* 4th ed. Philadelphia, PA: Lippincott, Williams & Wilkins; 2013.)

FIGURE 1-4 **DNA synthesis**

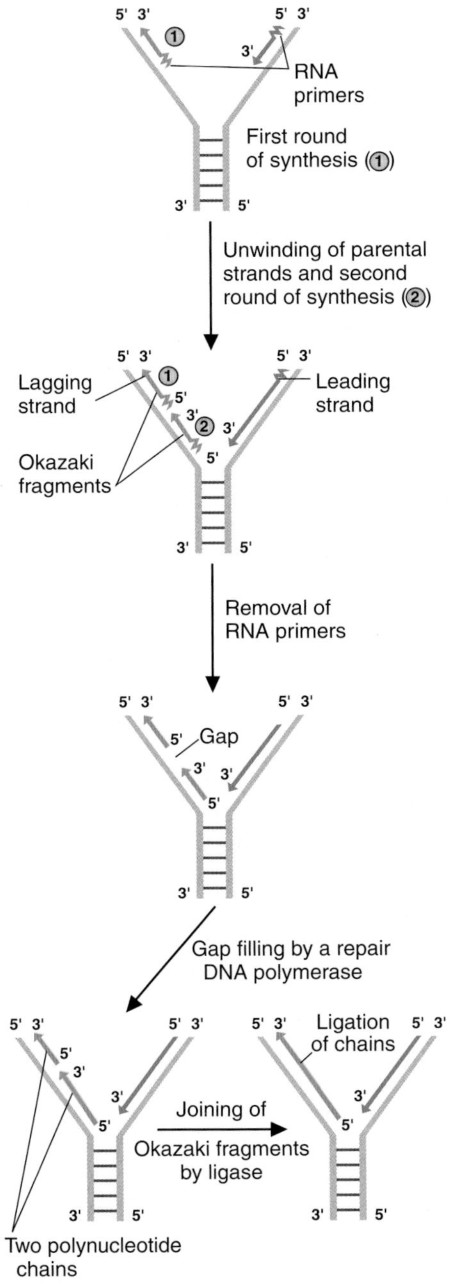
5' 3'
5' 3'
3'
RNA primers
First round of synthesis (1)
3'
5'
Unwinding of parental strands and second round of synthesis (2)
Lagging strand
Leading strand
Okazaki fragments
Removal of RNA primers
Gap
Gap filling by a repair DNA polymerase
Ligation of chains
Joining of Okazaki fragments by ligase
Two polynucleotide chains

(Reprinted with permission from Lieberman M, Marks AD. *Marks' Basic Medical Biochemistry: A Clinical Approach.* 4th ed. Philadelphia, PA: Lippincott Williams & Wilkins; 2013.)

- The leading strand of DNA is copied continuously from 5′ to 3′ in the direction of the replication fork.

b. Lagging strand
- The lagging strand of DNA is copied piecewise in the direction opposite of the replication fork.
- The lagging strand produces small pieces of new DNA with RNA interspersed, which are called Okazaki fragments.

3. The DNA chain is elongated by DNA polymerase III (in prokaryotes), which adds nucleotides with energy provided by breaking of the triphosphate bond.
4. When DNA strand synthesis is complete, it is proofread.
   a. The proofreading function of DNA polymerase III (3′-5′ exonuclease) allows it to correct mismatched base pairs.

b. The improperly placed base is hydrolytically removed and replaced with the appropriate one.

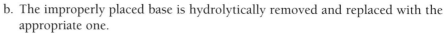

5. RNA primers are removed from the Okazaki fragments and leading strand.
   a. DNA polymerase I or III has **3′-5′ exonuclease** activity, which allows it to remove the RNA primer.
   b. Once the primer is removed, the space is filled with DNA.
6. The break in the strand backbone is sealed by **DNA ligase**.

F. Repair
1. Damage caused by ultraviolet light
   a. Ultraviolet light exposure results in pyrimidine dimers (especially thymine–thymine dimers).
   b. Dimers inhibit the replication process.
   c. Specialized **endonucleases** recognize a dimer and cleave it at its 5′ end.
   d. An **exonuclease** then excises the dimer and leaves a gap in the DNA strand.
   e. The gap is filled with the appropriate nucleotides by DNA polymerase I.
   f. The strand is resealed by DNA ligase.
2. Base alterations
   a. Bases may be changed spontaneously or slowly over time because of **alkylating agents** (cyclophosphamide and nitrosoureas).
   b. Specialized **glycosylases** remove the improper base and leave an empty (apyrimidinic or apurinic) space.
   c. The empty space is filled by specific endonucleases or polymerases in the same manner that dimers are repaired.
3. DNA repair defects
   a. **Xeroderma pigmentosum** – hypersensitivity to UV light, resulting in a 1,000-fold increased risk of skin cancers
   b. **Ataxia-telangiectasia** – sensitivity to ionizing radiation, immunodeficiency, and ataxia beginning at 1 to 2 yrs
   c. **Bloom syndrome** – hypersensitivity to sunlight; leukemias and lymphomas are common; average age of cancer onset is 25 years
   d. **Hereditary nonpolyposis colorectal cancer** (HNPCC) – caused by a defect in mismatch repair genes, leading to increased risk of colorectal and other cancers
   e. ***BRCA1* and *BRCA2*** gene products are important for repairing double-strand DNA breaks; mutations in these genes leads to an increased risk of breast and ovarian cancer

G. Drugs that affect replication
1. Fluoroquinolones – inhibit prokaryotic topoisomerase
2. Etoposide – inhibits eukaryotic topoisomerase

QUICK HIT

Xeroderma pigmentosum is a genetic disease in which cells cannot repair damaged DNA. People suffering from this disease cannot repair skin damage caused by sunlight and are predisposed to skin cancer.

III. DNA packaging

A. Owing to its incredible length, DNA must be properly coiled inside the cell.

B. **Histones** are a group of proteins designed to coil DNA.
1. The high content of arginine and lysine gives histones a positive charge, which attracts them to negatively charged DNA.
2. Histones organize themselves into a group of eight to make a **nucleosome** core; each core contains two each of types H2A, H2B, H3, and H4 histones.
3. DNA twists approximately twice around each core.
4. Between cores, a type H1 histone is attached to the DNA.
5. The arrangement of histones and DNA is called a nucleosome and produces a characteristic "beads-on-a-string" appearance.
6. The nucleosomes coil around themselves to produce nucleofilaments.
7. **Nucleofilaments** are further packaged and coiled into more compact structures when DNA is not being replicated.

IV. mRNA synthesis

A. Initiation of transcription is influenced by a variety of factors.
1. **RNA polymerase** binds to the promoter region of the DNA.
2. The TATAAT nucleotide sequence is a section of the promoter located upstream from the start of transcription; it is contained in the Hogness box of eukaryotes and the Pribnow box of prokaryotes.

QUICK HIT

In eukaryotes, different RNAs are synthesized by different RNA polymerases. RNA polymerase I synthesizes ribosomal RNA, RNA polymerase II synthesizes messenger RNA, and RNA polymerase III synthesizes transfer RNA.

3. The CAAT box, found in eukaryotes, and the -35 sequence, found in prokaryotes, are located farther upstream from the TATAAT sequence and have promoter function.

B. After recognition of the promoter region by RNA polymerase, elongation begins.
   1. Elongation of RNA occurs in a manner similar to DNA replication but does not require a primer for initiation.
   2. RNA polymerase does not have a proofreading function, so it cannot correct mismatched base pairs that may occur.

C. In eukaryotic cells, RNA undergoes **posttranslational** modification; in prokaryotic cells, transcription and translation occur simultaneously.
   1. RNA synthesized by eukaryotic **RNA polymerase II** is called **heterogeneous nuclear RNA (hnRNA)** and is found in the nucleus of the cell.
   2. This hnRNA is **capped at the 5′ end** by a 7-methylguanine molecule provided by S-adenosylmethionine (SAM).
   3. **A poly-A nucleotide tail is added to the 3′ end.**
   4. Introns are cleaved out.
   5. The molecule is now mature messenger RNA (mRNA) and is transported to the cytoplasm.

V. Protein synthesis *(Figure 1-5)*

A. Initiation is started with the binding of the ribosomal subunits to the mRNA.

B. The start codon **AUG** is the first codon to be recognized and translated; initiation factor 2 (**IF-2** in prokaryotes, **eIF-2** in eukaryotes) and guanosine 5′-triphosphate (GTP) are required.

C. A methionine is added as the first amino acid.

D. Elongation requires a transfer RNA (tRNA) with the appropriate **anticodon** to the codon on the mRNA, elongation factors, and GTP.

E. Termination requires a **UAA**, **UAG**, or **UGA** codon.

F. Regulation of RNA synthesis
   1. Eukaryotes
      a. Control is accomplished by gene **methylation**, **amplification**, and **rearrangement**.
      b. Histones play a role in gene suppression.
      c. Inducers activate gene expression.
      d. Some eukaryotic genes are regulated at transcription.
   2. Prokaryotes
      a. Protein synthesis is controlled at the level of transcription using operons.
      b. An **operon** is a set of adjacent genes that are activated or deactivated.
      c. Each operon has a **promoter** region upstream from the genes, an operator that activates or deactivates the genes, and a **repressor** protein that can bind to the operator and deactivate transcription (Figure 1-6).

QUICK HIT

Point mutations include **silent mutations** (the same amino acid), **missense** mutations (a new amino acid), and **nonsense mutations** (stop codon). Insertions are the addition of extra amino acids, and deletions are the loss of amino acids.

VI. Posttranslational folding of proteins

A. Newly synthesized proteins have a linear structure (**primary structure**).

B. On the basis of interactions between amino acids, these linear structures can assume **secondary structures**, such as an **α-helix** or a **β-pleated sheet**.

C. The **tertiary structure** incorporates the secondary structures into a complete three-dimensional configuration. This is the final conformation of many proteins.

D. A **quaternary structure** is formed when several tertiary structures are arranged together. This occurs in hemoglobin, for example, in which two α and two β globular proteins form the complete hemoglobin molecule.

E. In the Golgi apparatus and endoplasmic reticulum, **chaperone proteins** are important for the proper folding of polypeptides. Some chaperones are synthesized constantly and are involved in normal intracellular protein trafficking. Other chaperones are induced by stress such as heat (**heat shock proteins** hsp70 and hsp90). These chaperones "rescue" heat-stressed proteins from misfolding. If the folding process is not successful, the chaperones facilitate degradation of the damaged protein. This degradative process often involves **ubiquitin** (also a heat shock protein), which is added to the abnormal protein and marks it for degradation by the ubiquitin-proteasome complex.

QUICK HIT

Disulfide bonds play a major role in maintaining the tertiary structure of proteins.

FIGURE 1-5 **Protein synthesis**

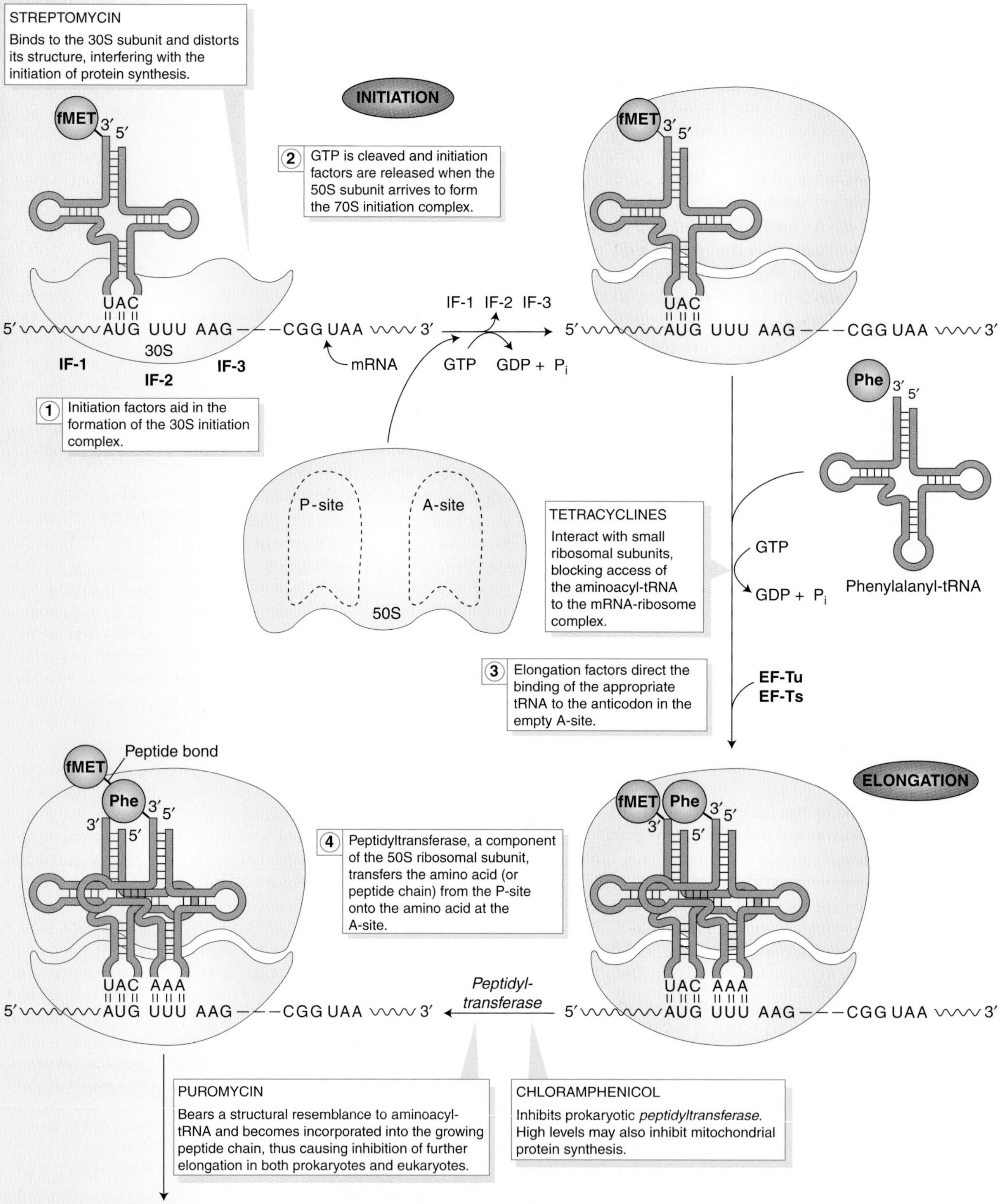
STREPTOMYCIN
Binds to the 30S subunit and distorts its structure, interfering with the initiation of protein synthesis.
INITIATION
fMET 3′ 5′
2 GTP is cleaved and initiation factors are released when the 50S subunit arrives to form the 70S initiation complex.
UAC
5′ AUG UUU AAG – – CGG UAA 3′
30S
IF-1
IF-2
IF-3
mRNA
IF-1 IF-2 IF-3
GTP GDP + P_i
1 Initiation factors aid in the formation of the 30S initiation complex.
Phe 3′ 5′
P-site
A-site
50S
TETRACYCLINES
Interact with small ribosomal subunits, blocking access of the aminoacyl-tRNA to the mRNA-ribosome complex.
GTP
GDP + P_i
Phenylalanyl-tRNA
3 Elongation factors direct the binding of the appropriate tRNA to the anticodon in the empty A-site.
EF-Tu
EF-Ts
Peptide bond
fMET Phe 3′ 5′ 3′ 5′
ELONGATION
4 Peptidyltransferase, a component of the 50S ribosomal subunit, transfers the amino acid (or peptide chain) from the P-site onto the amino acid at the A-site.
UAC AAA
5′ AUG UUU AAG – – CGG UAA 3′
Peptidyl-transferase
PUROMYCIN
Bears a structural resemblance to aminoacyl-tRNA and becomes incorporated into the growing peptide chain, thus causing inhibition of further elongation in both prokaryotes and eukaryotes.
CHLORAMPHENICOL
Inhibits prokaryotic peptidyltransferase. High levels may also inhibit mitochondrial protein synthesis.

Continued at top of next page

A, adenine; Arg, arginine; C, cytosine; EF, elongation factor; fMET, formyl methionine; G, guanine; GDP, guanine diphosphate; GTP, guanine triphosphate; IF, initiation factor; Phe, phenylalanine; P_i, inorganic phosphate; RF, release factor; T, thymine; tRNA, transfer RNA; U, uracil. (Adapted from Champe PC, Harvey RA. *Lippincott's Illustrated Reviews: Biochemistry.* 2nd ed. Philadelphia, PA: Lippincott-Raven Publishers; 1994:396–397. Used with permission of Lippincott Williams & Wilkins.)

FIGURE 1-5 *(Continued)*

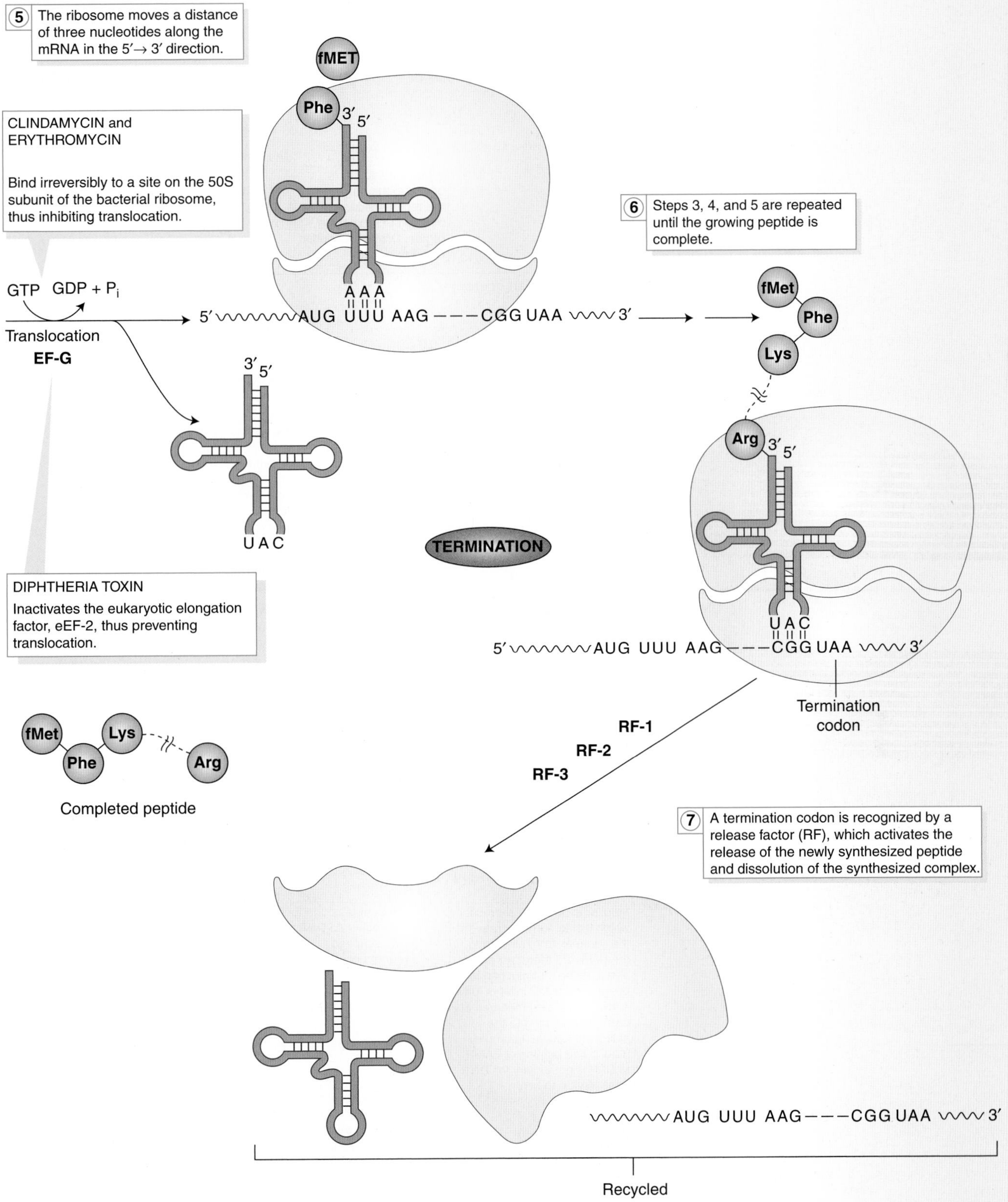

5 The ribosome moves a distance of three nucleotides along the mRNA in the 5′→ 3′ direction.
fMET
Phe
3′
5′
CLINDAMYCIN and ERYTHROMYCIN
Bind irreversibly to a site on the 50S subunit of the bacterial ribosome, thus inhibiting translocation.
GTP
GDP + P$_i$
Translocation
EF-G
A A A
5′ AUG UUU AAG – – – CGG UAA 3′
3′
5′
U A C
6 Steps 3, 4, and 5 are repeated until the growing peptide is complete.
fMet
Phe
Lys
Arg
3′
5′
TERMINATION
DIPHTHERIA TOXIN
Inactivates the eukaryotic elongation factor, eEF-2, thus preventing translocation.
U A C
5′ AUG UUU AAG – – – CGG UAA 3′
Termination codon
RF-1
RF-2
RF-3
fMet
Lys
Phe
Arg
Completed peptide
7 A termination codon is recognized by a release factor (RF), which activates the release of the newly synthesized peptide and dissolution of the synthesized complex.
AUG UUU AAG – – – CGG UAA 3′
Recycled

FIGURE 1-6 **Operons**

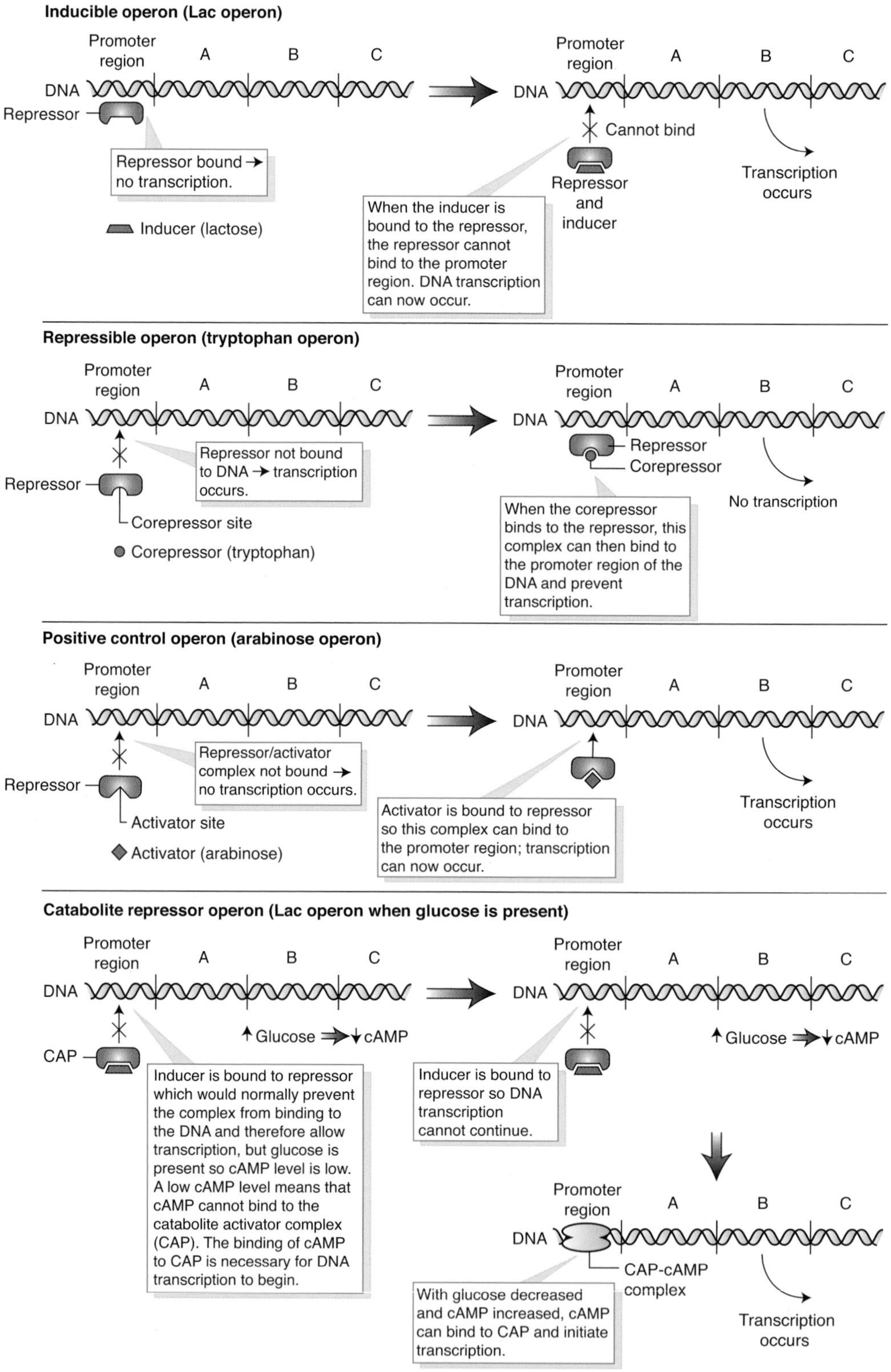
Inducible operon (Lac operon)
Promoter region
A
B
C
DNA
Repressor
Repressor bound → no transcription.
Inducer (lactose)
Cannot bind
Repressor and inducer
When the inducer is bound to the repressor, the repressor cannot bind to the promoter region. DNA transcription can now occur.
Transcription occurs
Repressible operon (tryptophan operon)
Repressor not bound to DNA → transcription occurs.
Corepressor site
Corepressor (tryptophan)
Repressor
Corepressor
When the corepressor binds to the repressor, this complex can then bind to the promoter region of the DNA and prevent transcription.
No transcription
Positive control operon (arabinose operon)
Repressor/activator complex not bound → no transcription occurs.
Activator site
Activator (arabinose)
Activator is bound to repressor so this complex can bind to the promoter region; transcription can now occur.
Transcription occurs
Catabolite repressor operon (Lac operon when glucose is present)
CAP
↑Glucose ⇒↓cAMP
Inducer is bound to repressor which would normally prevent the complex from binding to the DNA and therefore allow transcription, but glucose is present so cAMP level is low. A low cAMP level means that cAMP cannot bind to the catabolite activator complex (CAP). The binding of cAMP to CAP is necessary for DNA transcription to begin.
Inducer is bound to repressor so DNA transcription cannot continue.
CAP-cAMP complex
With glucose decreased and cAMP increased, cAMP can bind to CAP and initiate transcription.
Transcription occurs

cAMP, cyclic adenosine monophosphate.

BACTERIAL MORPHOLOGY AND GENETICS

I. Cell wall—the outermost component of all bacteria

A. Cell wall components
1. Peptidoglycan, which provides rigid support and protects against osmotic pressure changes, is thick and multilayered in gram-positive organisms and thin and single layered in gram-negative organisms.
2. Gram-positive outer membrane contains teichoic acid.
3. Gram-negative outer membrane contains lipid-A (toxic component of endotoxin) and polysaccharide (major surface antigen).
4. Cytoplasmic membrane is a lipoprotein bilayer without sterols—the site of oxidative and transport enzymes.

QUICK HIT

Peptidoglycan cross-linking is disrupted by penicillin and cephalosporins.

B. Bacterial stains
1. Gram stain separates most bacteria into two groups
 a. Gram-positive organisms stain blue/purple.
 b. Gram-negative organisms stain pink.
2. Giemsa stain – *Chlamydia, Chlamydophila, Borrelia*, and some fungi (*Histoplasma*) and protozoans (*Plasmodium, Trypanosoma*)
3. Silver stain – *Legionella pneumoniae, Pneumocystis jirovecii*
4. Ziehl-Neelsen stain (acid fast) – *Mycobacteria* spp.
5. Periodic acid-Schiff (PAS) – *Tropheryma whippelii*

II. Bacterial genome

A. Bacteria have a **haploid** genome, whereas humans have a **diploid** genome.
B. A typical bacterial cell has a **circular** DNA molecule.

III. Mutation

A. Several types of mutations occur that can alter the bacterial genome.
B. Mutation is an important factor in bacterial survival because it allows the bacteria to change and adapt to their environment.
C. Mutations may be caused by a mistake committed by DNA polymerase, a chemical mutagen, ultraviolet light, a virus, or another cause.
D. Types of mutations
1. **Base substitution**
 a. One base replaces another.
 b. Occurs at DNA replication.
 c. Can generate a missense mutation, which causes the wrong amino acid to be placed in the protein, or it can generate a nonsense mutation, which is read as a stop codon.
 d. Also occurs in eukaryotic cells but can be repaired by the processes described earlier.
2. **Frameshift mutation**
 a. One or more bases are added or removed (not a multiple of 3).
 b. The reading frame is shifted on the mRNA molecule, causing massive errors in translation.
 c. Often causes protein to end prematurely as a result of creation of a stop codon
 d. Also occurs in eukaryotic cells.
3. **Transposons** (Figure 1-7)
 a. They are called "jumping genes" because they transfer pieces of DNA from one bacterium to another.
 b. Transposons can integrate small pieces of DNA into the bacterial genome, plasmids, or bacteriophages.
 c. Integration of transposon DNA into the host genome can occur within a preexisting gene and render the host gene useless.
 d. Each transposon has four domains:
  - **Inverted repeats**—appear at the ends and mediate integration of the transposon into a DNA molecule

FIGURE 1-7 Transposons

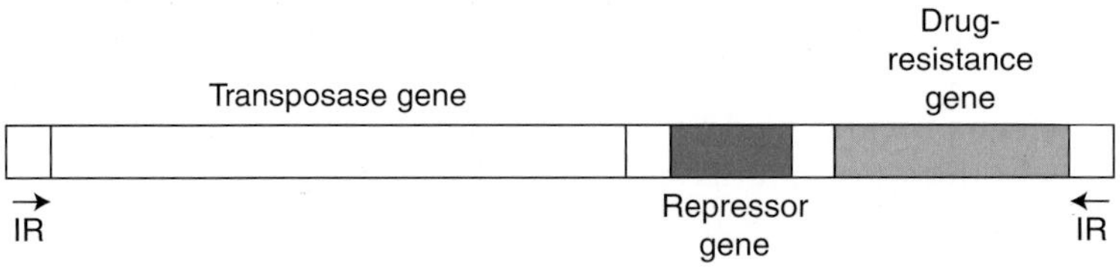
Drug-
resistance
gene
Transposase gene
IR
Repressor
gene
IR

IR, inverted repeats.

- **Transposase**—the enzyme that controls integration and removal of the transposon
- **Repressor gene**—controls synthesis of transposase and whichever gene is in the fourth domain
- **Drug-resistance gene**—often appears in the fourth gene domain

e. Transposons replicate with the host DNA and are not capable of independent replication.
f. When transposons integrate and remove themselves from a DNA molecule, they can cause profound mutations.

IV. Genetic transfer

A. Transfer within a cell
1. Transposons can transfer information between different areas of the same DNA molecule.
2. **Programmed rearrangements**
a. These are performed by certain organisms, including *Neisseria*, *Borrelia*, and trypanosomes.
b. Programmed rearrangements cause a silent gene to be expressed. Programmed rearrangements also allow the organism to evade the immune system.

B. Transfer between cells (Table 1-1)

QUICK HIT

Conjugation is performed by fertility plasmid (F plasmid). A bacterium containing the F plasmid (the male) has a sex pilus, which can attach to an F plasmid–deficient bacterium (the female). Once attached, the female is reeled in and DNA is transferred.

TABLE 1-1 Genetic Transfer in Prokaryotes

Mode	Mechanism	Notes
Conjugation	Transfer of DNA from one bacterium to another via contact and exchange	Can transfer either chromosomes or (mainly) **plasmids**; uses a sex pilus
Transduction	Transfer of DNA from one cell to another using a viral vector	Generalized transduction can transfer any gene and contains no viral DNA; specialized transduction can transfer only certain genes and contains viral DNA
Transformation	Uptake of DNA from the environment	Most commonly *Streptococcus pneumoniae*, *Haemophilus influenzae*, *Neisseria* spp.
Transposition	Excision and reinsertion of genetic material from one DNA molecule to another	Plasmid to plasmid, plasmid to chromosome, chromosome to chromosome

VIRAL GENETICS

- Comparison of Cells and Viruses (Table 1-2)

In contrast to infectious bacteria and fungi, viruses are not cells. They do not have a nucleus or organelles and are not capable of reproducing independently. Current antiviral agents, such as acyclovir and foscarnet, can only suppress viral replication. Viral elimination requires a functioning host immune response.

TABLE 1-2 **Comparison of Cells and Viruses**

	Eukaryotes	Prokaryotes	Viruses
Size (in μm)	7	2–6	0.01–0.2
Membrane-bound organelles	Present	Absent	Absent
Ribosomes	80S	70S	Absent
DNA	46 chromosomes	1 circular chromosome	DNA or RNA; circular, single-strand, or multiple segments
Replication	Mitosis or meiosis	Binary fission	Production and assembly

> **QUICK HIT**
>
> **Prions** lack most of the features associated with cells or viruses. Prions are thought to be abnormally folded proteins that are capable of catalyzing similar folding in the host's proteins. Accumulation of these abnormally folded proteins can cause spongiform diseases characterized by vacuolization of brain tissues, such as kuru or Creutzfeldt–Jakob disease.

I. Viral structure *(Figure 1-8)*

A. Nucleic acid
   1. May be DNA or RNA, but never both
   2. May be single or double stranded
   3. May be linear, segmented, or circular
   4. Most are haploid, but retroviruses are diploid

B. **Capsid**
   1. The protein coat around the nucleic acid core (the capsid) is composed of repeating units called **capsomeres**.
   2. The capsid assumes one of two shapes:
      a. **Helical**—hollow rod shape
      b. **Icosahedral**—multiple triangles arranged into a small sphere
   3. The capsid functions to protect the viral nucleic acid.

C. **Envelope**
   1. Surrounds the capsid of some viruses.
   2. Causes the virus to be more susceptible to drying and lipid solvents.
   3. Composed of virus-specific proteins and cell-derived lipids.
   4. Most **DNA viruses** derive their envelope from the host cell's **nuclear membrane**, whereas most **RNA viruses** derive their envelope from the host's **plasma membrane.**

> **QUICK HIT**
>
> Viral structure is highly variable among viruses but constant for each particular virus.

FIGURE 1-8 **Structure of viruses**

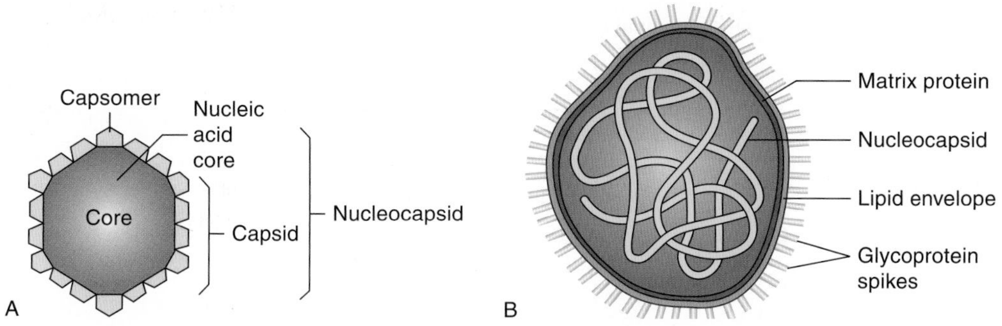
Capsomer
Nucleic acid core
Core
Capsid
Nucleocapsid
A
B
Matrix protein
Nucleocapsid
Lipid envelope
Glycoprotein spikes

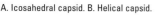

A. Icosahedral capsid. B. Helical capsid.

> **QUICK HIT**
>
> The duration of a viral multiplication cycle ranges from 6 h for poliovirus to 48 h for the papovavirus and adenovirus.

II. Replication

A. Attachment
   1. Viral surface proteins specifically attach to receptor proteins on the cell surface.
   2. The noncovalent interaction of proteins determines host range.

B. **Penetration**
  1. The virus may be engulfed by the host via a pinocytotic vesicle (**viropexis**).
  2. Nonenveloped viruses may slip through the host membrane by direct **translocation**.
  3. The viral **envelope may fuse with the host cell membrane**.

C. **Uncoating**
  1. DNA viruses partially uncoat in the cytoplasm and undergo final uncoating in the nucleus (to protect the DNA from endonucleases in the cytoplasm).
  2. RNA viruses uncoat in the cytoplasm.

QUICK HIT

The influenza virus is the only RNA virus that replicates in the nucleus.

D. **Expression and replication**
  1. DNA viruses replicate in the nucleus (except poxvirus) using the host cell's RNA polymerase and other proteins.
  2. **Positive single-stranded RNA viruses** contain an mRNA genome, which interacts **directly with host ribosomes** for translation of a viral RNA polymerase, which completes replication.
  3. **Negative single- and double-stranded RNA viruses** are packaged with a **viral RNA polymerase, which produces positive RNA** for transcription.
  4. Thousands of copies of viral proteins are produced.
  5. For the retrovirus life cycle, see discussion of HIV (Chapter 8).

E. **Assembly**
  1. DNA viruses are assembled in the nucleus (except for the pox viruses).
  2. RNA viruses are assembled in the cytoplasm (except for the influenza virus, which is assembled in the nucleus).

F. **Release**
  1. Nonenveloped viruses usually **rupture the host cell membrane**, which releases mature particles.
  2. Enveloped viruses are released via budding, in which each mature particle becomes surrounded by a portion of the host cell's membrane.

ENZYME KINETICS

QUICK HIT

Genetic mutations leading to inborn errors of metabolism may alter substrate bonding or enzyme activity on a substrate.

I. Enzymes

A. An enzyme is a protein or nucleic acid molecule that decreases the **energy of activation for a reaction** (Figure 1-9).
B. Enzymes interact specifically with substrates at an enzyme active site.
C. By lowering the energy of activation, enzymes increase the rate of reaction.
D. Enzymes **do not alter the equilibrium** of substrates and products, which is concentration dependent, or the free energy released from the reaction.

FIGURE 1-9 Enzyme effect on a chemical reaction

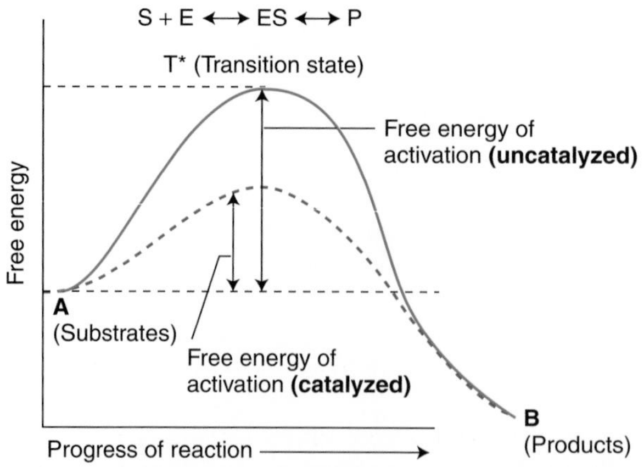
S + E ⟷ ES ⟷ P
T* (Transition state)
Free energy of activation (uncatalyzed)
Free energy
A (Substrates)
Free energy of activation (catalyzed)
B (Products)
Progress of reaction

An enzyme (E) acts as a catalyst to decrease the amount of free energy required to convert a substrate (S) to a product (P). An uncatalyzed reaction (represented by the solid blue line) requires a much higher amount of free energy than an enzyme-catalyzed reaction (dashed green line).

E. Enzymatic reactions generally require cofactors, such as metals, derivatives of vitamins, or small organic molecules. The vitamins and small organic molecules are often referred to as coenzymes.

II. Kinetics

A. **Velocity** (V) is the rate of reaction and is dependent on enzyme concentration, substrate concentration, temperature, and pH.
   1. Enzyme concentration: increased enzyme concentration leads to faster rate of reaction.
   2. Substrate concentration: increased concentration leads to increased rate of reaction until a maximum is reached when all enzyme receptor sites are saturated.
   3. Temperature: increased temperature leads to increased rate of reaction up to a maximum, after which enzymes denature.
   4. pH: velocity of a reaction is maximum at its optimal pH. A pH that is either too high or too low leads to a slower reaction or may denature the enzyme.

B. Michaelis–Menten equation
   1. Enzymatically catalyzed reactions can be characterized by the Michaelis–Menten equation:

      $V = V_{max} \times [S]/(K_m + [S])$

      where V is the velocity of the reaction.

      V_{max} is the maximum velocity of the reaction.
      $[S]$ is the substrate concentration.
      K_m is the Michaelis constant (the substrate concentration at which velocity is one-half of the maximum velocity of a given reaction; $V = V_{max}/2$)
   2. Effect of substrate concentration on reaction velocity (Figure 1-10)

FIGURE 1-10 Effect of substrate concentration on reaction velocity

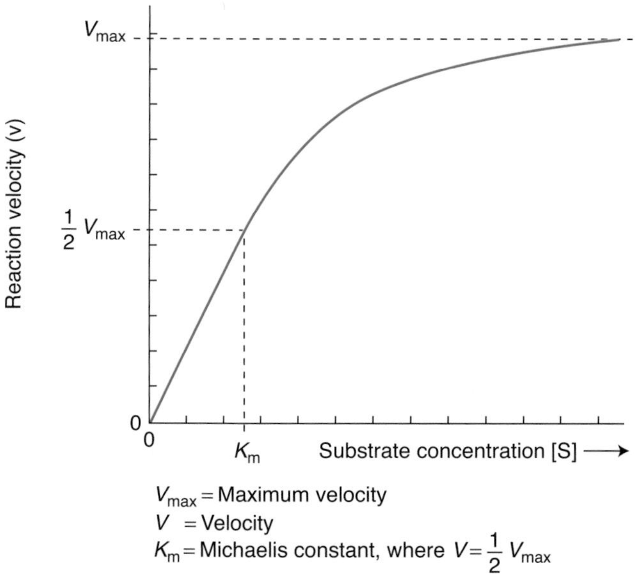
V_{max}
$\frac{1}{2} V_{max}$
Reaction velocity (v)
0
0
K_m
Substrate concentration [S] ⟶
V_{max} = Maximum velocity
V = Velocity
K_m = Michaelis constant, where $V = \frac{1}{2} V_{max}$

C. Lineweaver–Burk plots (Figure 1-11)
   1. A Lineweaver–Burk plot is a linear representation of the Michaelis–Menten equation, which allows for easier interpretation of the maximum velocity of an equation.
      a. Competitive inhibitors increase the K_m by competing with substrate binding to enzyme at the active site.
      b. Noncompetitive inhibitors decrease the V_{max} by bonding to the enzyme (E or ES) outside of the active site.
      c. Irreversible inhibitors inactivate the enzyme with kinetics similar to noncompetitive inhibition. Example: Aspirin inhibition of cyclooxygenases.
   2. Regulatory enzymes in metabolic pathways are influenced by allosteric interactions and will have nonlinear Lineweaver–Burk plots for their kinetics.

Basic Concepts

FIGURE 1-11 **Lineweaver–Burk plot**

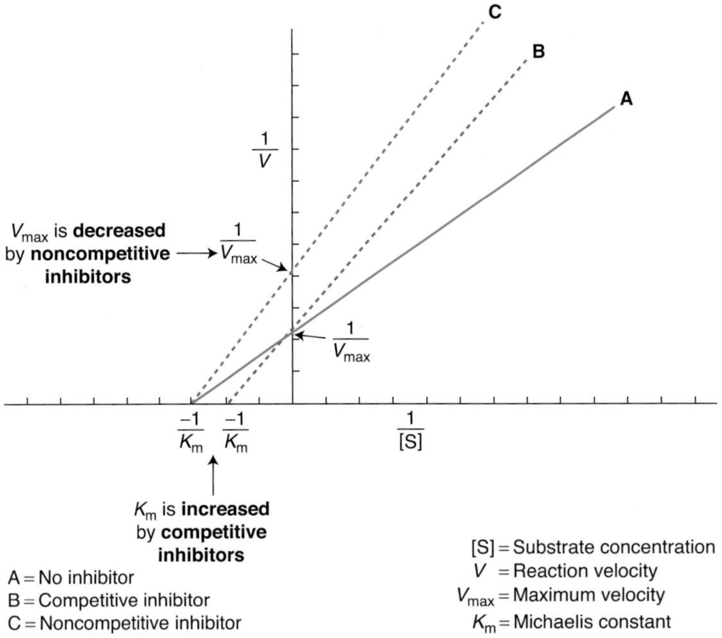
C
B
A
1/V
V_{max} is **decreased** by **noncompetitive inhibitors**
$\frac{1}{V_{max}}$
$\frac{1}{V_{max}}$
$\frac{-1}{K_m}$ $\frac{-1}{K_m}$
$\frac{1}{[S]}$
K_m is **increased** by **competitive inhibitors**
A = No inhibitor
B = Competitive inhibitor
C = Noncompetitive inhibitor
[S] = Substrate concentration
V = Reaction velocity
V_{max} = Maximum velocity
K_m = Michaelis constant

$\frac{1}{V_{max}}$ is where the plot crosses the *y*-axis

$\frac{-1}{K_m}$ is where the plot crosses the *x*-axis

QUICK HIT

When infusing a drug, it takes 4.3 half-lives to achieve 95% of the steady-state concentration.

CONCEPTS IN PHARMACOLOGY

I. Absorption

A. There are many routes of administration (Figure 1-12).

FIGURE 1-12 **Routes of drug administration**

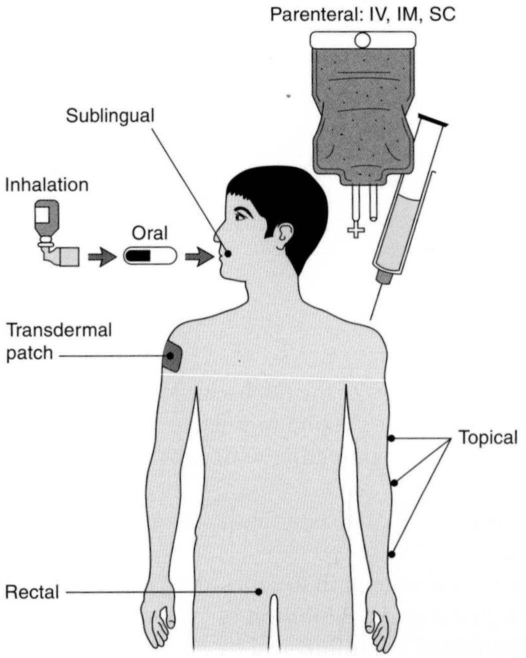
Parenteral: IV, IM, SC
Sublingual
Inhalation
Oral
Transdermal patch
Topical
Rectal

IM, intramuscular; IV, intravenous; SC, subcutaneous. (Adapted from Mycek M, Harvey RA, Champe PC. *Lippincott's Illustrated Reviews: Pharmacology.* 2nd ed. Philadelphia, PA: Lippincott-Raven Publishers; 1996:2. Used with permission of Lippincott Williams & Wilkins.)

B. Oral administration is the most common route.
C. Most drugs are absorbed in the **duodenum**.
   1. Drugs enter the portal circulation.
   2. They are subject to **first-pass metabolism** by the liver.
D. Other factors that affect absorption are
   1. Intestinal pH.
   2. Whether taken with food (slows transit allowing for further acid digestion).
   3. Whether the drug is a sustained-release preparation.
   4. Whether gastrointestinal diseases or malabsorption syndromes are present.

QUICK HIT

If a drug is rapidly metabolized by the liver, the amount reaching the target tissues is significantly reduced. Such drugs include propranolol, lidocaine, verapamil, and meperidine.

II. Distribution

$V_d = D/C$

A. V_d, volume of distribution; D, amount of drug in body; C, plasma concentration.
B. Distribution occurs more rapidly with high blood flow, high vessel permeability, and a **hydrophobic drug**.
C. Binding to **plasma proteins** (albumin and globulins) accelerates absorption into plasma but slows diffusion into tissues.
D. Many disease states alter distribution:
   1. Edematous states (e.g., cirrhosis, heart failure, nephrotic syndrome) prolong distribution and delay clearance.
   2. Obesity allows for greater accumulation of lipophilic agents within fat cells, increasing distribution and prolonging half-life.
   3. Pregnancy increases intravascular volume, thus increasing V_d.
   4. Hypoalbuminemia allows drugs that are protein bound to have increased availability because of lack of albumin for binding.

QUICK HIT

Charged species do not cross the gastrointestinal membrane as readily as uncharged species. Therefore, the percentage of drug in the uncharged state determines the rate of absorption.

$$pH = pK_a + \log \frac{\textit{pronated}}{\textit{unpronated species}}$$

QUICK HIT

Acidophilic drugs bind to albumin, whereas basophilic drugs bind to globulins. The administration of a drug that binds to sites already occupied by a drug can displace the first drug. This leads to a surge in free drug, which, in turn, leads to increased activity and elimination.

III. Pharmacokinetics

A. The effect an agonist has on its receptors depends on concentration.
B. **Efficacy** is a measure of the maximum effect a drug can produce.
C. **Potency** is a measure of the amount of drug needed to produce a given effect (Figure 1-13).
D. Effective dose (ED) and lethal dose (LD)
   1. ED is the dose of the drug that produces the desired effect.
   2. ED_{50} is the dose of the drug that produces the desired effect in 50% of the population.
   3. LD is the dose of the drug that produces death.

QUICK HIT

Efficacy is equivalent to maximum velocity (V_{max}) in enzyme kinetics.

FIGURE 1-13 Dose–response curve

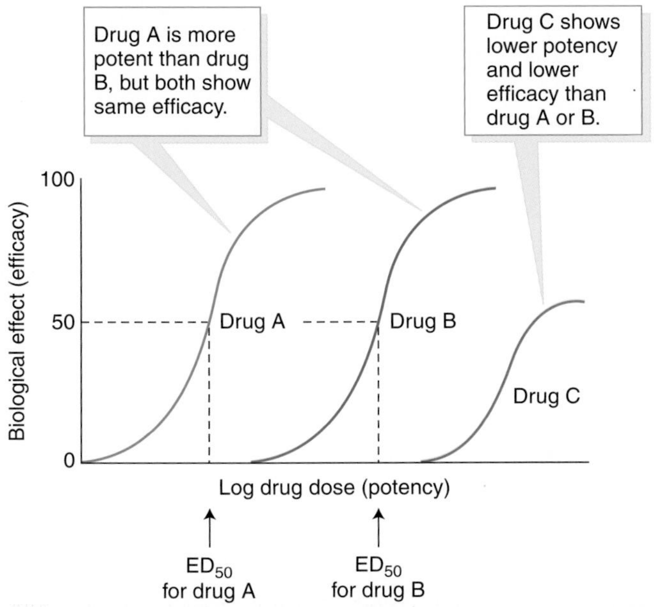
Drug A is more potent than drug B, but both show same efficacy.
Drug C shows lower potency and lower efficacy than drug A or B.
100
50
0
Biological effect (efficacy)
Drug A
Drug B
Drug C
Log drug dose (potency)
ED50 for drug A
ED50 for drug B

ED_{50}, dose effective in 50% of population.

FIGURE 1-14 Therapeutic range

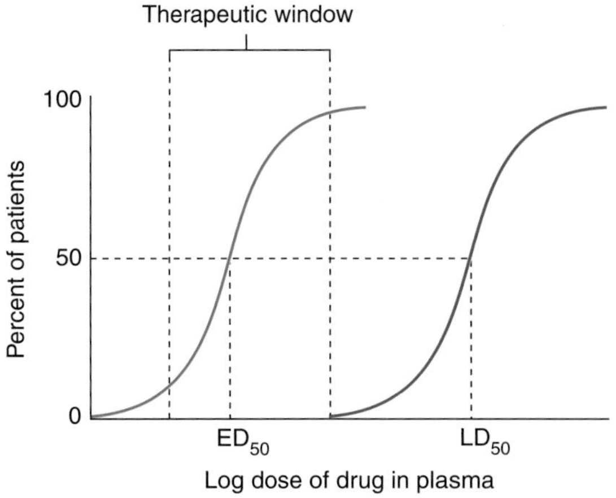
Therapeutic window
100
50
0
Percent of patients
ED50
LD50
Log dose of drug in plasma

ED_{50}, dose effective in 50% of population; LD_{50}, dose that is lethal in 50% of population.

4. LD_{50} is the dose of the drug that produces death in 50% of the population.
5. Separation of ED and LD determines therapeutic range (Figure 1-14).
6. A drug's **therapeutic index** (TI) is a measure of how safe it is to use.
   $TI = LD_{50}/ED_{50}$

E. Antagonists (Figure 1-15)
1. **Competitive antagonist**: competes for the same binding site as the agonist or drug
   a. Increases K_m
   b. Does not affect V_{max}
2. **Noncompetitive antagonist**
   a. Prevents binding of the agonist or drug to the receptor or prevents activation of the receptor by the agonist
   b. Decreases the efficacy of the agonist
   c. Decreases V_{max}, but does not affect K_m

FIGURE 1-15 Drug antagonism

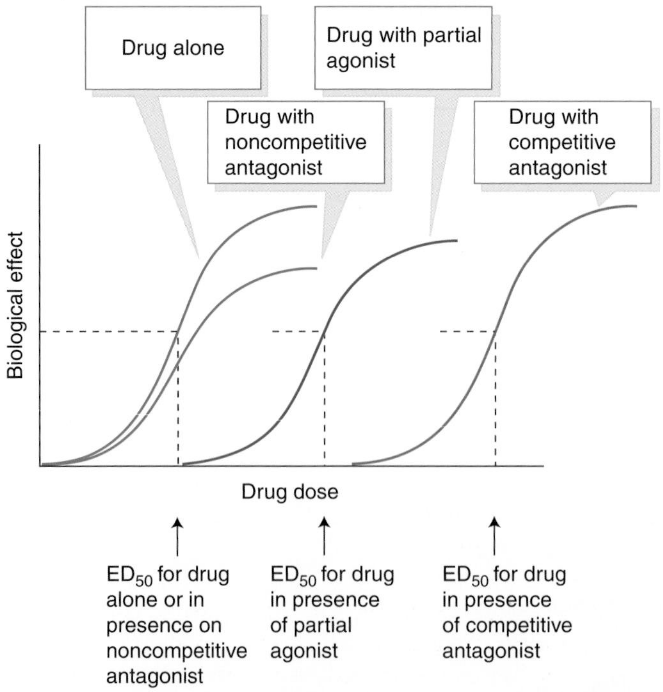
Drug alone
Drug with partial agonist
Drug with noncompetitive antagonist
Drug with competitive antagonist
Biological effect
Drug dose
ED50 for drug alone or in presence on noncompetitive antagonist
ED50 for drug in presence of partial agonist
ED50 for drug in presence of competitive antagonist

ED_{50}, dose effective in 50% of population.

3. **Complete antagonist**: prevents all pharmacologic action(s) of the agonist or drug
4. **Partial agonist**: binds to the same receptor site as the agonist or drug but has a lower efficacy

F. Pharmacokinetics is affected by disease states:
1. Hyperthyroidism increases the heart's sensitivity to catecholamines.
2. Patients with cirrhosis are more sensitive to sedative-hypnotics.
3. Patients with cirrhosis and congestive heart failure (CHF) will retain fluids if taking nonsteroidal anti-inflammatory drugs (NSAIDs) because of the role of prostaglandins in maintaining renal function.

IV. Metabolism

A. Drugs may be chemically altered, varying activity or aiding excretion.

B. The enzymatic transformation of drugs usually follows one of two kinetics:
1. **First-order kinetics**: a constant **fraction** of drug is metabolized in a certain unit of time, by far the most common. This arises because drugs have higher affinities for their receptors (K_d) than their metabolizing enzymes (K_m).
2. **Zero-order kinetics**: a constant **amount** of drug is metabolized in a certain unit of time (e.g., ethanol)—rare.

C. The liver is the primary site of metabolism and uses two sets of reactions:
1. **Phase 1**: drugs are modified or portions are removed (cytochrome P450 oxidation, enzymatic reduction, hydrolysis)
2. **Phase 2**: conjugation reactions add chemical groupings to the drug (e.g., glucuronidation, sulfate or glutathione conjugation, acetylation, methylation)

D. **Prodrugs** are drugs that are administered in an inactive form and are metabolically activated by the body.

E. Some drugs are metabolized to toxic products (e.g., acetaminophen).

QUICK HIT

Ethanol, barbiturates, and phenytoin induce cytochrome P450 enzymes, whereas cimetidine and ketoconazole inhibit cytochrome P450 enzymes, increasing and decreasing the metabolism of other drugs, respectively (e.g., warfarin). The macrolide antibiotics (e.g., erythromycin) inhibit cytochrome P450 enzymes and increase the cardiac toxicity of cisapride.

V. Elimination

A. Most drugs are eliminated in the urine or bile.

B. Volatile drugs (e.g., ethanol) can be eliminated through the lungs.

C. **Renal excretion**
1. Substances with a molecular weight (MW) $< 5{,}000$ that are free in the plasma are filtered in the glomerulus.
2. Higher concentrations of a substance within the tubules may favor some reabsorption.
3. The proximal convoluted tubule (PCT) may actively secrete a drug.
4. The urine pH, molecular size, lipid solubility, and negative logarithm of the acid ionization constant (pK_a) of the drug affect renal excretion.

D. Biliary excretion
1. Hepatocytes actively take up the drug from plasma, store it or metabolize it, and release it into the bile duct.
2. Some drugs are excreted in feces.
3. Some drugs are reabsorbed in the terminal ileum (enterohepatic cycling).

QUICK HIT

Filtration is dependent on the amount of free drug in the blood, whereas active secretion is dependent on the total plasma concentration (free and bound drug).

VI. Special circumstances

A. **Older patients**
1. These patients often use multiple prescriptions and over-the-counter medications.
2. Decreased body size, body water, and serum albumin, along with increased body fat, alter drug distribution.
3. **Decreased phase 1 reactions**, liver mass, and liver blood flow all slow metabolism.
4. Decreased kidney mass, renal blood flow, glomerular filtration rate, and tubular function hamper drug excretion.

B. **Pediatric patients**
1. **Most drugs cross the placenta** to some extent, and their possible effects on the fetus are ranked as category A, B, C, D, and X (A = no evidence of first trimester risk in well-controlled human studies, X = positive evidence of fetal risk, and the risks outweigh the potential benefits).

2. Absorption
   a. High gastric pH and delayed emptying affect enteral absorption.
   b. High surface area-to-volume ratio affects transdermal administration.
   c. Low muscle mass limits intramuscular (IM) administration to the **vastus lateralis** in infancy.
3. Albumin does not reach adult levels until 1 year of age.
4. Both phases of metabolism are deficient to varying degrees until 12 years of age.
5. Specific antibiotics avoided in childhood include **quinolones** (articular cartilage erosion and tendon damage) and **tetracycline** (depression of bone and teeth formation).

C. **Pharmacogenetics**
1. Acetylation of isoniazid
   a. **In patients who are slow acetylators**, there is increased incidence of neuropathy, bladder cancer, and familial Parkinson disease.
   b. **Patients who are rapid acetylators** are the majority of the population.
   c. It also affects metabolism of hydralazine, dapsone, and phenytoin.
2. Succinylcholine sensitivity
   a. Atypical **pseudocholinesterase** does not hydrolyze succinylcholine effectively.
   b. It leads to prolonged paralysis (succinylcholine apnea).
   c. It is **autosomal recessive**.
3. Ethanol metabolism
   a. Ethanol is metabolized by two enzymes:
      i. **Alcohol dehydrogenase** (converts ethanol to acetaldehyde)
      ii. **Aldehyde dehydrogenase** (converts acetaldehyde to acetate)
   b. Aldehyde dehydrogenase shows diminished activity in certain patients (e.g., approximately 30%–40% of Chinese and Japanese individuals have diminished activity).
   c. Acetaldehyde accumulation leads to facial flushing, headache, nausea, and vomiting.

D. Toxicology (Table 1-3)

ANTI-INFECTIVE AGENTS

I. Antibiotics *(Table 1-4)*

A. **β-Lactam agents**
1. Specific agents
   a. Penicillins (e.g., penicillin G, ampicillin, piperacillin)
   b. Cephalosporins (e.g., cefazolin, ceftriaxone)
   c. Monobactams (e.g., aztreonam)
   d. Carbapenems (e.g., meropenem)
2. Mechanism of action: bactericidal
   a. **Inhibit cell wall synthesis**
   b. Act on penicillin-binding proteins (PBPs) in bacterial cell walls
   c. Require active cell division for bactericidal effect
3. Spectrum of action varies for each particular drug
   a. Gram-positive and gram-negative aerobic bacteria
   b. Anaerobes and spirochetes
4. Side effects/adverse reactions
   a. **Allergic reactions** (especially a rash with penicillins)
   b. Neutropenia and thrombocytopenia
   c. Diarrhea
   d. Direct central nervous system (CNS) toxicity
   e. Superinfections including *Clostridium difficile* and yeasts such as *Candida* spp.
5. Mechanisms of resistance
   a. Inactivation by β-lactamase enzymes
   b. Failure to reach PBP targets
   c. Poor binding to PBPs

> **QUICK HIT**
> β-Lactam inhibitors, which have weak bactericidal activity but greatly inhibit β-lactamase, are used in combination with some penicillins to enhance their effectiveness (e.g., amoxicillin-clavulanate, ampicillin-sulbactam, piperacillin-tazobactam).

> **QUICK HIT**
> Remember the following drugs as **bacteriostatic**: tetracyclines, erythromycin, clindamycin, chloramphenicol, sulfonamides, and trimethoprim. Remember these drugs as **bactericidal:** penicillin, cephalosporin, vancomycin, aminoglycosides, fluoroquinolones, metronidazole, and polymyxin.

TABLE 1-3 **Toxicology**

Poison	Therapy
Acetaminophen	*N*-acetylcysteine
Amphetamine	Ammonium chloride (acidify urine)
Arsenic	Dimercaprol, succimer, penicillamine
Aspirin	Activated charcoal, sodium bicarbonate (alkalinize urine), dialysis
Atropine	Physostigmine
Benzodiazepines	Flumazenil
β-Blockers	Atropine, activated charcoal, glucagon, calcium chloride
Carbon monoxide	100% oxygen, hyperbaric oxygen
Cocaine	Supportive care, benzodiazepines, calcium channel blockers
Copper	Penicillamine
Cyanide	Sodium thiosulfate; amyl nitrite plus sodium nitrite
Digitalis	Activated charcoal, digoxin immune Fab, potassium (if serum potassium level is low), possibly atropine
Ethylene glycol (antifreeze)	Fomepizole, ethanol, dialysis
Heparin	Protamine sulfate
Iron	Deferoxamine
Isoniazid	Vitamin B_6
Isopropyl alcohol	Supportive care
Lead	Succimer, EDTA, dimercaprol
Mercury	Dimercaprol
Methanol	Fomepizole, ethanol, dialysis
Methemoglobin	Methylene blue
Opioids	Naloxone, naltrexone
Organophosphates	Atropine, pralidoxime
Sulfonylureas	Dextrose, octreotide
tPA, streptokinase	Aminocaproic acid
Tricyclic antidepressants	Gastric lavage, sodium bicarbonate (serum alkalinization), diazepam for seizures
Warfarin	Vitamin K, fresh frozen plasma

EDTA, ethylenediaminetetraacetic acid; tPA, tissue plasminogen activator.

B. **Aminoglycosides** (e.g., gentamicin, tobramycin, neomycin)
  1. Mechanism of action: bactericidal
    a. Bind to the **30S ribosomal subunits of bacteria**
    b. Subsequently interfere with protein synthesis
  2. Spectrum of action
    a. Broad-spectrum activity against gram-negative bacilli
    b. Some activity against gram-positive bacteria
    c. No anaerobic activity
  3. Side effects/adverse reactions
    a. Ototoxicity
    b. Nephrotoxicity

Basic Concepts

TABLE 1-4 Antibiotics

Therapeutic Agent (common name, if relevant) [trade name, where appropriate]	Class–Pharmacology and Pharmacokinetics	Indications	Side Effects or Adverse Effects	Contraindications or Precautions to Consider; Notes
Cell wall inhibitors				
Penicillin	**β-Lactam—binds PBP → inhibits transpeptidase** cross-linking of cell wall → **inhibits bacterial cell wall synthesis → activates autolytic enzymes;** bactericidal	**Gram-positive cocci, gram-positive rods, gram-negative cocci, some anaerobes, enterococci,** and **spirochetes**	**Hypersensitivity reactions, neutropenia, thrombocytopenia, hemolytic anemia, CNS effects, superinfection** (pseudomembranous colitis)	Not penicillinase resistant
Methicillin, nafcillin, oxacillin, dicloxacillin	**β-Lactam, penicillin derivative**—same mechanism as penicillin; distinguished by activity against **penicillinase-producing *Staphylococcus;*** bactericidal	***Staphylococcus* infections** (except MRSA)	**Hypersensitivity reactions,** interstitial nephritis (methicillin)	Penicillinase resistant; MRSA is resistant to methicillin because of altered PBP target site
Ampicillin, amoxicillin, ampicillin-sulbactam [Unasyn]**, amoxicillin-clavulanate** [Augmentin]	**β-Lactam penicillin derivative**—same mechanism as penicillin; distinguished by activity against **gram-negative rods;** bactericidal	Gram-positive cocci, gram-positive rods, gram-negative cocci, and **gram-negative rods extended spectrum:** *Escherichia coli, Proteus, Salmonella, Shigella, Haemophilus influenzae*	**Hypersensitivity reaction, rash when given to mononucleosis patients**	Not effective against penicillin-resistant *Staphylococcus*, **can be combined with clavulanic acid** (β-lactamase inhibitor) to enhance spectrum. Amoxicillin is used as oral agent and ampicillin as IV agent
Ticarcillin, carbenicillin, piperacillin, piperacillin-tazobactam [Zosyn]**, ticarcillin-clavulanate** [Timentin]	**β-Lactam penicillin derivative**—same mechanism as penicillin; distinguished by activity against ***Pseudomonas*;** bactericidal	**Extended spectrum**—*Pseudomonas, Proteus, Enterobacter* species	**Hypersensitivity reactions,** decreased platelet function	Not effective against penicillin-resistant *Staphylococcus*, **can be combined with clavulanic acid** (β-lactamase inhibitor) to enhance spectrum; administered IV.
Cephalosporins	**β-Lactam**—same mechanism as penicillin, **from first generation to third generation:** a. **Gram-positive** coverage **decreases** b. **Gram-negative** coverage **increases** c. **CNS penetration increases** d. β-Lactamase **resistance increases**; bactericidal	**First generation: gram-positive cocci and PEcK** (*Proteus mirabilis, E. coli*, and *Klebsiella*) **Second generation:** same as first generation + **HENPEcK** (*H. influenzae, Enterobacter, and Neisseria*) **Third generation: cephalosporins are used for meningitis, *Klebsiella,* Lyme disease, and gram-negative bacteria**	**Hypersensitivity reaction, pain at injection site, intolerance to alcohol** (cefamandole, cefotetan, moxalactam, cefoperazone), **hypothrombinemia** (cefamandole, cefoperazone, moxalactam due to vitamin K inhibition), **thrombophlebitis, positive Coombs test**	**First generation:** cefazolin, cephalexin; **second generation:** cefaclor, cefoxitin, cefuroxime; **third generation:** ceftriaxone, cefotaxime, ceftazidime; **fourth generation:** cefepime; ***Pseudomonas* coverage:** ceftazidime, cefepime; **cross-hypersensitivity with penicillins occurs in 5%–10% of patients**

(continued)

TABLE 1-4 **Antibiotics** *(Continued)*

Therapeutic Agent (common name, if relevant) [trade name, where appropriate]	Class–Pharmacology and Pharmacokinetics	Indications	Side Effects or Adverse Effects	Contraindications or Precautions to Consider; Notes
Aztreonam [Azactam]	**Monocyclic β-lactam**—same mechanism as penicillin (binds to PBP3); bactericidal	**Gram-negative bacteria, esp. *Pseudomonas, Klebsiella, Serratia,* and Enterobacteriaceae No activity against gram-positives or anaerobes.**	Skin rash, GI distress (nausea, vomiting)	**Does not cross-react with penicillin; synergistic with aminoglycosides;** can be used in patients with **penicillin allergies** and **renal insufficiency who cannot take aminoglycosides**
Imipenem/cilastatin [Primaxin]	**Carbapenem**—same mechanism as penicillin; bactericidal	**Broad spectrum—gram-positive cocci** (MSSA and *Streptococcus*), **gram-negative rods** (*Pseudomonas* and *Enterobacter* species), **anaerobes**	Hypersensitivity reaction, **seizure,** confusion state	Significant side effects; limit use to when other drugs have failed or in the case of life-threatening infections; always administered with cilastatin (inhibits renal dehydropeptidase) to reduce inactivation in renal tubules
Meropenem [Merrem]	**Carbapenem—same** mechanism as penicillin; bactericidal	**Broad spectrum—gram-positive cocci** (MSSA and *Streptococcus*), **gram-negative rods** (*Pseudomonas* and *Enterobacter* species), **anaerobes**	Reduced risk of seizure compared to imipenem	Stable to dehydropeptidase I, unlike imipenem
Vancomycin	**Cell wall inhibitor—binds** to D-alanyl-D-alanine portion of cell wall → inhibits cell wall glycopeptide polymerization → stops bacterial cell wall synthesis; usually bactericidal	**Serious infections by gram-positive bacteria: *Streptococcus, Staphylococcus,* and some anaerobes (especially *Clostridium difficile*)**	**Ototoxicity, nephrotoxicity, thrombophlebitis, diffuse flushing—"red man syndrome"; caused by histamine release**	Can prevent red man syndrome by pretreatment with antihistamines and slow infusion; resistance occurs when bacteria change amino acid in cell wall to D-alanyl-D-alanine
Protein synthesis inhibitors				
Streptomycin, gentamicin, tobramycin, amikacin, spectinomycin	**Aminoglycosides—irreversibly bind 30S ribosome** subunits; **bacteriostatic** at low concentration; **bactericidal** at high concentration	**Broad-spectrum—**gram-negative rods; good for **bone** and **eye** infections; *Proteus, Pseudomonas, Enterobacter, Klebsiella, E. coli;* also used for tuberculosis	**Ototoxicity, renal toxicity, neuromuscular blockade,** nausea, vomiting, vertigo, allergic skin rash	

(continued)

Basic Concepts

TABLE 1-4 **Antibiotics** *(Continued)*

Therapeutic Agent (common name, if relevant) [trade name, where appropriate]	Class–Pharmacology and Pharmacokinetics	Indications	Side Effects or Adverse Effects	Contraindications or Precautions to Consider; Notes
Tetracycline, doxycycline, demeclocycline, minocycline	**Tetracyclines—bind 30S ribosome subunits** → prevent attachment of tRNA; bacteriostatic	**Broad-spectrum including atypical pathogens: *Chlamydia, Rickettsia, Mycoplasma pneumoniae, Vibrio cholerae, Ureaplasma urealyticum,* tularemia, *Helicobacter pylori, Borrelia burgdorferi* (Lyme disease)**	**Liver toxicity, GI distress, depression of bone/teeth development** (less with doxycycline), **photosensitivity** (less with doxycycline), **Fanconi syndrome**	**Contraindicated in pregnancy and children; divalent cations inhibit gut absorption, therefore cannot be taken with milk, antacids, or iron-containing preparations. Tetracycline is renally eliminated; doxycycline is fecally eliminated**
Erythromycin, clarithromycin [Biaxin], **azithromycin** [Zithromax]	**Macrolide**—binds to the 23S RNA of the 50S ribosome subunits → block translocation → prevents protein synthesis; bacteriostatic	**First choice for cell wall–deficient bugs: *Mycoplasma, Rickettsia, Chlamydia, Legionella, Corynebacterium diphtheria;*** gram-positive **cocci** (*Streptococcus*)	GI discomfort, **acute cholestatic hepatitis, skin rashes;** increases concentration of **oral anticoagulants** and theophyllines	Can be used in patients with **streptococcal infections** and **penicillin allergies**
Chloramphenicol antifungal agents	**Protein synthesis inhibitor—inhibits 50S peptidyltransferase activity; bacteriostatic,** but bactericidal versus *H. influenzae* and *Neisseria meningitidis*	Meningitis (*H. influenza, N. meningitidis, Streptococcus pneumoniae*), typhoid fever, *Salmonella; Rickettsia* (Rocky Mountain spotted fever in children), *Bacteroides*	**Fatal aplastic anemia, bone marrow suppression, gray baby syndrome** (cyanosis, vomiting, green stools, vasomotor collapse due to insufficient glucuronidase in neonatal liver)	Interacts with phenytoin, warfarin, or coumadin; inhibits cytochrome P450; used to treat serious infections after other antibiotics have failed given side effects
Clindamycin [Cleocin]	**Protein synthesis inhibitor—binds to 50S subunits** → blocks peptide bond formation; bacteriostatic or bactericidal depending on concentration, site, and organism	**Gram-positive bacteria (*Streptococcus, Staphylococcus*), treat anaerobic infections**	Severe diarrhea, **potentially fatal pseudomembranous colitis caused by *C. difficile***	
DNA synthesis inhibitors				
Sulfamethoxazole, sulfisoxazole, sulfadiazine	**Sulfonamide—competitive inhibitor of dihydropteroate synthetase (blocks folic acid synthesis);** bacteriostatic	**Broad-spectrum—gram-positive UTI, *Chlamydia* infection of genital tract and eye, treatment of nocardiosis**	**Form crystals in kidney and bladder causing damage; hypersensitivity reaction; photosensitivity; kernicterus (in infants); hemolysis (in G6PD deficiency)**	Displaces other drugs such as warfarin from albumin
Trimethoprim [Proloprim, Trimpex]	**Antibiotic—competitive inhibition of dihydrofolate reductase** (blocks folic acid synthesis); bacteriostatic	**Gram-negative UTI, combined with sulfonamides to treat UTI, otitis media, chronic bronchitis, shigellosis, *Salmonella*, and PCP**	Megaloblastic anemia, leukopenia, granulocytopenia	Supplementation with folic acid may help pancytopenia

(continued)

TABLE 1-4 **Antibiotics** *(Continued)*

Therapeutic Agent (common name, if relevant) [trade name, where appropriate]	Class–Pharmacology and Pharmacokinetics	Indications	Side Effects or Adverse Effects	Contraindications or Precautions to Consider; Notes
Ciprofloxacin [Cipro], **norfloxacin, ofloxacin, levofloxacin** [Levaquin], **moxifloxacin** [Avelox]	**Quinolone antibiotic—inhibits DNA gyrase** (topoisomerase II) and **topoisomerase IV** → blocks DNA synthesis; bactericidal	**Gram-negative infections (esp. UTI and bone): *Pseudomonas*, *Enterobacteriaceae*, *Neisseria*; gram-positive infections** (*Staphylococcus*, *Streptococcus*); **intracellular: *Legionella***	**GI disturbances, headache, dizziness, phototoxicity, cartilage damage (children, fetus), tendonitis and tendon rupture (adults), myalgias (children)**	**May elevate theophylline to toxic levels causing seizure; contraindicated in pregnant women. Divalent cations inhibit gut absorption, therefore cannot be taken with milk, antacids, or iron-containing preparations.**
Metronidazole [Flagyl]	**Antibiotic, antiprotozoal**—penetrates cell membrane and gives off nitro moiety → forms toxic metabolites → react and damage DNA; bactericidal	***Bacteroides fragilis*** (esp. for endocarditis and CNS), **Pseudomembranous colitis** (*C. difficile*), **amebiasis, giardiasis, trichomoniasis, bacterial vaginosis** (*Gardnerella vaginalis*), **peptic ulcer disease** (part of *H. pylori* triple therapy)	Nausea, vomiting, **disulfiram-like reaction to alcohol,** metallic taste, paresthesia, stomatitis, carcinogenic and mutagenic	**Contraindicated in pregnancy**
Cell membrane inhibitor				
Polymyxins (colistin)	**Antibiotic—bind to cell membranes** → disrupt osmotic properties; bactericidal	**Gram-negative bacteria: *Pseudomonas* and coliforms, usually topical, can be used IV or nebulized for difficult-to-treat gram-negative infections**	**Neurotoxic, nephrotoxic** (acute renal tubular necrosis)	

CNS, central nervous system; G6PD, glucose-6-phosphate dehydrogenase; GI, gastrointestinal; IV, intravenous; MRSA, methicillin-resistant *Staphylococcus aureus*; MSSA, methicillin-sensitive *S. aureus*; PBP, penicillin-binding protein; PCP, ; tRNA, transfer RNA; UTI, urinary tract infection.

4. Mechanisms of resistance
    a. Enzymatic modification of the aminoglycoside
    b. Altered ribosome binding sites
    c. Altered antibiotic uptake

C. **Tetracyclines** (e.g., tetracycline, demeclocycline, doxycycline)
1. Mechanism of action: **bacteriostatic**
    a. Reversibly bind to the 30S ribosomal subunit
    b. Prevent the addition of new amino acids onto growing peptide chain
2. Spectrum of action: broad-spectrum activity
    a. Gram-positive and gram-negative bacteria, anaerobes, spirochetes, mycoplasmas, rickettsiae, and chlamydiae
    b. Some protozoa
3. Side effects/adverse reactions
    a. Teeth discoloration
    b. **Depression of skeletal growth**
    c. Gastrointestinal distress (most common side effect)

QUICK HIT

Tetracyclines are contraindicated in pregnancy and in children because of their effect on the teeth and bones.

Basic Concepts

QUICK HIT

Avoid the following drugs in pregnancy: aminoglycosides (ototoxicity), **tetracyclines** (tooth discoloration and decreased bone growth), **clarithromycin** (embryotoxic), **chloramphenicol** (gray baby syndrome), **sulfonamides** (kernicterus), **fluoroquinolones** (cartilage damage), **metronidazole** (mutations), **ribavirin** (teratogenic), **griseofulvin** (teratogenic).

d. **Hepatotoxicity**
e. Photosensitivity
4. Mechanisms of resistance
a. Reduction of tetracycline influx
b. Active tetracycline export from within the bacterial cell

D. **Chloramphenicol**
1. Mechanism of action: usually bacteriostatic but bactericidal in some organisms
a. Binds to the 50S ribosomal subunit
b. Prevents the addition of new amino acids onto growing peptide chain
2. Spectrum of action
a. Gram-positive and gram-negative bacteria
b. Spirochetes, rickettsiae, chlamydiae, and mycoplasmas
3. Side effects/adverse reactions: chloramphenicol is rarely a first choice because of its adverse reactions
a. **Aplastic anemia**
b. Reversible bone marrow depression
c. **Gray baby syndrome**: abdominal distention, vomiting, flaccidity, cyanosis, circulatory collapse, and death
4. Mechanisms of resistance
a. Impermeability of bacteria to drug
b. Production of enzymes that inactivate the antibiotic

QUICK HIT

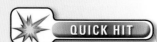

Although clindamycin is typically associated with pseudomembranous colitis (*Clostridium difficile* infection), cephalosporins cause more cases of pseudomembranous colitis because of their greater use.

E. **Macrolides** (e.g., erythromycin, azithromycin, clarithromycin) and lincosamides (e.g., clindamycin)
1. Mechanism of action: bactericidal activity is relative to dose, and these agents are generally considered bacteriostatic.
a. Bind to the bacterial 50S ribosomal subunit
b. Consequently inhibit RNA-dependent protein synthesis
2. Spectrum of action: broad-spectrum activity
a. Gram-positive and gram-negative bacteria. **Clindamycin is especially effective against anaerobes**.
b. Treponemes, mycoplasmas, chlamydiae, and rickettsiae. Erythromycin is a good choice for cell wall–deficient organisms such as *Mycoplasma, Chlamydia,* and *Legionella.*
3. Side effects/adverse reactions
a. Gastrointestinal distress
b. Allergic reactions
c. Superinfections
- Candida with erythromycin
- *C. difficile* (pseudomembranous colitis) with clindamycin
4. Mechanisms of resistance
a. Decreased permeability into bacterial cells
b. Active efflux out of cells
c. Alteration in a 50S ribosomal protein
d. Enzymatic inactivation of antibiotic

QUICK HIT

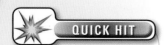

The **sulfa-containing drugs** are sulfonamides, sulfasalazine, sulfonylureas, thiazide diuretics, and furosemide. These drugs should not be given in patients with sulfa drug allergies.

F. **Sulfonamides** (e.g., sulfamethoxazole) and trimethoprim
1. Mechanism of action: The **bacteriostatic** action is potentiated when sulfonamides and trimethoprim are used together.
a. Competitively inhibits dihydrofolate reductase (trimethoprim)
b. Competitively inhibits dihydropteroate synthetase (sulfonamides)
c. **Blocks folic acid synthesis** in this way
2. Spectrum of action: broad-spectrum activity
a. Gram-positive and gram-negative bacteria, *Chlamydia*
b. *Actinomyces, Plasmodium, Toxoplasma, Pneumocystis*
3. Side effects/adverse reactions
a. Gastrointestinal distress
b. Acute hemolytic anemia, aplastic anemia, agranulocytosis, and thrombocytopenia in individuals with glucose-6-phosphate dehydrogenase (G6PD) deficiency

QUICK HIT

Sulfamethoxazole–trimethoprim is used primarily for urinary tract infections.

c. Hypersensitivity reactions, including erythema multiforme (Stevens–Johnson syndrome)
4. Mechanisms of resistance
a. Bacterial mutation resulting in microbial overproduction of folic acid precursors
b. Structural change in bacterial enzymes, with lowered affinity for sulfonamides and trimethoprim
c. Decreased bacterial cell permeability

G. **Quinolones** (e.g., ciprofloxacin, levofloxacin, moxifloxacin, gatifloxacin)
1. Mechanism of action: bactericidal
a. **Inhibit DNA gyrase** and DNA topoisomerase
b. Block DNA synthesis in this way
2. Spectrum of action: aerobic gram-negative bacilli and gram-negative cocci
3. Side effects/adverse reactions
a. Gastrointestinal distress
b. Headache, dizziness
c. Phototoxicity
d. **Damages developing cartilage and tendons (contraindicated in children and pregnancy)**
e. Risk of tendinopathy and tendon rupture in adults
f. Some prolong QT_c interval
4. Mechanisms of resistance
a. Mutation of bacterial enzymes
b. Decreased permeability of bacterial wall to antibiotic

H. **Other agents**: vancomycin, teicoplanin, and the streptogramins quinupristin/dalfopristin
1. Mechanism of action
a. Vancomycin and teicoplanin: **inhibit cell wall assembly**
b. Quinupristin/dalfopristin: can be bactericidal or bacteriostatic depending on the organism; bind to the 50S bacterial ribosomal subunit
2. Spectrum of action
a. Vancomycin and teicoplanin: serious gram-positive infections and some anaerobic infections
b. Quinupristin/dalfopristin: serious infections caused by *Staphylococcus* or *Enterococcus*
3. Side effects/adverse reactions
a. Vancomycin and teicoplanin
(1) **Red man syndrome** (flushing of the face, neck, and torso)
(2) Fever, chills, and phlebitis at injection site
b. Quinupristin/dalfopristin
(1) Gastrointestinal distress
(2) Pain at injection site
(3) Arthralgia, muscle weakness
4. Mechanisms of resistance
a. Vancomycin and teicoplanin: gene-mediated alteration in cell wall peptidoglycans
b. Quinupristin/dalfopristin
(1) Drug-modifying enzymes
(2) Efflux of antibiotic out of bacterial cell

II. Antimycobacterial agents

A. Drugs active against *Mycobacterium tuberculosis* (Table 1-5)
B. **First-line agents**: isoniazid, rifampin, pyrazinamide, ethambutol, and streptomycin
C. Bactericidal, except for ethambutol
D. Initial therapy: three first-line agents for **6 to 9 months**

QUICK HIT

Quinolones are a good choice for urinary tract infections, respiratory infections, and gastrointestinal infections.

QUICK HIT

"-floxacin" suffix = quinolone derivative. Ciprofloxacin, norfloxacin, ofloxacin = second generation; Levofloxacin = third generation; Moxifloxacin = fourth generation

QUICK HIT

Methicillin-resistant *Staphylococcus aureus* (MRSA) is often treated with vancomycin.

QUICK HIT

Isoniazid therapy requires vitamin B_6 as an adjunct.

QUICK HIT

Isoniazid, rifampin, ethambutol, and **pyrazinamide** are used in the treatment of **tuberculosis. Azithromycin, rifampin, ethambutol,** and **streptomycin** are used in the treatment of **MAC. Dapsone, rifampin,** and **clofazimine** are used in the treatment of **leprosy.**

QUICK HIT

Isoniazid is used as a solo agent to treat latent *M. tuberculosis* (TB) infection. **Azithromycin** is used as a solo agent for *M. avium intracellulare* (MAC) prophylaxis.

TABLE 1-5 Antimycobacterials

Therapeutic Agent (common name, if relevant) [trade name, where appropriate]	Pharmacology and Pharmacokinetics	Indications	Side Effects or Adverse Effects	Contraindications or Precautions to Consider; Notes
Isoniazid [INH, Nydrazid]	Inhibits synthesis of mycolic acids	***Mycobacterium*** **treatment (*M. tuberculosis* and *M. kansasii*), *M. tuberculosis* prophylaxis**	**Peripheral and CNS effects as a result of pyridoxine deficiency, liver damage, hemolytic anemia in G6PD deficiency, SLE-like syndrome**	Pyridoxine (vitamin B_6) can prevent neurotoxicity
Rifampin [Rifadin]	**Inhibits DNA-dependent RNA polymerase**	***Mycobacterium;*** **reduces resistance to dapsone when used in treatment of leprosy; prophylaxis in close contacts of people with *N. meningitidis* meningitis**	**Turns body fluid orange in color; liver damage**	**Interferes with birth control pills by increasing estrogen metabolism; induces cytochrome P450**
Ethambutol [Myambutol]	Unknown mechanism	*Mycobacterium*	**Optic neuropathy (red–green color blindness);** tolerance develops	
Streptomycin	**Aminoglycoside; binds 30S ribosome subunits; bacteriostatic at low concentration; bactericidal at high**	**Tuberculosis and other mycobacteria**		
Pyrazinamide	Postulated mechanism involves inhibition of enzyme pyrazinamidase → inhibition of fatty acid synthesis	*Mycobacterium*	Impairs liver function	

CNS, central nervous system; G6PD, glucose-6-phosphate dehydrogenase; SLE, systemic lupus erythematosus.

MNEMONIC

To remember the **mechanism of action of griseofulvin,** think "**greasy tubes.**"

MNEMONIC

To remember the **side effects of amphotericin** B think, "**shake and bake**": shaking, chills, and fever.

QUICK HIT

Both acyclovir and ganciclovir are effective against herpes virus, but ganciclovir is also effective against cytomegalovirus.

III. Antifungal agents *(Table 1-6)*

1. **Amphotericin B**
   a. Disrupts fungal membrane, leading to increased permeability
   b. Used for serious systemic fungal infections
   c. **Nephrotoxic**
2. Triazoles (e.g., fluconazole)
   a. **Disrupt synthesis of ergosterol**, which is necessary for fungal membranes
   b. Fluconazole is used for candida infections and cryptococcal meningitis

IV. Antiviral agents *(Table 1-7)*

A. **Antiretrovirals** (see Chapter 8)
   1. Reverse transcriptase inhibitors (e.g., zidovudine [AZT], tenofovir [TDF], efavirenz)
      a. Act as either nucleoside/nucleotide analogs or inhibit the reverse transcriptase enzyme itself
      b. **Prevent creation of DNA copy of viral RNA**
   2. Protease inhibitors (e.g., lopinavir, atazanavir)
      a. **Block the cleavage of viral polyproteins**
      b. Result in the production of immature, defective viral particles

B. **Acyclovir and ganciclovir**
   1. Inhibit viral DNA polymerase, which blocks viral DNA synthesis
   2. **Suppress symptoms of herpes simplex virus infections** but are **not a cure**

TABLE 1-6 **Antifungals**

Therapeutic Agent (common name, if relevant) [trade name, where appropriate]	Pharmacology and Pharmacokinetics	Indications	Side Effects or Adverse Effects	Contraindications or Precautions to Consider; Notes
Amphotericin B [Fungizone]	**Binds to cell membrane sterols** (esp. ergosterol); forms pores in membrane; fungicidal	**Wide spectrum fungal coverage: *Candida, Histoplasma, Cryptococcus*, *Blastomyces, Aspergillus*, *Coccidioides*, *Sporothrix, Mucor***	**Impaired renal function, hypersensitivity, flushing, fever, shaking chills,** hypotension, thrombophlebitis, anemia, arrhythmias, hypokalemia	**Penetrates CNS poorly;** poor GI absorption so given IV
Nystatin [Mycostatin]	**Binds to cell membrane sterols** (esp. ergosterol) → disrupting fungal membranes	**Mucosal *Candida* infections** (skin, vaginal, GI)	Few	Used topically or as mouth rinse; too toxic for systemic use
Ketoconazole [Nizoral]	**Inhibits ergosterol synthesis,** preventing cell membrane formation; **inhibits adrenal and gonadal steroid synthesis**	**Chronic mucocutaneous candidiasis,** blastomycosis, histoplasmosis, coccidioidomycosis, **prostate carcinoma, hypercortisolism**	**GI irritation, gynecomastia, thrombocytopenia, hepatotoxic, rash, fever, chills**	**Inhibits cytochrome P450**
Fluconazole [Diflucan]	**Inhibits ergosterol synthesis,** preventing cell membrane formation	**Cryptococcal meningitis, mucosal candidiasis, coccidioidomycosis**	**Abdominal pain, nausea, hepatotoxicity**	
Itraconazole [Sporanox]	**Inhibits ergosterol synthesis,** preventing cell membrane formation	Oral for dermatophytoses and onychomycosis; **drug of choice for histoplasmosis, blastomycosis, sporotrichosis, paracoccidioidomycosis**	**GI disturbances, hepatotoxicity**	
Voriconazole [Vfend]	**Inhibits ergosterol synthesis,** preventing cell membrane formation	Serious invasive fungal infections (**invasive aspergillosis**, invasive candidiasis)	**Vision disturbances (blurred vision, light sensitivity)**, GI disturbances, hepatotoxicity	
Miconazole [Monistat IV], **clotrimazole** [Lotrimin, Mycelex]	**Inhibits ergosterol synthesis**, preventing cell membrane formation	**Topical use against yeasts, dermatophytes, ringworm, fungi, mold, and oral candidiasis in AIDS**	Burning, itching, and redness when used topically; nausea; vomiting; anaphylaxis when used IV	
Flucytosine [Ancobon]	Competitive inhibitor of thymidylate synthetase; impairs DNA synthesis	*Candida, Cryptococcus*	Nausea, vomiting, diarrhea, rash, bone marrow and liver toxicity, enterocolitis	Imported in the fungus via permease
Caspofungin	Inhibits cell wall synthesis	Invasive aspergillosis or *Candida*	GI irritation, flushing	Administered IV
Terbinafine [Lamisil]	Inhibits squalene-2, 3-epoxidase	Orally for onychomycosis; topically for dermatophytes	Hepatotoxicity	
Griseofulvin [Fulvicin, Grifulvin, Grisactin]	**Inhibits cell mitosis by disrupting mitotic spindles; binds to tubulin**	**Dermatophytes (esp. *Trichophyton rubrum*)**	**Headache, confusion, rash, GI irritation, hepatotoxicity, photosensitivity, carcinogenic, teratogenic**	Increases **cytochrome P450** and warfarin metabolism

CNS, central nervous system; GI, gastrointestinal; IV, intravenous.

Basic Concepts

TABLE 1-7 **Antivirals**

Therapeutic Agent (common name, if relevant) [trade name, where appropriate]	Pharmacology and Pharmacokinetics	Indications	Side or Adverse Effects	Contraindications or Precautions to Consider; Notes
Amantadine [Symmetrel]	Inhibits fusion of lysosomes; inhibits viral penetration and uncoating; also increases release of endogenous dopamine	**Influenza A** (prophylaxis and treatment), **Parkinson disease**	**CNS effects** (ataxia, dizziness, slurred speech, nervousness, seizure), **anticholinergic,** orthostatic hypotension, **livedo reticularis** (skin rash)	Rarely used for influenza because of widespread resistance; mechanism of viral resistance is mutated M2 protein
Zanamivir [Relenza], **oseltamivir** [Tamiflu]	**Inhibits neuraminidase** → decreases release of progeny viruses	**Influenza A and B treatment and prophylaxis**		Begin within 2 days of onset of flu symptoms to decrease duration and intensity of symptoms
Ribavirin	**Guanosine analog;** inhibits IMP dehydrogenase → decreases synthesis of guanine nucleotides	**RSV in children; hepatitis C when given with interferon**	**Hemolytic anemia, elevated bilirubin, teratogen**	
Acyclovir [Zovirax]	**Guanosine analog;** monophosphorylated by **viral thymidine kinase;** triphosphorylated form **inhibits viral DNA polymerase**	**HSV, VZV, EBV, CMV** (at high doses); **HSV-induced mucocutaneous genital lesions,** and **encephalitis**	**Side effects depend on route of administration: IV—neurotoxicity, renal problems,** tremor **Oral—diarrhea,** headache **Topical—local skin irritation**	**Resistant forms lack thymidine kinase**
Valacyclovir [Valtrex]	**Antiviral—guanosine analog;** inhibits DNA polymerase	**HSV, VZV, EBV, and CMV at high doses**	**GI disturbances, CNS and renal problems, headache, tremor, rash**	**Longer lasting than acyclovir**
Ganciclovir [Cytovene]	**Antiviral—guanosine analog;** inhibits viral DNA polymerase	**CMV (esp. CMV retinitis in AIDS)**	**Bone marrow suppression** (leukopenia, neutropenia, thrombocytopenia), **renal impairment, seizures**	**Resistance from lack of thymidine kinase or mutation of viral DNA polymerase; more toxic than acyclovir**
Foscarnet [Foscavir]	**Antiviral—** nonnucleoside inhibitor of DNA polymerase	**CMV retinitis (resistant to ganciclovir), HSV (resistant to acyclovir)**	Hypocalcemia; CNS, cardiac, and **renal toxicity;** anemia	**Does not require activation by viral kinase**
Interferon α-2a (Roferon A), α-2b (Intron A), and α-n3 (Alferon-N)	**Antiviral—glycoproteins → block viral RNA, DNA, and protein synthesis**	**Genital warts, chronic hepatitis B and C, AIDS-related Kaposi sarcoma, laryngeal papillomatosis, hairy cell leukemia**	**Flulike symptoms, neutropenia, depression**	
Interferon β	**Antiviral—glycoproteins → block viral RNA, DNA, and protein synthesis**	**Multiple sclerosis**	**Flulike symptoms, neutropenia, depression**	
Interferon γ	**Antiviral—glycoproteins → block viral RNA, DNA, and protein synthesis**	**Chronic granulomatous disease**	**Flulike symptoms, neutropenia**	

CMV, cytomegalovirus; CNS, central nervous system; EBV, Epstein–Barr virus; GI, gastrointestinal; HSV, herpes simplex virus; IMP, inosine 5′monophosphate; RSV, respiratory syncytial virus; VZV, varicella-zoster virus.

C. **Amantadine and rimantadine**
   1. Inhibit the replication of influenza A
   2. Can be used prophylactically and therapeutically, although resistance is prevalent

D. **Ribavirin**
   1. Alters viral messenger RNA formation
   2. Used to treat chronic hepatitis C infection

E. **Interferons (IFNs)**
   1. Most cells produce IFN-α and IFN-β in response to viral infection.
   2. IFN-γ mediates the inflammatory response and has less antiviral action.
   3. IFNs are not directly antiviral but stimulate cellular mechanisms of viral resistance.
   4. IFNs also may cause some of the symptoms and tissue damage associated with viral infections.
   5. Used for hepatitis B, hepatitis C, and some types of cancer.

BIOSTATISTICS AND EPIDEMIOLOGY

I. Sensitivity and specificity *(Table 1-8)*

QUICK HIT

High-sensitivity tests are better suited for screening purposes, whereas high-specificity tests are used as confirmatory tests.

TABLE 1-8 Sensitivity and Specificity

		Disease	
		Yes	**No**
Test Results:	**Positive**	True Positive (A)	False Positive (B)
	Negative	False Negative (C)	True Negative (D)

Terminology	Equation	Definition
Sensitivity (positive in disease)	$\frac{A}{(A+C)}$	Probability that a person having a disease will be correctly identified
Specificity (negative in healthy)	$\frac{D}{(D+B)}$	Probability that a person who does not have a disease will be correctly identified
Positive predictive value (PPV)	$\frac{A}{(A+B)}$	Probability that an individual who tests positive has the disease
Negative predictive value (NPV)	$\frac{D}{(C+D)}$	Probability that an individual who tests negative does not have the disease
Prevalence	$\frac{A+C}{(A+B+C+D)}$ Generally calculated by incidence × duration of disease	Total number of cases in a population at a given time
Incidence	Generally calculated by number of new cases/susceptible population	Number of new cases of disease in the population over a given time

QUICK HIT

For chronic conditions (e.g., diabetes or cirrhosis), the prevalence is higher than the incidence because the long length of the disease process increases prevalence. For conditions that resolve quickly (e.g., strep throat) or are rapidly fatal (e.g., pancreatic cancer), the incidence and prevalence are approximately equal.

QUICK HIT

A screening test is more useful in a population where the disease is highly prevalent. As prevalence increases, PPV increases, and clinical usefulness is reflected in PPV.

II. Incidence and prevalence *(Table 1-8)*

A. Incidence is the number of new individuals who develop an illness in a given time period divided by the total number of individuals at risk for the illness.

B. Prevalence is the number of individuals in the population who have an illness divided by the total population.

C. Example: **Incidence** is the number of IV drug abusers newly diagnosed with HIV in 2007 divided by the number of HIV-negative IV drug abusers in the population in 2007. **Prevalence** is the number of IV drug users in the United States who are currently HIV-positive divided by the total population of IV drug users.

III. Key relationships among statistical variables

A. **Sensitivity (Sn), false-negative ratio (FNR), negative predictive value**
1. Sn and FNR are inversely related: Sn = 1 − FNR.
2. Therefore, increasing the sensitivity of a test decreases the FNR (the number of false negatives) and increases the negative predictive value.
3. Example: An FBS >126 mg/dL is used to diagnose diabetes. If we lower the threshold to 110 mg/dL, then we will catch more individuals with diabetes. Statistically, this means decreasing the number of false negatives (those individuals who test negative but actually have the disease) and increasing sensitivity.

B. **Specificity (Sp), false-positive ratio (FPR), positive predictive value (PPV)**
1. Sp and FPR are inversely related: Sp = 1 − FPR
2. Therefore, increasing the specificity of a test decreases the FPR (the number of false positives) and increases the positive predictive value.
3. Example: Western blot testing is used as a confirmatory test for HIV because of its high specificity. The initial screening test is highly sensitive (catches all true positives, plus some false positives). Western blot is specific, therefore the false positives on the first test are shown to be true negatives on the Western blot test.

C. **Specificity and sensitivity**
1. Sp and Sn are inversely related: as Sp increases, Sn decreases and vice versa.

D. **Treatment**
1. Treatment decreases prevalence by shortening duration (remember that prevalence = incidence × duration of disease) (Table 1-8).
2. Treatment has no effect on incidence.
3. Adherence, therapy, physician access, early detection → decreases duration → decreases prevalence.

MNEMONIC

To remember which statistical variables affect each other, think of the rule of Ns and Ps: Sensitivity and false-negative ratio are inversely related. Specificity and false-positive ratio are inversely related.

IV. Research study designs *(Table 1-9)*

A. **Cohort studies**
1. Observational and can be prospective or retrospective
2. After assessment of exposure to a risk factor, subjects are compared with each other for a period of time
3. Clinical treatment trial
   a. Highest quality cohort study
   b. Compares the therapeutic benefits of two or more treatments
4. **Relative risk**
   a. Calculated only for cohort studies
   b. Compares incidence rate in exposed group with incidence rate in unexposed individuals

B. **Case-control studies**
1. Retrospective and observational
2. Subjects with and without disorder are identified, and information on exposure to risk factors is assessed
3. **Odds ratio**
   a. Calculated in case-control studies; approximates the relative risk
   b. Based on disease occurring with or without exposure
   c. Odds ratio = (A × D)/(B × C) = (A/C)/(B/D) = (A/B)/(C/D)

QUICK HIT

The most rigorous form of a clinical trial is the **double-blind study**, in which neither the subject nor the examiner knows which drug the subject is receiving. Single-blind, double-blind, randomized, crossover, and placebo studies are done to reduce bias.

Where

	Disease	
	Yes	**No**
Exposure: Yes	A	B
No	C	D

TABLE 1-9 **Research Study Designs**

Study	Purpose	Notes
Case series	A study reporting on a consecutive collection of patients treated in a similar manner; no control group	
Case-control	Retrospective study designed to determine the association between an exposure and outcome: patients are sampled by outcome (e.g., patients with the disease are compared to patients without the disease); the investigator then examines the proportion of patients with the exposure in the two groups	Information reported as odds ratio. Example: Individuals with and without lung cancer are identified (outcome = lung cancer). The number of individuals who smoke within each group are counted (exposure = smoking)
Cohort	Prospective study of the factors that might cause a disorder; begins with identification of a specific population (cohort) free of outcome; one cohort is exposed to the putative cause and compared with a concurrent cohort not exposed to the putative cause; both cohorts are then followed to compare the incidence of the outcome of interest	Information reported as relative risk. Example: Two groups are made: one is exposed to UV radiation, the other is not (exposure = UV radiation). The number of individuals developing skin cancer is then counted within each group (outcome = skin cancer)
Crossover	A study design in which all patients receive both experimental and control treatments in sequence	Subjects act as own control
Cross-sectional	Provide information on possible risk factors and health status of a group of individuals at one specific point in time	Assess prevalence
Meta-analysis	Pooling data from several studies to achieve greater statistical power: often done via literature searches	
Controlled trial	Type of cohort study in which a cohort receiving one treatment/intervention is compared with a cohort receiving a different treatment or placebo	Example: Two groups are made: one is applied sunscreen, the other is applied a placebo cream (intervention = sunscreen). The number of individuals developing skin cancer is then counted within each group (outcome = skin cancer)

V. Biases—A systematic tendency to produce an outcome that differs from the underlying truth

A. **Sampling bias**—Volunteer subjects in a study may not be representative of the population being studied; as a consequence, the results of the study may not be generalizable to the entire population.

B. **Selection bias**—Occurs when there is a systematic difference in the way study groups are chosen. One method of decreasing this bias is randomization.

C. **Expectancy bias**—Occurs when a physician knows which patients are in treatment versus placebo group, causing the physician to draw conclusions supporting the expected outcome. One method of decreasing this bias is a double-blind design.

D. **Late-look bias**—Results from information being gathered too late to draw conclusions about the disease or exposure of interest from the entire study population. For instance, the more severe cases may have already died.

E. **Measurement bias**—Describes how information gathered affects information collected. For example, the Hawthorne effect describes how people act differently when being watched.

F. **Proficiency bias**—This is an issue when comparing the effects of different treatments administered at multiple sites. Physicians at one site may have more skill, thereby providing better treatment.

G. **Recall bias**—Patients who experience an adverse outcome have a different likelihood of recalling an exposure than do patients who do not have an adverse outcome, independent of the true extent of the exposure.

VI. Disease prevention

A. **Primary prevention** stops disease occurrence; for example, encouraging use of sun protection to prevent skin cancer.

B. **Secondary prevention** detects disease early; for example, physician checking for suspicious growths.

C. **Tertiary prevention** decreases devastating complications of the disease; for example, administering insulin to a diabetic.

VII. Testing and statistical methods

A. **Reliability versus validity**
   1. **Reliability** refers to the reproducibility of test results, which reflects the absence of random variation. Also known as precision.
   2. **Validity** refers to the appropriateness of a test's measurements; that is, how closely the test results reflect the truth. Also known as accuracy.
   3. **Sensitivity** and **specificity** are measures of validity.

B. Bell curve (Figure 1-16)
   1. In a normal distribution, the mean, median, and mode are equal.
      a. Mean: average
      b. Median: middle value in a sequentially ordered group of numbers
      c. Mode: number that appears most often in a group
   2. A bimodal distribution has two peaks.
   3. Skew refers to the way a peak may be offset.
      a. **Positive skew**: peak is to the left (most scores at low end; mean > median > mode)

FIGURE 1-16 Bell curve

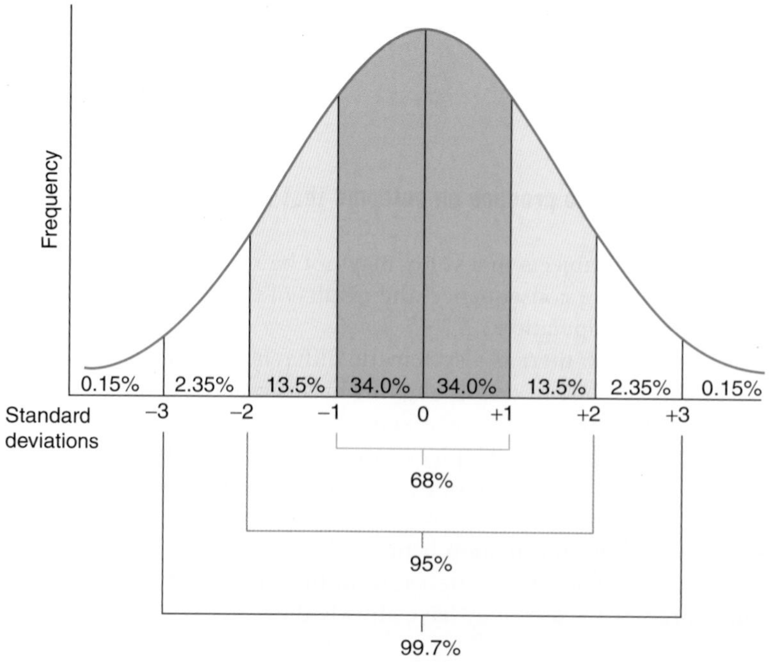
Frequency
0.15%
2.35%
13.5%
34.0%
34.0%
13.5%
2.35%
0.15%
Standard deviations
−3
−2
−1
0
+1
+2
+3
68%
95%
99.7%

b. **Negative skew**: peak is to the right (most scores at high end; mean < median < mode)

C. The **null hypothesis** (H_0)
1. Postulates that there is no significant difference between groups.
2. A **type I error** occurs when the null hypothesis is rejected when it is true. The α is the probability of making a type I error.
   a. The α value is set by the investigator, usually at 0.05.
   b. The ***p* value** is the probability that the study results occurred due to chance alone, given the null hypothesis is true.
   c. If p is less than α (usually 0.05), the results are considered "significant," and the null hypothesis is rejected.
3. A **type II error** occurs when the null hypothesis is accepted when it is not true. The β is the probability of making a type II error.
4. **Power** is the probability of rejecting the null hypothesis when the null hypothesis is false. Power $= 1 - \beta$. Increasing the sample size increases power. If $p < 0.05$, then the null hypothesis can be rejected.
5. Example
   a. A study is conducted on the influence of medical school on dating frequency.
   b. The null hypothesis would be that medical school students, when compared with 22- to 26-year-olds in the working population, have no difference in dating frequency.
   c. If the p value of the study is less than 0.05 (meaning that there is a statistical difference), then the null hypothesis can be rejected. Thus, it can be stated that medical school decreases dating frequency.

2 The Nervous System

> **QUICK HIT**
>
> Symptoms of a disc herniation are referred to the myotome and dermatome **below** the lesion. For example, a herniation of the C4–C5 disc would cause impingement of the C5 nerve root.

DEVELOPMENT

I. Central nervous system (CNS)

A. The CNS includes the **brain** and **spinal cord**.
B. The CNS forms from the neural tube.
  1. The **basal plate** of the neural tube forms **motor neurons**.
  2. The **alar plate** of the neural tube forms **sensory neurons**.
  3. The basal and alar plates are **separated** by the sulcus **limitans**.
C. **Oligodendrocytes** are responsible for **myelination**, which begins 4 months after conception and is completed by the second year of life.
D. The distal end of the spinal cord, the conus medullaris, is at the level of the third lumbar vertebra (**L3**) at **birth**. As the body grows, the cord "ascends" to its final resting position at the first lumbar vertebra (**L1**) (Figure 2-1).

FIGURE 2-1 Adult derivatives of embryonic structures in the nervous system

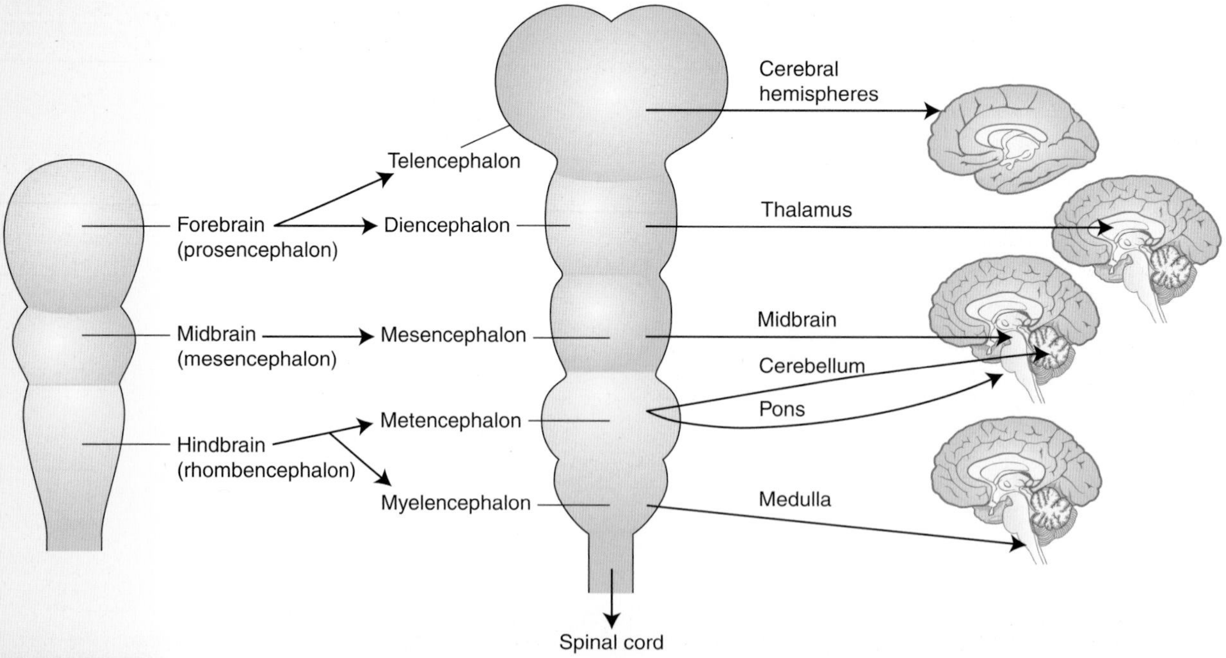
Forebrain
(prosencephalon)
Midbrain
(mesencephalon)
Hindbrain
(rhombencephalon)
Telencephalon
Diencephalon
Mesencephalon
Metencephalon
Myelencephalon
Spinal cord
Cerebral
hemispheres
Thalamus
Midbrain
Cerebellum
Pons
Medulla

> **QUICK HIT**
>
> Each oligodendrocyte can myelinate several axons, whereas each Schwann cell can only myelinate one axon.

II. Peripheral nervous system (PNS)

A. The PNS includes the **peripheral nerves** and the **autonomic** and **sensory ganglia**.
B. It is **derived from neural crest cells**, which give rise to:
  1. Schwann cells
  2. Pseudounipolar cells of the spinal and cranial nerve (CN) ganglia

3. Multipolar cells of the autonomic ganglia
4. Pia and arachnoid mater (not part of PNS)
5. Melanocytes (not part of PNS)
6. Epinephrine-producing chromaffin cells of the adrenal gland (not part of PNS)

C. **Schwann cells** are responsible for **myelination**, which begins 4 months after conception and is completed by the second year of life.

CONGENITAL MALFORMATIONS OF THE NERVOUS SYSTEM

Abnormal development of the embryonal components of the nervous system can result in some of the malformations described in Table 2-1.

TABLE 2-1 **Congenital Malformations of the Nervous System**

Condition	Clinical Features
Fetal alcohol syndrome	• **Most common cause of mental retardation** • **Cardiac septal defects** • Facial malformations including widely spaced eyes and long philtrum • Growth retardation

Spina bifida	• Improper closure of posterior neuropore
	• Several forms
	  • **Spina bifida occulta** (mildest form)—failure of vertebrae to close around spinal cord (tufts of hair often evident)
	  • Spinal meningocele (spina bifida cystica)—meninges extend out of defective spinal canal
	  • Meningomyelocele—meninges and spinal cord extend out of spinal canal
	  • Rachischisis (most severe form)—neural tissue is visible externally

Hydrocephaly	• Accumulation of CSF in ventricles and subarachnoid space • Caused by congenital blockage of cerebral aqueducts • May be caused by **cytomegalovirus** or **toxoplasma infection** • Increased head circumference in neonates
Dandy–Walker malformation	• Dilation of fourth ventricle, leading to hypoplasia of cerebellum • Failure of foramina of Luschka and Magendie to open • May result from riboflavin inhibition, posterior fossa trauma, or viral infection
Anencephaly	• Failure of brain to develop • Caused by lack of closure of anterior neuropore • Associated with increased maternal α-fetoprotein (AFP) • Decreased head circumference in neonates
Arnold–Chiari malformation	• Herniation of the **cerebellar vermis** through the foramen magnum • Hydrocephaly • Myelomeningocele

CSF, cerebrospinal fluid.

QUICK HIT

The risk of spina bifida can be decreased by taking folate supplements prior to conception and during pregnancy.

QUICK HIT

Noncommunicating (obstructive) hydrocephalus refers to increased intracranial pressure caused by a block in cerebrospinal fluid (CSF) flow. In communicating (nonobstructive) hydrocephalus, there is a normal flow of CSF but with abnormal absorption.

QUICK HIT

Syringomyelia is associated with formation of Arnold–Chiari malformation.

MAJOR RECEPTORS OF THE NERVOUS SYSTEM

I. Receptors of the sympathetic and parasympathetic nervous systems

A. The sympathetic and parasympathetic nervous systems exert their effects via various receptors scattered throughout the body (Table 2-2).

B. These effects are mediated by the substances shown in Figure 2-2.

II. Neurotoxins and their effects *(Figure 2-3)*

TABLE 2-2 **Receptors of the Sympathetic and Parasympathetic Nervous Systems**

	Sympathetic Nervous System		Parasympathetic Nervous System	
Site of Action	**Receptor**	**Effect on Site**	**Receptor**	**Effect on Site**
Smooth muscle, skin and viscera	α_1	Contract	Muscarinic	Relax
Smooth and skeletal muscle	α_1 β_2	Contract Relax	Muscarinic	Relax
Smooth muscle of the lung	β_2	Relax	Muscarinic	Contract
Smooth muscle of the gastrointestinal tract	β_2 α_1	Relax intestinal wall Contract sphincters	Muscarinic	Contract intestinal wall, relax sphincter
Heart, SA node	β_1	Increase heart rate	Muscarinic	Decrease heart rate
Heart, ventricles	β_1	Increase contractility and conduction velocity	Muscarinic	Small decrease in contractility
Eye, radial muscle	α_1	**Mydriasis** (dilation of pupil)	N/A	N/A
Eye, sphincter muscle	N/A	N/A	Muscarinic	**Miosis** (constriction of pupil)
Eye, ciliary muscle	β_2	**Relax**	Muscarinic	**Contract** (near vision)
Bladder	β_2 α_1	Relax wall Contract sphincter	Muscarinic	Contract wall, relax sphincter
Uterus	α_1 β_2	Contract Relax	Muscarinic	Contract
Penis	α_2	Emission, ejaculation	Muscarinic	Erection
Sweat glands	Muscarinic	Secrete	N/A	N/A
Pancreas	α_2 β_2	**Decrease insulin secretion** **Increase insulin secretion**	N/A N/A	N/A N/A
Liver	α_1, β_2	Glycolysis, gluconeogenesis	N/A	N/A
Adipose tissue	β_1, β_3	Lipolysis	N/A	N/A

N/A, not applicable; SA, sinoatrial.

FIGURE 2-2 **Major receptors of the nervous system**

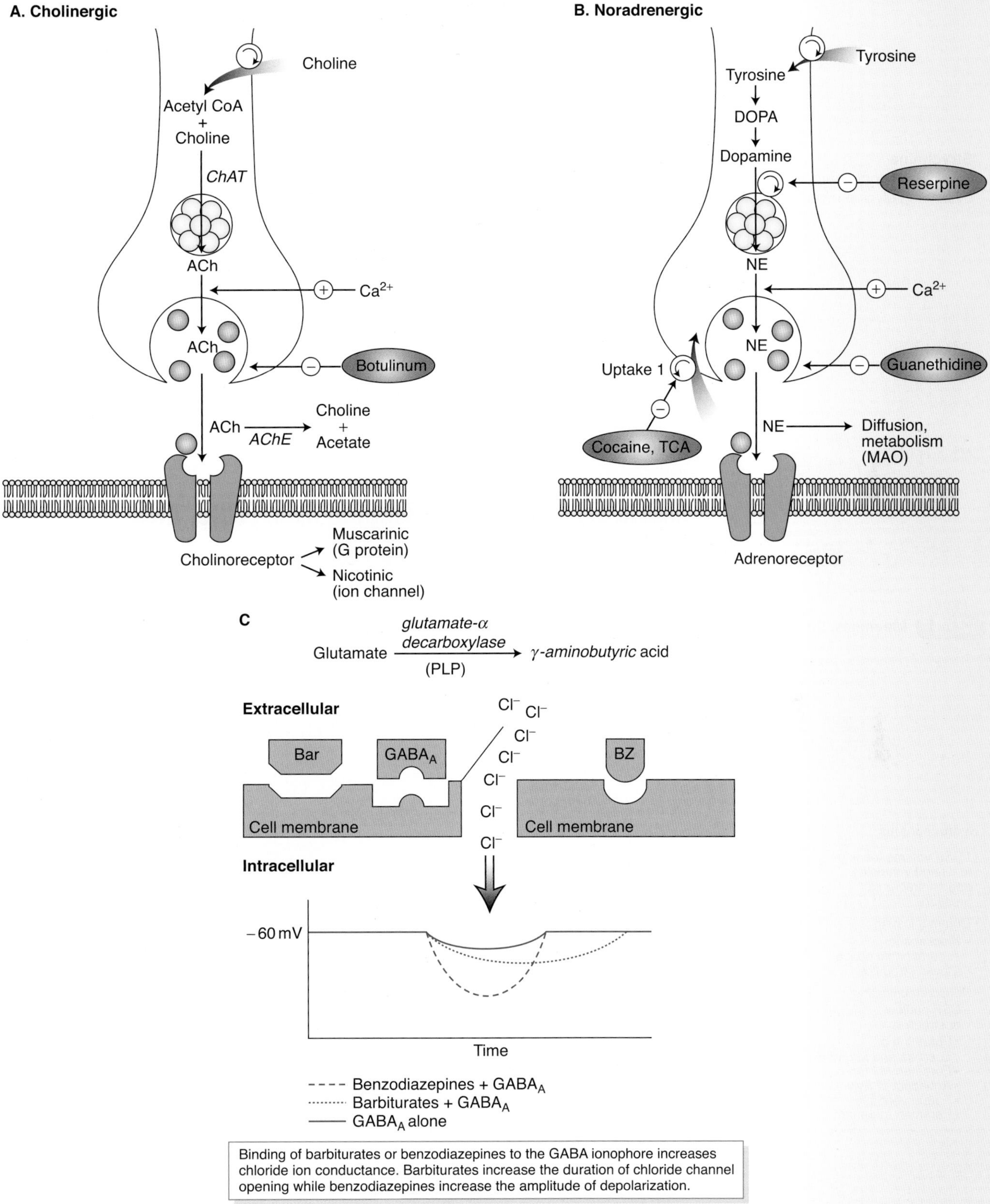
A. Cholinergic
Choline
Acetyl CoA
+
Choline
ChAT
ACh
Ca2+
ACh
Botulinum
ACh
AChE
Choline
+
Acetate
Cholinoreceptor
Muscarinic
(G protein)
Nicotinic
(ion channel)
B. Noradrenergic
Tyrosine
Tyrosine
DOPA
Dopamine
Reserpine
NE
Ca2+
NE
Uptake 1
Guanethidine
Cocaine, TCA
NE
Diffusion,
metabolism
(MAO)
Adrenoreceptor
C
Glutamate
glutamate-α decarboxylase
(PLP)
γ-aminobutyric acid
Extracellular
Bar
GABAA
BZ
Cell membrane
Cell membrane
Intracellular
–60 mV
Time
Benzodiazepines + GABAA
Barbiturates + GABAA
GABAA alone
Binding of barbiturates or benzodiazepines to the GABA ionophore increases chloride ion conductance. Barbiturates increase the duration of chloride channel opening while benzodiazepines increase the amplitude of depolarization.

Ach, acetylcholine; AChE, acetylcholinesterase; Bar, barbiturates; BZ, benzodiazepine; ChAT, choline acetyltransferase; CoA, coenzyme A; DOPA, dihydroxyphenylalanine; GABA, γ-aminobutyric acid; MAO, monoamine oxidase; NE, norepinephrine; PLP, pyridoxal phosphate; TCA, tricyclic antidepressant.

FIGURE 2-3 **Neurotoxins and their effects**

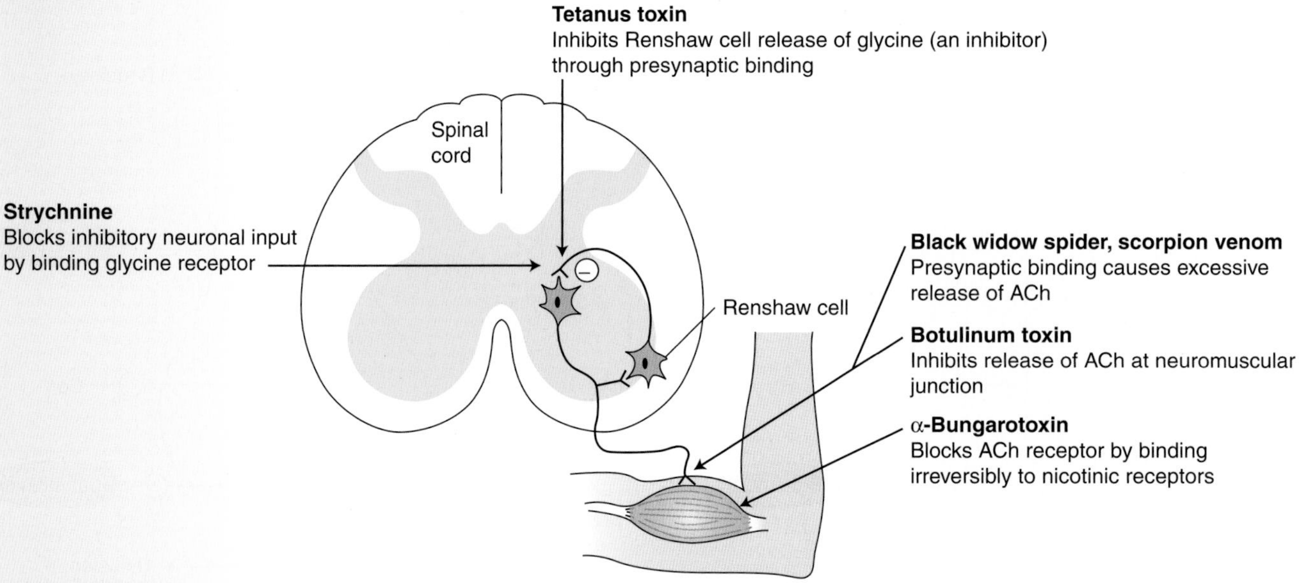
Tetanus toxin
Inhibits Renshaw cell release of glycine (an inhibitor) through presynaptic binding
Spinal cord
Strychnine
Blocks inhibitory neuronal input by binding glycine receptor
Renshaw cell
Black widow spider, scorpion venom
Presynaptic binding causes excessive release of ACh
Botulinum toxin
Inhibits release of ACh at neuromuscular junction
α-Bungarotoxin
Blocks ACh receptor by binding irreversibly to nicotinic receptors

ACh, acetylcholine.

MENINGES, FLOW OF CEREBROSPINAL FLUID, AND PATHOLOGIC TRAUMA *(Figure 2-4)*

FIGURE 2-4 **Meninges, flow of cerebrospinal fluid, and pathologic trauma**

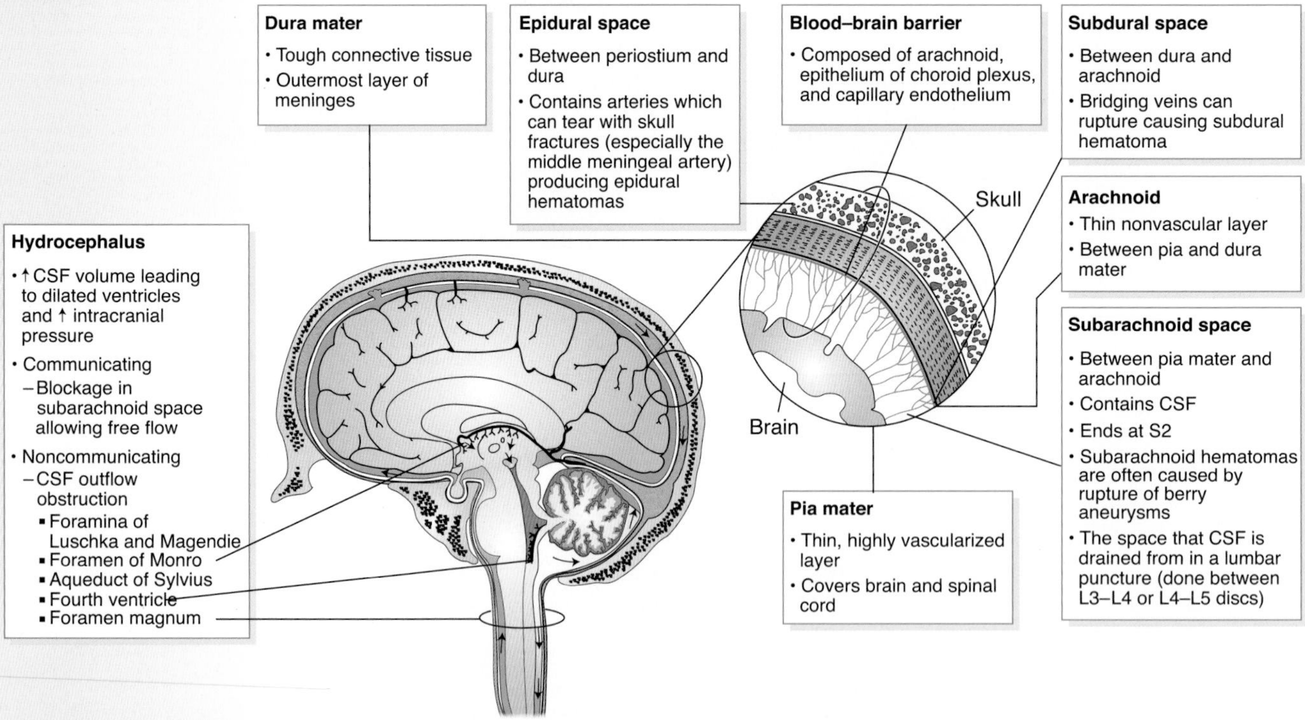
Dura mater
• Tough connective tissue
• Outermost layer of meninges
Epidural space
• Between periostium and dura
• Contains arteries which can tear with skull fractures (especially the middle meningeal artery) producing epidural hematomas
Blood–brain barrier
• Composed of arachnoid, epithelium of choroid plexus, and capillary endothelium
Subdural space
• Between dura and arachnoid
• Bridging veins can rupture causing subdural hematoma
Skull
Arachnoid
• Thin nonvascular layer
• Between pia and dura mater
Subarachnoid space
• Between pia mater and arachnoid
• Contains CSF
• Ends at S2
• Subarachnoid hematomas are often caused by rupture of berry aneurysms
• The space that CSF is drained from in a lumbar puncture (done between L3–L4 or L4–L5 discs)
Brain
Pia mater
• Thin, highly vascularized layer
• Covers brain and spinal cord
Hydrocephalus
• ↑ CSF volume leading to dilated ventricles and ↑ intracranial pressure
• Communicating
– Blockage in subarachnoid space allowing free flow
• Noncommunicating
– CSF outflow obstruction
▪ Foramina of Luschka and Magendie
▪ Foramen of Monro
▪ Aqueduct of Sylvius
▪ Fourth ventricle
▪ Foramen magnum

CSF, cerebrospinal fluid.

BLOOD SUPPLY TO THE BRAIN *(Figure 2-5)*

Cerebrovascular disease is the most common cause of CNS pathology and the third major cause of death in the United States (Table 2-3).

FIGURE 2-5 Blood supply to the brain

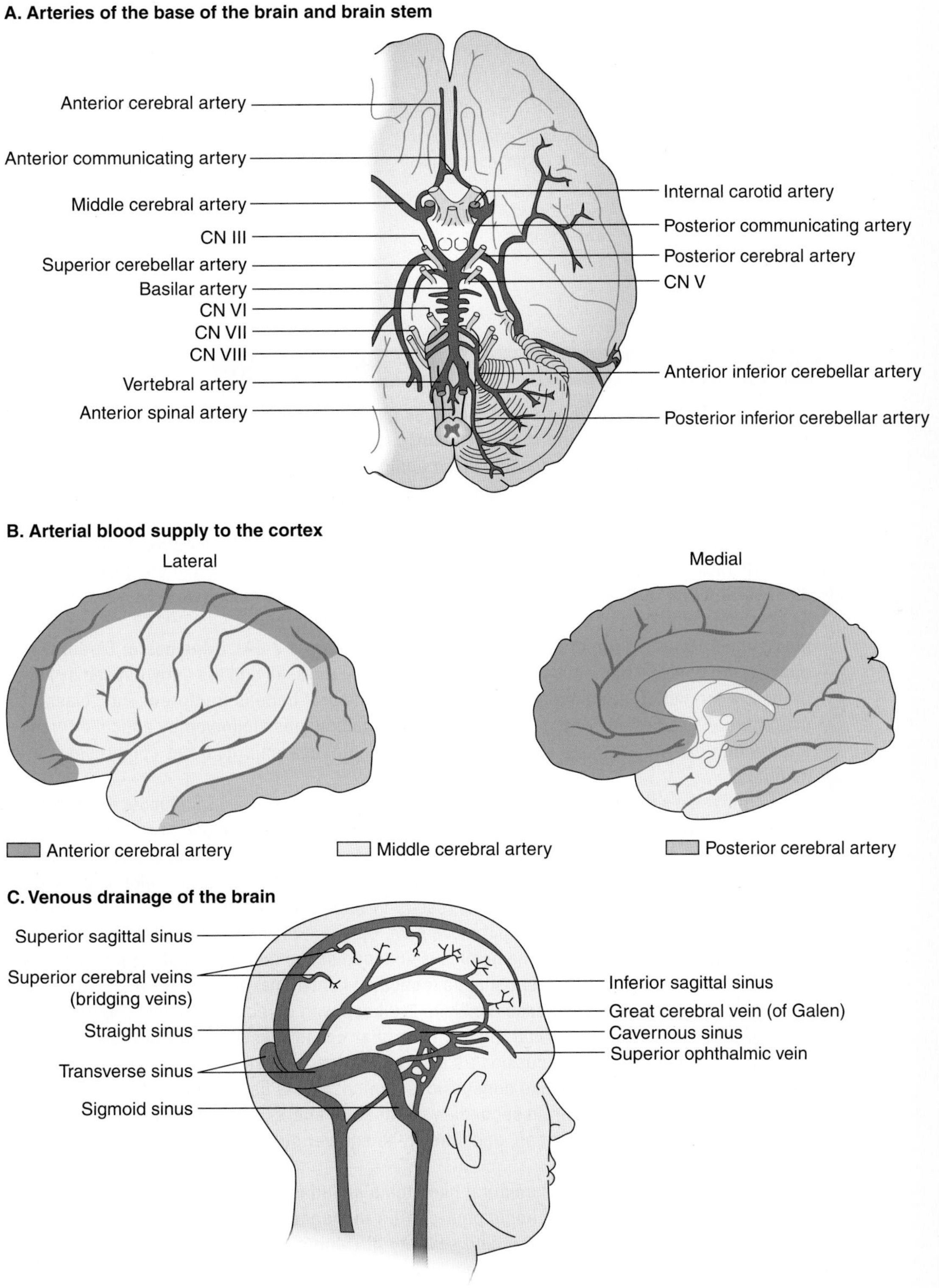
A. Arteries of the base of the brain and brain stem
Anterior cerebral artery
Anterior communicating artery
Middle cerebral artery
CN III
Superior cerebellar artery
Basilar artery
CN VI
CN VII
CN VIII
Vertebral artery
Anterior spinal artery
Internal carotid artery
Posterior communicating artery
Posterior cerebral artery
CN V
Anterior inferior cerebellar artery
Posterior inferior cerebellar artery
B. Arterial blood supply to the cortex
Lateral
Medial
Anterior cerebral artery
Middle cerebral artery
Posterior cerebral artery
C. Venous drainage of the brain
Superior sagittal sinus
Superior cerebral veins (bridging veins)
Straight sinus
Transverse sinus
Sigmoid sinus
Inferior sagittal sinus
Great cerebral vein (of Galen)
Cavernous sinus
Superior ophthalmic vein

CN, cranial nerve.

TABLE 2-3 Cerebrovascular Disease

Disease	Predisposing Factor	Common Sites
Infarction (more frequent than hemorrhage)		
Thrombosis	Atherosclerosis	Arterial obstruction of internal and external carotid arteries in neck, vertebral and basilar arteries, and vessels branching from circle of Willis to middle cerebral artery
Embolus	Cardiac mural thrombi Valvular vegetation Fat emboli	Middle cerebral artery: leads to contralateral paralysis, motor and sensory deficits, aphasias Smaller vessels: leads to **lacunar strokes**
Hemorrhage		
Intracerebral (bleeding into brain substance)	Hypertension, coagulation disorders, hemorrhage within tumor	Rupture of **Charcot–Bouchard** aneurysms (long-standing hypertension), basal ganglia, pons, frontal lobe, cerebellum
Subarachnoid (bleeding into subarachnoid space)	Associated with **berry aneurysm** in circle of Willis	Circle of Willis, bifurcation of middle cerebral artery

Clinical Vignette 2-1

CLINICAL PRESENTATION: A 26-year-old man was pushed down a flight of stairs in a fight. He **briefly lost consciousness,** then regained consciousness and went to dinner. **After 1 hour** at the restaurant, the man lost consciousness again. He was rushed to the emergency room, and after airway, breathing, and circulation were assessed and secured, a computerized tomography (CT) scan of the head was performed. The scan (Figure 2-6A) showed a convex mass over the right parietal lobe. An eye exam showed a fixed and dilated **right pupil**.

DIFFERENTIALS: Epidural hematoma, subdural hematoma, concussion, brain stem herniation

DIAGNOSTIC TESTS: A **CT scan of the head** is essential for diagnosis in patients with a history of head trauma with loss of consciousness. **An epidural hematoma** is seen on CT as a **convex mass,** which overlays the brain with high attenuation (Figure 2-6A). **(Mnemonic: Epidural = convEx).** An epidural hematoma is a blood clot between the skull and the dura, caused by laceration of the **middle meningeal artery** when the temporal bone is fractured. The "classic" presentation is a patient who has a brief loss of consciousness followed by a lucid interval, after which the patient goes into a coma as the hematoma enlarges and compresses the midbrain.

In contrast, a **subdural** hematoma forms between the dura and the brain (under the dura). It results from **venous bleeding** (as opposed to arterial in epidural hematomas) after blunt head trauma. The movement of brain relative to the skull causes rupture of **bridging veins.** Patients at higher risk for incurring a subdural hematoma after trauma are alcoholics and elderly patients. This is because of brain atrophy, which results in more "space" for the superficial bridging veins to move in response to rapid movement, thus increasing the risk of vessel rupture. Another risk factor for a subdural hematoma is anticoagulation therapy. A subdural hematoma on a CT scan appears as a crescent-shaped (**concave**) hematoma, which is usually less dense than an epidural hematoma because the blood is diluted with cerebrospinal fluid (Figure 2-6B).

CONCUSSION: Brain injury following blunt trauma that usually results in a brief loss of consciousness. Some refer to concussion as a "brain bruise." Those at increased risk include patients with a history of previous concussions. Concussion is caused by dysfunction of the electrophysiology of the midbrain secondary to impact. Patients experience confusion, dizziness, problems with concentration, and inability to answer questions (or a delay in answering) after awakening.

MANAGEMENT: Treatment for an epidural hematoma includes rapid surgical decompression. Conversely, an acute subdural hematoma can be managed by observation or craniotomy with evacuation, depending on size and severity of symptoms. There is no treatment for a concussion.

FIGURE 2-6 **A. Epidural hematoma**

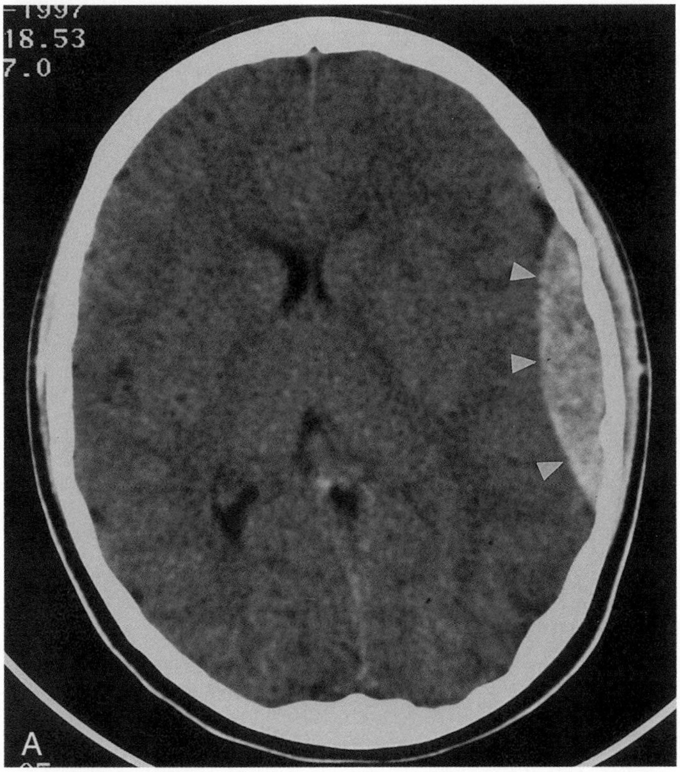

(Reproduced from Daffner RH, Ed. *Clinical Radiology: The Essentials.* 2nd ed. Philadelphia, PA: Lippincott Williams & Wilkins; 1999:513, with permission.)

B. Subdural hematoma

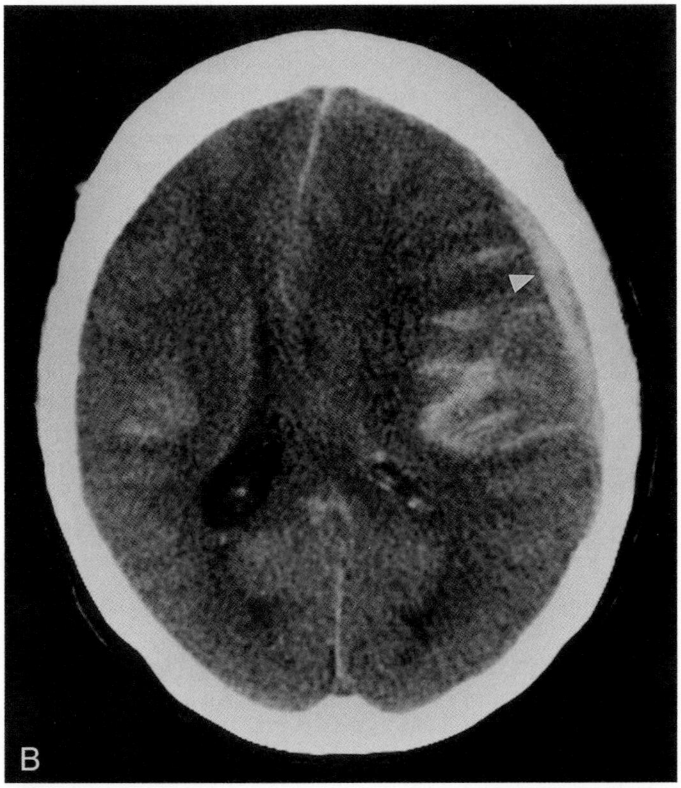
B

(Reproduced from Daffner RH, Ed. *Clinical Radiology: The Essentials.* 2nd ed. Philadelphia, PA: Lippincott Williams & Wilkins; 1999: 513.9, with permission.)

LESIONS OF THE CEREBRAL CORTEX (*Figure 2-7*)

FIGURE 2-7 **Lesions of the cerebral cortex**

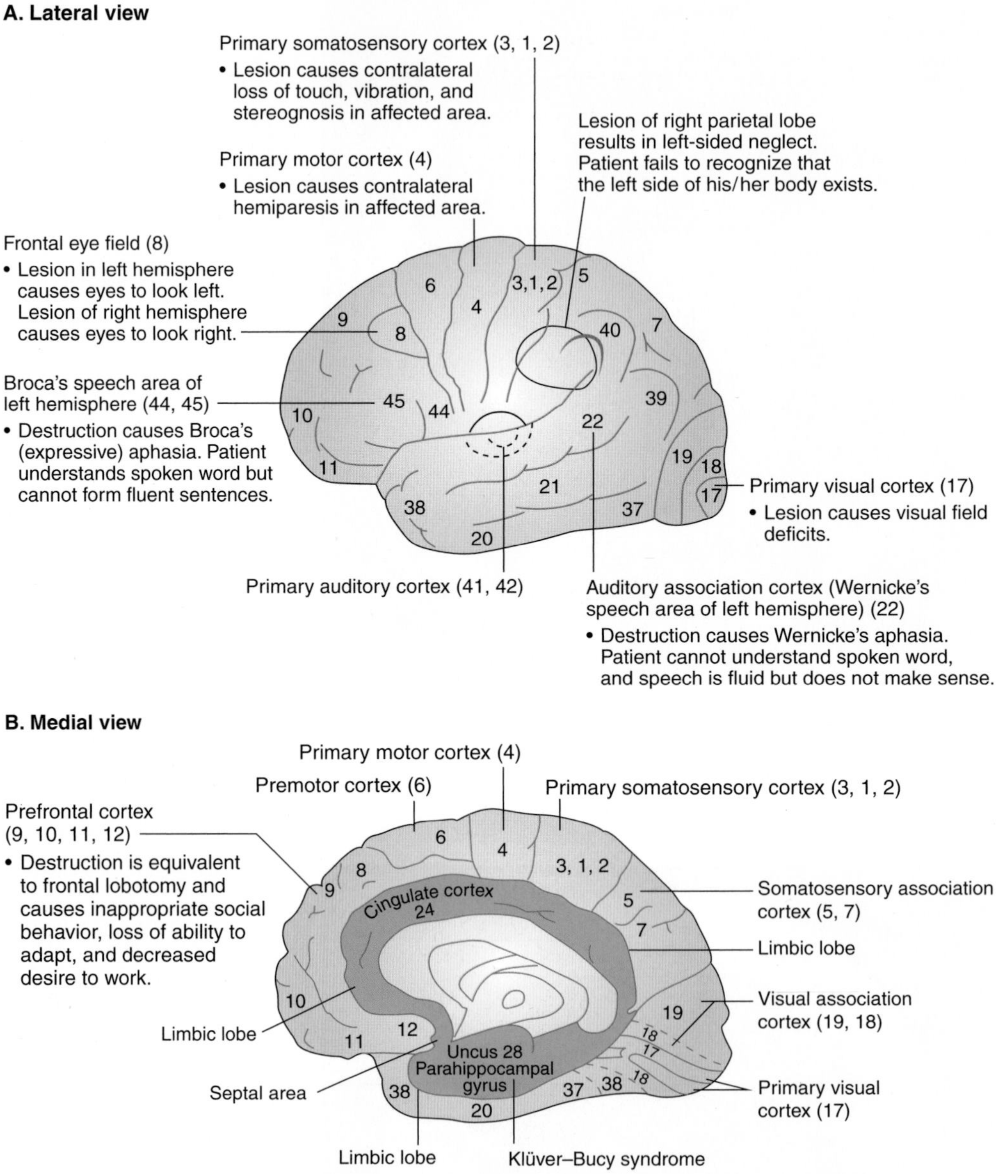
A. Lateral view
Primary somatosensory cortex (3, 1, 2)
• Lesion causes contralateral loss of touch, vibration, and stereognosis in affected area.
Primary motor cortex (4)
• Lesion causes contralateral hemiparesis in affected area.
Lesion of right parietal lobe results in left-sided neglect. Patient fails to recognize that the left side of his/her body exists.
Frontal eye field (8)
• Lesion in left hemisphere causes eyes to look left. Lesion of right hemisphere causes eyes to look right.
Broca's speech area of left hemisphere (44, 45)
• Destruction causes Broca's (expressive) aphasia. Patient understands spoken word but cannot form fluent sentences.
Primary visual cortex (17)
• Lesion causes visual field deficits.
Primary auditory cortex (41, 42)
Auditory association cortex (Wernicke's speech area of left hemisphere) (22)
• Destruction causes Wernicke's aphasia. Patient cannot understand spoken word, and speech is fluid but does not make sense.
B. Medial view
Primary motor cortex (4)
Premotor cortex (6)
Primary somatosensory cortex (3, 1, 2)
Prefrontal cortex (9, 10, 11, 12)
• Destruction is equivalent to frontal lobotomy and causes inappropriate social behavior, loss of ability to adapt, and decreased desire to work.
Cingulate cortex 24
Somatosensory association cortex (5, 7)
Limbic lobe
Visual association cortex (19, 18)
Uncus 28
Parahippocampal gyrus
Septal area
Primary visual cortex (17)
Limbic lobe
Klüver–Bucy syndrome

(Adapted from Fix JD. *High-Yield Neuroanatomy.* Baltimore, MD: Lippincott Williams & Wilkins; 1995:102, with permission.)

QUICK HIT

Klüver–Bucy syndrome is a bilateral lesion of the amygdala nuclei. It results in hypersexuality, docility, and hyperorality.

QUICK HIT

Muscle spindles function as the afferent limb of the myotactic (stretch) reflex (e.g., tapping knee with reflex hammer). Ventral horn motor neurons function as the efferent limb.

QUICK HIT

Muscle spindles are arranged **in parallel** with the extrafusal muscle fibers; **Golgi tendon organs** are arranged in **series**.

IMPORTANT PATHWAYS OF THE SPINAL CORD (*Figure 2-8*)

I. Posterior white column (dorsal column medial lemniscus pathway)

A. The posterior white column is the ascending pathway that conveys **discriminatory touch (two-point touch)**, **vibration**, **proprioception**, and **stereognosis**.

B. The posterior white column receives information at all spinal cord levels from pseudounipolar cells of dorsal root ganglia. This information is conveyed from a variety of receptors:

1. Meissner corpuscles (rate of applied stimulus)
2. **Pacinian corpuscles (vibration stimulus)**
3. Joint receptors (joint position; proprioception)

FIGURE **2-8** **Important pathways of the spinal cord**

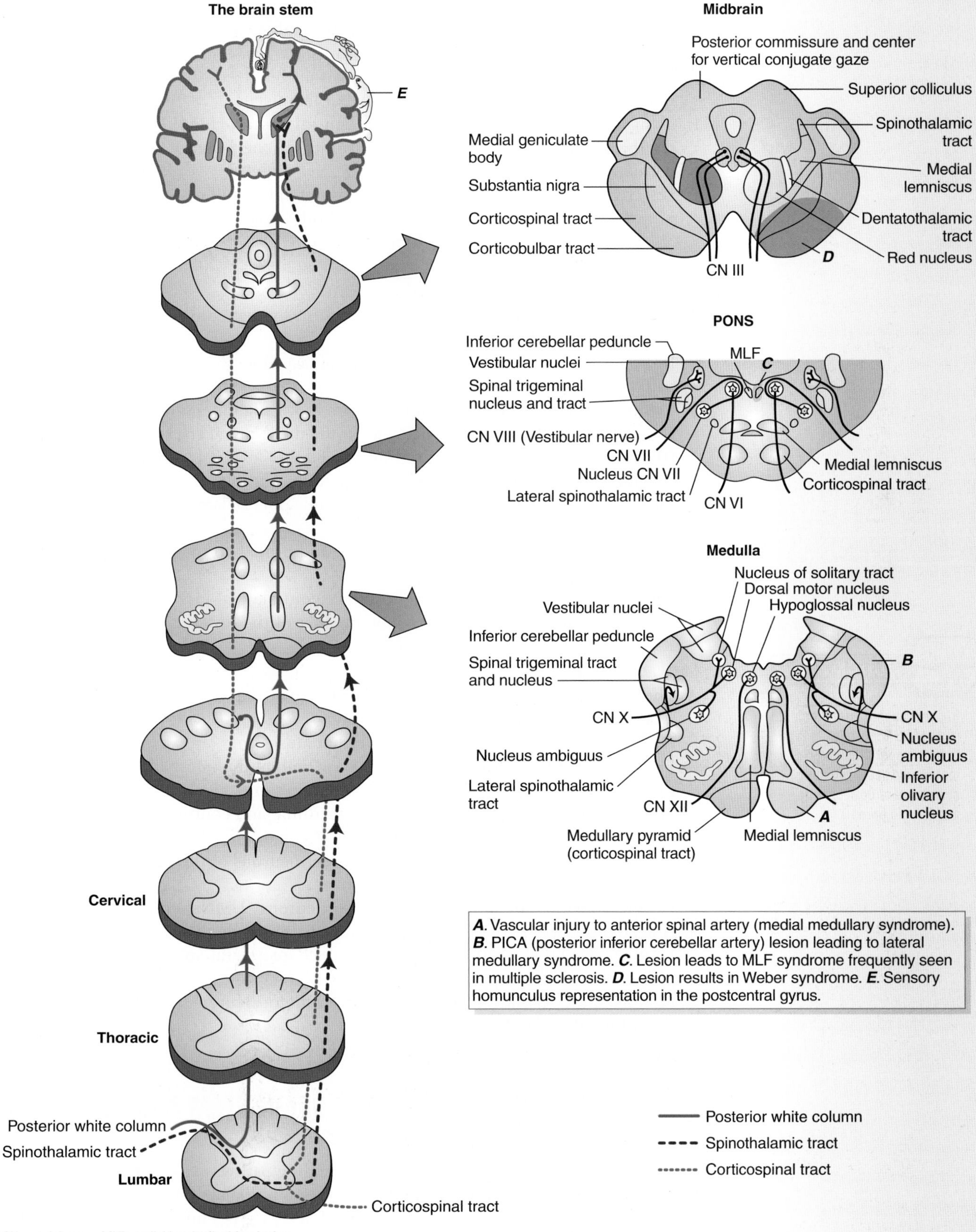
The brain stem
E
Cervical
Thoracic
Posterior white column
Spinothalamic tract
Lumbar
Corticospinal tract
Midbrain
Posterior commissure and center for vertical conjugate gaze
Superior colliculus
Spinothalamic tract
Medial geniculate body
Medial lemniscus
Substantia nigra
Dentatothalamic tract
Corticospinal tract
Corticobulbar tract
D
Red nucleus
CN III
PONS
Inferior cerebellar peduncle
MLF
C
Vestibular nuclei
Spinal trigeminal nucleus and tract
CN VIII (Vestibular nerve)
CN VII
Nucleus CN VII
Medial lemniscus
Corticospinal tract
Lateral spinothalamic tract
CN VI
Medulla
Nucleus of solitary tract
Dorsal motor nucleus
Hypoglossal nucleus
Vestibular nuclei
Inferior cerebellar peduncle
B
Spinal trigeminal tract and nucleus
CN X
CN X
Nucleus ambiguus
Nucleus ambiguus
Inferior olivary nucleus
Lateral spinothalamic tract
CN XII
A
Medullary pyramid (corticospinal tract)
Medial lemniscus
Posterior white column
Spinothalamic tract
Corticospinal tract

A. Vascular injury to anterior spinal artery (medial medullary syndrome). ***B***. PICA (posterior inferior cerebellar artery) lesion leading to lateral medullary syndrome. ***C***. Lesion leads to MLF syndrome frequently seen in multiple sclerosis. ***D***. Lesion results in Weber syndrome. ***E***. Sensory homunculus representation in the postcentral gyrus.

CN, cranial nerve; MLF, medial longitudinal fasciculus.

4. Muscle spindles (length of a muscle)
5. **Golgi tendon organs** (**tension** on a muscle)

C. First-order neurons of the dorsal root ganglia enter at the dorsal horn, ascend in the **fasciculus gracilis (lower limb)** and **fasciculus cuneatus (upper limb)**, and synapse in the nucleus gracilis and cuneatus.
D. Second-order neurons arise from these two nuclei, decussate at the level of the inferior medulla, and ascend as the **medial lemniscus**.
E. Medial lemniscus fibers synapse in the **ventral posterolateral (VPL) nucleus** of the thalamus, and third-order neurons project to the **primary somatosensory cortex**.
F. Lesions below the decussation produce ipsilateral loss of discriminatory touch, proprioception, and vibration, whereas lesions above the decussation produce contralateral loss of these sensations.

II. Spinothalamic tract

A. The spinothalamic tract is the ascending pathway that conveys **pain** and **temperature** from the body.
B. It receives input from free nerve endings of fast (A-type) and slow (C-type) pain fibers.
C. First-order neurons originate in the dorsal root ganglion, enter the spinal cord, and synapse on second-order neurons in the dorsolateral tract of Lissauer (thoracic vertebra level 2 [T2] to lumbar vertebra level 3 [L3]).
D. Second-order neurons ascend while decussating through the **ventral white commissure** and continue to ascend in the lateral spinothalamic tract, terminating in the VPL nucleus of the thalamus.
E. Third-order neurons originate in the VPL and project to the primary somatosensory **cortex**.
F. Lesions of the spinothalamic tract produce contralateral loss of pain and temperature sensation beginning **one level below that of the lesion**.

QUICK HIT

In amyotrophic lateral sclerosis (ALS), there is damage to both upper and lower motor neurons, producing symptoms of both spastic and flaccid paresis.

III. Corticospinal tract

A. The corticospinal tract is the descending pathway that originates in the **primary motor cortex**.
B. It mediates **voluntary movement** of striated muscle.
C. First-order neurons project to the posterior limb of the internal capsule, descend through the middle three-fifths of the midbrain's **crus cerebri** and base of the pons, **decussate in the pyramids of the medulla**, and continue down the spinal cord as the corticospinal tract.
D. Corticospinal fibers synapse on second-order neurons of the ventral horn via interneurons.
E. Lesions above the pyramids (upper motor neurons [**UMNs**]) produce **contralateral spastic paresis** and a positive Babinski sign (upgoing toes).
F. Lesions below the pyramids (**UMNs**) produce **ipsilateral spastic paresis** and a positive Babinski sign.
G. Lesions of the second-order neurons (lower motor neurons [**LMNs**]) produce **flaccid paralysis** and fasciculations.

IMPORTANT PATHWAYS OF THE BRAIN STEM AND CEREBRUM

I. Trigeminothalamic pathway

A. The trigeminothalamic pathway is the ascending pathway that conveys **pain** and **temperature from the face** (analogous to the spinothalamic tract).
B. It receives input from free nerve endings of fast (A-type) and slow (C-type) pain fibers.
C. First-order neurons originate in the **trigeminal** ganglion and synapse on second-order neurons in the spinal trigeminal nucleus (ventral trigeminothalamic tract)

or principal sensory nucleus of the trigeminal nerve (dorsal trigeminothalamic tract).

D. Second-order neurons of the ventral tract decussate while ascending; however, the dorsal tract neurons remain uncrossed, with termination in the ventral posteromedial (VPM) nucleus of the thalamus.

E. Third-order neurons originate in the VPM nucleus and project to the **primary somatosensory cortex**.

II. Corticobulbar tract

A. The corticobulbar tract is the descending pathway that originates in the **primary motor cortex**.

B. It mediates voluntary movement of the **muscles of facial expression** (analogous to the corticospinal tract).

C. First-order neurons project to the genu of the **internal capsule**, descend through the anterior one-third of the midbrain's crus cerebri, and synapse in the nucleus of CN VII (facial nucleus).

D. Second-order neurons innervate the muscles of facial expression (orbicularis oculi, orbicularis oris, buccinator, frontalis, and platysma) via the **facial** nerve.

E. The **upper face** (orbicularis oculi and frontalis muscles) receives **bilateral input** from the UMN and therefore is unaffected by unilateral cortical lesions.

F. The **lower face** (buccinator, orbicularis oris, and platysma) receives only **contralateral input**.

III. Cerebellar pathway

A. The cerebellar pathway controls posture and balance, maintains muscle tone, and coordinates motor activity.

B. The **dentatothalamic** tract is the major cerebellar tract.

1. It originates in the dentate nucleus of the cerebellum.
2. It projects to the **ventrolateral** nucleus of the thalamus (not the VPL nucleus) via the superior cerebellar peduncle.
3. Thalamic fibers within the tract project to area 4 (primary motor cortex; see Figure 2-7A).
4. Cerebral fibers within the tract project to corticospinal neurons.
5. The pons receives cerebral fibers and sends fibers to the cerebellum, where they terminate on mossy fibers.

C. Damage to one side of the vestibulocerebellum results in ipsilateral findings. Patient will fall toward the affected side (**positive Romberg sign**).

IV. Vestibulocochlear pathways

A. Auditory pathway

1. The auditory pathway originates from hair cells in the organ of Corti in the cochlea.
2. Signals are sent down bipolar cell axons and are then relayed to the cochlear nuclei of the pons via the spiral ganglion.
3. Signals are sent to higher CNS areas and relayed to the cerebral hemisphere via the **medial geniculate body of the thalamus**.
4. Fibers terminate in the transverse temporal gyri.
5. Because of the bilateral projection of information in the auditory pathway, one-sided lesions of this pathway at any point beyond the cochlear nuclei do not produce hearing loss.
6. Lesions of the cochlear nerve itself will produce ipsilateral hearing loss.

B. Vestibular pathway

1. Hair cells of the three **semicircular canals** encode **angular acceleration** and **deceleration**.
2. Hair cells of the **utricle** encode **linear acceleration**.
3. Information is passed via the vestibular nerve to the vestibular nuclei of the low pons.

QUICK HIT

Bell palsy is an **LMN lesion** of the **facial nerve**. This lesion results in complete facial paralysis on the affected side and is characterized by loss of the nasolabial fold, drooling, and ptosis. It is often idiopathic and usually resolves spontaneously.

QUICK HIT

In **Friedreich ataxia** (autosomal recessive), the most common congenital ataxia, the brain shows diffuse neuronal loss involving the posterior white columns, the dentate nuclei, and the spinocerebellar tract. These patients commonly have diabetes and heart disease.

QUICK HIT

Tonotopic localization of sound in the cochlea is caused in part by the increasing thickness of the basilar membrane as it ascends toward the helicotrema. The **base** of the cochlea (closest to the oval window) is sensitive to **high-frequency sounds.** The **apex** of the cochlea is sensitive to **low-frequency sounds.**

QUICK HIT

Linear acceleration sensed by the utricle and saccule can cause nausea and vomiting. Dimenhydrinate and scopolamine can prevent motion sickness. These drugs work best if used before the onset of symptoms.

MNEMONIC

Remember **COWS: c**old **o**pposite, **w**arm **s**ame side for the direction of movement during fast phase of caloric nystagmus.

TABLE 2-4 **Direction of Movement in Types of Nystagmus**

Form of Nystagmus	Direction of Movement during Fast Phase	Direction of Movement during Slow Phase
Rotary nystagmus (i.e., while spinning in a circle)	Same as direction of rotation	Opposite direction of rotation
Postrotary nystagmus (i.e., after spinning in a circle)	Opposite direction of rotation	Same as direction of rotation
Caloric nystagmus		
• Warm water placed in one ear	**Toward the ear with warm water placed in it**	**Away from the ear with warm water placed in it**
• Cold water placed in one ear	**Away from the ear with cold water placed in it**	**Toward the ear with cold water placed in it**

4. Fibers then project to:
   a. The spinal cord
   b. The cerebellum
   c. The thalamus
   d. CNs III, IV, and VI via the medial longitudinal fasciculus (MLF)
5. **Nystagmus** is mediated by the vestibular and oculomotor nuclei, the MLF, and the muscles of ocular movement controlled by CNs III, IV, and VI (Table 2-4).

V. Visual pathways and vision abnormalities *(Figure 2-9)*

A. Muscles of the eye (Figure 2-10)

B. **Horner syndrome**
   1. It is caused by a lesion of the sympathetic trunk in the neck.
   2. Clinical features of the syndrome include ipsilateral **ptosis**, **anhydrosis**, **flushing of skin**, and **miosis**.

C. **Argyll Robertson pupil**
   1. A pupil that **accommodates** to near objects but **does not react to light**
   2. Seen in syphilis, systemic lupus erythematosus (SLE), and diabetes mellitus

D. **Marcus Gunn pupil** (aka afferent defect)
   1. It is caused by a relative deficit in the afferent portion of the light reflex pathway.
   2. Shining a light in the affected pupil causes minimal bilateral constriction, but shining light in the unaffected pupil causes normal constriction of both pupils.

E. **MLF syndrome**
   1. Caused by a lesion of the MLF and can be unilateral or bilateral.
   2. **Clinical features**
      a. The ipsilateral eye (the eye on the side of the MLF lesion) is unable to adduct, and the contralateral eye (the opposite eye) has nystagmus. For example, in the cases of right MLF lesions, the right eye is unable to adduct and the left eye has nystagmus when looking left.
      b. Convergence is unaffected.
   3. Often seen in **multiple sclerosis (MS)** and may be seen in stroke.

F. **Uncal herniation**
   1. The uncus of the temporal lobe is forced through the opening of the tentorium.
   2. Clinical features include (Figure 2-9):
      a. Compression of CN III occurs, leading to fixed and dilated ("blown") pupil on ipsilateral side
      b. Ophthalmoplegia (paralysis of one or more of the ocular muscles)
      c. Compression of the corticospinal tract leading to ipsilateral hemiparesis
      d. Compression of the posterior cerebral artery leading to contralateral homonymous hemianopsia

QUICK HIT

Injury to CN III (oculomotor) results in **ptosis** because of loss of the levator palpebrae superioris muscle, **exotropia** because of the unopposed pull of the lateral rectus, **dilation** of the pupil because of unopposed pull of the dilator pupillae muscle, and **impairment of near vision** as a result of loss of accommodation of the ciliary muscle.

QUICK HIT

Horner syndrome is often caused by **Pancoast tumor**, a lung neoplasm that invades the cervical sympathetic chain.

QUICK HIT

The Marcus Gunn pupil can be diagnosed using the **swinging flashlight test.** Shining a flashlight in the normal pupil causes constriction of both pupils. Swinging the flashlight quickly to the affected eye causes paradoxical dilation of the pupils.

FIGURE 2-9 Visual pathways.

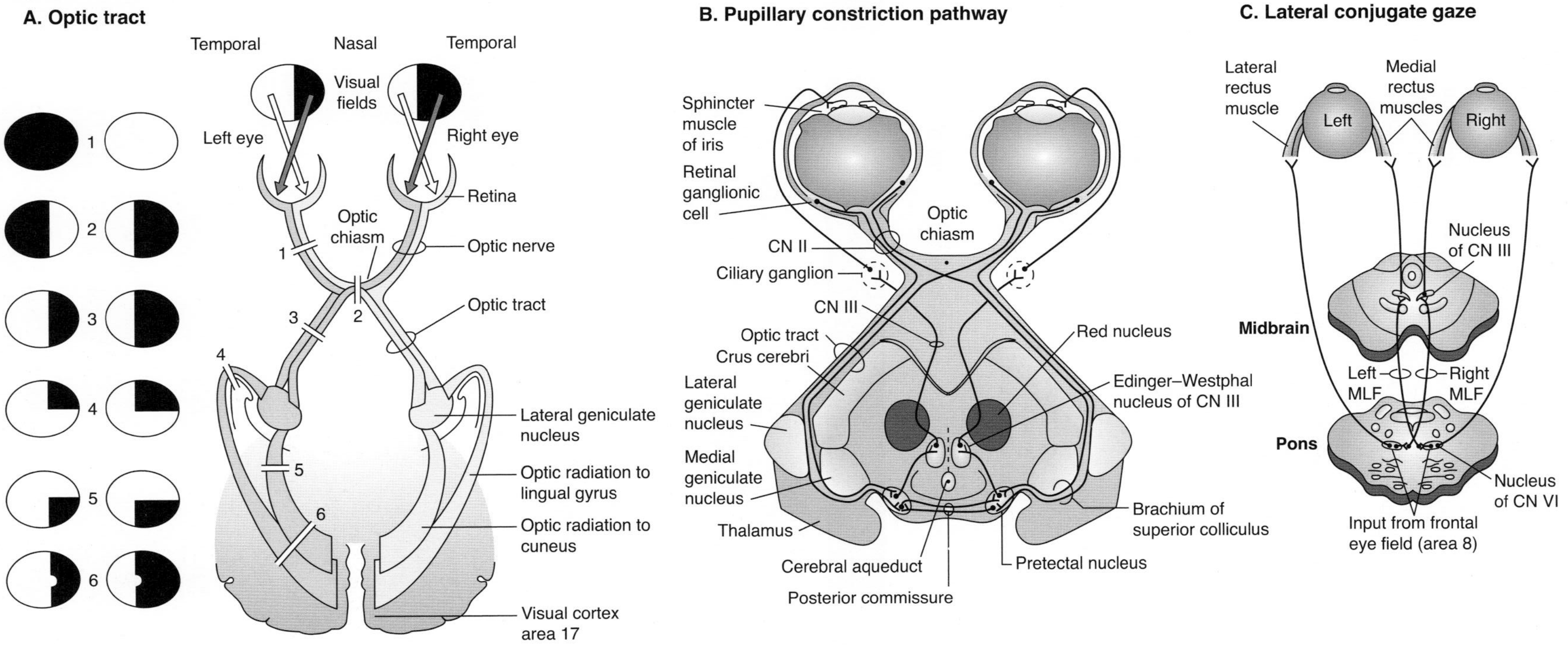
A. Optic tract
Temporal
Nasal
Temporal
Visual fields
Left eye
Right eye
Retina
Optic chiasm
Optic nerve
Optic tract
Lateral geniculate nucleus
Optic radiation to lingual gyrus
Optic radiation to cuneus
Visual cortex area 17
1
2
3
4
5
6
B. Pupillary constriction pathway
Sphincter muscle of iris
Retinal ganglionic cell
CN II
Ciliary ganglion
CN III
Optic tract
Crus cerebri
Lateral geniculate nucleus
Medial geniculate nucleus
Thalamus
Cerebral aqueduct
Posterior commissure
Pretectal nucleus
Brachium of superior colliculus
Edinger–Westphal nucleus of CN III
Red nucleus
Optic chiasm
C. Lateral conjugate gaze
Lateral rectus muscle
Medial rectus muscles
Left
Right
Nucleus of CN III
Midbrain
Left MLF
Right MLF
Pons
Nucleus of CN VI
Input from frontal eye field (area 8)

A. Legend for lesions: (1) total blindness; (2) bitemporal hemianopsia—common lesion caused by superiorly growing pituitary tumor; (3) right hemianopsia; (4) right upper quadrantanopia; (5) right lower quadrantanopia; (6) right hemianopsia with macular sparing. **B.** Light shined in one eye causes constriction of both pupils. **C.** Abduction of one eye results in adduction of the other eye in individuals with an intact medial longitudinal fasciculus and normal lateral conjugate gaze. CN, cranial nerve; MLF, medial longitudinal fasciculus. (Adapted from Chung, Kyung Won. *BRS Gross Anatomy.* 2nd ed. Baltimore, MD: Lippincott Williams & Wilkins; 1991:302, with permission.)

FIGURE 2-10 **Muscles of the eye**

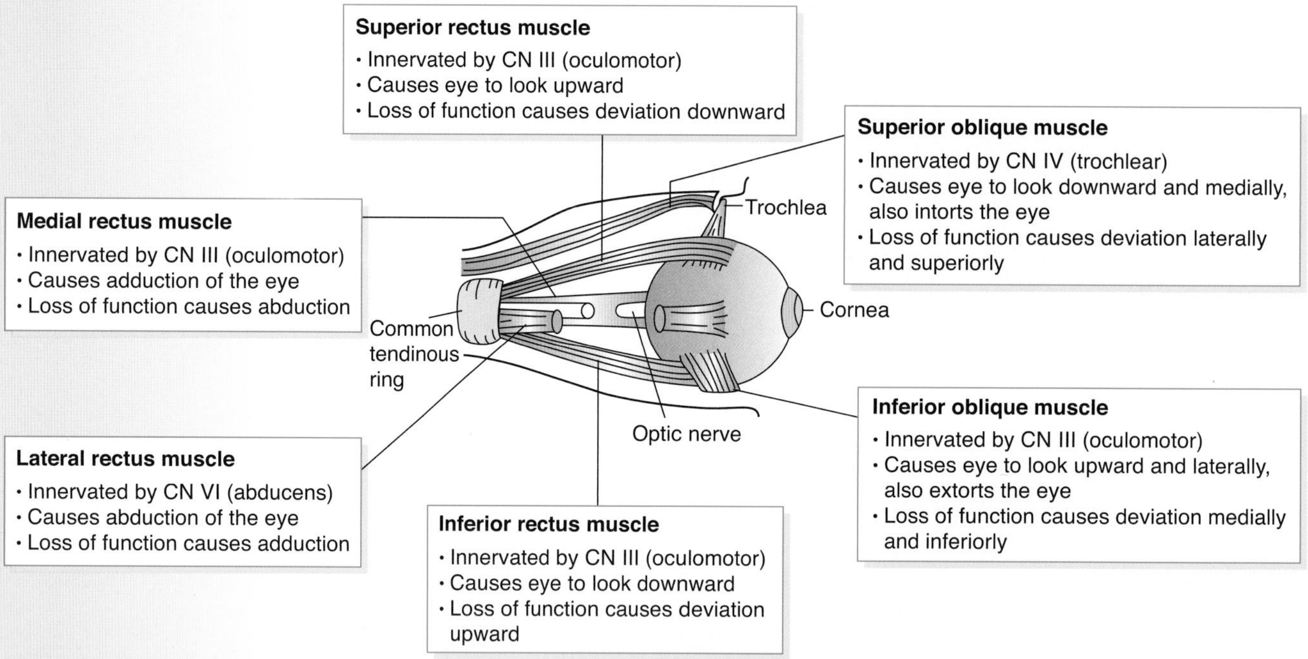
Superior rectus muscle
• Innervated by CN III (oculomotor)
• Causes eye to look upward
• Loss of function causes deviation downward
Superior oblique muscle
• Innervated by CN IV (trochlear)
• Causes eye to look downward and medially, also intorts the eye
• Loss of function causes deviation laterally and superiorly
Trochlea
Medial rectus muscle
• Innervated by CN III (oculomotor)
• Causes adduction of the eye
• Loss of function causes abduction
Cornea
Common tendinous ring
Inferior oblique muscle
• Innervated by CN III (oculomotor)
• Causes eye to look upward and laterally, also extorts the eye
• Loss of function causes deviation medially and inferiorly
Optic nerve
Lateral rectus muscle
• Innervated by CN VI (abducens)
• Causes abduction of the eye
• Loss of function causes adduction
Inferior rectus muscle
• Innervated by CN III (oculomotor)
• Causes eye to look downward
• Loss of function causes deviation upward

CN, cranial nerve. (Adapted from Chung, Kyung Won. *BRS Gross Anatomy.* 2nd ed. Baltimore, MD: Lippincott Williams & Wilkins; 1991:302, with permission.)

TABLE 2-5 **Common Ocular Pathology**

Disorder	Etiology	Pathology	Clinical Features
Diabetic retinopathy	Proposed mechanism: accumulation of sorbitol in capillary pericytes results in loss of function, leading to retinal ischemia	Nonproliferative type observes microaneurysms, flame hemorrhages, dot and blot hemorrhages, soft exudates (cotton-wool spots), hard exudates (deposits of protein that have leaked from damaged capillaries), venous beading; proliferative type also observes neovascularization and fibrosis	Loss of visual acuity; advanced disease is the major cause of blindness
Age-related macular degeneration	Proposed mechanism: genetic	Pigmentary changes (drusen), macular hemorrhage or edema	Loss of central vision
Cataract	Aging, diabetes, galactosemia, Hurler disease, congenital causes (trisomy, myotonic dystrophy, hypoglycemia, TORCH infections)	Opacity of lens as a result of precipitation of sorbitol (diabetes), galactitol (galactosemia), mucopolysaccharide (Hurler disease), lens proteins (senile)	Decreased visual acuity, glare
Hypertensive retinopathy	High blood pressure → damages capillary walls	Copper wiring, flame hemorrhages, arteriovenous nicking, optic disc swelling (acute rise in blood pressure)	
Atherosclerosis	Atherosclerotic plaque from carotid artery embolizes into ipsilateral retinal artery	Hollenhorst plaque, copper wiring, flame hemorrhages, arteriovenous nicking	Amaurosis fugax (transient loss in vision, classically described as "shade falling over eye")
Papilledema	Increased intracranial pressure	Optic disc swelling (bilateral)	Headache; no changes in visual acuity until advanced disease
Angle-closure glaucoma	Acutely increased intraocular pressure	The lens abuts the posterior surface of the iris, pushing the iris forward and blocking the flow of aqueous humor	Acutely red, painful, rock-hard eye; decreased vision; halos around lights
Open-angle glaucoma	Chronically increased intraocular pressure	Less well understood; may be due to degeneration of the trabecular meshwork and canal of Schlemm	Gradual onset of loss of peripheral vision

TORCH, toxoplasmosis, other infections, rubella, cytomegalovirus, and herpes simplex virus.

FIGURE 2-11 **Age-related macular degeneration**

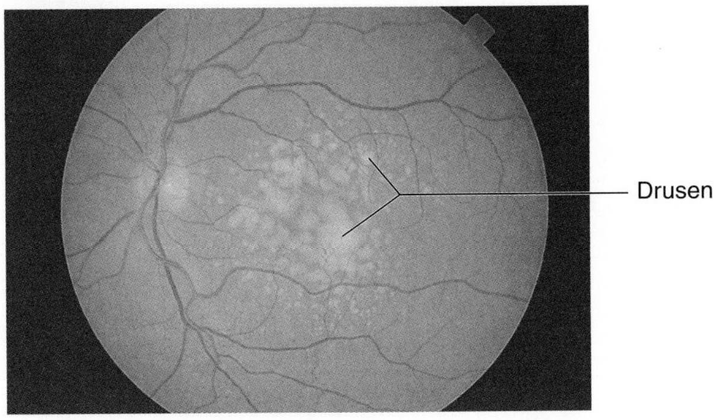
Drusen

(Reproduced from Tasman W, Jaeger E. *The Wills Eye Hospital Atlas of Clinical Ophthalmology.* 2nd ed. Baltimore, MD: Lippincott Williams & Wilkins; 2001, with permission.)

FIGURE 2-12 **Diabetic retinopathy**

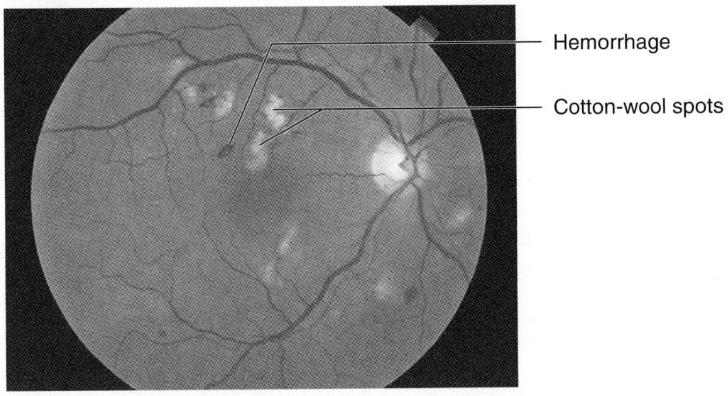
Hemorrhage
Cotton-wool spots

(Reproduced from Tasman W, Jaeger E. *The Wills Eye Hospital Atlas of Clinical Ophthalmology.* 2nd ed. Baltimore, MD: Lippincott Williams & Wilkins; 2001, with permission.)

VI. Taste

A. The **solitary** nucleus of the medulla receives taste sensation via the solitary tract from three sources:
   1. The anterior two-thirds of the tongue via the **chorda tympani** nerve of the facial nerve (CN VII)
   2. The posterior third of the tongue via the **glossopharyngeal** nerve (CN IX)
   3. The epiglottic region of the pharynx via the **vagus** nerve (CN X)

B. Neurons carrying taste sensations ascend in the ventral tegmental tract to the VPM nucleus of the thalamus.

C. The VPM nucleus of the thalamus sends fibers to the parietal lobe.

VII. Limbic system

A. Mediates behavior and emotion, specifically:
   1. Feeding
   2. Feeling (emotions)
   3. Fighting
   4. Fleeing
   5. Sexual activity

B. Primarily controlled by the hypothalamus and autonomic nervous system

C. Primary components
   1. Anterior nucleus of thalamus
   2. Cingulate gyrus
   3. Mammillary bodies
   4. Septal area
   5. Hippocampus
   6. Amygdala (Table 2-5 and Figs. 2-11 and 2-12)

QUICK HIT

Lesions of the mammillary bodies occur in thiamine deficiency, commonly seen in chronic alcoholism due to malnutrition. Damage results in **Korsakoff syndrome,** characterized by confusion, severe memory impairment, and confabulation, which is **irreversible.**

CLASSIC LESIONS OF THE SPINAL CORD *(Figure 2-13)*

FIGURE 2-13 Classic lesions of the spinal cord

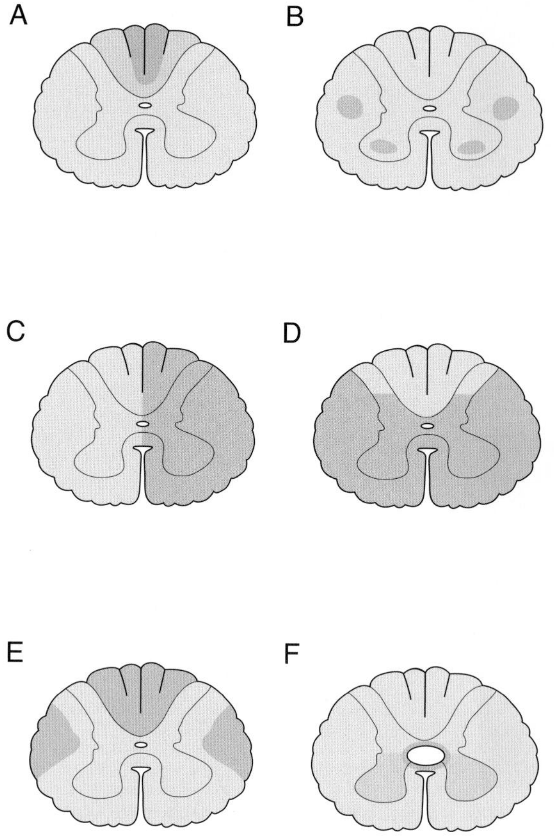
A
B
C
D
E
F

Tabes dorsalis
- Seen in tertiary syphilis
- Bilateral loss of touch, vibration, and tactile sense from lower limbs due to lesion of fasciculus gracilis

Amyotrophic lateral sclerosis
- Combined UMN and LMN lesion of corticospinal tract
- Spastic paresis (UMN sign)
- Flaccid paralysis with fasciculations (LMN)

Brown–Séquard syndrome
- Ipsilateral loss of touch and vibration and tactile sense below lesion due to posterior white column lesion
- Contralateral loss of pain and touch due to loss of spinothalamic tract
- Ipsilateral spastic paresis below lesion due to lesion of corticospinal tract
- Ipsilateral flaccid paralysis at level of lesion due to loss of LMN
- If lesion occurs above T1, Horner syndrome on side of lesion will result

Spinal artery infarct
- Bilateral loss of pain and temperature one level below lesion due to loss of spinothalamic tract
- Bilateral spastic paresis below lesion due to lesion of corticospinal tract
- Bilateral flaccid paralysis at level of lesion due to loss of LMN
- Loss of bladder control due to lesion of corticospinal tract innervation of S2–S4 parasympathetics
- Bilateral Horner syndrome if above T2

Subacute combined degeneration (Vitamin B_{12} deficiency)
- Bilateral loss of touch, vibration, and tactile sense due to posterior white column lesion
- Bilateral spastic paresis below lesion due to lesion of corticospinal tracts

Syringomyelia
- Bilateral loss of pain and temperature one level below due to lesion of ventral white commissure (spinothalamic tract)
- Bilateral flaccid paralysis of level of lesion due to loss of LMN

LMN, lower motor neuron; UMN, upper motor neuron.

HYPOTHALAMUS *(Figure 2-14)*

FIGURE 2-14 Hypothalamus

Paraventricular and supraoptic nuclei
- Regulate water balance
- Produce ADH and oxytocin
- Destruction causes diabetes insipidus

Anterior commissure

Anterior nucleus
- Thermal regulation (dissipation of heat)
- Stimulates parasympathetic NS
- Destruction results in hyperthermia

Preoptic area
- Contains sexual dimorphic nucleus
- Regulates release of gonadotropic hormones

Suprachiasmatic nucleus
- Receives input from retina
- Controls circadian rhythms

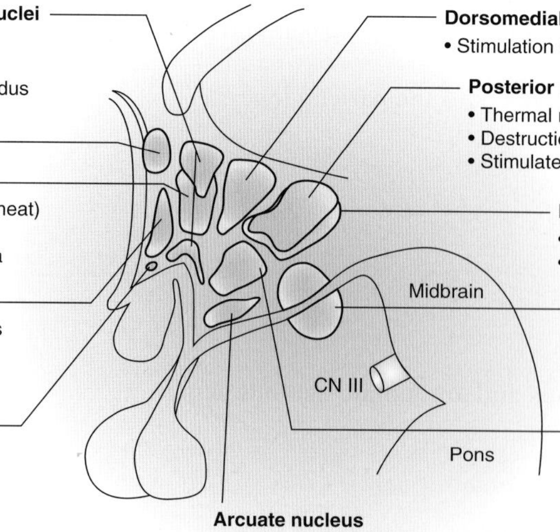
Midbrain
CN III
Pons

Dorsomedial nucleus
- Stimulation results in obesity and savage behavior

Posterior nucleus
- Thermal regulation (conservation of heat)
- Destruction results in inability to thermoregulate
- Stimulates the sympathetic nervous system

Lateral nucleus
- Stimulation induces eating
- Destruction results in starvation

Mammillary body
- Receives input from hippocampal formation
- Contains hemorrhagic lesions in Wernicke encephalopathy

Ventromedial nucleus
- Satiety center
- Destruction results in obesity and savage behavior

Arcuate nucleus
- Produces hypothalamic-releasing factors
- Contains DOPA-nergic neurons that inhibit prolactin release

ADH, antidiuretic hormone; CN, cranial nerve; NS, nervous system. (Redrawn from Fix JD. *High-Yield Neuroanatomy.* Baltimore, MD: Lippincott Williams & Wilkins; 1995:84, with permission.)

CONTENTS OF THE CAVERNOUS SINUS *(Figure 2-16)*

FIGURE
2-16 Contents of the cavernous sinus

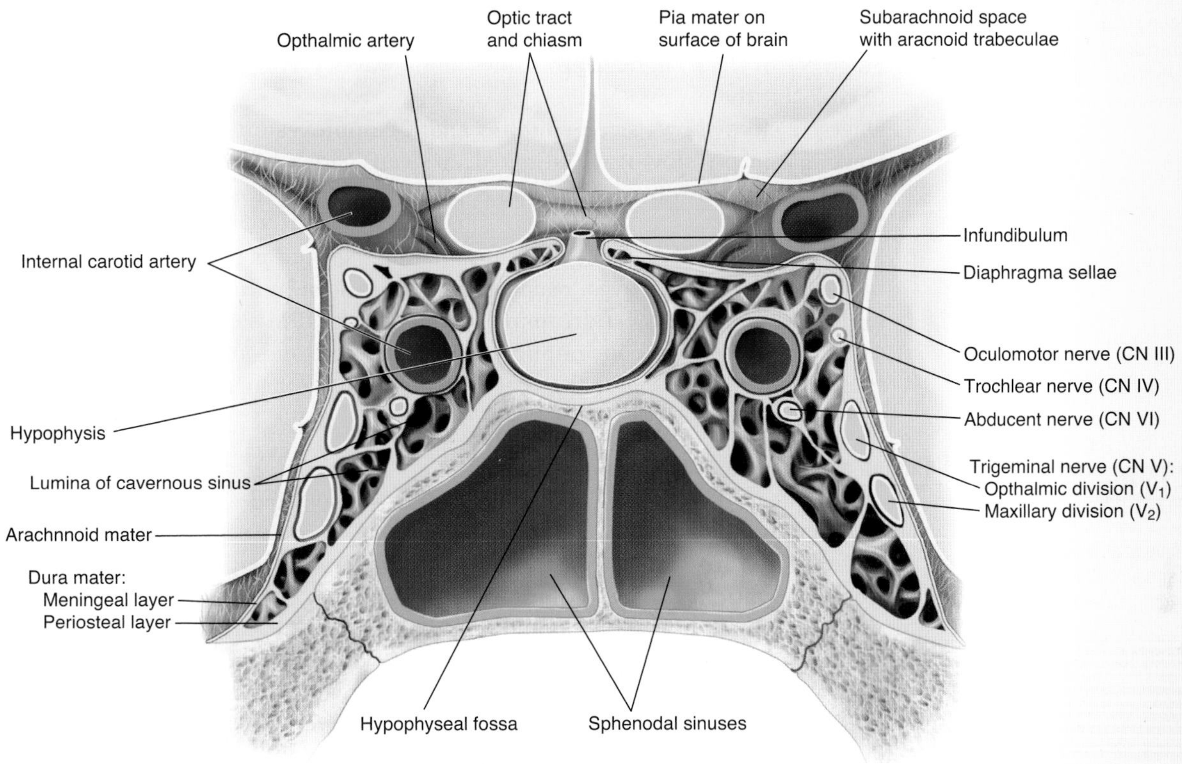
Opthalmic artery
Optic tract and chiasm
Pia mater on surface of brain
Subarachnoid space with aracnoid trabeculae
Infundibulum
Diaphragma sellae
Internal carotid artery
Oculomotor nerve (CN III)
Trochlear nerve (CN IV)
Abducent nerve (CN VI)
Hypophysis
Trigeminal nerve (CN V):
Opthalmic division (V1)
Maxillary division (V2)
Lumina of cavernous sinus
Arachnnoid mater
Dura mater:
Meningeal layer
Periosteal layer
Hypophyseal fossa
Sphenodal sinuses

CN, cranial nerve. (Adapted from Bushan V, Le T, Amin C. *First Aid for the USMLE Step 1.* Stamford, CT: Appleton & Lange; 1999:110, with permission.)

SLEEP *(Figure 2-17)*

FIGURE
2-17 The sleep cycle

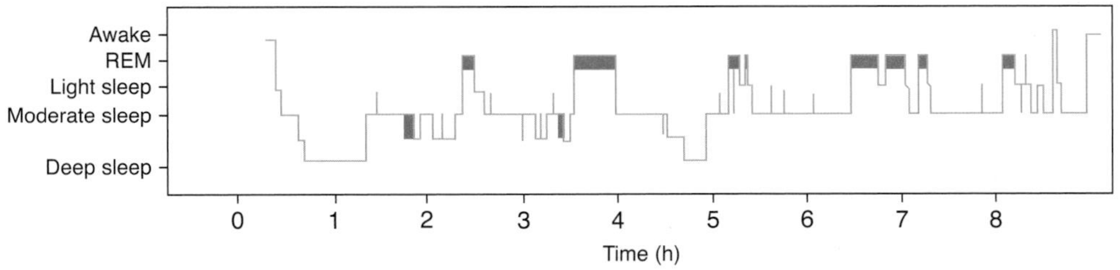
Awake
REM
Light sleep
Moderate sleep
Deep sleep
0
1
2
3
4
5
6
7
8
Time (h)

Stages of rapid eye movement (REM) sleep in the young adult. As sleep progresses, slow-wave sleep decreases and REM sleep episodes increase in duration and frequency. In the elderly, there is decreased slow-wave sleep, increased awakenings, early sleep onset, and early morning awakenings. Solid bars indicate REM sleep.

QUICK HIT

The time spent in stage N3 sleep decreases with age and with the use of some drugs (e.g., benzodiazepines).

I. Sleep–wake cycles

A. Based on circadian rhythms controlled by the suprachiasmatic nucleus of the hypothalamus

B. **Serotonin** (5-HT) released from the raphe nuclei of the brain stem is important in initiating sleep, whereas the **reticular activating system** maintains alertness.

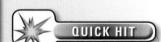

C. Sleep is divided in the three non–rapid eye movement (REM) stages (N1, N2, and N3), and REM sleep.
1. An awake, alert individual shows low amplitude, high-frequency (12 to 30 Hz) **beta** waves on electroencephalograph (EEG).
2. A relaxed individual (still awake but with eyes closed, in preparation for sleep) shows lower frequency (8 to 12 Hz) **alpha** waves.
3. **Stage N1** of sleep (light sleep) shows alpha waves giving way to low-frequency (4 to 7 Hz) **theta** waves.
4. Stage N2 sleep shows **sleep spindles** and **K-complexes** on EEG.
5. Stage N3 sleep ("slow-wave sleep," deep sleep) shows very low-frequency (0 to 4 Hz) **delta** waves. Dreaming is possible (though less common than in REM sleep).
6. REM sleep normally occurs at 90-minute intervals and is characterized by high-frequency **beta** waves, which mirror those seen in the alert individual in the waking state. Most dreaming occurs during REM sleep along with increased brain oxygen consumption, nocturnal erections, and loss of skeletal muscle tone. REM sleep is thought to be important for memory processing and consolidation.

> **QUICK HIT**
> Slow-wave sleep, which is the deepest, most relaxed sleep, is the sleep stage in which night terrors, enuresis (bed-wetting), and sleepwalking occur.

II. Common sleep disorders

A. Insomnia affects 30% of the U.S. population. It is associated with anxiety and leads to daytime sleepiness.

B. Restless leg syndrome is the sensation of unpleasant paresthesias that compels the patient to have voluntary, spontaneous, continuous leg movements. It is usually a primary idiopathic disorder, but it can occur secondary to iron deficiency, end-stage renal disease, diabetic neuropathy, Parkinson disease, pregnancy, rheumatic diseases, varicose veins, and excessive caffeine intake.

C. Nightmares versus night terrors
1. Nightmares are frightening dreams that occur during REM sleep, and patients actually awake from sleep.
2. Night terrors occur during non-REM sleep, and patients may appear to be awake (frightened/screaming, tachycardic, and diaphoretic) but are not actually fully awake. They are often difficult to arouse and usually fall right back to sleep after the episode.

D. Central sleep apnea, affecting less than 0.5% of the population, involves an absence of respiratory effort (for a discussion of obstructive sleep apnea, see Chapter 4).

E. Narcolepsy is seen in 0.04% of the population and is characterized by sudden onset of sleep with rapid onset of REM sleep. It may be associated with hallucinations and cataplexy (sudden loss of muscle tone).

F. Nocturnal enuresis is overnight bed-wetting after 5 years of age (developmental age), when daytime bladder control has been achieved. It is often familial.
1. Treatment is usually delayed until the child is at least 7 years of age.
2. Behavioral interventions are usually first-line, including motivational therapy (e.g., star charts), nighttime fluid restriction, scheduled wakening, and enuresis alarms (most effective long-term therapy).
3. Pharmacologic interventions are usually second-line and may include short-term imipramine, oral desmopressin, or indomethacin. There is a high likelihood of recurrence upon discontinuation.

> **QUICK HIT**
> Narcolepsy can be associated with hypnagogic hallucinations upon going to sleep and hypnopompic hallucinations upon awakening.

> **QUICK HIT**
> Status epilepticus (characterized by continuous or rapidly recurring seizures with no return of consciousness) can be caused by any type of seizure and is potentially fatal. Treatment is intravenous diazepam.

SEIZURE TYPES

Seizures are paroxysmal events caused by abnormal and excessive discharges from CNS neurons triggered by a variety of causes (Table 2-7).

The antiepileptic agents, which include several different medications, affect **ion channels** (Table 2-8). The side effects of these agents are often significant. Because it is frequently necessary to take these agents for long periods, it is important to understand these side effects.

> **QUICK HIT**
> Barbiturates and benzodiazepines are **sedative-hypnotics** that are often used to treat seizure activity. The more common examples are flurazepam, phenobarbital, temazepam, triazolam, and zolpidem.

TABLE 2-7 **Seizure Types**

Type	Patient	Presentation	Pathology	Treatment
Simple partial seizures	All ages	Malfunction of one muscle or muscle group No loss of consciousness Sensory distortions	Single focus in brain No spread, localized muscular manifestations With chronicity, may progress to generalized muscular manifestations	Phenytoin, carbamazepine
Jacksonian seizures	All ages (subtype of simple partial)	Expanding area of motor malfunction	Original focus spreads to adjacent areas of cortex	Carbamazepine
Complex partial seizures	First seizure during first two decades of life may be caused by fever in children 6 months to 5 years of age (febrile seizure)	Incontinence Jaw movements (or other automatisms) Loss of consciousness Elaborate sensory distortions	Single focus	Phenytoin, carbamazepine (febrile seizures do not require antiseizure medication)
Absence (petit mal) seizures	Begin at 2–3 years of age Often end with puberty	1–5 second loss of consciousness Several episodes per day Blank stare with rapid blinking	Original focus rapidly spreads across both hemispheres	Ethosuximide, valproic acid
Tonic–clonic (grand mal) seizures	Most common type Encountered in different clinical settings, often in patients with metabolic disorders	Sudden loss of consciousness Loss of postural control and continence Tonic phase (static extension) Clonic phase (jerking movements) Recovery period with exhaustion and disorientation	Original focus rapidly spreads across both hemispheres	Phenytoin, carbamazepine

The Nervous System

TABLE 2-8 **Antiepileptic Agents**

Drug	Mechanism of Action	Type(s) of Seizure(s) Controlled	Side Effects	Notes
Carbamazepine	Blocks voltage-gated **sodium channels** by increasing the refractory period	Tonic–clonic (grand mal), partial, Jacksonian	Liver enzyme induction, ataxia, diplopia, blood dyscrasias (agranulocytosis, aplastic anemia), teratogenesis, **induction of cytochrome P450**	Can be used to treat trigeminal neuralgia
Ethosuximide	Inhibits certain **sodium channels,** particularly in certain parts of thalamus that produce cyclic cortical discharges	Absence	Headache, lethargy, diarrhea, urticaria, Stevens–Johnson syndrome	
Phenytoin	Blocks voltage-gated **sodium channels** by increasing refractory period	Tonic–clonic (grand mal), partial	Liver enzyme induction, ataxia, diplopia, megaloblastic anemia, lupus-like syndrome, nystagmus, sedation, teratogenesis (fetal hydantoin syndrome), peripheral neuropathy, **hirsutism, gingival hyperplasia, induction of cytochrome P450,** malignant hyperthermia (rare)	
Valproic acid	May affect **potassium channels** to cause hyperpolarization of neuronal membranes	Absence, tonic–clonic (grand mal), partial	Liver enzyme induction, diarrhea, rarely hepatotoxic, tremor, weight gain, neural tube defects in fetus (spina bifida)	Contraindicated in pregnancy
Phenobarbital (barbiturate)	Increase inhibitory effects of γ-aminobutyric acid (GABA) by increasing **duration of chloride channel** opening	Tonic–clonic (grand mal), partial	Liver enzyme induction, sedation, tolerance, dependence, induction of cytochrome P450	First line in pregnant women, children

(continued)

TABLE 2-8 **Antiepileptic Agents** *(Continued)*

Drug	Mechanism of Action	Type(s) of Seizure(s) Controlled	Side Effects	Notes
Benzodiazepines (diazepam, lorazepam)	Increase inhibitory effects of GABA by increasing **frequency of chloride channel** opening	First line for acute **status epilepticus**	Sedation, tolerance, dependence	Used for seizures of eclampsia
Lamotrigine	Blocks voltage-gated sodium channels	Tonic–clonic (grand mal), partial	Stevens–Johnson syndrome	
Gabapentin	Increases GABA release	Tonic–clonic (grand mal), partial	Sedation, ataxia	Used for peripheral neuropathy
Topiramate	Blocks sodium channels, increases GABA action	Tonic–clonic (grand mal), partial	Sedation, weight loss, nephrolithiasis	Also used for migraine prophylaxis

DEGENERATIVE DISEASES

Degeneration in specific parts of the CNS can lead to focal or systemic loss of function. Many of the degenerative diseases affecting the CNS are irreversible and are listed in Table 2-9.

Parkinson disease, a movement disorder, results from deterioration of the **basal ganglia**. **Dopamine** production decreases, which in turn increases the relative effects of **acetylcholine**. Treatment is symptomatic and is aimed at trying to restore the balance between the two hormones (Table 2-10).

TABLE 2-9 **Degenerative Diseases**

Disease	Etiology	Clinical Manifestation	Notes
Vitamin B_{12} deficiency	Strict vegetarian diet, **pernicious anemia,** fundal gastritis type A, *Diphyllobothrium latum*	**Megaloblastic anemia, peripheral neuropathy, myelin degeneration of posterior white columns** and lateral corticospinal tracts	Megaloblastic anemia component of vitamin B_{12} deficiency can be treated with folate; however, this will not resolve the peripheral neuropathy component of the deficiency
Parkinson disease	**Decrease in dopamine** caused by depletion of cells of substantia nigra and locus coeruleus; similar symptoms may be caused by depression, hydrocephaly, MPTP intoxication	**Resting tremors, masked facies, muscular rigidity,** shuffling gait, **Lewy bodies**	Usually appears after 55 years of age; therapy with dopamine precursors or ACh inhibitors
Poliomyelitis	Poliovirus (RNA); fecal–oral; replicates in pharynx; spreads to CNS	Aseptic meningitis, **death of anterior horn cells** in spinal cord, paralysis	Killed (Salk) and live-attenuated (Sabin) vaccine available; Sabin vaccine given to children because of IgA response, longer action, and availability of oral form
Rabies	**Rhabdovirus** (RNA); spread via saliva	Laryngeal spasm resulting in fear of water, CNS excitability, **Negri body** inclusions, hippocampal degeneration	Treatment via passive and active immunization at distant sites
Spongiform encephalopathies (a) Animals – Scrapie (sheep) – Bovine spongiform encephalopathy (BSE; cows; aka mad cow disease)	Prions: an abnormally folded variant of a normal cell protein; only infectious agent with no nucleic acid	Vacuolization of brain tissue, dementia, ataxia, depositions of the abnormal protein, long incubation (years), rapid death after onset (months)	Diagnosed at autopsy; no treatment; new-variant CJD acquired by eating BSE-contaminated meat; Kuru spread by nonalignment of neurologic tissue; CJD has been spread by corneal transplant and on contaminated neurosurgical equipment

(continued)

TABLE 2-9 **Degenerative Diseases** *(Continued)*

Disease	Etiology	Clinical Manifestation	Notes
(b) Humans – Creutzfeldt–Jakob disease (CJD) – New-variant CJD – Kuru			
Tay–Sachs disease	Autosomal recessive; **deficiency of hexosaminidase A** with increase in G_{M2}, ganglioside seizures	Mental retardation, **cherry-red spot on macula,** muscular weakness	Fatal, prenatal diagnosis possible, usually affects cells of CNS
Thiamine deficiency	Severe malnutrition (may be secondary to alcoholism)	**Degeneration of mammillary bodies,** Wernicke–Korsakoff syndrome—psychosis manifested with confusion, ataxia, and confabulation Dry beriberi—polyneuropathy with peripheral sensorimotor loss Wet beriberi—dry beriberi with cardiovascular symptoms	**Wernicke** encephalopathy **(reversible)** and **Korsakoff** syndrome **(irreversible)** are both secondary to deficiency caused by alcoholism
Wilson disease	Autosomal recessive; **decreased ceruloplasmin**	Copper accumulation, asterixis, dementia, liver cirrhosis, **Kayser–Fleischer ring** in cornea	Hepatolenticular **degeneration of the basal ganglia**

Ach, acetylcholine; CNS, central nervous system; IgA, immunoglobulin A; MPTP, 1-methyl-4-phenyl-1,2,3,6-tetrahydropyridine.

The Nervous System

TABLE 2-10 **Antiparkinsonian Agents**

Drug	Mechanism of Action	Side Effects	Notes
Levodopa (L-dopa) (dopamine precursor)	More readily **crosses the blood–brain barrier;** converted to dopamine in the brain by DOPA decarboxylase	Dyskinesias (following dose), akinesia (between doses), postural hypotension, anorexia, depression, psychosis, arrhythmia	Development of tolerance, wildly varying effectiveness **(on–off phenomenon),** often necessitates drug holidays
Carbidopa	Inhibits conversion of L-dopa to dopamine in the periphery by **DOPA decarboxylase**	Decreases systemic side effects of L-dopa such as anorexia and nausea	Given with L-dopa, **does not cross the blood–brain barrier;** inhibition of systemic conversion of L-dopa, which reduces L-dopa dosing approximately 75%
Amantadine	Unclear; may stimulate dopamine receptors, stimulate dopamine release, or inhibit its reuptake	Agitation, restlessness, psychosis, urinary retention	Rapid deterioration of effectiveness over a period of weeks
Selegiline	Selectively and irreversibly **inhibits MAO type B,** which metabolizes dopamine	Dyskinesias, hepatic conversion to amphetamine causes insomnia and anorexia	In high doses, inhibition of MAO type A, which is prevalent in the gut, allowing absorption of ingested amines, which can cause **hypertensive crises**
Entacapone, tolcapone	Inhibits COMT which metabolizes dopamine	Nausea, dyskinesia, orthostatic hypotension	Administered with levodopa/carbidopa to reduce "wearing off" symptoms at the end of dosing interval
Bromocriptine	Acts as a **dopamine receptor agonist**	Anorexia, nausea, vomiting, postural hypotension, psychosis	Given as an adjuvant with L-dopa, inhibits release of prolactin and growth hormone and is therefore used for **prolactinomas** and **acromegaly**
Pramipexole, ropinirole	Dopamine receptor agonist	Postural hypotension/syncope, dizziness, sedation, fatigue, hallucinations, abnormal dreams	Also used to treat restless leg syndrome
Benztropine	Blocks **muscarinic acetylcholine receptors**	**Atropine-like** side effects, inattention, psychosis	Used in combination with dopamine agonists and L-dopa, **improves tremor and rigidity** but has little effect on bradykinesia

COMT, catechol-*O*-methyltransferase; MAO, monoamine oxidase.

DEMYELINATING DISEASES

Loss of the neuronal sheath can lead to impaired nerve conduction, which, in turn, causes deficits and disease (Table 2-11).

DISEASES THAT CAUSE DEMENTIA

Dementia is a chronic progressive deterioration in cognitive ability in which mental faculties, such as executive function, attention span, judgment, memory, mood, and behavior, are affected (Table 2-12).

ACUTE MENINGITIS

Meningitis is an infection of the meninges resulting in an inflammatory reaction characterized by severe headache, fever, photophobia, and positive Kernig and Brudzinski signs. Meningitis in immunocompetent adults is generally caused by *Streptococcus pneumoniae* or

QUICK HIT

CNS stimulants, which are at the other end of the spectrum from the sedative-hypnotics, usually cause sympathetic stimulation, resulting in increased alertness. They can also lower the seizure threshold. Common drugs of this type are amphetamine, caffeine, cocaine, dextroamphetamine, ephedrine, and methylphenidate.

QUICK HIT

Tay–Sachs disease and Niemann–Pick disease, a deficiency of sphingomyelinase, can both present with a **cherry-red spot** on the macula.

QUICK HIT

Amantadine, used in the treatment of Parkinson disease, also has antiviral effects and is sometimes used in the prevention and treatment of **influenza A.**

QUICK HIT

The triad of jaundice, right upper quadrant pain, and fever is also known as the Charcot triad and is associated with cholangitis.

QUICK HIT

Werdnig–Hoffmann disease is an infantile, autosomal recessive, and lower motor neuron disease similar to ALS.

QUICK HIT

Progressive multifocal leukoencephalopathy is a demyelinating disease caused by JC virus infection of oligodendrocytes. It is seen in patients with immune deficiency.

TABLE 2-11 **Demyelinating Diseases of the Nervous System**

Disease	Etiology	Clinical Manifestation	Notes
Amyotrophic lateral sclerosis (ALS, Lou Gehrig disease)	No specific pattern of inheritance, although autosomal dominant in 5% of cases (similar symptoms with some heavy metal poisonings, infections, or tumors)	**Both upper and lower motor neuron signs;** loss of lateral corticospinal tracts and anterior motor neurons leading to muscle atrophy	Most common motor neuron disease; rapidly fatal course
Guillain–Barré syndrome	Postviral autoimmune reaction involving peripheral nerves	Muscle weakness and paralysis **ascending upward** from the lower extremities	Young adults; **albuminocytologic dissociation is** pathognomonic (high albumin, low cell count)
Huntington disease	Chromosome 4; **CAG triple-base repeat** with anticipation	Degeneration of **caudate nucleus,** onset at 30–40 years of age, athetoid movements, muscular deterioration, dementia	Usually involves acetylcholine (ACh) and γ-aminobutyric acid (GABA) neurons
Krabbe disease	Autosomal recessive; decrease in β-galactocerebrosidase	Loss of myelin from globoid cells and peripheral nerves, mental retardation, blindness, paralysis, **globoid bodies** in white matter	Usually affects infants; **rapidly fatal**
Metachromatic leukodystrophy	Autosomal recessive defect of arylsulfatase A	Progressive paralysis and dementia, loss of myelin, accumulation of sulfatides, nerves stain **yellow-brown** in color, ataxia	Fatal in first decade
Multiple sclerosis (MS)	Unknown; more common in northern Europe; more common in women	Multiple focal areas of demyelination; variable course; **Triad of MS:** intention tremor, scanning speech, nystagmus	Most common demyelinating disease; increased cerebrospinal fluid (CSF) immunoglobulin

Clinical Vignette 2-2

CLINICAL PRESENTATION: A 28-year-old female presents to the emergency department complaining of numbness in her right leg that lasted several hours, which worsened when she took a **warm** shower. She also complained of feeling fatigued lately and she remembered that 1 year ago she had an episode of **transient unilateral vision loss** that resolved and never recurred. Vital signs: temperature = 97.0° F; blood pressure = 122/75 mm Hg; heart rate = 76 bpm; respiration rate = 18 breaths/min. Physical exam is significant for **nystagmus, scanning speech,** and diminished sensation in the right leg but normal strength.
DIFFERENTIALS: Multiple sclerosis (MS), Guillain–Barré syndrome.
DIAGNOSTIC STUDIES: Order magnetic resonance imaging (MRI) of the brain and a lumbar puncture (LP). MS should be suspected in young adults with relapsing and remitting neurologic signs and symptoms that do not seem associated to the same area of CNS white matter. MRI shows **demyelinating lesions (plaques)** at the **angles of the lateral ventricles** (which is the classic location of plaques in MS). MS is caused by selective demyelination of the spinal cord and brain, sparing PNS and gray matter. There are no laboratory tests specific for MS, but LP and CSF analysis will show **oligoclonal bands of IgG in** 90% of patients with MS. Transient sensory deficits are a common presenting feature of MS, as are visual disturbances caused by optic neuritis. Optic neuritis presents as monocular visual loss, pain on movement of eyes, central scotoma (black spot in center of vision), or decreased pupillary reaction to light. Also, be aware of the **Charcot triad:** intention tremor, nystagmus, and scanning speech.
MANAGEMENT: Treat this patient with **high-dose intravenous (IV) corticosteroids,** which can shorten an **acute** attack. After treatment of an acute attack, manage patient with **interferon therapy,** which should be started early in the course of disease. Treat symptoms of muscle spasticity with baclofen and carbamazepine or gabapentin for neuropathic pain.

QUICK HIT

Subacute sclerosing panencephalitis is a demyelinating disease caused by the measles virus. Infection is chronic but progressive and ultimately fatal.

QUICK HIT

Dementia is a chronic loss of cognitive function without an altered level of consciousness. Delirium is an acute altered level of consciousness accompanied by disordered cognition.

Neisseria meningitidis. Conditions predisposing an individual to acute bacterial meningitis as a result of pneumococcus include distant foci of infection (such as otitis, sinusitis, or pneumonia), sickle cell disease (secondary to splenic autoinfarction), alcoholism, or trauma with loss of meningeal integrity. Patients with a deficiency of complement components C5 to C8 are at a greater risk of developing meningococcal meningitis. *Haemophilus*

MNEMONIC

To recall the features of Alzheimer disease, remember **RONALD** Reagan:
Reduced acetylcholine
Old age
Neurofibrillary tangles
Amyloid plaques; **A**trophy of cerebral cortex
Language impairment
Dementia/**D**own syndrome

TABLE 2-12 **Diseases That Cause Dementia**

Disease	Etiology	Clinical Manifestation	Notes
Alzheimer dementia	Unknown; possibly **chromosome 21,** degeneration of nucleus basalis of Meynert, decreased choline acetyltransferase	Progressively worsening memory loss, **neurofibrillary tangles, senile plaques** (amyloid **β/A4** protein)	**Most common cause of dementia;** age of onset is usually 65 years (younger in patients with Down syndrome)
Multi-infarct dementia	Cerebral atherosclerosis	Stepwise decline of function, signs of dementia and possible motor deficits	**Second most common cause of dementia**
Primary HIV dementia	Macrophages, infected with HIV, enter CNS	Onset before immunodeficiency, slow thinking, ataxia, *Toxoplasma gondii* on autopsy	**Most common CNS manifestation of HIV**
Frontotemporal dementia (Pick disease)	Unknown; may be familial	Dementia plus personality/behavioral changes; possibly progressive aphasia	
Lewy body dementia	Unknown; combination of genetics and environmental factors	Dementia plus parkinsonian features, visual hallucinations, syncope/falls	More common in men

CNS, central nervous system.

QUICK HIT

Toxoplasma gondii can infect the immunocompromised individual via three routes: undercooked meat, cat feces, or in utero. It is the most common CNS infection in patients with AIDS.

QUICK HIT

Prevnar is a pneumococcal conjugate vaccine that is being given to children. The goal is to prevent invasive pneumococcal infections. There are two pediatric formulations: one with 7 serotypes, and one with 13 serotypes. The serotypes used to make the immunization are thought to be responsible for the majority of severe, invasive pneumococcal infections. Common, less invasive infections, such as otitis media, are unlikely to be affected because many other serotypes are not included in the vaccine.

QUICK HIT

Tumors of the CNS are usually intracranial, with **adult tumors** commonly **supratentorial** and **childhood tumors** usually **infratentorial**.

TABLE 2-13 Common Causes of Meningitis in Various Age Groups

Age Group	Causes
Newborns	Group B streptococci *Escherichia coli* *Listeria*
Children	*Haemophilus influenzae* b (declining since Hib vaccine introduced) *Streptococcus pneumoniae* *Neisseria meningitidis* Enteroviruses
Adolescents and young adults	Enteroviruses *N. meningitidis* *S. pneumoniae* Herpes simplex virus
Elderly	*S. pneumoniae* Gram-negative rods *Listeria*

influenzae type B was once a common cause of meningitis in children, although these numbers have decreased because of widespread vaccination (Table 2-13).

Lumbar puncture (LP) is often performed to confirm a suspected diagnosis of meningitis. The LP usually shows increased neutrophils, increased protein, and decreased glucose if bacterial in origin. Also, organisms may be seen on Gram stain. However, if the CSF contains increased lymphocytes and a normal glucose level, viral agents such as enterovirus, HIV, and herpes simplex virus should be considered (Table 2-14). If the LP shows organisms with a thick capsule when stained with India ink, this suggests *Cryptococcus neoformans;* and the infected individual is most likely immunocompromised as a result of HIV infection. Adults who are immunocompromised are also at risk for developing meningitis caused by *Listeria monocytogenes.*

NERVOUS SYSTEM TUMORS

Nearly 50% of the tumors occurring within the nervous system are metastases to the brain from tumors elsewhere in the body. The other 50% are primary nervous system tumors. Tables 2-15 and 2-16 list the most common nervous system tumors in adults and children. Seventy percent of adult brain tumors are supratentorial; 70% of childhood brain tumors are infratentorial.

TABLE 2-14 Evaluation of Cerebrospinal Fluid to Determine Cause of Meningitis

Laboratory Test	Bacterial	Viral	Fungal
Opening CSF pressure	↑	N	↑
Lymphocytes	N	↑	↑
Neutrophils	↑	N	N
Glucose	↓	N	↓
Protein	↑	N	↑

↑, Increased; ↓, decreased; CSF, cerebrospinal fluid; N, normal.

TABLE 2-15 Nervous System Tumors in Adults

Tumor	Presentation	Significant Features
Metastatic neoplasms	Headache, focal defects, formation of discrete nodules in brain	Nearly half of all intracranial neoplasm; usually bloodborne; commonly from lung, breast, gastrointestinal, thyroid, kidney, genitourinary, and melanoma
Glioblastoma (grade IV astrocytoma)	Cerebral hemisphere tumor, irregular mass with necrotic center surrounded by edema seen on CT	**Most common primary intracranial neoplasm;** poor prognosis; neural tube origin; **pseudopalisading** arrangement of cells; astrocytes stain with GFAP
Meningioma	**Psammoma bodies,** slowly growing, originates in arachnoid cells, follows sinuses	Second most common primary CNS tumor; usually occurs in women; resectable; neural crest origin
Schwannoma	Tinnitus and hearing loss, ataxic gait, positive Romberg sign, increased intracranial pressure, hydrocephalus, benign	Third most common primary intracranial tumor; neural crest origin; usually occurs in the cerebellopontine angle and involves CN VIII; seen **bilaterally in neurofibromatosis type 2 (NF-2)**
Oligodendroglioma	Slow-growing frontal lobe tumor	Rare; clearing of the cytoplasm around the nuclei **(perinuclear halo)** give tumor cells a **"fried egg" appearance**

CN, cranial nerve; CNS, central nervous system; CT, computed tomography; GFAP, glial fibrillary acidic protein.

QUICK HIT

Psammoma bodies are also seen in papillary adenocarcinoma of the thyroid, serous papillary cystadenocarcinoma of the ovary, and malignant mesothelioma.

TABLE 2-16 Nervous System Tumors in Children

Tumor	Presentation	Significant Features
Pilocytic astrocytoma (grade I astrocytoma)	Benign, usually posterior fossa, good prognosis	**Most common primary brain tumor in children;** astrocytes stain with GFAP; eosinophilic Rosenthal fibers
Medulloblastoma	Cerebellar mass, may compress the fourth ventricle (**noncommunicating hydrocephalus**), ataxic gait, projectile vomiting	**Most common malignant primary brain tumor of childhood;** neural tube origin; **Homer-Wright rosettes** (circular arrangement of tumor cells around a central tangle of fibrils)
Ependymoma	May compress the fourth ventricle (**noncommunicating hydrocephalus**)	Neural tube origin; **perivascular rosettes** (circular arrangement of tumor cells around a central vessel)
Craniopharyngioma	Endocrine abnormalities, papilledema, **bitemporal hemianopsia** due to compression of optic chiasm	Enlarged sella turcica; **most common supratentorial brain tumor in children; ectodermal origin** (Rathke pouch)

GFAP, glial fibrillary acidic protein.

MNEMONIC

ClAssic migraines have an Aura, common migraines are without aura.

HEADACHE *(Table 2-17)*

TABLE 2-17 Primary Headache Syndromes

Type	General Characteristics	Clinical Features	Treatment
Tension	Worsens throughout the day; precipitated by stress, anxiety, and depression; more frequent in women	Tight, **bandlike** pain encircling the entire head; most intense around the neck or back of head; tenderness in posterior neck muscles	Stress reduction, NSAIDs, acetaminophen, and aspirin if mild/moderate; if severe, TCAs or SSRIs
Cluster	Usually occurs in **middle-aged men; episodic**—lasts 2–3 months, with remissions of months to years; occurs around bedtime and lasts 30–90 min	Excruciating periorbital pain **("behind the eye"), unilateral; stabbing or deep, burning pain;** accompanied by ipsilateral lacrimation, nasal congestion or discharge, facial flushing	Acute: **sumatriptan, oxygen inhalation**; Prophylaxis: **verapamil** taken daily—drug of choice (alternatives: ergotamine, methyllithium, methyl sergide, corticosteroids)
Migraine	**Inherited;** caused by serotonin depletion; women > men; family history subtypes: **1. Classic:** migraine with **aura** (aura usually visual such as flashing lights, scotoma, visual distortions) **2. Common:** migraine without aura **3. Menstrual**	Prodromal phase; severe **throbbing or dull achy unilateral headaches,** may be generalized; lasts for 4–72 h; pain is **aggravated by coughing, physical activity, and bending down;** other symptoms include nausea and vomiting, photophobia, and increased sensitivity to smell	Acute: NSAIDs, dihydroergotamine, sumatriptan; Prophylaxis: first line—TCAs and propranolol; second line—verapamil, valproic acid, and methysergide

NSAID, nonsteroidal anti-inflammatory drug; SSRI, selective serotonin reuptake inhibitor; TCA, tricyclic antidepressant.

PSYCHIATRY AND BEHAVIORAL SCIENCE

I. Nonpharmacologic therapeutic modalities *(Table 2-18)*

TABLE 2-18 Nonpharmacologic Therapeutic Modalities

Therapy	Characteristics	Notes
Biofeedback	Gaining control over physiology via continuous information; motivation and practice required	Used for hypertension, migraine headaches, and tension headaches
Classical conditioning	**A reflexive, natural behavior** is elicited in **response to a learned stimulus** (e.g., ringing of a bell causing salivation)	**Aversive conditioning** pairs an unwanted response to a painful stimulus; stages include acquisition, extinction, and recovery
Cognitive therapy	**Negative thinking** is reorganized into self-affirming, positive thoughts	Short-term psychotherapy used to treat depression and anxiety
Electroconvulsive therapy (ECT)	Electric current introduced into brain to alter neurotransmitter function; improvement seen faster than with pharmacologic regimens	Used for **major depression;** safe; effective; retrograde amnesia is a major side effect
Operant conditioning	Behavior that is not part of the natural repertoire is learned by altering the reward **(reinforcement)**	Reinforcement can be positive or negative; reward schedule includes continuous, fixed, or variable
Psychoanalysis	Intensive treatment based on recovering and integrating past experiences from the unconscious via free association; based on **Freud's theories**	**Id**—sexual drives and aggression; **ego**—controls instinct and interacts with the world; **superego**—morality and conscience
Systematic desensitization	Classical conditioning technique in which relaxation procedures are combined with increasing doses of anxiety-provoking stimuli	Used to **eliminate** phobias
Token economy	Positive reinforcement in which a reward is used to elicit a desired response	Seen often in mental hospitals or parents dealing with children

II. Eating disorders *(Table 2-19)*

TABLE 2-19 Eating Disorders

Disorder	Characteristics	Treatment	Notes
Anorexia nervosa	Body weight <85% of ideal, **distorted body image,** intense fear of gaining weight	Supportive care, counseling, cognitive behavioral therapy, family therapy, **pharmacotherapy is typically ineffective**	Higher incidence in female adolescents, **upper-middle socioeconomic classes;** amenorrhea; decreased libido
Bulimia nervosa	Binge eating, followed by some inappropriate behavior to prevent weight gain (e.g., purging; abuse of laxatives); **normal weight**	Psychotherapy; pharmacotherapy; with **fluoxetine** (first line), other SSRIs, TCAs, or MAOIs; bupropion is contraindicated due to risk of seizures	Normal libido; no amenorrhea (unlike anorexics); erosion of tooth enamel; hypokalemic hypochloremic metabolic alkalosis (due to vomiting); hypertrophy of parotid glands
Binge eating disorder	Binge eating as an expression of deeper psychological problems; no purging; excessive weight gain	Psychotherapy, cognitive behavioral therapy, SSRIs	Patients may have negative attitudes toward food
Compulsive eating	Binge eating; constant preoccupation with and fantasizing about food	SSRIs, SNRIs, cognitive behavioral therapy	A form of obsessive-compulsive disorder
Obesity	BMI >30	Dieting and exercise; strict fad dieting ineffective; bariatric surgery may be useful in selected patients with good dietary compliance	Lower socioeconomic groups; genetics plays a role; increased risk of disease

BMI, body mass index; MAOI, monoamine oxidase inhibitor; SNRI, serotonin-norepinephrine reuptake inhibitor; SSRI, selective serotonin reuptake inhibitor; TCA, tricyclic antidepressant.

QUICK HIT

Substance abuse is defined as use of psychoactive substances for at least 1 month with interference in the user's life but without meeting the criteria for dependence. Substance dependence involves craving, withdrawal, and tolerance.

III. Drugs of abuse and dependence *(Table 2-20)*

TABLE 2-20 Drugs of Abuse and Dependence

Drug	Mechanism	Intoxication Effect	Withdrawal Effects
Alcohol	Unknown; possible effect at GABA receptor directly on membranes	Sedation, hypnosis, slurred speech, ataxia, loss of motor coordination, Wernicke–Korsakoff syndrome	Malaise, tachycardia, tremors, seizures, **delirium tremens,** death
Amphetamine	Release of intracellular stores of catecholamines	Insomnia, irritability, tremor, hyperactive reflexes, arrhythmias, anorexia, psychosis	Lethargy, depression, hunger, craving for drug resulting in bizarre psychological behavior, anxiety
Barbiturates	**Potentiation of GABA** action on chloride by **increase of duration** of chloride channel opening	Mental sluggishness, anesthesia, hypnosis	Restlessness, anxiety, tremor, death

(continued)

QUICK HIT

Alcohol is the most widely used drug, followed by nicotine. Caffeine is the most often used psychoactive substance, followed by nicotine.

QUICK HIT

Dependence is mediated by **dopamine**, the neurotransmitter linked to the pleasure and reward center.

TABLE 2-20 Drugs of Abuse and Dependence *(Continued)*

Drug	Mechanism	Intoxication Effect	Withdrawal Effects
Benzodiazepines	**Potentiation of GABA** action on chloride by **increase of frequency** of chloride channel opening	Sedation, ataxia, mild respiratory depression	Tremors, anxiety, psychosis, **seizures**
Caffeine	Translocation of Ca^{2+}, inhibition of phosphodiesterase (increase in cAMP, cGMP)	Insomnia, anxiety, agitation	Lethargy, irritability, headache
Cocaine	Blockade of norepinephrine, 5-HT, and dopamine reuptake	Hallucinations, anxiety, arrhythmias, nasal problems, sudden death	Craving, depression, excessive sleeping, fatigue
Lysergic acid diethylamide (LSD)	5-HT agonist action in the midbrain	Pupillary dilation, increased blood pressure and body temperature, piloerection, hallucinations	Flashbacks
Marijuana	Unknown; tetrahydrocannabinol (THC) is active compound; possible endogenous receptors in brain	Increased appetite, visual hallucinations, increased heart rate, decreased blood pressure Impairment of short-term memory and mental activity	Fatigue, hypersomnia, psychomotor retardation
Nicotine	Low doses—ganglionic stimulation; high doses—ganglionic blockade	**Increased heart rate and blood pressure,** irritability, tremors, intestinal cramps	Irritability, anxiety, restlessness, headaches, insomnia, difficulty in concentrating
Opioids (heroin)	Inhibition of adenylate cyclase by opioid receptors within the CNS	Constipation, **pinpoint pupils,** potentially lethal via **respiratory depression,** sedation	Insomnia, diarrhea, sweating, fever, piloerection
Phencyclidine (PCP)	Inhibition of dopamine, serotonin, and norepinephrine reuptake	Hostile, bizarre behavior; nystagmus hypersalivation; anesthesia	Sudden onset of violent behavior

cAMP, cyclic adenosine monophosphate; cGMP, cyclic guanosine monophosphate; CNS, central nervous system; GABA, γ-aminobutyric acid; 5-HT, serotonin.

IV. Schizophrenia

A. Diagnostic features
   1. Hallucinations (usually auditory)
   2. Delusions
   3. Disorganized speech
   4. Disorganized or catatonic behavior
   5. Negative symptoms: flattened affect, social withdrawal, lack of motivation, thought blocking, poor grooming

B. Neurotransmitters involved: increased dopamine may be implicated

C. Other features
   1. Usually first presents in young adulthood
   2. Marijuana use during teenage years is a risk factor
   3. Enlarged lateral ventricles and third ventricle

D. Subtypes of schizophrenia
   1. Paranoid
   2. Disorganized

3. Catatonic
4. Undifferentiated
5. Residual

V. Schizophrenia-related disorders

A. Brief psychotic disorder
1. Symptoms of schizophrenia for <1 month
2. Usually stress related

B. Schizophreniform disorder—symptoms of schizophrenia for 1 to 6 months

C. Schizoaffective disorder—schizophrenia/psychosis as the primary disorder, in addition to a secondary mood disorder (either bipolar disorder or depression)

D. Delusional disorder
1. Characterized by non-bizarre delusions that are more than simply overvalued ideas
2. Absence of hallucinations
3. Functioning is not impaired, and behavior is not odd

VI. Antipsychotics *(Table 2-21)*

Experts theorize that an excess of **dopamine** in certain areas of the brain is in some way responsible for psychosis. The development of psychosis as a common side effect of treatment of Parkinson disease with dopamine and dopamine agonists supports this theory. It is thought that most antipsychotics exert their effect by blocking **dopamine receptors**.

Antipsychotic drugs have several particular side effects in common. The side effects may be grouped into the following categories: (1) **extrapyramidal**, (2) **anticholinergic**, (3) **alpha-blocking effect**, and (4) **histamine receptor effects**. Extrapyramidal side effects

QUICK HIT

The timeline for extrapyramidal side effects is:
4 hours—acute dystonia
4 days—akinesia
4 weeks—akathisia
4 months—tardive dyskinesia.

QUICK HIT

In its most severe form, extrapyramidal effects may develop into **neuroleptic malignant syndrome,** a potentially fatal combination of severe rigidity, decreased perspiration, hyperpyrexia, and autonomic instability. Treatment involves immediate discontinuation of antipsychotic medications, supportive measures, and administration of **dantrolene**.

TABLE 2-21 **Antipsychotics**

Drug	Clinical Uses	Side Effects	Notes
Typical antipsychotics (traditional neuroleptics)			
High potency			
Haloperidol, fluphenazine	**Schizophrenia, psychosis**; haloperidol is often used off-label for acute agitation and delirium	**EPS** (dystonia, akinesia, akathisia, tardive dyskinesia); toxicity results in **NMS** (rigidity, myoglobinuria, autonomic instability, hyperpyrexia); anticholinergic side effects are less common; **prolonged QT syndrome**	NMS is treated with dantrolene and dopamine agonists
Droperidol	Postoperative nausea and vomiting	*Same as haloperidol*	Rarely used because of QT prolongation and risk of arrhythmia
Trifluoperazine, thiothixene, loxapine, perphenazine	Schizophrenia, psychosis	*Same as haloperidol*; variable QT prolongation	These are sometimes inconsistently classified as "moderate potency" neuroleptics
Typical antipsychotics (traditional neuroleptics)			
Low potency			
Chlorpromazine	Schizophrenia, psychosis	**Anticholinergic side effects** (dry mouth, constipation); weight gain; some alpha blockade (hypotension) and histamine blockade (sedation); EPS and NMS are less common.	
Thioridazine		*Same as chlorpromazine*, plus high risk of QT prolongation and arrhythmias	Not commonly used
Atypical antipsychotics			
Clozapine	Schizophrenia, useful for both positive and negative symptoms	**Agranulocytosis, weight gain, diabetes,** low risk of anticholinergic side effects; EPS and NMS occur at lower rates than with typicals	Second-line agent used for refractory schizophrenia, check weekly blood counts due to risk of agranulocytosis
Olanzapine, quetiapine, risperidone, ziprasidone, paliperidone, sertindole, aripiprazole	**Schizophrenia, bipolar disorder**	**Weight gain, diabetes,** low risk of anticholinergic side effects; EPS and NMS occur at lower rates than with typicals	Of these drugs, olanzapine has the highest risk of weight gain and diabetes

EPS, extrapyramidal symptoms; NMS, neuroleptic malignant syndrome.

refer to acute dystonia, akinesia, and akathisia. **Dystonia** presents acutely within a few hours of starting the medication as a muscular spasm, stiffness, and oculogyric crisis. **Akinesia** presents within a few days of starting the medication as parkinsonian symptoms. **Akathisia** presents within a few weeks of starting the medication as restlessness. **Tardive dyskinesia** presents after a few months of starting the medication with stereotypic oral facial movements, likely due to dopamine receptor sensitization. Tardive dyskinesia is often irreversible and is most common in older women who have received long-term treatment with high doses. **Anticholinergic side effects** include dry mouth and constipation. **Alpha-blocking effects** include hypotension. **Histamine receptor effects** include sedation. **Atypical antipsychotics** such as clozapine, olanzapine, risperidone, quetiapine, aripiprazole, and ziprasidone have a lower incidence of extrapyramidal and anticholinergic side effects. Finally, antipsychotics also may be **antiemetic** and have a tendency to **lower the seizure threshold**.

VII. Depression

A. Major depressive disorder (MDD)
   1. Diagnostic features **(SIG E CAPS):** sleep disturbances, loss of interest in formerly pleasurable things (anhedonia), guilt, low energy, poor concentration, appetite changes, psychomotor retardation or agitation, suicidal ideation, and depressed mood
   2. Symptoms must be present for at least 2 weeks.
   3. Neurotransmitters involved: decreased norepinephrine (NE) and 5-HT
   4. Decreased REM latency (rapid onset of REM sleep) is commonly seen.
   5. Treatment
      a. Pharmacotherapy: selective serotonin reuptake inhibitors (SSRIs), serotonin-norepinephrine reuptake inhibitors (SNRIs), tricyclic antidepressants (TCAs), monoamine oxidase inhibitors (MAOIs)
      b. Nonpharmacologic therapies: cognitive behavioral therapy, electroconvulsive therapy (ECT)

B. Atypical depression
   1. Features include hypersomnia, overeating and weight gain, mood reactivity, rejection hypersensitivity
   2. Treatment: MAOIs or SSRIs

C. Postpartum depression
   1. Depression in the postpartum period that exceeds 2 weeks and may persist for longer than a year
   2. Treatment: same as for MDD

D. Dysthymia—A milder form of depression with the same diagnostic features as MDD that lasts at least 2 years

E. Seasonal affective disorder
   1. A form of major depression that occurs during the winter season due to a deficiency of retinal stimulation with light
   2. Treatment: supplemental light therapy daily

F. SAD PERSONS scale—assessment of likelihood of suicide completion
   1. S – Sex (male > female)
   2. A – Age (teenagers and elderly)
   3. D – Depression
   4. P – Previous attempt
   5. E – Ethanol or other drug use
   6. R – Rational thinking is lost
   7. S – Sickness (major medical illness, or three or more prescription medications)
   8. O – Organized plan
   9. N – No spouse
   10. S – Social support lacking

> **QUICK HIT**
>
> Amitriptyline is somewhat more potent than imipramine and nortriptyline, which means that it often has more significant side effects.

> **QUICK HIT**
>
> The use of the combination of selective serotonin reuptake inhibitors (SSRIs) and monoamine oxidase inhibitors (MAOIs) may produce a **"serotonin syndrome."** This constellation of hyperpyrexia, muscle spasm, and mental status changes can be fatal.

VIII. Antidepressants *(Table 2-22)*

The "**amine theory**" attributes mood to levels of certain amines such as NE and 5-HT. It is theorized that low levels of these hormones lead to depression, and many of the antidepressants **boost amine levels**. The sites of action of the antidepressants are represented graphically (Figure 2-18).

TABLE 2-22 **Antidepressants**

Class of Antidepressant (Specific Agent)	Mechanism of Action	Clinical Uses	Side Effects	Notes
Selective serotonin reuptake inhibitors (SSRIs) (e.g., fluoxetine, paroxetine, sertraline, citalopram)	Inhibit **reuptake** of 5-HT at neuronal synapses	Major depression, OCD, anxiety disorders, bulimia nervosa	Inhibits liver enzymes, nausea, agitation, **sexual dysfunction** (anorgasmia), dystonic reactions	Contraindicated with **MAOIs** secondary to **serotonin syndrome** (hyperthermia, muscle rigidity, cardiovascular collapse). Allow time for antidepressant effect; usually takes 2–3 weeks
Serotonin-norepinephrine reuptake inhibitors (SNRIs) (venlafaxine, desvenlafaxine, duloxetine, milnacipran, sibutramine)	Inhibit **reuptake** of NE and 5-HT at neuronal synapses	Major depression, anxiety disorders, neuropathic pain (duloxetine), fibromyalgia (milnacipran), obesity (sibutramine)	Sedation, nausea, constipation, hypertension, mild sexual dysfunction	Sibutramine is used only as an appetite suppressant for morbid obesity
Tricyclic antidepressants (TCAs) (amitriptyline, imipramine, nortriptyline, desipramine, clomipramine, doxepin, amoxapine)	Inhibit **reuptake** of NE and 5-HT at neuronal synapses	Major depression, OCD (clomipramine), nocturnal enuresis (imipramine), panic disorder	Sedation, **α-blocking effects** (orthostatic hypotension), **anticholinergic** (tachycardia, dry mouth, urinary retention), hallucinations (in elderly), confusion (elderly) Overdose toxicity results in **convulsions, coma, cardiotoxicity** (arrhythmias), respiratory depression, hyperpyrexia	Desipramine is the least sedating Used off-label for insomnia
Monoamine oxidase inhibitors (MAOIs) (isocarboxazid, phenelzine, tranylcypromine)	Inhibit **degradation** of NE and 5-HT at neuronal synapses	**Atypical depression** (with hypersomnia, anxiety, sensitivity to rejection, hypochondriasis)	**Hypertensive episodes** with ingestion of tyramine-containing foods or beta agonists, hyperthermia, convulsions	Contraindicated with **SSRIs** and **meperidine** secondary to **serotonin syndrome** (hyperthermia, muscle rigidity, cardiovascular collapse)
Other antidepressants				
Bupropion	Inhibits reuptake of NE and dopamine	Major depression, smoking cessation	Tachycardia, insomnia, headache, seizure (especially patients with bulimia)	Does not have sexual side effects
Mirtazapine	α_2-antagonist → increases release of NE and 5-HT	Major depression (especially with insomnia)	**Weight gain**, dry mouth, increased appetite, sedation	
Maprotiline	Blocks NE uptake	Major depression	Sedation, orthostatic hypotension	
Trazodone	Inhibits 5-HT reuptake	Major depression (especially with insomnia), insomnia	Sedation, nausea, **priapism**, postural hypotension	

5-HT, serotonin; OCD, obsessive-compulsive disorder; NE, norepinephrine.

QUICK HIT

An **overdose** of a tricyclic antidepressant (TCA) causes delirium, coma, seizures, respiratory depression, and arrhythmias and is potentially fatal and difficult to treat. The large volume of distribution of a TCA makes dialysis relatively ineffective.

FIGURE 2-18 Antidepressant sites of action

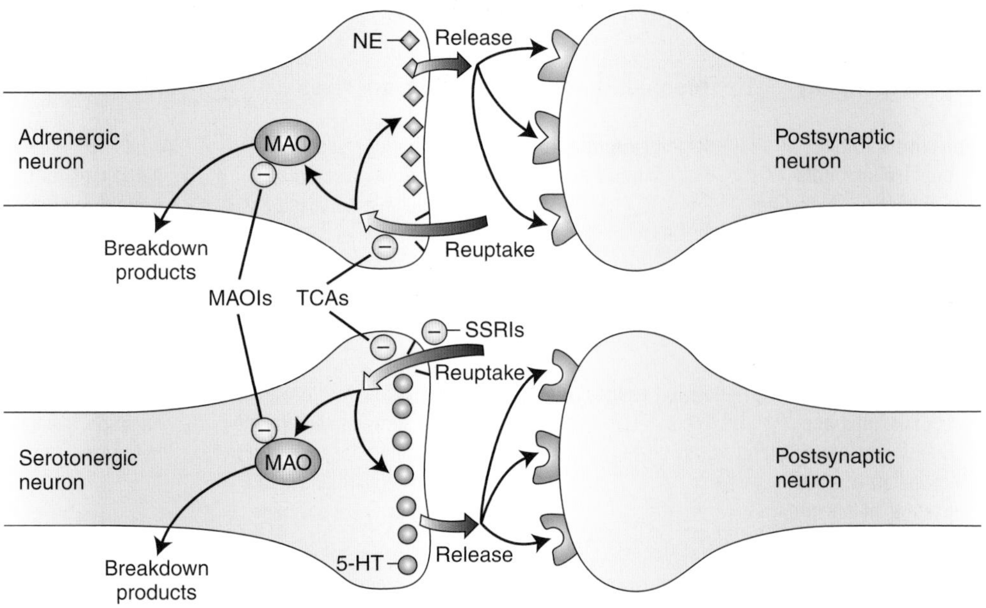
NE
Release
Adrenergic neuron
MAO
Postsynaptic neuron
Breakdown products
Reuptake
MAOIs
TCAs
SSRIs
Reuptake
Serotonergic neuron
MAO
Postsynaptic neuron
Breakdown products
5-HT
Release

5-HT, 5-hydroxytryptamine (serotonin); MAO, monoamine oxidase; MAOI, monoamine oxidase inhibitor; NE, norepinephrine; SSRIs, selective serotonin reuptake inhibitors; TCAs, tricyclic antidepressants.

IX. Anxiety disorders *(Table 2-23)*

TABLE 2-23 Anxiety Disorders

Disorder	Characteristics	Neurotransmitter(s) Involved	Treatment	Notes
Panic disorder	Discrete, episodic periods of intense anxiety or discomfort; palpitations; chest pain; sweating; fear of dying	Decreased serotonin, norepinephrine, GABA	Imipramine; behavioral therapy	Associated with mitral valve prolapse; young women predominantly affected; genetic component
Generalized anxiety disorder	Generalized, persistent anxiety; tension; insomnia; irritability	Decreased serotonin, norepinephrine, GABA	**SSRIs,** buspirone (Table 2-25), benzodiazepines	Anxiety for more than **6 months**
Posttraumatic stress disorder (PTSD)	Result of trauma, hypervigilance, nightmares, flashbacks	Decreased serotonin, norepinephrine, GABA	Counseling, group therapy, benzodiazepines for symptoms	For the first 3 months after the trauma, it is called acute PTSD; symptoms lasting longer than 3 months is chronic PTSD
Obsessive-compulsive disorder	Recurrent thoughts and actions; patients are distressed by repetitive actions	Decreased serotonin	Behavioral therapy, clomipramine, trazodone, SSRIs	
Phobias	Irrational, situational fear	Decreased serotonin, norepinephrine, and GABA	Systematic desensitization; propranolol useful for physiologic manifestations	EEG changes

EEG, electroencephalogram; GABA, γ-aminobutyric acid; SSRI, selective serotonin reuptake inhibitor.

X. Other neuropsychiatric disorders and other psychiatric drugs *(Table 2-24, Table 2-25)*

QUICK HIT

Dissociative disorders result in retrograde amnesia, whereas head trauma results in anterograde amnesia.

QUICK HIT

Munchausen syndrome is a factitious disorder in which the patient fakes illness in order to receive medical attention, such as a nurse purposely injecting himself or herself with insulin to receive medical attention. **Munchausen syndrome by proxy** is a syndrome wherein the attention seeker feigns or creates illness in another, usually his or her child, to gain medical attention. It is considered a form of abuse.

TABLE 2-24 **Other Neuropsychiatric Disorders**

Disorder	Characteristics	Treatment	Notes
Bipolar disorder	Rapid speech, decreased need for sleep, hyperenergetic state, impaired judgment followed by a state of depression	**Lithium** (Table 2-25), certain anticonvulsants, atypical antipsychotics	
Cyclothymia	Alternating between dysthymia and hypomania, lasting at least 2 years	Same as bipolar disorder	
Delirium	Impaired cognitive processes, diurnal variation in mood (worse at **night—"sundowning"**), illusions and hallucinations	Treat the underlying cause	**Most common** problem in hospitalized patients with psychiatric disorders
Dissociative disorders	Psychological factors resulting in memory loss and loss of function	Psychotherapy, hypnotherapy, medication for associated symptoms	Includes amnesia, fugue, dissociative identity disorder, depersonalization
Somatoform disorders	Symptoms of disease occur without related pathology	Psychotherapy and therapeutics may help; variable response	Patients truly believe in having illness, whereas factitious disorders are the result of faking illness
Factitious disorder	Patient consciously produces signs or symptoms of illness without a conscious motive or external incentive	Treatment of self-induced illness; avoid unnecessary tests and procedures	
Malingering	Patient consciously produces signs or symptoms of illness for secondary gain (avoiding work, obtaining money, drugs, shelter)	Avoid unnecessary tests and procedures	Patients often leave when confronted
Attention deficit hyperactivity disorder (ADHD)	Hyperactive, poor attention span, highly sensitive to stimuli	Amphetamines (methylphenidate—see Table 2-25)	More common in **male children**
Tourette syndrome	Involuntary **motor and vocal** movements (need both)	Haloperidol, clonidine	Onset occurs in childhood

TABLE 2-25 **Other Psychiatric Drugs**

Class/Drug	Mechanism of Action	Clinical Uses	Side Effects	Notes
Lithium	Unclear; inhibits regeneration of IP_3 and DAG; important for many second-messenger systems	**Bipolar disorder,** acute mania	Tremor, hypothyroidism, teratogenesis **nephrogenic diabetes insipidus**	**Requires close monitoring** of serum levels due to narrow therapeutic window
Buspirone	5-HT receptor agonist	**Generalized anxiety disorder**	Dizziness, drowsiness, headache, nausea	
Varenicline	Partial agonist of nicotinic receptor	Smoking cessation	Nausea, headache, insomnia, abnormal dreams	
Methylphenidate	CNS stimulant—blocks presynaptic reuptake of NE and dopamine	Attention deficit hyperactivity disorder, narcolepsy	Insomnia, restlessness	Contraindicated in patients with heart disease or hypertension

5-HT, serotonin; CNS, central nervous system; DAG, diacylglycerol; IP_3, inositol triphosphate; NE, norepinephrine.

The Nervous System

XI. Defense mechanisms *(Table 2-26)*

TABLE 2-26 **Defense Mechanisms**

Mechanism	Characteristics	Example
Immature mechanisms		
Acting out	Stress is dealt with through actions	After the death of his brother, a priest breaks all the windows in his church.
Denial	Not accepting the reality of a situation	A woman refuses to consider the possibility of pregnancy after having unprotected intercourse and missing two periods.
Displacement	Feelings for causal source are transferred to another object	A man kicks his dog after getting fired from his job.
Dissociation	Loss of memory or change in personality as a result of stressor	A woman who was sexually abused as a child develops another personality.
Identification	Behavior patterned after another	A teenager smokes pot because his favorite rock star does.
Intellectualization	Reason is used to cope with anxiety	A physician starts reading textbooks and journal articles about her father's cancer.
Isolation of affect	Events are separated from emotion	An airline passenger describes an emergency landing to his family without any emotion.
Projection	One's own characteristics are applied to another	A flirtatious man accuses his wife of cheating.
Rationalization	Analytical reason is used to justify unacceptable feelings	A man claims that his driving under the influence arrest would never have happened if his softball team had won.
Reaction formation	Feelings are denied and opposite actions are performed	A woman who wants to cheat on her husband instead buys him a new car.
Regression	Stress-induced behavior that involves returning to a childlike state	Medical students have a food fight during their lunch break on the day of board examinations.
Repression	Holding back an unacceptable feeling or idea from reaching consciousness	A recent widower feels no sense of loss.
Splitting	Feelings or stressors are placed in distinct, opposite compartments (i.e., either all good or all bad)	A man in a doctor's office describes how much he hates the nurses but loves the receptionist.
Mature mechanisms		
Altruism	One unselfishly assists others	A woman donates her entire estate to her favorite charities upon her death.
Humor	Humor is used to reduce stress	While stuck in an elevator, a young man makes jokes to ease the tension.
Sublimation	Unacceptable impulse is directed into a socially accepted action	A boy who got into a lot of fights as a kid decides to become a professional boxer.
Suppression	Conscious effort to suppress thoughts or feelings	A recent widower actively refuses to think about his deceased wife while packing her things away.

XII. Personality disorders *(Table 2-27)*

TABLE 2-27 Personality Disorders

Disorder	Characteristics	Example
CLUSTER A		
Paranoid	Hostile, suspicious, mistrustful, usually male	A patient being prepared for surgery yells at the doctors on rounds because he feels they are gossiping about him.
Schizoid	**Voluntarily** socially withdrawn without psychological problems; usually male	A 52-year-old computer programmer lives alone, is not married, has no friends, and is contented.
Schizotypal	Odd behavior, thoughts, and appearance without psychosis	A woman wears many-layered clothing and inappropriately applied makeup and only talks to people with brown-colored hair.
CLUSTER B		
Histrionic	Dramatic, overemotional, sexually provocative, unable to maintain close friendships, usually female	A woman exaggerates her suffering over a mild cold and behaves seductively toward the physician.
Narcissistic	Grandiosity, hypersensitivity to criticism, and lack of empathy	A resident refuses to operate with anyone but the best surgeon in the hospital because he feels it is beneath his talent.
Antisocial	Inability to conform to societal rules; criminal behavior; more often male; requires diagnosis of conduct disorder as child	A multiple rapist has no concern for his victims or the law.
Borderline	Unstable, impulsive, suicide attempts, vulnerable to abandonment, usually female, uses splitting	After an argument with her boyfriend, a woman chases him out of her home and later calls him and tells him she cannot live without him.
CLUSTER C		
Avoidant	Shy, **involuntarily** (compare to schizoid) withdrawn because fears rejection, usually female	A businesswoman defers speaking during presentations to her project partner and has few friends
Obsessive-compulsive	Rigid, perfectionist, stubborn, orderly; found twice as often in males	A businessman works long hours on a project, holding up both the project deadline and his personal life in vain attempts to make it perfect.
Dependent	Defers decision making; not comfortable with an authority position; insecure; has the ability to make long-lasting relationships (unlike avoidant); usually female	A third-year resident often accepts on-call duty for other residents, never speaks up when talked down to by the junior residents, and has trouble writing orders.
Passive–aggressive	Obstinate, inefficient, procrastinating, noncompliant	School student intentionally does poorly on homework because he does not like his teacher.

QUICK HIT

Schizotypal is a personality disorder characterized by odd beliefs or magical thinking. **Schizoid** is a personality disorder characterized by voluntary social isolation. Neither of these meets the diagnostic criteria for schizophrenia, but both are risk factors for the development of schizophrenia.

ETHICS AND THE ROLE OF THE PHYSICIAN

The role of the nervous system in the manifestation of psychological problems is under debate. The occurrence of certain psychopathology has been linked to neurotransmitters and the lack of regulation in certain parts of the CNS.

Communication skills are essential to determine a patient's physical and psychological problems. Establishing trust and confidence via facilitation, reflection, and an open-ended clinical interview allows the physician to gather physical, psychological, and social information. If an individual suffers from psychopathology, proper steps must be taken not to alienate, offend, or judge the patient. On the other hand, the individual's problems must be dealt with directly.

When presenting therapeutic options or advice, the physician should be forthright, direct, and honest. In making an assessment of any patient, the physician needs to be sensitive to problems affecting certain populations. For instance, it is important to remember that in elderly patients, sexual changes occur (i.e., men may have slower erections and women may have increased vaginal dryness and decreased vaginal length, though libido is not necessarily affected), sleep may decrease, suicide rate may increase, and depression becomes more prevalent.

Although the physician must be **nonmaleficent** (not intending to do harm) and **beneficent** (doing what is best for the patient), **physician autonomy** and **patient autonomy** ultimately prevail in making the final decision about treatment. The physician must consider the patient's ability to make decisions based on communication skills, level of understanding about medicine, stability, consistency, and soundness of mind. Physicians have a **duty** to provide medical care to their patients, and if **breach** of this duty directly leads to **damage**, the physician has been **negligent** and therefore is **liable** for malpractice. The breach of duty owing to negligence and the damages caused by it represent a **tort**.

Before making a final decision regarding patient care, physicians should make an effort to obtain an **informed consent**, which indicates that the patient understands the risks and benefits of therapy. Treatment of minors requires consent of the parent (or other responsible adult), with certain exceptions:

- Emancipated minors (≥16 years old, living on his or her own, and managing his or her own finances)
- Treatment of sexually transmitted infections
- Treatment related to pregnancy (other than abortion)
- Treatment of drug addiction/dependency
- Treatment of the child *of* a minor
- Treatment of minor serving a sentence of confinement
- Emergency situations where parental consent cannot be obtained

Disheartening as it may be, terminal disease may require the physician to explain to the patient and his family that further intervention is inappropriate inasmuch as maximal treatment has failed and it seems to be a reasonable conclusion that the goals of care will not be reached. **Advance directives** from the patient, either written or oral, may assist the physician in coming to a conclusion about when to terminate treatment measures.

Information about the patient must remain **confidential** unless the patient poses a risk to self or to others; information concerning the patient's own disease, diagnosis, or prognosis cannot be withheld from the patient, despite the wishes of the family.

The Cardiovascular System

3

DEVELOPMENT

I. Heart

A. The cardiovascular system is derived from the **mesoderm**.
B. Paired endocardial heart tubes form in the **cephalic region** of the embryo.
C. Lateral and cephalocaudal folding causes the heart tubes to join together and lie in a **ventral location** between the primitive mouth and the foregut.
D. The **primitive heart** dilates into five areas, as shown in Figure 3-1. The five embryologic regions and their adult derivatives are as follows:
   1. **Truncus arteriosus** → proximal aorta and proximal pulmonary artery
   2. **Bulbus cordis** → smooth parts of the right ventricle (conus arteriosus) and left ventricles
   3. **Primitive ventricle** → right and left ventricles (trabeculated parts)
   4. **Primitive atrium** → right and left atria
   5. **Sinus venosus** → smooth part of right atrium, the coronary sinus, and oblique vein
E. The lumen of the truncus arteriosus and bulbus cordis is divided into the aorta and **pulmonary trunk** by the aorticopulmonary septum.
F. The septum primum, septum secundum, and atriovenous (AV) cushion form the **atrial septum**.
G. The **foramen ovale** is a communication between the right and left atria, which is formed by the walls of the septum primum and septum secundum.
   1. It allows blood to flow from the venous side of the circulation to the arterial side without passing through the lungs as a result of **higher pressure on the venous side during gestation**.
   2. **After birth**, the foramen ovale closes because of **increased arterial pressure** that pushes the septum primum against the atrial septum.

QUICK HIT

In dextrocardia, the heart is located on the right side in the thorax. An isolated, misplaced heart is often accompanied by multiple anomalies. If all of the body's organs are transposed (situs inversus—associated with Kartagener syndrome; immotile cilia caused by a defect in the dynein arms resulting in lung disease and male sterility), the heart is often normal.

FIGURE 3-1 Embryologic development of the heart

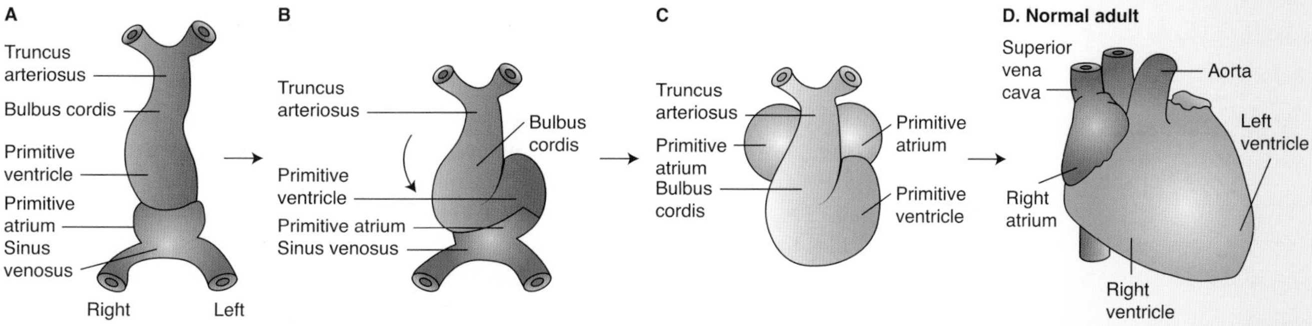
A
Truncus arteriosus
Bulbus cordis
Primitive ventricle
Primitive atrium
Sinus venosus
Right
Left
B
Truncus arteriosus
Bulbus cordis
Primitive ventricle
Primitive atrium
Sinus venosus
C
Truncus arteriosus
Primitive atrium
Bulbus cordis
Primitive atrium
Primitive ventricle
D. Normal adult
Superior vena cava
Aorta
Left ventricle
Right atrium
Right ventricle

Folding of the developing heart **(A–C)** during weeks 5–8 into the normal adult heart **(D)**

QUICK HIT

Aberrant development of the aorticopulmonary septum is responsible for tetralogy of Fallot, transposition of the great vessels, and persistent truncus arteriosus.

H. The aorticopulmonary septum (also called the spiral septum, derived from neural crest cells), the right and left bulbar ridges, and the AV cushion form the **interventricular septum**.

II. Arterial vessels

A. **Aortic arches (pharyngeal arch arteries)**: Initially, there are six paired aortic arches. Arches 3, 4, and 6 play a significant role in the adult. Arch 5 degenerates early in fetal development.
   1. **Arches 1 and 2** give rise to the maxillary artery and stapedial artery, respectively.
   2. **Arch 3** helps form the adult common carotid arteries bilaterally.
   3. **Arch 4** helps form the aorta on the left and the proximal subclavian artery on the right.
   4. **Arch 6** helps form the ductus arteriosus and part of the pulmonary trunk.

B. Paired dorsal aortae are paired vessels that run along the length of the embryo. They coalesce to form the **descending aorta**.

III. Venous vessels

A. The paired vitelline, umbilical, and cardinal veins form the definitive adult structures.

B. The **vitelline veins** help form the ductus venosus and hepatic sinusoids, the inferior vena cava, the portal vein, and the superior and inferior mesenteric veins.

C. **Umbilical veins**
   1. No adult vascular structures are formed by these veins.
   2. The left umbilical vein connects to the ductus venosus and carries oxygenated blood from the placenta to the fetus.
   3. **Left umbilical vein** gives rise to ligamentum teres hepatis.
   4. **Right umbilical vein** regresses.

D. **Cardinal veins**
   1. The **anterior cardinal veins** help form the internal jugular vein and the superior vena cava.
   2. The **posterior cardinal veins** help form the inferior vena cava, common iliac veins, azygos vein, and renal veins.

IV. Fetal circulation *(Figure 3-2)*

V. Congenital defects of the heart and great vessels *(Table 3-1)*

QUICK HIT

Conduction velocity depends on the rate of depolarization (represented by upstroke of the action potential), not on action potential duration.

PHYSIOLOGY AND PATHOLOGY OF HEART FUNCTION

Properly timed and integrated myocyte contraction is essential to normal heart function. Cardiac myocytes have gap junctions that allow for rapid relay of electrical signals between them. Electrical impulses are transmitted via the electrical conduction system composed of the sinoatrial (SA) node, atrioventricular (AV) node, and His–Purkinje cells (Figure 3-3). Normally, the SA node is the pacemaker of the heart. The node exhibits automaticity, in which spontaneous phase 4 depolarization generates rhythmic action potentials (APs). These electrical signals propagate from the SA node through the atrial tissue and cause it to contract. Further propagation leads to excitation of the AV node, the ventricular bundles, and, lastly, the ventricular tissue. The nodal tissues are dependent on Ca^{2+} for their phase 0 depolarization, whereas the cardiac muscular tissue uses Na^{+} for phase 0 depolarization. The AV node transmits APs more slowly than do the other cardiac tissues. This feature allows the atria to contract before the ventricles, with time for the ventricles to repolarize, fill with blood, and prepare to receive their next electrical signal. Furthermore, it also prevents excessively rapid beats from reaching and damaging the ventricular tissue. The conduction system of the heart can best be visualized on an

FIGURE 3-2 Fetal circulation

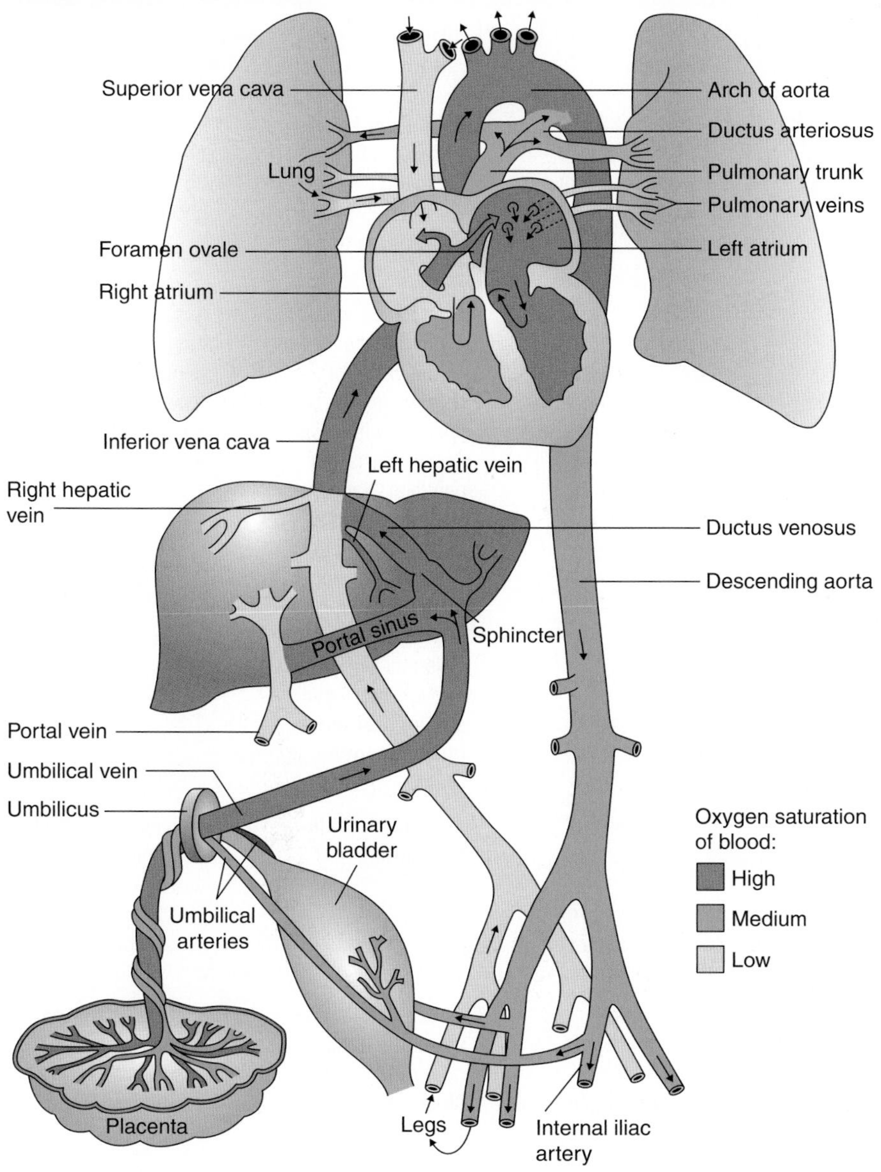
Superior vena cava
Arch of aorta
Ductus arteriosus
Lung
Pulmonary trunk
Pulmonary veins
Foramen ovale
Left atrium
Right atrium
Inferior vena cava
Left hepatic vein
Right hepatic vein
Ductus venosus
Descending aorta
Portal sinus
Sphincter
Portal vein
Umbilical vein
Umbilicus
Urinary bladder
Oxygen saturation of blood:
High
Medium
Low
Umbilical arteries
Placenta
Legs
Internal iliac artery

electrocardiogram (ECG). ECG plots can determine disturbances, such as arrhythmias, along the cardiac conduction path.

Multiple mechanisms can affect the intrinsic mechanical properties of the heart. Chronotropic effects on the heart cause a change in heart rate by affecting the rate of depolarization of the SA node. Inotropic effects cause a change in contractility of the heart. Greater contractility allows the heart to squeeze harder and increase cardiac output. Increased intracellular Ca^{2+}, either drug mediated (e.g., cardiac glycosides, diltiazem, verapamil, and nifedipine) or as a result of sympathetic β-receptor stimulation, allows for an increased inotropic effect. The preload and afterload also affect the function of the heart. Increased preload as a result of increased filling of the ventricles lengthens the myocytes, which induces stronger contraction, up to a certain point, after which the myocytes are too stretched to contract effectively. Afterload of the left ventricle is equivalent to aortic pressure. It is influenced by the total peripheral resistance. A higher afterload means the left ventricle must work harder or cardiac output will fall. The cardiovascular system is constantly working to maintain homeostatic equilibrium.

QUICK HIT

The umbilical circulation is one of the only places in the body (along with the pulmonary circulation) where an artery does not carry oxygenated blood. The paired umbilical arteries carry deoxygenated blood to the placenta, whereas the umbilical vein brings oxygenated blood back to the fetus.

QUICK HIT

The ductus arteriosus closes in the first days of life. Exposure to oxygenated blood alters the production of prostaglandins (PGs). Indomethacin (PG synthesis inhibitor) induces closure of a patent ductus arteriosus (PDA), whereas alprostadil (PGE1) therapy maintains patency.

QUICK HIT

Congenital cardiac defects with the **letter D** are initially **left-to-right shunts** (PDA, VSD, AVSD, and ASD), whereas those cardiac defects without the letter D are right-to-left shunts.

QUICK HIT

The baroreceptor reflex greatly affects total peripheral resistance. The carotid sinus baroreceptors, located at the bifurcation of the carotid arteries, sense arterial pressure. Afferent signals via cranial nerve (CN) IX induce efferent signals via CN X to influence heart rate. Increased arterial pressure causes an increase in vagal output and a reduction of heart rate and blood pressure. A decrease in arterial pressure causes a decrease in vagal output, resulting in an increase in heart rate and blood pressure.

QUICK HIT

The most common type of atrial septal defect (ASD) is a patent foramen ovale.

QUICK HIT

Eisenmenger syndrome is the change from a left-to-right shunt to a right-to-left shunt, secondary to increasing pulmonary hypertension; it usually occurs as a result of a chronic, adaptive response to preexisting left-to-right shunts, such as a VSD.

QUICK HIT

Cyanosis occurs in right-to-left shunts: tetralogy of Fallot and transposition of the great vessels (TGA). Cyanosis can lead to clubbing, hypertrophic osteoarthropathy, and polycythemia. Initial left-to-right shunts are not cyanotic: ASD, VSD, PDA, and atrioventricular septal defect (AVSD).

TABLE 3-1 Congenital Defects of the Heart and the Great Vessels

Anomaly	Pathology	Clinical Presentation	Notes
Atrial septal defect (ASD)	**Secundum ASD** (defect of septum primum or septum secundum) Primum ASD (low), sinus venosus ASD (high)	**Left-to-right shunt,** asymptomatic into the fourth decade, murmur, right ventricular hypertrophy	Much higher incidence in females (3:1); 75%–80% are secundum type
Coarctation of the aorta	Infantile (proximal to PDA); adult (constriction at closed ductus arteriosus, distal to the origin of left subclavian artery)	Symptoms depend on the extent of narrowing; infant presents with lower limb cyanosis and right heart failure at birth; adult asymptomatic with upper limb hypertension, rib notching on radiograph from collateral circulation through intercostal arteries, and **weak pulses in lower limbs**	Much higher incidence in males (3:1) and females with **Turner syndrome**
Patent ductus arteriosus (PDA)	Failure of closure of the ductus arteriosus; may be caused by premature birth with **hypoxemia** or structural defects	Continuous **machinery murmur**	Second most common congenital heart defect
Tetralogy of Fallot	Defective development of the infundibular septum; results in **overriding aorta, VSD, pulmonary stenosis, and hypertrophy of the right ventricle**	Cyanosis (may not be present at birth), right-to-left shunt, **"boot-shaped heart"**	Survival to adulthood possible; patient assumes squatting position to relieve symptoms
Transposition of the great vessels	Aorta drains right ventricle; pulmonary artery from left ventricle; **separate pulmonary and systemic circuits**	Incompatible with life unless shunt present; cyanosis (present at birth)	Mother with diabetes
Ventricular septal defect (VSD)	Membranous VSD, Single muscular VSD	Left-to-right shunt; **loud holosystolic murmur means small defect,** large defects can present as heart failure at birth; small defects can close spontaneously	Much higher incidence in males; most common congenital heart defect (33%); 90% are membranous type

FIGURE 3-3 **Heart anatomy and signal conduction**

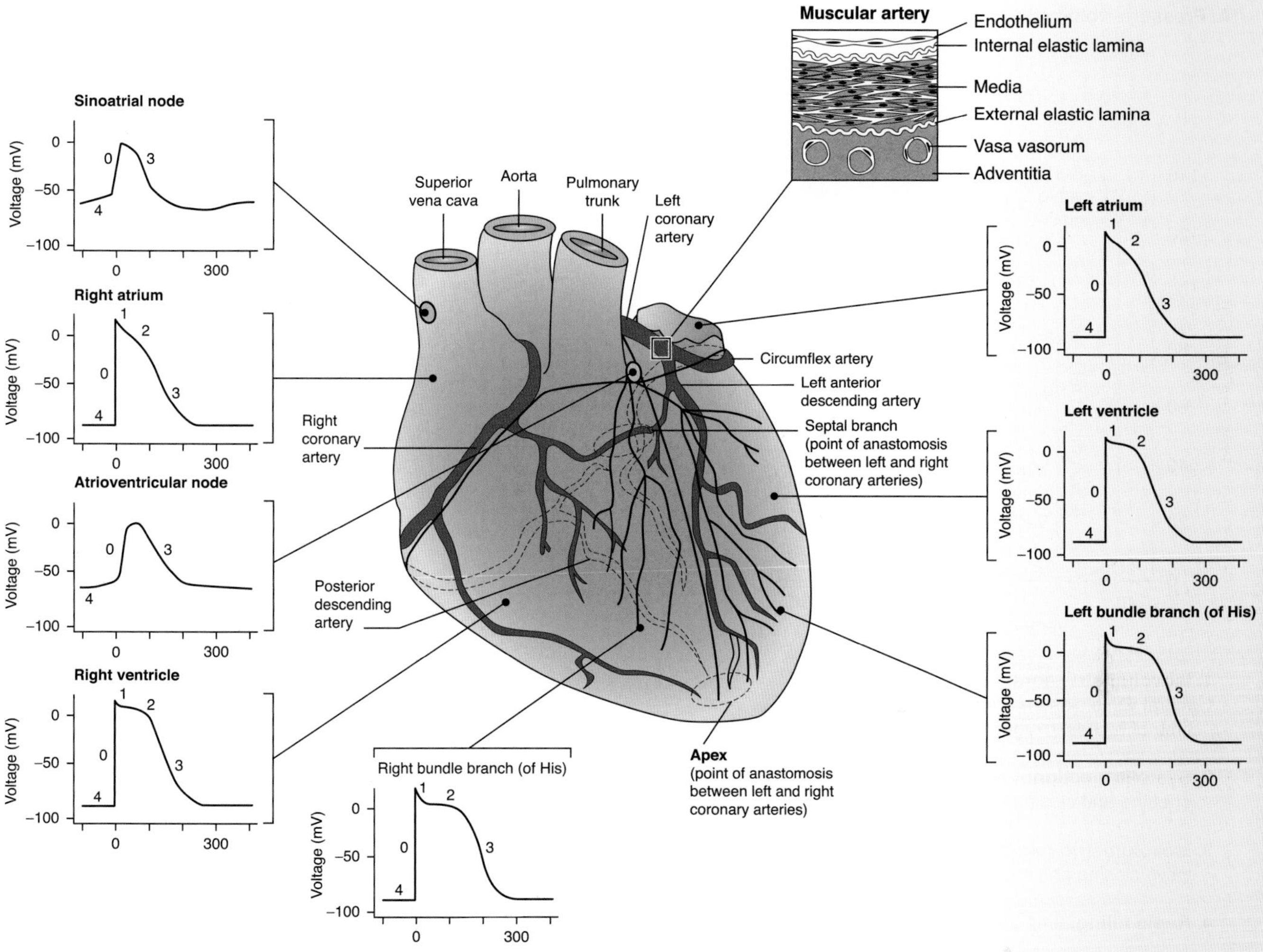
Muscular artery
Endothelium
Internal elastic lamina
Media
External elastic lamina
Vasa vasorum
Adventitia
Sinoatrial node
Right atrium
Atrioventricular node
Right ventricle
Right bundle branch (of His)
Left atrium
Left ventricle
Left bundle branch (of His)
Voltage (mV)
Superior vena cava
Aorta
Pulmonary trunk
Left coronary artery
Circumflex artery
Left anterior descending artery
Septal branch (point of anastomosis between left and right coronary arteries)
Right coronary artery
Posterior descending artery
Apex (point of anastomosis between left and right coronary arteries)

Hormonal systems also respond to changes in homeostasis. A major influence on the cardiovascular system is exerted by the renin-angiotensin-aldosterone (RAA) axis. Whereas the baroreceptors attempt to maintain adequate pressures in the vascular system over a short-term period, the RAA system helps to regulate pressure over a longer period of time. The RAA axis responds to changes in arterial pressure by altering salt and water retention by the kidneys. Low blood pressure causes an increased release of renin, which converts angiotensinogen from the liver to angiotensin I. Angiotensin I travels to the lung, where it is cleaved to angiotensin II (Ang II) by angiotensin-converting enzyme (ACE). Ang II stimulates constriction of arterioles and increases release of aldosterone (salt and water retention; see Chapter 6), both of which increase blood pressure. Atrial natriuretic peptide (ANP) also responds to blood pressure changes. An increase in blood pressure causes stretch of atrial myocytes, which then release ANP. ANP lowers blood pressure by relaxing smooth muscle, increasing salt and water excretion, and inhibiting renin release. Antidiuretic hormone (ADH), also known as arginine vasopressin (AVP), is involved in the response to changes in blood pressure. When released from the pituitary, it acts on the kidney to reduce urine output and retain water while simultaneously constricting arterioles to increase total peripheral resistance (Figure 3-4).

The physiologic function of the heart can be represented in several ways (e.g., pressure–volume loops and the cardiac cycle) (Figure 3-5). The effects of cardiac output, total peripheral resistance, contractility, preload, and afterload are represented on the Frank–Starling curve. Cardiac output is measured using the Fick principle (Figure 3-6), and normal output is approximately 5 L/min.

FIGURE 3-4 Cardiac physiology

A. Pressure–volume loop

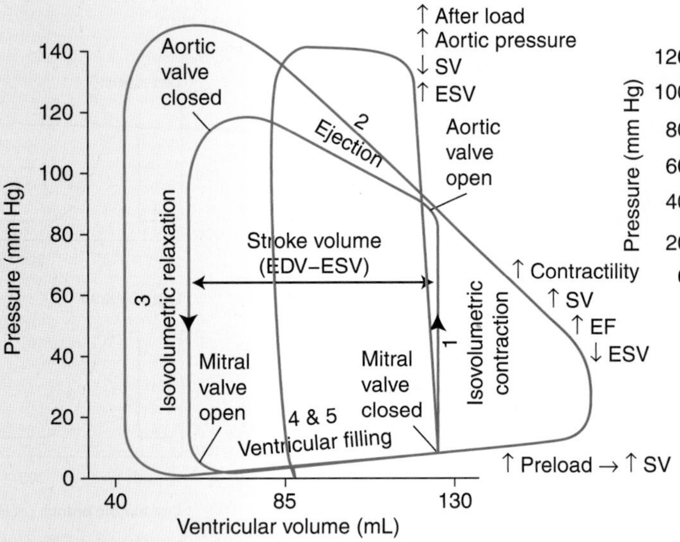

↑ After load
↑ Aortic pressure
↓ SV
↑ ESV
Aortic valve closed
2 Ejection
Aortic valve open
Stroke volume (EDV–ESV)
↑ Contractility
↑ SV
↑ EF
↓ ESV
3 Isovolumetric relaxation
1 Isovolumetric contraction
Mitral valve open
Mitral valve closed
4 & 5 Ventricular filling
↑ Preload → ↑ SV
Pressure (mm Hg)
Ventricular volume (mL)

1. **Isovolumetric contraction:** time between mitral valve closure and aortic valve opening; time of highest oxygen consumption
2. **Systolic ejection:** time between aortic valve opening and closing
3. **Isovolumetric relaxation:** time between aortic valve closing and mitral valve opening
4. **Rapid filling:** time after mitral valve opening
5. **Reduced filling:** time right before mitral valve closing

B. The cardiac cycle

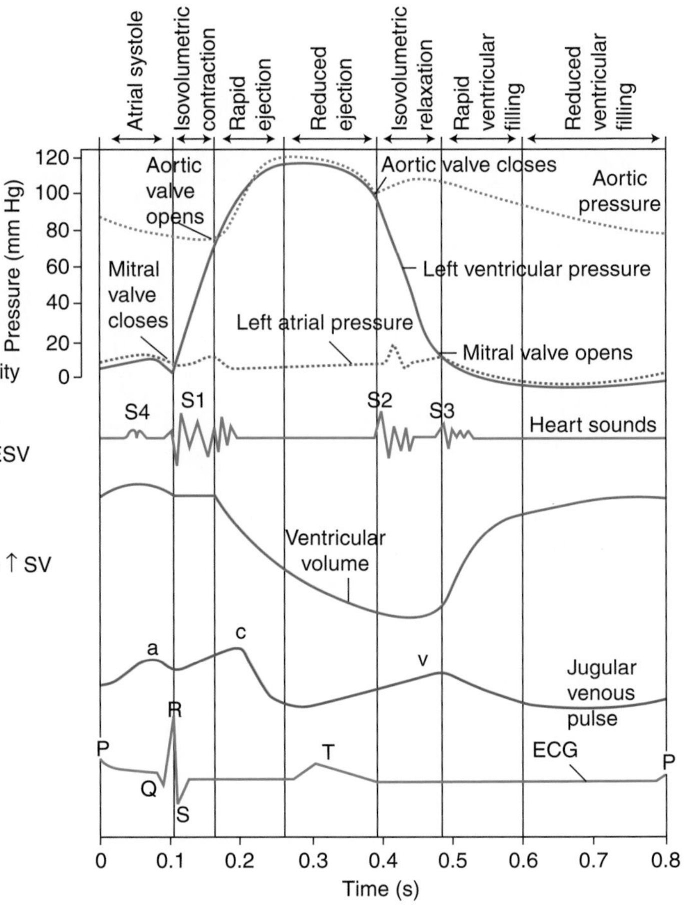

Atrial systole
Isovolumetric contraction
Rapid ejection
Reduced ejection
Isovolumetric relaxation
Rapid ventricular filling
Reduced ventricular filling
Aortic valve opens
Aortic valve closes
Aortic pressure
Left ventricular pressure
Mitral valve closes
Left atrial pressure
Mitral valve opens
Pressure (mm Hg)
S4 S1 S2 S3
Heart sounds
Ventricular volume
a c v
Jugular venous pulse
P Q R S T P
ECG
Time (s)

a wave—atrial contraction
c wave—contraction of right ventricle; peak due to tricuspid valve bulging into atrium
v wave—increased atrial pressure secondary to filling against closed tricuspid valve

C. Progression of the action potential through cardiac muscle cells

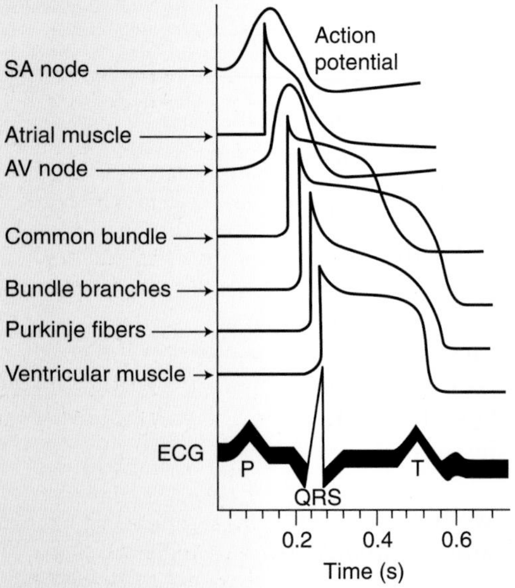

SA node
Atrial muscle
AV node
Common bundle
Bundle branches
Purkinje fibers
Ventricular muscle
ECG
Action potential
P
QRS
T
Time (s)

D. Frank–Starling relationship

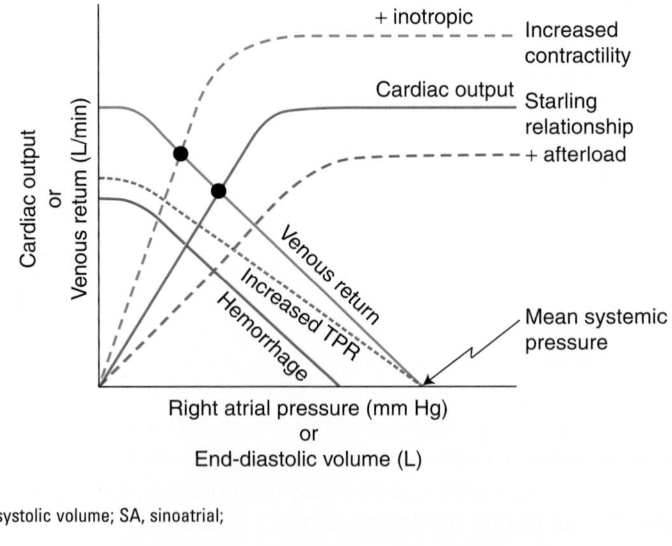

+ inotropic
Increased contractility
Cardiac output
Starling relationship
+ afterload
Venous return
Increased TPR
Hemorrhage
Mean systemic pressure
Cardiac output or Venous return (L/min)
Right atrial pressure (mm Hg) or End-diastolic volume (L)

AV, atrioventricular; ECG, electrocardiogram; EDV, end-diastolic volume; ESV, end-systolic volume; SA, sinoatrial; TPA, total peripheral resistance.

FIGURE 3-5 Physiologic cardiovascular relationships

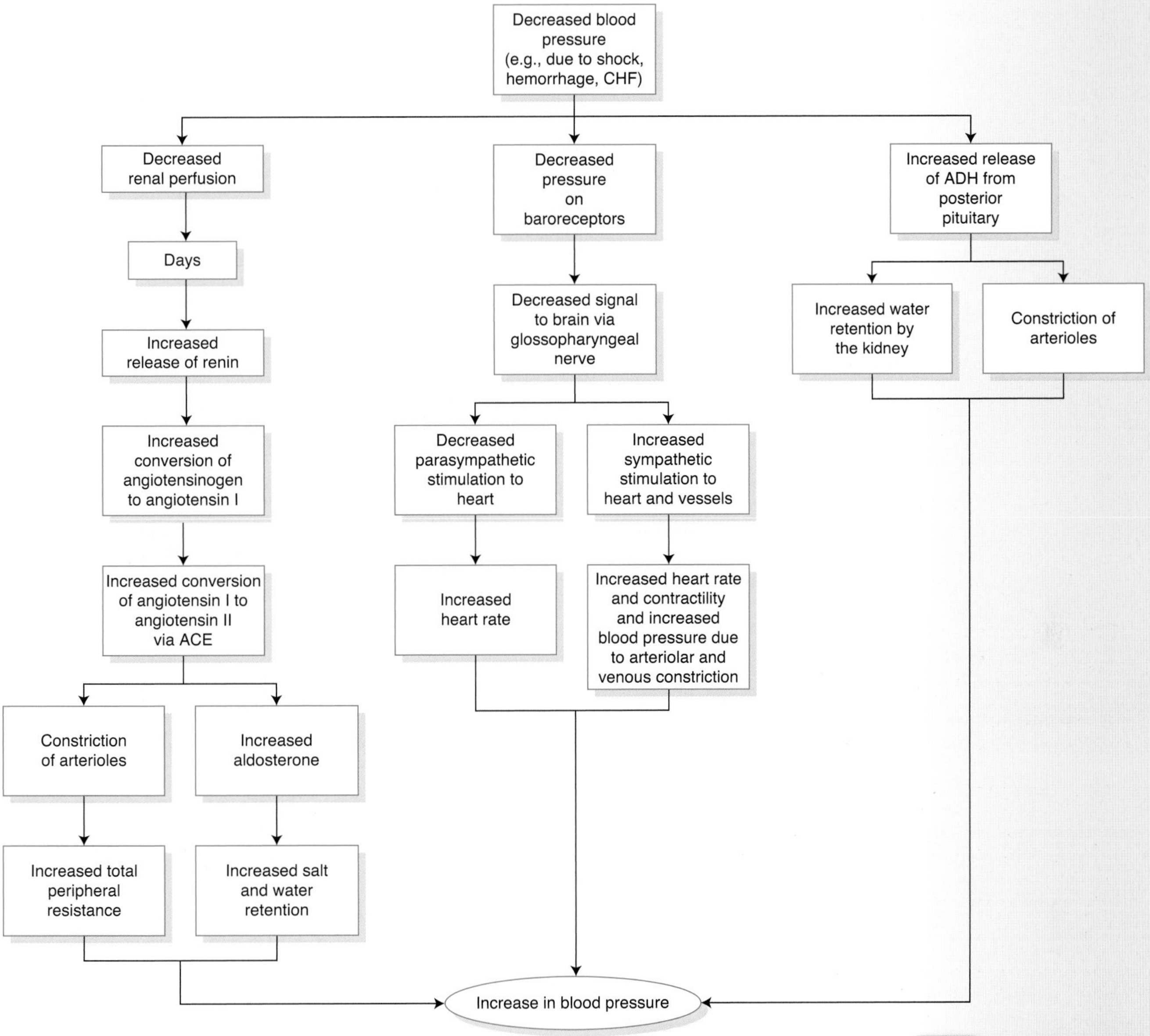
Decreased blood pressure (e.g., due to shock, hemorrhage, CHF)
Decreased renal perfusion
Days
Increased release of renin
Increased conversion of angiotensinogen to angiotensin I
Increased conversion of angiotensin I to angiotensin II via ACE
Constriction of arterioles
Increased aldosterone
Increased total peripheral resistance
Increased salt and water retention
Decreased pressure on baroreceptors
Decreased signal to brain via glossopharyngeal nerve
Decreased parasympathetic stimulation to heart
Increased sympathetic stimulation to heart and vessels
Increased heart rate
Increased heart rate and contractility and increased blood pressure due to arteriolar and venous constriction
Increased release of ADH from posterior pituitary
Increased water retention by the kidney
Constriction of arterioles
Increase in blood pressure

ACE, angiotensin-converting enzyme; ADH, antidiuretic hormone; CHF, congestive heart failure.

> **QUICK HIT**
> Chronic atrial fibrillation can lead to clots in the atrium that may embolize to the systemic circulation. Treatment is to prevent emboli with anticoagulation such as warfarin.

ARRHYTHMIAS *(Figure 3-7) (Table 3-2)*

Arrhythmias can be organized into tachycardias and bradycardias. The ECGs of important arrhythmias can be seen in Figure 3-7, and features of the heart blocks are described in Table 3-2.

> **QUICK HIT**
> Class IB agents (lidocaine, tocainide, mexiletine, and phenytoin) all have central nervous system (CNS) side effects. Long-term control using tocainide can also cause neutropenia and thrombocytopenia.

ANTIARRHYTHMICS *(Figure 3-8) (Table 3-3)*

Antiarrhythmics work to change different phases of depolarization and repolarization. They also alter the conduction velocity, change the effective refractory period (ERP), and alter the AP duration. The treatment options for arrhythmias are as follows:

I. Atrial fibrillation

A. **Rate control** (with β-blockers, diltiazem, verapamil, or digoxin) is generally preferred over rhythm control.

FIGURE 3-6 Important cardiovascular equations

$CO = \frac{O_2 \text{ consumption}}{([O_2] \text{ pulmonary vein} - [O_2] \text{ pulmonary artery})}$	**The Fick equation** is used to calculate either cardiac output (CO) or oxygen (O_2) consumption
$CO = SV \times HR$	CO = cardiac output SV = stroke volume HR = heart rate
$R \propto \frac{1}{r^4}$	This relationship shows how arteriolar diameter can effectively control systemic resistance. For instance, if the radius (r) is increased by 2, the resistance (R) drops 16-fold.
$\dot{Q} = \frac{\Delta P}{R}$	$\dot{Q}$ = flow ΔP = Aortic pressure–right atrial pressure or pressure difference R = resistance
$MBP = CO \times TPR$	MBP = mean blood pressure (equivalent to ΔP) CO = cardiac output (equivalent to $\dot{Q}$) TPR = total peripheral resistance (equivalent to R)
Series resistance: $R_{total} = R_1 + R_2 + R_3 + R_4 \ldots$	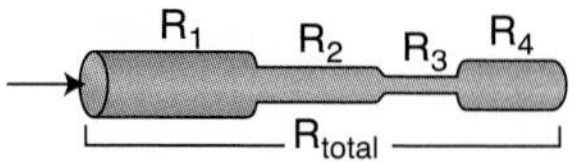R_1 R_2 R_3 R_4 R_{total}
Parallel resistance: $\frac{1}{R_{total}} = \frac{1}{R_1} + \frac{1}{R_2} + \frac{1}{R_3} + \frac{1}{R_4} \ldots$	This relationship lowers resistance when the body recruits unused parallel vessels (especially in capillary beds) 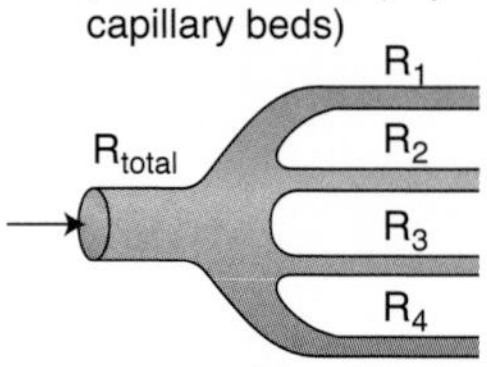R_1 R_2 R_3 R_4 R_{total}

B. Conversion to sinus rhythm (if indicated) may be achieved with electrical cardioversion or antiarrhythmic drugs (most commonly, amiodarone), although reversion to atrial fibrillation is common.

II. Supraventricular tachycardia

A. Adenosine (diagnostic purposes)
B. Verapamil (long-term control)

III. Ventricular fibrillation

A. Lidocaine or amiodarone

QUICK HIT

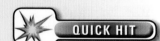

Of the antiarrhythmics, class II and class III agents decrease mortality, whereas other antiarrhythmics can be proarrhythmics, so carefully monitor a patient.

IV. Ventricular tachycardia

A. **Digoxin**

V. Digitalis toxicity

A. Activated charcoal in repeated doses (every 4 to 6 hours for 24 hours)
B. **Digoxin immune Fab** (only if one of the following is present):
  1. Hemodynamic instability
  2. Life-threatening arrhythmias or severe bradycardia (even if responsive to atropine)
  3. Plasma potassium level >5 mEq/L in an acute overdose
  4. Plasma digoxin level >10 ng/mL
  5. Ingestion of >10 mg of digoxin in adults (or >4 mg in children)
  6. Presence of a digoxin-toxic rhythm in the setting of an elevated digoxin level
C. Treat hyperkalemia only if it is causing ECG disturbances and avoid calcium, which can worsen intracellular hyperkalemia in these particular patients.
D. Atropine, if bradycardia is present

QUICK HIT

Class II agents (β-blockers) work at nodal tissue, so use these to control ventricular rate affected by atrial fibrillation, atrial flutter, and excess catecholamines.

VI. Torsades de pointes

A. Intravenous (IV) Mg^{2+}

FIGURE **3-7** **ECGs of important arrhythmias**

Normal ECG

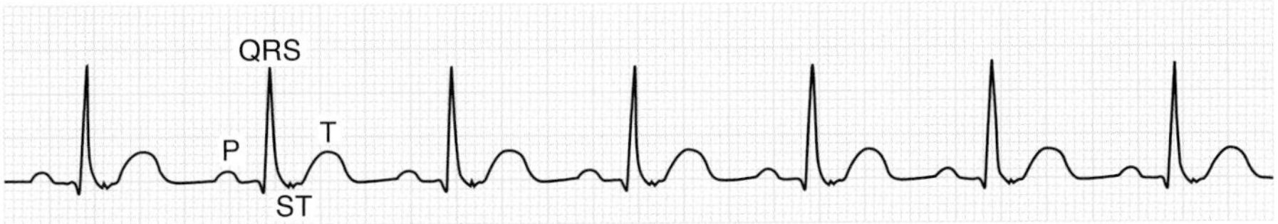
QRS
P
T
ST

- P wave is atrial depolarization (atrial repolarization usually occurs during the QRS and remains unseen in ECG).
- PR interval (0.12–0.2 s) measures time between atrial and ventricular depolarization.
- QRS interval (normally less than 0.1 s) reflects the duration of ventricular depolarization.
- T wave is ventricular repolarization.

Sustained ventricular tachycardia

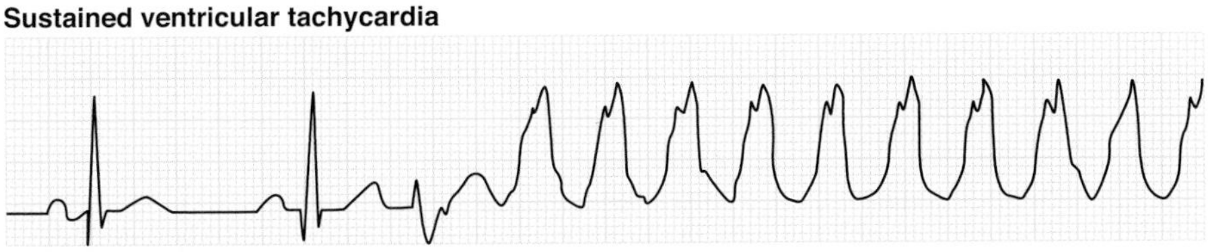

- Constant QRS morphology and fairly regular cycle length
- Initiating beat morphology may differ from ongoing VT
- AV dissociation a hallmark but not always present, nor easy to identify when present

Ventricular fibrillation

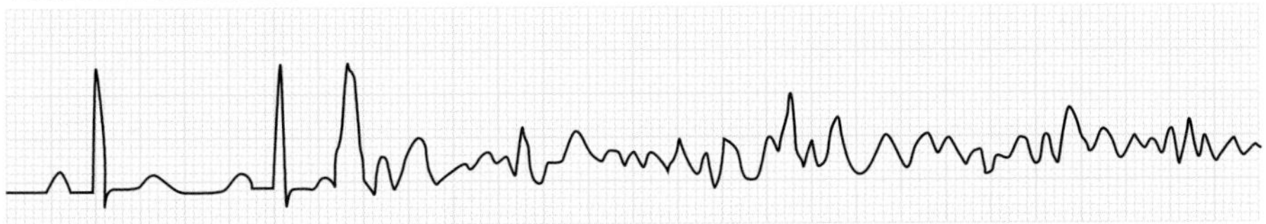

- Undulating baseline, no organized electrical activity
- Incompatible with life
- Atria may be dissociated, still in sinus rhythm

Atrial flutter

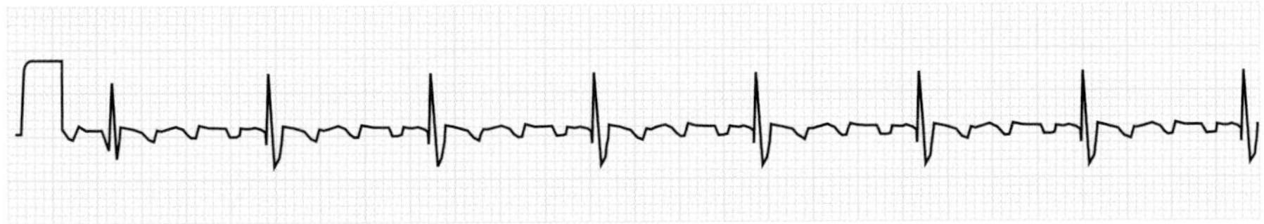

- A regular, saw-toothed pattern of atrial activity, usually very near 300/min
- Discrete, organized atrial activity on intracardiac electrograms
- Usually even-numbered AV conduction ratio (2:1, 4:1)

Atrial fibrillation

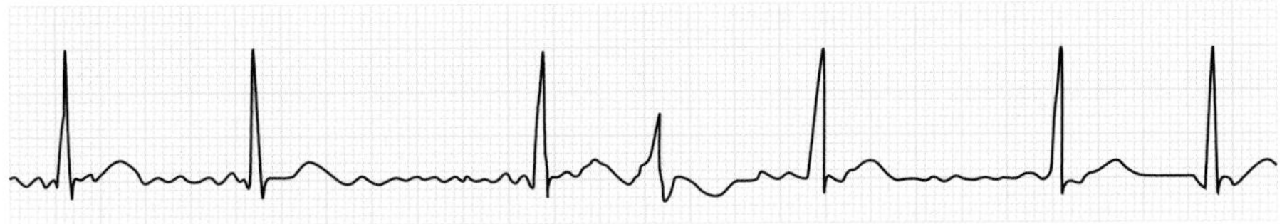

- Undulating, low amplitude atrial activity on ECG
- Intracardiac electrogram shows chaotic rapid spikes
- Variable conduction pattern as AV node is constantly bombarded with impulses; "long-short" sequences yield wide QRS complexes (aberrant, "Ashman" beats)

Wolff–Parkinson–White syndrome

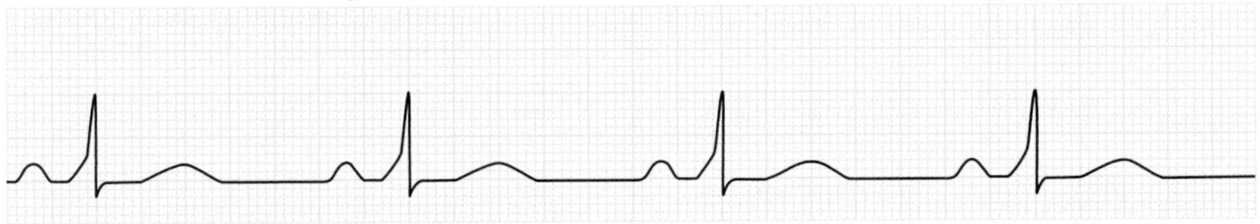

- Accessory atrioventricular conductions
- Anterograde or retrograde conduction
- Tachyarrhythmias
- Blurred QRS (referred to as δ-wave)

AV, atrioventricular; ECG, electrocardiogram; VT, ventricular tachycardia.

QUICK HIT

Torsades de pointes (twisting of the points): ventricular tachycardia often caused by antiarrhythmic drugs, especially quinidine. It is characterized by a long QT interval and a "short-long-short" sequence before the inception of tachycardia. The ECG shows a series of upward-pointing QRS complexes followed by a series of downward-pointing complexes.

QUICK HIT

Diltiazem can be used to control the ventricular response rate in atrial fibrillation because it slows AV nodal conduction.

QUICK HIT

Down syndrome is associated with endocardial cushion defects, which may manifest as ASD or VSD.

QUICK HIT

Paradoxical emboli are emboli that originate in the venous circulation and pass through a patent foramen ovale or ASD to produce symptoms on the arterial side.

QUICK HIT

Myocardial infarctions (MIs) can cause both second-degree and third-degree heart block.

TABLE 3-2 Conduction Anomalies

Anomaly	Pathology	Notes	ECG
First-degree heart block	Atrioventricular nodal anomaly **lengthens PR interval** (greater than 0.2 seconds)	May be caused by drugs (e.g., β-blockers, digitalis, and calcium channel blockers)	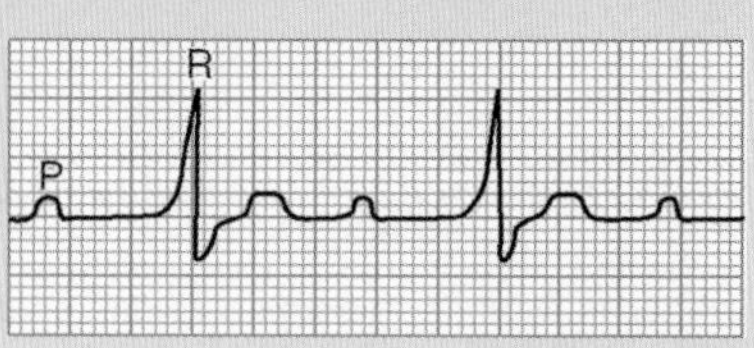 R P
Second-degree heart block: Mobitz type 1 (Wenckebach)	Defect in atrioventricular node; progressively **increasing PR interval until QRS wave is lost**	Relatively common; usually **does not require treatment**	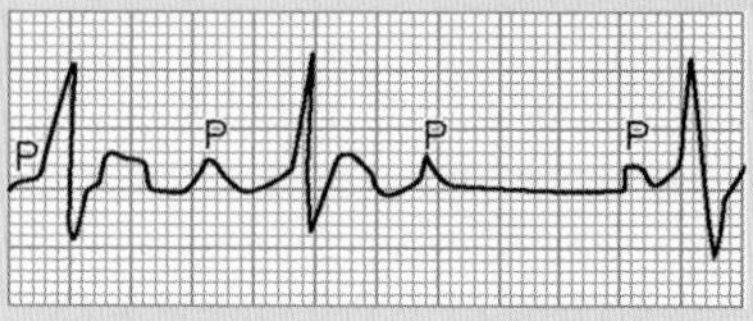 P P P P
Second-degree heart block: Mobitz type 2	**Defect in His–Purkinje system;** constant PR interval with random dropped QRS complexes	Less common and more dangerous than Mobitz type 1; **pacemaker**	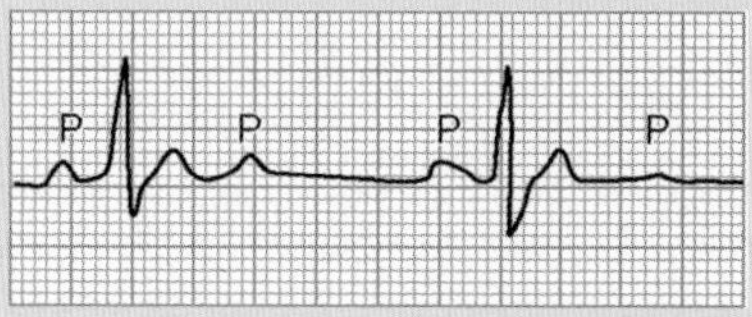 P P P P
Third-degree heart block	No electrical connection between atria and ventricles; **atria and ventricles contract independently**	His–Purkinje system sets the rate of ventricular contraction; pacemaker may be necessary	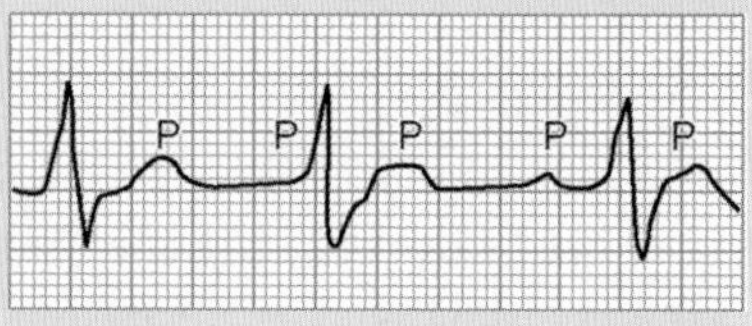 P P P P P

FIGURE 3-8 Antiarrhythmic drugs

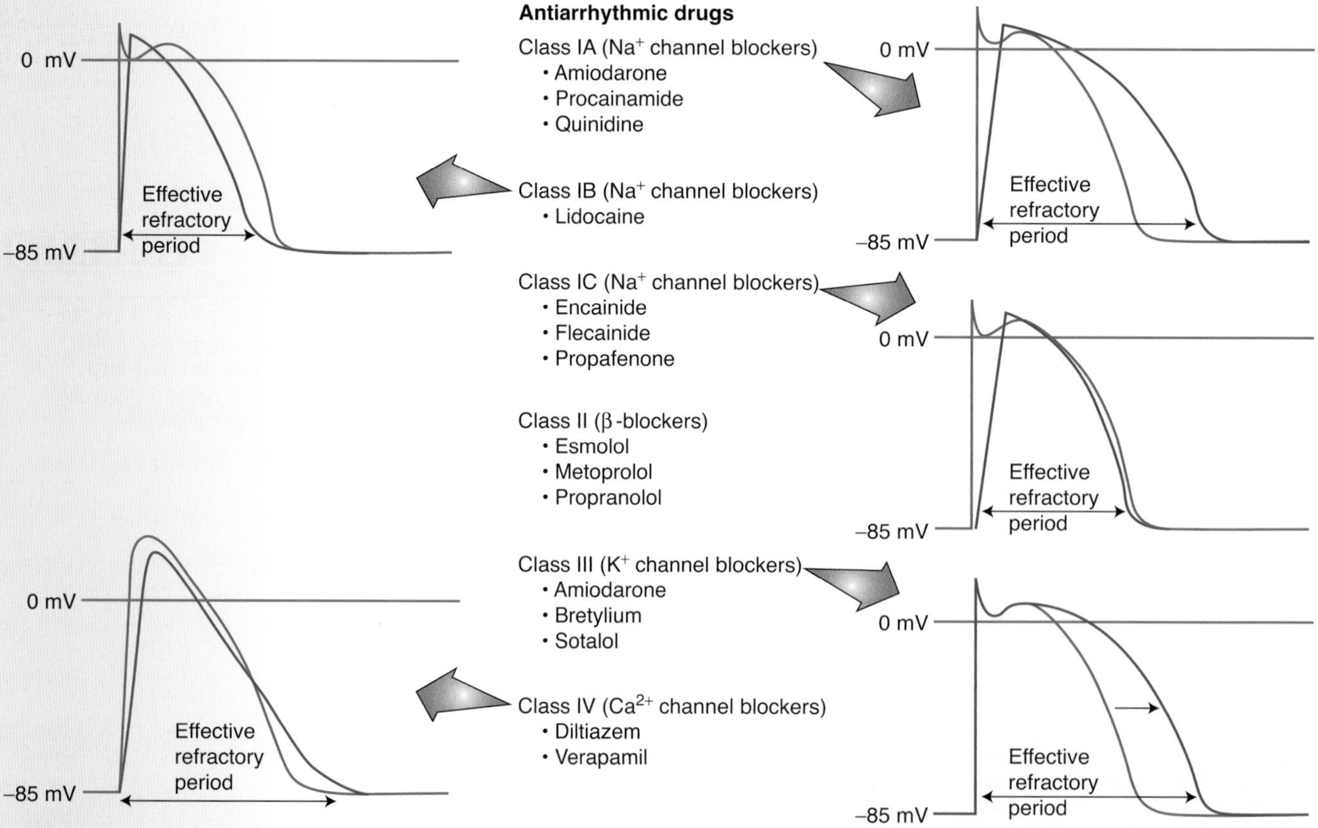
Antiarrhythmic drugs
Class IA (Na+ channel blockers)
• Amiodarone
• Procainamide
• Quinidine
Class IB (Na+ channel blockers)
• Lidocaine
Class IC (Na+ channel blockers)
• Encainide
• Flecainide
• Propafenone
Class II (β-blockers)
• Esmolol
• Metoprolol
• Propranolol
Class III (K+ channel blockers)
• Amiodarone
• Bretylium
• Sotalol
Class IV (Ca2+ channel blockers)
• Diltiazem
• Verapamil
0 mV
–85 mV
Effective refractory period

Class IA (slows phase 0, prolongs phase 3); class IB (shortens phase 3); class IC (markedly slows phase 0); class II (suppresses phase 4 depolarization rate); class III (prolongs phase 3); class IV (slows the action potential).

The Cardiovascular System

TABLE 3-3 **Antiarrhythmics**

Therapeutic Agent (common name, if relevant) [trade name, where appropriate]	Class–Pharmacology and Pharmacokinetics	Indications	Side Effects or Adverse Effects	Contraindications or Precautions to Consider; Notes
Digoxin	**Inotropic agent—cardiac glycoside; inhibits Na/K/ATPase → indirect inhibition of Na^+/Ca^{2+} exchanger → increases Ca^{2+} → increases cardiac contractility**	**Severe left ventricular systolic dysfunction** (increases contractility), **atrial fibrillation** (decreases conduction at AV node and depresses SA node)	**Progressive dysrhythmia,** anorexia, nausea, vomiting, headache, fatigue, **confusion, blurred vision, altered color perception, halos around dark objects**	Contraindicated in patients with right-sided heart failure and diastolic failure; **ECG changes: increases PR, decreases QT, depresses ST, and inverts T; toxicities of digoxin are increased by renal failure** (decreases excretion), **hypokalemia** (potentiates the drug's effects), and **quinidine** (decreases clearance and displaces digoxin)
Sodium channel blockers (Class I)				
Quinidine, procainamide, disopyramide	**Class IA—sodium channel blocker; increases AP duration, ERP, QT interval**	**Atrial and ventricular arrhythmia** (especially reentrant and ectopic supraventricular and ventricular tachycardia)	**Torsades de pointes;** reversible lupus-like syndrome (procainamide); **Cinchonism—**headache, tinnitus, thrombocytopenia (quinidine)	Hyperkalemia increases toxicity
Lidocaine, mexiletine, tocainide	**Class IB—sodium channel blocker; decreases AP duration**	**Acute ventricular arrhythmias** (especially post-MI), digitalis-induced arrhythmia; **local anesthesia**	**CNS stimulation and depression, cardiovacular depression**	**Hyperkalemia increases toxicity**
Flecainide, propafenone	**Class IC—sodium channel blocker; no effect on AP duration**	**Ventricular tachycardia progressing to ventricular fibrillation, intractable supraventricular tachycardia,** last resort in ventricular arrhythmias	**Proarrhythmic (especially post-MI), prolongs refractory period in AV node**	**Hyperkalemia increases toxicity**

(continued)

QUICK HIT

Drugs that are used to treat arrhythmias may also cause them, especially when their use is stopped suddenly. This is an important consideration for digoxin, class IA (quinidine, disopyramide, and procainamide), class IC (propafenone, flecainide, and encainide), and class II (propranolol) drugs.

TABLE 3-3 **Antiarrhythmics** *(Continued)*

Therapeutic Agent (common name, if relevant) [trade name, where appropriate]	Class–Pharmacology and Pharmacokinetics	Indications	Side Effects or Adverse Effects	Contraindications or Precautions to Consider; Notes
β-blockers (Class II)				
Propranolol, esmolol, metoprolol, atenolol, timolol	β-blocker—decreases cAMP and calcium currents → increases PR interval, suppresses abnormal pacemakers, especially in AV node	**Ventricular tachycardia, supraventricular tachycardia,** slowing the ventricular rate during **atrial fibrillation and atrial flutter**	**Impotence, exacerbation of asthma, bradycardia,** AV block, CHF, sedation, sleep alteration, dyslipidemia (metoprolol)	Esmolol (very short acting)
Potassium channel blocker (Class III)				
Sotalol, ibutilide, bretylium, amiodarone	**Potassium channel blocker—increases AP duration, ERP, and QT interval**	**Wolff–Parkinson–White syndrome; used when other antiarrythmics fail**	**Torsades de pointes,** excessive beta block, and hypotension; amiodarone-**pulmonary fibrosis,** corneal deposits, **hepatotoxicity,** skin deposits, photodermatitis, neurologic effects, constipation, bradycardia, CHF, heart block, and **hypothyroidism/hyperthyroidism**	
Calcium channel blockers (Class IV)				
Verapamil, diltiazem	**Calcium channel blocker—decreases conduction velocity of AV nodal cells, increases ERP, PR interval**	**Prevent nodal arrhythmias (supraventricular tachycardia)**	Constipation, **flushing, edema,** CHF, AV block, sinus node depression, torsades de pointes	
Other				
Adenosine	**Increases potassium efflux → hyperpolarizes the cell**	**Diagnosis and treatment of AV nodal-arrhythmias**	**Flushing, hypotension, and chest pain**	Very short acting
Potassium	**Depresses ectopic pacemaker in hypokalemia**	**Digoxin toxicity**		

AP, action potential; ATPase, adenosine triphosphatase; AV, atrioventricular; cAMP, cyclic adenosine monophosphate; CHF, congestive heart failure; CNS, central nervous system; ECG, electrocardiogram; ERP, effective refractory period; MI, myocardial infarction; SA, sinoatrial.

ATHEROSCLEROSIS

I. Atherosclerosis is a disease of large and medium-sized vessels, characterized by the formation of atheromas (i.e., lesions that have a central lipid-rich core surrounded by fibrous tissue) deposited in the intima of arteries. It is the leading cause of mortality in the United States.

II. Risk factors

A. Major risk factors
1. Dyslipidemia: high blood cholesterol, high low-density lipoproteins (LDLs), high triglycerides, and decreased high-density lipoproteins (HDLs; <45 mg/dL) (Table 3-4)
2. Diabetes mellitus
3. Cigarette smoking
4. Hypertension
5. Obesity

B. Minor risk factors
1. Lack of physical activity
2. Male sex
3. Increased age
4. Family history
5. Oral contraceptives, decreased estrogens, or premature menopause
6. Type A personality
7. Elevated homocysteine level

III. Pathogenesis

A. Atheroma formation
1. Monocytes adhere to vessel walls, enter tissue, and become macrophages.
2. Macrophages are transformed into foam cells after engulfing oxidized LDLs.
3. Foam cells accumulate in the intima.
4. Foam cells release factors that cause the aggregation of platelets, the release of fibroblast growth factor, and the accumulation of smooth muscle.
5. After formation of plaque, calcification occurs.
6. The central core of the plaque consists mainly of cholesterol.

B. Complications
1. Plaque rupture
2. Ischemic heart disease or MI
3. Stroke
4. Renal arterial ischemia
5. Death

QUICK HIT

Although amiodarone has class I, II, III, and IV activity, it has a number of side effects: pulmonary fibrosis, photodermatitis, thyroid changes (mostly hypothyroid), CNS effects (rare), and decreased liver function (rare).

QUICK HIT

Adenosine terminates reentry pathways, so it is the drug of choice for acute paroxysmal supraventricular tachycardia (PSVT). It can also help diagnose whether ventricular tachycardia was induced supraventricularly or ventricularly.

QUICK HIT

Frequency of fibrous plaques: abdominal aorta > proximal coronary artery > popliteal artery > descending thoracic aorta > internal carotid artery > renal artery.

FAMILIAL DYSLIPIDEMIAS *(Table 3-4)*

TABLE 3-4 **Selected Familial Dyslipidemia**

Familial Dyslipidemias	Elevated	Blood Lipid Levels	Pathology (see Chapter 5)	Clinical Picture	Treatment
Hypercholesterolemia IIa	LDL	↑ Cholesterol	**Decreased LDL receptors**	Greatly increased vascular and heart disease; **xanthomas**	Cholestyramine/colestipol, lovastatin (and niacin for homozygotes)

(continued)

QUICK HIT

Type IIb and type IV are the two most common dyslipidemias.

QUICK HIT

HDL works to remove cholesterol from tissues and plaques, thereby exerting a protective effect. HDL is increased by exercise.

TABLE 3-4 **Selected Familial Dyslipidemia** *(Continued)*

Familial Dyslipidemias	Elevated	Blood Lipid Levels	Pathology (see Chapter 5)	Clinical Picture	Treatment
Dysbetalipoproteinemia III	VLDL	↑ TG, ↑ Cholesterol	Altered apolipoprotein E	Increased vascular and heart disease; xanthomas	Niacin and clofibrate or lovastatin
Hypertriglyceridemia IV	VLDL	↑↑ TG, normal to ↑ cholesterol	Hepatic overproduction (with possible decreased clearance) of VLDL	Increased vascular and heart disease; obese, **diabetic, pregnant,** and **alcoholic** patients	Weight loss, low-fat diet, niacin and clofibrate or lovastatin (if necessary)

LDL, low-density lipoproteins; TG, triglycerides; VLDL, very low-density lipoproteins.

LIPID-LOWERING AGENTS *(Table 3-5)*

TABLE 3-5 **Lipid-Lowering Agents**

Therapeutic Agent (common name, if relevant) [trade name, where appropriate]	Class–Pharmacology and Pharmacokinetics	Indications	Side Effects or Adverse Effects	Contraindications or Precautions to Consider; Notes
Lovastatin, pravastatin, simvastatin, atorvastatin	**HMG-CoA reductase inhibitors**—inhibits the synthesis of cholesterol precursor mevalonate; **decreases LDL, increases HDL, and decreases TG**	**High LDL, preventative after thrombotic event (e.g., MI, stroke)**	Reversible increase in LFTs, myositis	
Niacin	**Inhibits lipolysis** in fat tissue, **reduces** hepatic **VLDL secretion** into circulation; decreases **LDL, increases HDL, and decreases TG**	**Increased LDL, decreased HDL**	Flushing (decreased by aspirin or long-term use)	
Cholestyramine, colestipol	**Bile acid resin/cholesterol absorption blocker**—binds bile acids → prevents intestinal reabsorption of bile acid and therefore cholesterol; **decreases LDL and increases HDL**	**Increased LDL**	**Tastes like sand, GI irritation,** and decreased absorption of fat-soluble vitamins	
Ezetimibe	**Cholesterol absorption blocker**—prevents cholesterol reabsorption at brush border in the small intestine; **decreases LDL; no effect on HDL or TG**	**Increased LDL**	Increased LFT (rarely)	No proven clinical benefit; may increase plaque thickness
Gemfibrozil, clofibrate, bezafibrate, fenofibrate	**Upregulates lipoprotein lipase (periphery) → increases TG clearance; decreases LDL, increases HDL, and decreases TG**	**Increased TG, increased LDL**	Myositis, increased LFTs	Reduces TG more than other agents

GI, gastrointestinal; HDL, high-density lipoprotein; HMG-CoA, 3-hydroxy-3-methylglutaryl-coenzyme A; LDL, low-density lipoprotein; LFT, liver function test; MI, myocardial infarction; TG, triglyceride; VLDL, very low-density lipoprotein.

HYPERTENSION

I. Essential

A. Most common type (95% of cases)
B. Unknown etiology
C. Risk factors
  1. Family history
  2. Race (more common in Blacks)
  3. Obesity
  4. Cigarette smoking
  5. Physical inactivity
D. Characteristics
  1. Blood pressure greater than 140/90 mm Hg on three separate occasions, with the patient comfortably sitting and arm at the level of the patient's heart.
E. Chronic complications
  1. Hypertrophy of left ventricle
  2. Onion skinning of vessel walls
  3. Retinal hemorrhages
F. Essential hypertension predisposes to ischemic heart disease (see next section).

II. Secondary hypertension refers to elevated systemic arterial pressure associated with a condition known to cause hypertension

A. Renal diseases are the most common cause of secondary hypertension.
  1. Renal parenchymal disorders (chronic kidney disease)
  2. Unilateral renal artery stenosis
    a. Atherosclerosis (more common in Black males and older individuals)
    b. Fibromuscular dysplasia (more common in White females and younger individuals)
  3. Renin–angiotensin axis activated
B. Endocrine causes
  1. Primary aldosteronism
  2. Pheochromocytoma
  3. Hyperthyroidism
  4. Acromegaly
  5. Cushing syndrome
C. Coarctation of the aorta

III. Malignant hypertension

A. **Hypertensive urgency** is blood pressure ≥180/120 mm Hg without symptoms and without evidence of end-organ damage.
B. **Hypertensive emergency** (malignant hypertension) is blood pressure ≥180/120 mm Hg with evidence of end-organ damage.
  1. Cardiovascular—vascular damage, aortic dissection
  2. Pulmonary—pulmonary edema
  3. Renal—"flea-bitten kidneys," azotemia
  4. Ocular—fundal hemorrhages, papilledema
  5. Central nervous system—encephalopathy, seizures, coma
C. This type of hypertension causes early death because of cerebrovascular accident (CVA).
D. Young Black males are the usual victims of this type of hypertension.

ANTIHYPERTENSIVE AGENTS *(Table 3-6)*

I. α-Blockers

A. α-Adrenergic receptors are the primary controllers of vascular tone, blockers are used primarily to lower blood pressure.
  1. α_1-Selective agents commonly used in the treatment of hypertension include prazosin, doxazosin, and terazosin.

QUICK HIT

Hypertrophy of the left ventricle is also caused by left-sided valvular disease such as aortic stenosis and mitral regurgitation.

QUICK HIT

Fibromuscular dysplasia of the renal artery causes a "beads-on-a-string" sign on radiograph.

QUICK HIT

Treatment for malignant hypertensive emergency (systolic blood pressure greater than 220 mm Hg or diastolic pressure greater than 120 mm Hg) commonly includes IV sodium nitroprusside or IV enalapril. It is dangerous to give pure β-blockers because of unopposed α stimulation. Therefore, an α/β-blocker such as labetalol can be given.

QUICK HIT

β-Blockers mask many of the symptoms of hypoglycemia (tremors, sweating, palpitations, etc.) that are mediated by epinephrine. This, as well as the endocrine effects, puts individuals with insulin-dependent diabetes taking β-blockers at increased risk for profound hypoglycemia.

TABLE 3-6 Antihypertensive Agents

Therapeutic Agent (common name, if relevant) [trade name, where appropriate]	Class—Pharmacology and Pharmacokinetics	Indications	Side Effects or Adverse Effects	Contraindications or Precautions to Consider; Notes
Diuretics				
Hydrochlorothiazide	Thiazide diuretic—inhibits transport of Na^+ and Cl^- into the cells of DCT	**Hypertension, CHF,** idiopathic hypercalciuria, nephrogenic diabetes insipidus	**Hypokalemia, metabolic alkalosis, mild hyperlipidemia, hyperuricemia,** malaise, **hypercalcemia,** hyperglycemia, hyponatremia	Do not give in patients with sulfa drug allergy
Furosemide	Loop diuretic—prevents cotransport of Na^+, K^+, and Cl^- in **thick ascending limb**	**Hypertension, CHF,** cirrhosis, nephrotic syndrome, **pulmonary edema,** and hypercalcemia	**Potassium wasting, metabolic alkalosis,** hypotension, dehydration, **ototoxicity,** nephritis, and gout	Do not give in patients with **sulfa drug allergy**
RAA system				
Captopril, enalapril, fosinopril, lisinopril, quinapril	ACE inhibitor → inhibits conversion of angiotensin (Ang) I to II → decreases Ang II levels → prevents vasoconstriction from Ang II	**Hypertension, CHF, post-MI agent, prevention/treatment of diabetic nephropathy**	**Cough, angioedema, hyperkalemia,** renal insufficiency (especially in bilateral renal artery stenosis)	Contraindicated in pregnancy (fetal renal malformation)
Losartan, valsartan, irbesartan, olmesartan, candesartan	ARBs → prevents vasoconstriction from Ang II	**Hypertension**	Fetal renal toxicity, **hyperkalemia**	
Sympathoplegics				
Metoprolol, atenolol, acebutolol, esmolol, propranolol, timolol, carvedilol, labetalol	β_1-Blocker (metoprolol, atenolol, acebutolol, esmolol), β_1- and β_2-blocker (propanolol, timolol), carvedilol, and labetalol (α- and β-blocker)	**Hypertension, angina, MI, antiarrhythmic**	**Bronchospasm, bradycardia,** AV block, heart failure, sedation, and sleep alterations	
Prazosin, terazosin, doxazosin	**α_1-Blocker** → vasodilation → decreases total peripheral resistance	**Pheochromocytoma, hypertension, benign prostatic hyperplasia**	**Orthostatic hypotension,** dizziness, and headache	First-dose orthostatic hypotension
Clonidine	Centrally acting sympathetic agent (α_2-agonist) → decreases sympathetic outflow from CNS → decreases peripheral resistance	**Hypertension**, heroin, and cocaine withdrawal	Drowsiness, **dry mouth, and rebound hypertension after abrupt withdrawal**	
Methyldopa	Centrally acting sympathetic agent (α-agonist) → decreases sympathetic outflow from CNS	**Hypertension** (most commonly used in pregnancy)	Sedation and hemolytic anemia	**Positive Coombs test**
Hexamethonium	Nicotinic ganglionic blocker	Hypertensive emergency	Severe orthostatic hypotension, blurred vision, constipation, and sexual dysfunction	
Reserpine	Prevents the storage of monoamines in synaptic vesicle	Hypertension	**Mental depression**, sedation, nasal stuffiness, and diarrhea	

(continued)

TABLE 3-6 **Antihypertensive Agents** *(Continued)*

Therapeutic Agent (common name, if relevant) [trade name, where appropriate]	Class—Pharmacology and Pharmacokinetics	Indications	Side Effects or Adverse Effects	Contraindications or Precautions to Consider; Notes
Guanethidine	Interferes with norepinephrine release	**Severe hypertension**	Orthostatic hypotension, exercise hypotension, impotence, and diarrhea	**Contraindicated in patients taking TCAs**
Vasodilators				
Hydralazine	Increases cGMP → smooth muscle relaxation → vasodilates arterioles → afterload reduction	**Severe hypertension, CHF**	**Compensatory tachycardia**, fluid retention, and **lupus-like syndrome**	**First-line therapy for hypertension in pregnancy**, used with methyldopa; contraindicated in angina/CAD because of compensatory tachycardia
Minoxidil	**K^+ channel opener** → hyperpolarizes and relaxes vascular smooth muscle	**Severe hypertension**	**Hypertrichosis** and pericardial effusion	
Nifedipine, felodipine, amlodipine	**Dihydropyridine Ca^{2+} channel blockers** block voltage-gated Ca^{2+} channels of **vascular** smooth muscle	**Hypertension, angina pectoris, Prinzmetal angina, Raynaud phenomenon**	Peripheral edema, **flushing, dizziness**, and constipation	
Diltiazem, verapamil	**Non-dihydropyridine Ca^{2+} channel blockers**—block voltage-gated Ca^{2+} channels of **cardiac** smooth muscle	**Hypertension, angina pectoris, arrhythmia**	Cardiac depression, peripheral edema, **flushing, dizziness**, and constipation	
Nitroprusside	Direct release of NO → increases cGMP → vasodilator (arterial dilation)	**Hypertensive emergency, CHF, and angina**	Cyanide toxicity, hypotension	Short acting
Diazoxide	**K^+ channel opener**—hyperpolarizes and relaxes vascular smooth muscle	**Hypertension**	Hypoglycemia (reduces insulin release) and hypotension	

ACE, angiotension-converting enzyme; ARB, angiotensin II receptor blocker; AV, atrioventricular; CAD, coronary artery disease; cGMP, cyclic guanosine monophosphate; CHF, congestive heart failure; CNS, central nervous system; DCT, distal convoluted tubule; MI, myocardial infarction; NO, nitric oxide; RAA, renin-angiotensin-aldosterone; TCA, tricyclic antidepressant.

2. They have little impact on the heart, but they do have selective effects that allow them to have other clinical uses (such as treatment for benign prostatic hypertrophy).

B. Side effects
1. Postural hypotension with reflex tachycardia (most common)
2. Nasal congestion and headache
3. Rebound hypertension if stopped abruptly

C. Phenoxybenzamine and phentolamine are nonselective α-blockers that can be used in the diagnosis and treatment of the symptoms of pheochromocytoma.

II. β-Blockers

A. β-Blockers can be divided into four subgroups:
1. Nonselective β-blockers (β_1 and β_2): propranolol, timolol, and nadolol
2. β_1-Selective agents: metoprolol, atenolol, acebutolol, and esmolol

3. β_2-Selective agents (discussed in Chapter 4)
4. α/β-Blockers (carvedilol, labetalol)

B. This important class of drugs has many clinical uses:
1. Cardiac uses (most common)
   a. Hypertension
   b. Stable angina
   c. Prophylaxis after an MI
2. Less common uses
   a. Symptomatic treatment of hyperthyroidism
   b. Prophylaxis against migraine headaches
   c. Anxiety disorder

C. Therapeutic effects of β-blockers on various organ systems are listed in Table 3-7.

D. Adverse effects
1. Sexual dysfunction in males
2. Arrhythmias if the drug is stopped abruptly
3. Bronchoconstriction
4. Blocking hypoglycemic response in a diabetic

III. Calcium channel blockers

A. Second-line antihypertensive agents

B. Act by binding to the L-type calcium channel of vascular smooth muscle cells and myocytes

C. Block the entry of calcium into these cells

D. These agents affect both vascular tone and the heart itself. Effects on the heart include negative inotropy and slowing of the conduction system.

E. Calcium channel blockers are often divided into two groups:
1. Dihydropyridines
   a. Examples: nifedipine and amlodipine
   b. Greater effect on vascular smooth muscle than on the heart
2. Non-dihydropyridines
   a. Examples: diltiazem and verapamil
   b. Increasingly greater effects on the myocardium

F. Adverse effects include hypotension, headache, constipation, peripheral edema, and exacerbation of gastroesophageal reflux and bradycardia.

IV. Other antihypertensive agents

A. Clonidine
1. Along with α-methyldopa, a centrally acting antihypertensive agent
2. This agent acts as an agonist at presynaptic α_2 receptors, thereby decreasing central sympathetic tone.

TABLE 3-7 Therapeutic Effects of β-blockers

Organ System	Effect	Clinical Implication
Cardiac (β_1)	Negative inotropic and chronotropic effects; slowing of SA and atrioventricular nodes	Decreases cardiac output; bradycardia can limit dosing; atrioventricular nodal slowing is useful in supraventricular tachycardia
Pulmonary (β_2)	Constriction of airway smooth muscle	β-Blockers are contraindicated in patients with chronic obstructive pulmonary disease
Endocrine	Decreased glycogenolysis, decreased glucagon release	β-Blockers must be used with caution in patients with diabetes taking insulin who are at risk for hypoglycemia
Ocular	Decreased aqueous humor production by processes of ciliary body	β-Blockers, such as timolol, can be used topically for glaucoma

Note: Those effects known to be predominantly caused by either β_1- or β_2-blockers are listed as such. SA, sinoatrial.

3. Adverse effects include sedation and rebound hypertension if the drug is stopped abruptly.

B. Sodium nitroprusside
1. Given intravenously, this agent is the drug of choice for hypertensive emergencies.
2. Given orally, this drug is toxic because it results in cyanide production.
3. It affects both arterial and venous smooth muscle.

C. Vasodilators (hydralazine, minoxidil)
1. Dilate both arteries and veins (predominantly arteries), lowering blood pressure
   a. Reflex tachycardia that results can actually precipitate attacks of angina.
   b. These agents are not first-line agents for hypertension.
   c. These are often used along with β-blockers and diuretics.
2. Adverse reactions to hydralazine include headache, arrhythmias, and a lupus-like reaction.
3. Adverse effects of minoxidil include sodium retention and hypertrichosis.

QUICK HIT

Berry aneurysms are commonly associated with adult polycystic kidney disease, an autosomal dominant disease; the gene is located on chromosome 16.

ANEURYSMS *(Table 3-8)*

TABLE 3-8 **Aneurysms**

Type of Aneurysm	Etiology	Characteristics
Arteriovenous fistula	Abnormal communication between arteries and veins; usually secondary to **trauma**	Ischemic changes, aneurysm formation, **high-output cardiac failure**
Atherosclerotic	**Atherosclerotic** disease, coronary artery disease	Usually in the **abdominal** aorta; located between renal arteries and iliac bifurcation
Berry	Congenital medial weakness at the bifurcations of the cerebral arteries	Saccular lesions in cerebral vessels (especially at the **circle of Willis**), hemorrhage into the **subarachnoid** space
Dissecting	**Hypertension,** cystic medial necrosis, **Marfan syndrome**	**Tearing pain;** longitudinal separation of tunica media of aortic wall
Syphilitic	Tertiary syphilis, obliteration of the vasa vasorum, necrosis of the media	Involves **ascending** aorta and aortic root; aortic valve insufficiency
Mycotic (infectious)	Inflammation secondary to bacterial infection; usually salmonella	Involves abdominal aorta

I. Abdominal aortic aneurysm (AAA)

A. Focal dilation of the aorta, generally thought to be due to atherosclerosis

B. The most common location is the infrarenal aorta. Therefore, an AAA may be palpated superior to the umbilicus because the aorta bifurcates at the level of the umbilicus.

C. Presentation
1. Usually asymptomatic until late in the course. May cause some abdominal pain.
2. The most common diagnosis mistaken for AAA in the emergency setting is kidney stones.
3. The most dangerous complication is rupture, which presents as a triad of **hypotension, abdominal pain, and pulsatile mass** in the abdomen. Hypertension increases the risk of rupture of an AAA.

D. All men aged 65 to 75 years with any history of smoking should be screened for AAA with a one-time abdominal sonogram.

E. Treatment is surgical repair for any of the following:
1. Aneurysm diameter ≥5.5 cm
2. Diameter increasing ≥0.5 cm in a 6-month interval
3. Any symptomatic AAA

Clinical Vignette 3-1

CLINICAL PRESENTATION: A 59-year-old male presents to the emergency room with **sudden, severe, and constant low back pain.** Past medical history is significant for **hypertension, hyperlipidemia, emphysema,** coronary artery disease, stable angina, and a 25-pack-year history of **smoking.** The patient was hospitalized for a cerebrovascular accident 7 years ago. Physical examination revealed a 5.8 cm **pulsatile mass** superior to the umbilicus in the abdomen. Temperature = 98.5°F; **blood pressure = 150/90 mm Hg;** heart rate = 80 bpm; and respiration rate = 23 breaths/min.

DIFFERENTIALS: Abdominal aortic aneurysm (AAA), aortic dissection, pyelonephritis/nephrolithiasis, prostatitis, and pancreatitis. Given that this pain developed suddenly and the presence of an abdominal pulsatile mass, this patient most likely has an AAA.

LABORATORY STUDIES: Proper follow-up for this patient would include an **abdominal ultrasound** and/or **computerized tomography (CT) scan with contrast.** The typical diameter for abdominal aorta is **2 cm**; therefore, any size greater than this indicates presence of an aneurysm. Advantages of an ultrasound are that it is quick, easy, and inexpensive; however, it is very operator dependent, less useful in obese individuals, and does not provide information about the iliac arteries, which could also be aneurysmal. **CT angiogram** can also be helpful in describing the anatomy of the aorta prior to surgery, but it is not commonly done in clinical practice. All patients with AAA should also undergo cardiac evaluation because patients with AAA often have underlying vascular pathology. In these patients, **cardiac catheterization** should also be performed to assess cardiac risk and potentially revascularize the patients prior to operation.

MANAGEMENT: As an aneurysm becomes larger than 5.5 cm, the risk of rupture increases exponentially; an aneurysm smaller than 5.5 cm in diameter is less likely to rupture, and risk-to-benefit ratio of surgery is less supportive. Therefore, if an AAA is **smaller than 5.5 cm** in diameter and asymptomatic, the patient can be followed with ultrasound or CT surveillance every 6 months. If the aneurysm is **larger than 5.5 cm** in diameter and symptomatic, the patient should be taken to the operating room. A patient with a ruptured AAA is taken to the operating room.

> **QUICK HIT**
>
> Syphilis is a sexually transmitted disease caused by *Treponema pallidum* (a spirochete) that is characterized initially (primary stage) by a painless, hard chancre. Untreated syphilis progresses to secondary and tertiary stages, which are characterized by rashes, lymphadenopathy, condylomata lata, Argyll Robertson pupils (pupils constrict with accommodation but not with light), and aortic root aneurysms.

II. Thoracic aortic dissection

A. A tear in the intima of the aorta, with blood forcing its way into the media and forming a false lumen

B. The most common risk factor is **hypertension**. Other risk factors can include trauma, syphilis aortitis, Marfan syndrome, and Ehlers–Danlos syndrome.

C. Most commonly found in the thoracic aorta
   1. Stanford A dissection involves any part of the ascending aorta and is treated surgically.
   2. Stanford B dissection is confined to the descending aorta (distal to the left subclavian artery).

D. Presentation
   1. Acute, "tearing" chest pain, radiating through to the back
   2. Widened mediastinum on chest x-ray.
   3. Dissections that involve other vessels may cause MI, stroke symptoms or syncope, or decreased peripheral pulses.

E. Management
   1. First, stabilize the blood pressure with β-blockers (labetalol) or nitroprusside.
   2. Surgical repair for Stanford A dissections or Stanford B dissections with rupture or other complications

> **QUICK HIT**
>
> Exercise tolerance testing (stress testing) is a good way to diagnose subacute coronary occlusion. Thallium-201 scans reveal perfusion defects. Technetium (^{99m}Tc) scans are useful for imaging MIs.

> **QUICK HIT**
>
> Risk factors for coronary artery disease: smoking; diabetes; ↑ LDL, ↓ HDL; family history; men or postmenopausal women; sedentary lifestyle; hypertension; ↑ age; ↑ homocysteine; obesity.

ISCHEMIC HEART DISEASE

I. It is defined as an inadequate supply of oxygen relative to demand.

II. Ischemic heart disease is most often caused by atherosclerosis.

III. There are four types of ischemic heart diseases.

A. Angina pectoris

1. Paroxysmal attacks of retrosternal pain, heaviness, and pressure-like or squeezing chest pain occur and may radiate to the neck, jaw, left shoulder, or arm. Angina pectoris is often associated with diaphoresis and nausea.
2. Imbalance between cardiac perfusion and cardiac demand is characteristic. Ninety percent occlusion of coronary vessel produces symptoms.
3. Three types of angina pectoris:
   a. **Stable angina**
      - Most common form
      - Induced by exercise
      - Relieved by rest
      - Results from chronic stenosis of coronary arteries

   b. **Prinzmetal (variant) angina**
      - Episodic pain occurs at rest.
      - Attacks are unrelated to activity, blood pressure, or heart rate but are related to coronary artery vasospasm.
      - Significant artery stenosis is often present.

   c. **Unstable angina**
      - This type occurs at both rest and activity.
      - It is usually preceded by decreasing physical activity or gradual increase in stable anginal symptoms.
      - It produces pain of increasing duration.
      - It is induced by ruptured atherosclerotic plaque with subsequent platelet-mediated thrombosis, which partially occludes the vessel. This results in ischemia and angina, but there is no myocardial necrosis.
4. Treatment of stable angina
   a. Nitrates
      - These drugs are converted within the cell to nitric oxide, a smooth muscle relaxant.
        (1) The relaxation of vascular smooth muscle causes widespread venous dilation.
        (2) This lowers preload and therefore reduces the workload and oxygen demand of the heart.
        (3) To a lesser extent, the relaxation of coronary arteries provides ischemic myocardium with increased oxygen.
      - Sublingual nitroglycerin is the treatment of choice for acute episodes of angina.
      - A long-acting nitrate such as isosorbide dinitrate can be used for angina prophylaxis.
      - Unwanted side effects of nitrate therapy include headache and tachyphylaxis, postural hypotension, and facial flushing.

   b. Calcium channel
   c. β-Blockers

B. **MI**

1. Lack of adequate perfusion to cardiac tissue leads to myocyte death in affected area.
2. MI is most often caused by atherosclerosis with plaque rupture and thrombus.
3. The subendocardium is most vulnerable to ischemia (because of decreased blood flow during systole) and thus most likely to infarct.
4. In a transmural infarct (see below), the full thickness of the ventricular wall is affected within 35 hours.
5. Two types of MI are possible:
   a. Non-ST elevation MI (NSTEMI)
      - Formerly called "nontransmural" or "non–Q-wave" infarct
      - As in unstable angina, atherosclerotic plaques rupture.
      - Platelet-mediated thrombosis completely occludes the vessel, resulting in loss of perfusion to inner one-third of muscular wall of ventricle occurs. Clot lysis limits the depth of infarction.

QUICK HIT

Angina pectoris causes ST depression on ECGs, but this is only observed during the attack, which lasts 2 to 5 min.

QUICK HIT

Anticoagulants (heparin, low-molecular-weight heparin, and aspirin), nitrates, and β-blockers can be used to treat unstable angina. Do *not* use calcium channel blockers or tissue plasminogen activator to treat unstable angina.

QUICK HIT

Cocaine use can also result in coronary vasospasm resulting in myocardial ischemia. In general, cocaine works by inhibiting the reuptake of endogenous catecholamines (dopamine, norepinephrine, epinephrine, and serotonin). Conversely, amphetamines stimulate the release of endogenous catecholamines.

QUICK HIT

The left anterior descending artery is the most common artery involved in acute MI. Infarcts of this artery affect the left ventricle near its apex or the anterior portion of the interventricular septum.

MNEMONIC

When remembering the sequence of histopathologic changes after an MI, think of the 1-3-1-3 rule: 1 day (**neutrophils** predominate), 3 days (**macrophages** infiltrate), 1 week (**fibroblasts** infiltrate), and 3 weeks (**granulation** tissue most prominent).

FIGURE 3-9 **Myocardial infarction enzyme release and timeline of histologic changes**

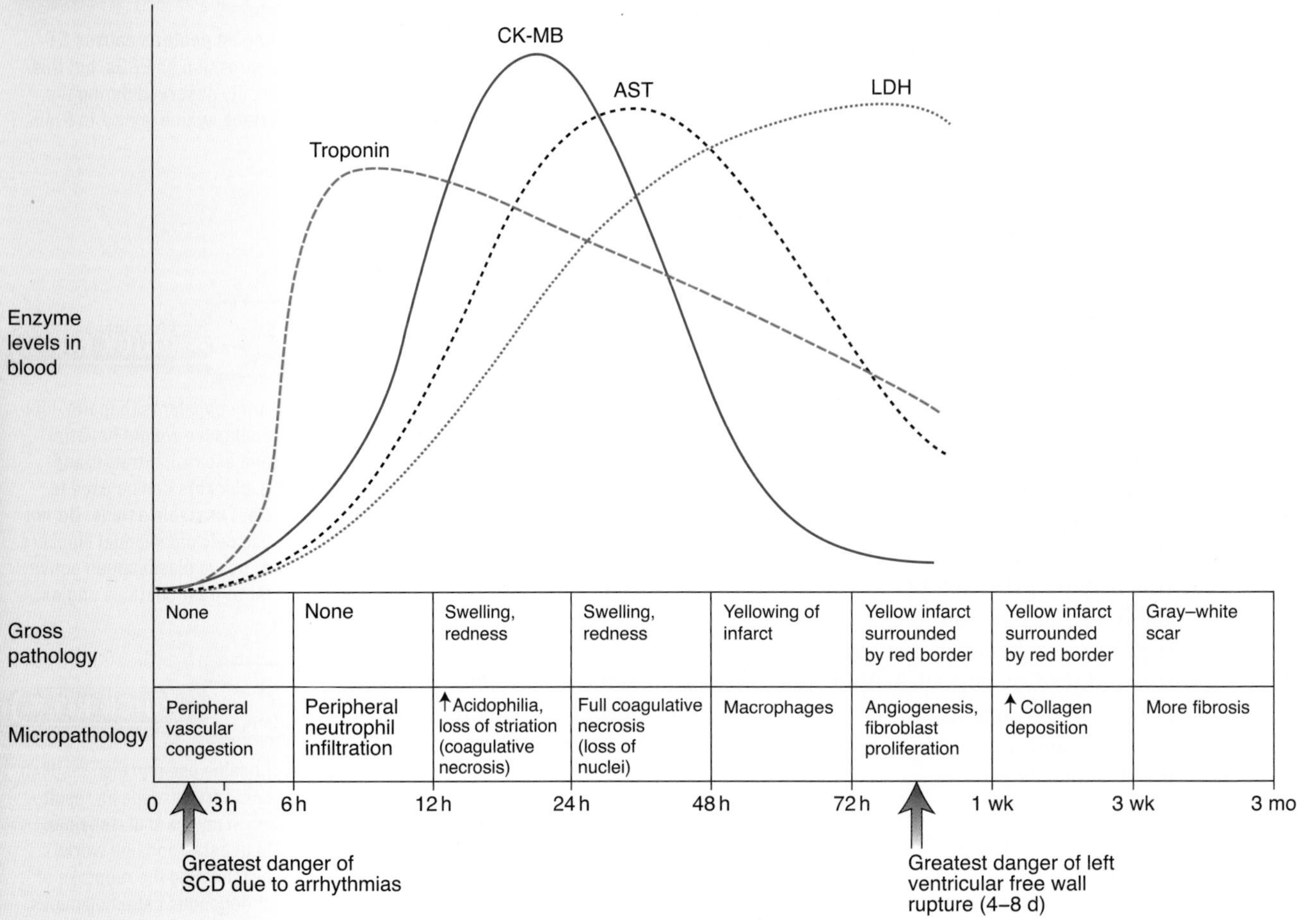
CK-MB
AST
LDH
Troponin
Enzyme levels in blood
Gross pathology
Micropathology
None
None
Swelling, redness
Swelling, redness
Yellowing of infarct
Yellow infarct surrounded by red border
Yellow infarct surrounded by red border
Gray–white scar
Peripheral vascular congestion
Peripheral neutrophil infiltration
↑Acidophilia, loss of striation (coagulative necrosis)
Full coagulative necrosis (loss of nuclei)
Macrophages
Angiogenesis, fibroblast proliferation
↑Collagen deposition
More fibrosis
0
3 h
6 h
12 h
24 h
48 h
72 h
1 wk
3 wk
3 mo
Greatest danger of SCD due to arrhythmias
Greatest danger of left ventricular free wall rupture (4–8 d)

CK-MB, creatine kinase-MB; AST, aspartate transaminase; LDH, lactate dehydrogenase; SCD, sudden cardiac death.

- Tissue infarction and myocardial necrosis lead to release of cardiac enzymes (Figure 3-9).
- ST-segment depression (but no ST elevation) is seen on ECG. Q waves do not develop.

b. ST elevation MI (STEMI)
- Formerly called "transmural" or "Q-wave" infarct
- As in NSTEMI, atherosclerotic plaques rupture, and platelet-mediated thrombosis completely occludes the vessel. There is no clot lysis, so the infarction extends to the entire muscular wall.
- Tissue infarction and myocardial necrosis lead to release of cardiac enzymes (Figure 3-9).
- ST-segment elevation is seen on ECG, and Q waves eventually develop.

6. Complications
   a. Arrhythmia—especially **ventricular fibrillation** (the primary cause of death in the first hour post-MI) heart block
   b. Papillary muscle rupture—presents as acute mitral regurgitation 2 to 7 days post-MI
   c. Myocardial rupture—rare, occurs most commonly 2 to 7 days post-MI
   d. **Dressler syndrome**—pericardial inflammation occurring **2 to 6 weeks post-MI**; presents with fever, malaise, pleuritic chest pain, pericardial friction rub, and elevated erythrocyte sedimentation rate (ESR)
   e. Ventricular aneurysm—usually due to anterior wall MI

QUICK HIT

Because of state-dependent block, lidocaine works on slightly depolarized or ischemic tissue more so than normal tissue. Therefore, use lidocaine (IV) to suppress acute MI-associated ventricular arrhythmias.

MNEMONIC

For the acute management of an MI, think **MONA B** (**m**orphine, **o**xygen, **n**itrates, **a**spirin, and **β**-blockers).

Clinical Vignette 3-2

CLINICAL PRESENTATION: A 45-year-old male was brought to the emergency department complaining of **crushing chest pain of 1-hour duration,** which he described as "a belt closed **tightly** around my chest." He indicated the location of the pain with a closed fist in the substernal region. The morning of admission, the patient was feeling ill and then experienced pain in the chest, which **radiated to his jaw, left shoulder, and down the left arm.** The pain was associated with **nausea;** the patient denied conditions that improved or worsened the pain. The patient's past medical history was significant for **hyperlipidemia** and **hypertension.** The patient stated that **his father recently underwent coronary artery bypass.** Past social history was significant for a 35-pack-year history of **smoking** and social drinking. On physical examination, the patient was found to be in acute distress and diaphoretic. Temperature = 97.6° F; blood pressure = 145/90 mm Hg; **heart rate = 101 bpm; and respiration rate =** 23 breaths/min.

DIFFERENTIALS: Acute myocardial infarction (MI), angina pectoris, aortic dissection, gastroesophageal reflux disease (GERD), pancreatitis and biliary tract disease, pericarditis, and pulmonary embolism (PE). Given the patient's description of pain and family history of coronary artery disease, he most likely has suffered from an acute MI.

LABORATORY STUDIES: An acute MI would be diagnosed via (a) **blood chemistry** showing elevated cardiac enzymes or (b) **ECG** showing ST elevation if transmural or ST depression if subendocardial. With these changes, aortic dissection, GERD, and PE can be ruled out. In an aortic dissection, we would expect a widened mediastinum on **chest radiograph,** confirmed by **CT scan;** also, an **aortogram** showing a double lumen would be diagnostic. Stable angina can be ruled out because it typically lasts a few minutes, and although it can precede an MI, this pain is characteristically **relieved by rest or nitroglycerin.** Other laboratory studies that would be done in this patient include **amylase, lipase, alkaline phosphatase** (elevated in pancreatitis), and **echocardiography** (to rule out pericarditis). Interestingly, pericarditis presents with chest pain that radiates to the trapezoid region, worsens with inspiration, and is relieved by sitting up/leaning forward.

MANAGEMENT: Revascularization, if done early, is beneficial via **thrombolytics** or **angioplasty.** Patients should also receive **morphine** (reduces pain and is a vasodilator), **heparin** (to prevent formation of thrombus), and **nitrates.** This patient should be started and maintained on **aspirin** (shown to decrease mortality), **α-blockers** (prevent remodeling), **ACE inhibitors** (prevent remodeling), and **statins** (lower cholesterol and decrease risk of future coronary events).

f. Mural thrombus with possible embolization
g. Progressive ischemic cardiomyopathy and congestive heart failure

7. Remodeling and scar formation occur over a period of 36 months after an infarct (Figure 3-9).

C. Chronic ischemic heart disease (CIHD)
1. Congestive heart failure (CHF) that results from ischemic cardiac damage leads to CIHD.
2. Hypertrophy of the heart and cardiac decompensation occur as a result of infarction.
3. CIHD is most often found in the elderly.

D. Sudden cardiac death
1. This is unexpected death from cardiac failure occurring within 2-hour post-MI.
2. This is caused less commonly by a congenital anomaly.
3. Marked atherosclerosis is usually present.
4. The mechanism of death is almost always because of arrhythmia.

QUICK HIT

Cor pulmonale is right-sided heart failure secondary to lung disorders that lead to pulmonary arterial hypertension.

QUICK HIT

Idiopathic dilated cardiomyopathy is the most common form of cardiomyopathy. Treatment includes digitalis, ACE inhibitors, heart transplant, and sometimes chronic anticoagulation.

CONGESTIVE HEART FAILURE *(Table 3-9 and Figures 3-9 to 3-11)*

CHF is a clinical diagnosis in which the heart is unable to pump an adequate amount of blood to meet the metabolic needs of the body. A number of factors play a role in CHF, including hormonal changes (RAA and sympathetic activation), peripheral vasoconstriction, and myocardial dysfunction. One of the final common pathways in CHF is

TABLE 3-9 **Congestive Heart Failure**

	Etiology	Clinical Manifestations
Left-sided congestive heart failure (CHF)	Ischemia (coronary artery disease) Systemic hypertension Left-sided valvular disease Myocarditis Cardiomyopathy Congenital heart disease Pericardial disease	**Pulmonary edema** Dyspnea on exertion/fatigue **Orthopnea** Paroxysmal nocturnal dyspnea Hyperventilation Reduction in renal perfusion (activates renin-angiotensin-aldosterone axis) **S3**
Right-sided CHF	Left-sided heart failure Left-sided lesions **Cor pulmonale** Myocarditis Cardiomyopathy Right-sided valvular disease	Hepatomegaly/ascites **(nutmeg liver)** Splenomegaly **Peripheral edema** (especially pitting edema of the ankles) **Distention of neck veins** Renal hypoxia

hypoperfusion of the kidneys and activation of the RAA axis, which leads to sodium and water retention. Treatment is directed at either blocking the RAA axis or increasing the cardiac performance and, therefore, renal perfusion. Therapeutic agents in CHF treatment include ACE inhibitors, angiotensin II receptor blockers (ARBs), digitalis, diuretics, and dobutamine.

I. ACE inhibitors

A. First-line treatment for CHF
B. ACE inhibitors are able to lower blood pressure (lower afterload), improve cardiac performance, and prevent the aldosterone-mediated salt and water retention typical of CHF.
C. Specific agents:
   1. Enalapril decreases mortality in CHF.
   2. Other ACE inhibitors include captopril and lisinopril.
D. Adverse effects of ACE inhibitors:
   1. Reversible renal failure
   2. Angioedema, hyperkalemia, dry cough, and orthostatic hypotension
   3. ACE inhibitors are fetotoxic and contraindicated in pregnancy.

II. ARBs

A. These agents block the RAA axis at the Ang II receptor, producing the same benefits as ACE inhibitors.
B. Examples of ARBs are losartan and valsartan.
C. These drugs have all the same effects as the ACE inhibitors except that, unlike the ACE inhibitors, they do not increase levels of bradykinin and hence do not cause cough as a side effect.

III. Digitalis

A. Treats CHF by increasing cardiac performance; digitalis treats CHF by increasing the intracellular concentration of calcium in cardiac myocytes, thus increasing contractility.
B. Blocks sodium–potassium pump:
   1. This increases the intracellular sodium concentration.
   2. Activity of a sodium–calcium antiporter is decreased.
   3. Decreased activity of this antiporter raises intracellular calcium levels.
C. Digitalis improves the symptoms of CHF, but unlike ACE inhibitors, it has not been shown to decrease mortality.
D. Digitalis also has a low therapeutic index, which means that the toxic dose is closer to the therapeutic dose.

FIGURE 3-10 **Congestive heart failure**

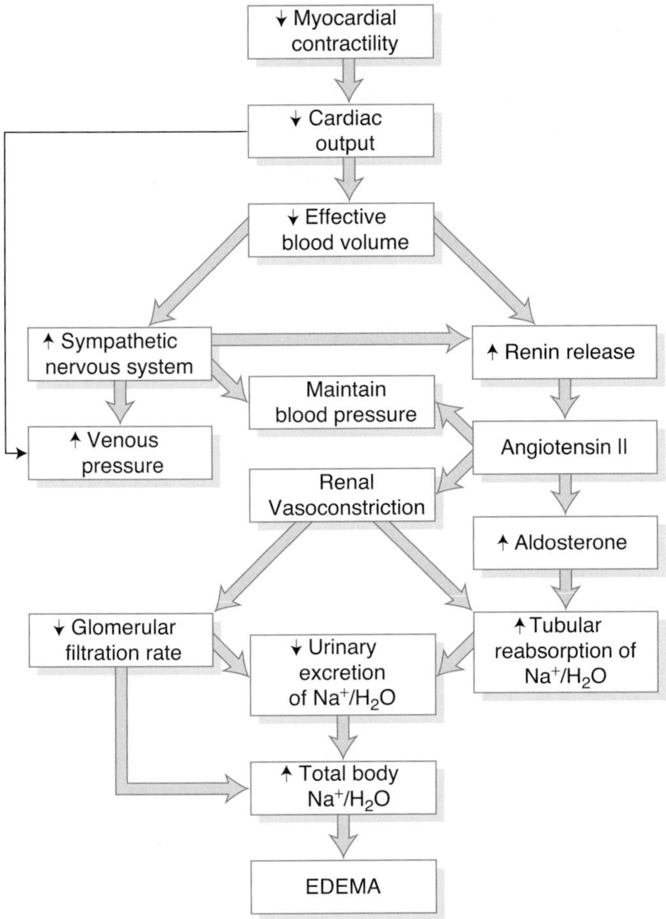
↓ Myocardial contractility
↓ Cardiac output
↓ Effective blood volume
↑ Sympathetic nervous system
↑ Renin release
Maintain blood pressure
↑ Venous pressure
Angiotensin II
Renal Vasoconstriction
↑ Aldosterone
↓ Glomerular filtration rate
↓ Urinary excretion of Na+/H2O
↑ Tubular reabsorption of Na+/H2O
↑ Total body Na+/H2O
EDEMA

FIGURE 3-11 **A chest radiograph showing congestive heart failure and pulmonary edema**

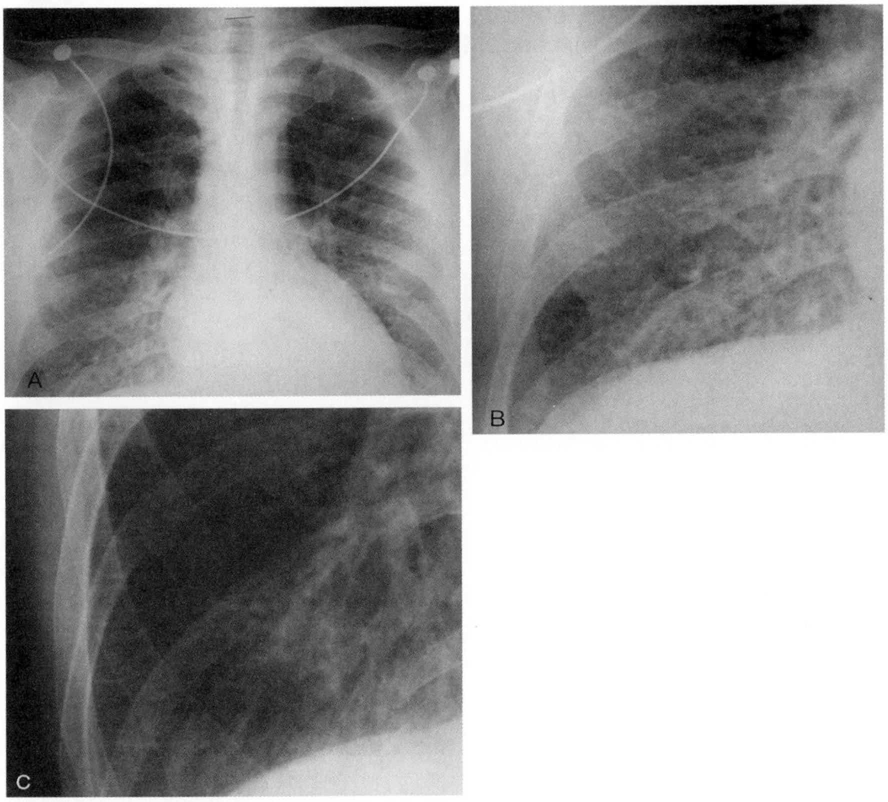
A
B
C

(Reproduced with permission from Daffner RH. *Clinical Radiology: The Essentials*. 2nd ed. Baltimore, MD: Williams & Wilkins; 1999.)

Clinical Vignette 3-3

CLINICAL PRESENTATION: A 67-year-old female complains to her primary care physician of **easy fatigue** and that each night, she has to **wake up to urinate (nocturia).** She also mentions that each night, her **ankles swell,** and she **sleeps with her head elevated on two to three pillows (orthopnea),** otherwise she finds herself waking to **catch her breath (paroxysmal nocturnal dyspnea).** Her past medical history is significant for **hypertension**; however, the patient has been noncompliant with medication. Physical examination reveals congestion; **1+ pitting edema,** an **enlarged liver,** and **elevated jugular venous pressure (JVP).** Other findings include **cold and clammy skin and S3 and S4 heart sounds.** Temperature = 98.5° F; **blood pressure = 165/100 mm Hg; heart rate = 92 bpm; and respiration rate = 34 breaths/min.**
DIFFERENTIALS: CHF and renal failure. Given the patient's history and classic presentation, this patient likely has CHF secondary to chronic hypertension.
LABORATORY STUDIES: Proper follow-up for suspect CHF would be (a) **chest radiograph** showing cardiomegaly (Figure 3-11), interstitial edema in the lungs, and pleural effusion; (b) **echocardiogram** (determines the cause of CHF, whether systolic or diastolic; quantifies ejection fraction [EF]); (c) **ECG** showing evidence of chamber enlargement or presence of ischemic disease; (d) **radionuclide ventriculography using ^{99m}Tc** (quantifies EF when echo suboptimal as in chronic obstructive pulmonary disease [COPD]); (e) **cardiac catheterization;** (f) **stress testing;** (g) **urine analysis** (elevated protein would suggest renal failure); and (h) **blood chemistry** (blood urea nitrogen [BUN] and creatinine [Cr] slightly elevated in CHF and markedly elevated in renal failure).
MANAGEMENT: Diastolic dysfunction is treated symptomatically. Systolic dysfunction should be managed by (a) **sodium restriction,** (b) **diuretics** (congestive symptoms), (c) **ACE inhibitors** (decrease preload, afterload, decrease mortality), and (d) **digitalis** (symptomatic relief; use in severe CHF). Note: If the patient cannot tolerate ACE inhibitors, use **ARBs, hydralazine,** and **isosorbide dinitrates.** Also, **α-blockers** have been proven to decrease mortality in post-MI CHF.

E. Common adverse reactions:
   1. Nausea and headache
   2. Arrhythmias (more serious)

IV. Diuretics, the other major treatment modality for CHF, are not discussed here (see Chapter 6).

INTRINSIC DISEASES OF THE HEART

I. Myocarditis

A. This is defined as inflammation of the cardiac muscle.
B. Etiology
   1. Viral etiology is the most common cause (usually coxsackie B virus, parvovirus B19, and human herpes virus [HHV]-6).
   2. HIV (via toxoplasmosis and metastasis of Kaposi sarcoma) may cause myocarditis.
   3. Bacterial causes include *Staphylococcus aureus, Corynebacterium diphtheriae,* and tuberculosis.
   4. Chagas disease
   5. Lyme disease
   6. Hypersensitivity reactions
   7. Sarcoidosis
C. Physical examination
   1. Muffled S1
   2. Audible S3 heart sound
   3. Murmur of mitral regurgitation
   4. Cardiomegaly

QUICK HIT

Trypanosoma cruzi causes Chagas disease and is transmitted by the reduviid bug (kissing bug).

QUICK HIT

Borrelia burgdorferi, a spirochete, causes Lyme disease and is transmitted by the Ixodes tick. Stage 1 is marked by erythema chronicum migrans. Stage 2 is marked by cardiac and neurologic involvement. Stage 3 involves arthritis.

QUICK HIT

Coxsackievirus B is the number one cause of neonatal myocarditis.

QUICK HIT

Prosthetic valves predispose individuals to endocarditis caused by *Staphylococcus epidermidis.*

II. Endocarditis

A. Inflammation of the heart lining and connective tissue

B. Causes

1. Rheumatic heart disease—endocarditis may be caused by rheumatic fever (see below).
2. Infective endocarditis
   a. Etiology
      - Gram-positive cocci are the most common cause. Rarely, the cause is fungi (*Aspergillus* and *Candida*) or gram-negative bacteria.
      - Damage, surgical repair, prosthetic heart valves, or congenital abnormalities are predisposing conditions.
      - Vegetative growth (usually on atrial surface of valves) can throw septic thrombi to brain or peripheral circulation.
      - Endocarditis is complicated by perivalvular abscesses or rupture of chordae tendineae.

   b. Characteristics
      - Clinical features
      - Mucosal petechiae
      - Janeway lesions (peripheral hemorrhages with slight nodular character)
      - Osler nodes (small, tender nodules on fingers and toe pads)
      - Splinter hemorrhages (subungual linear streaks)
      - Roth spots (retinal hemorrhages)
      - Splenomegaly
      - The mitral and aortic valves are frequently involved.
      - Right-sided valvular lesions (usually of the tricuspid) suggest IV drug abuse and are associated with septic pulmonary emboli.

C. Types

1. Acute endocarditis
   a. The cause is most often *S. aureus*.
   b. Onset is rapid.
   c. Clinical features include fever, anemia, embolic events, and heart murmur.
   d. Treatment is with IV antibiotics.
2. Subacute endocarditis
   a. The cause is most often the viridans streptococci.
   b. It results from poor dentition or oral surgery in patients with preexisting heart disease (and preexisting damage to heart valves).
   c. Onset is over a period of 6 months.
   d. Treatment is with IV antibiotics.
3. Nonbacterial (marantic) endocarditis
   a. This type is associated with metastatic cancer.
   b. Sterile fibrin deposits appear on valves.
   c. Sterile emboli can cause cerebral infarct.
4. Libman–Sacks endocarditis
   a. This is a manifestation of systemic lupus erythematosus (SLE).
   b. It is caused by autoantibody damage to valves.
   c. Vegetations form on both sides of the valve.
5. Carcinoid syndrome
   a. This syndrome is characterized by increased serotonin and other secretory products from a carcinoid tumor.
   b. Plaque builds on right-sided valves of the heart.

III. Rheumatic heart disease

A. This is a systemic inflammatory disorder with cardiac manifestations.

B. Pathogenesis

1. Acute rheumatic heart disease usually occurs 2 to 4 weeks after a bout of pharyngitis caused by group A β-hemolytic streptococci.

QUICK HIT

Associate acute endocarditis with Staphylococcal spp., and subacute endocarditis with viridans Streptococci. Associate endocarditis in intravenous drug abuse with *Staphylococcus aureus*.

QUICK HIT

If an endocarditis is caused by *Streptococcus bovis*, look for signs and symptoms for gastrointestinal carcinoma in the patient.

QUICK HIT

Culture-negative endocarditis can result from the HACEK group of organisms: *Haemophilus aphrophilus, Actinobacillus actinomycetemcomitans, Cardiobacterium hominis, Eikenella corrodens,* and *Kingella kingae.*

2. Antigenic mimicry occurs between streptococcal antigens and human antigens in the heart.
3. This results in immunologic origin for rheumatic heart disease.

C. Epidemiology
1. Children 5 to 15 years of age have the highest incidence of rheumatic fever.
2. Incidence is decreasing since the advent of penicillin.

D. Cardiac manifestations of rheumatic fever include the following conditions:
1. Pancarditis—inflammation of all structures of the heart
2. Pericarditis with effusions
3. Myocarditis
   a. Leads to cardiac failure
   b. Most common cause of early death in rheumatic fever
4. Endocarditis
   a. Usually afflicts the mitral and aortic valves (areas of high stress and turbulent flow)
   b. Mitral—aortic—tricuspid—pulmonary shows the order in which the valves become involved.
   c. Early nonembolic vegetations occur.
   d. With fibrosis and calcification, valvular damage leads to chronic rheumatic heart disease.

E. Other manifestations of rheumatic fever include:
1. Migratory polyarthritis
2. Sydenham chorea
3. Subcutaneous nodules
4. Erythema marginatum
5. Recent infection by group A streptococci (indicated by elevated antistreptolysin-O titers)
6. Aschoff body
   a. Lesion characterized by focal interstitial myocardial inflammation
   b. Fragmented collagen/fibrinoid material
   c. Anitschkow myocytes: large activated histiocytes
   d. Aschoff cells: granuloma with giant cells

QUICK HIT

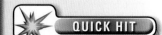

Systemic thromboembolism may develop in dilated cardiomyopathy, mitral valve prolapse, or from fragmented vegetations associated with infective endocarditis. Stasis of blood in the ventricle or atria leads to formation of mural thrombi as seen in dilated cardiomyopathy and mitral valve prolapse, respectively.

IV. Cardiomyopathies *(Table 3-10)*

QUICK HIT

Senile amyloidosis is derived from transthyretin. Primary amyloidosis is caused by the amyloid light chain (AL) protein from immunoglobulin light chains. This is seen in plasma cell disorders (see Chapter 10.

TABLE 3-10 Cardiomyopathies

	Pathology	Etiology	Clinical Manifestations	Notes
Dilated (systolic or contractile dysfunction)	Dilated ventricles, right and left heart failure, pulmonary edema	**Idiopathic,** alcoholics, thiamine deficiency, peripartum, **coxsackievirus** B, *Trypanosoma cruzi,* tricyclic antidepressants, lithium, doxorubicin, pregnancy associated	Premature ventricular contractions, **decreased ejection fraction,** JVP, cardiomegaly, hepatomegaly	**Most common** form

(continued)

TABLE 3-10 **Cardiomyopathies** *(Continued)*

	Pathology	Etiology	Clinical Manifestations	Notes
Restrictive (diastolic dysfunction or loss of compliance)	**Stiffened heart muscle;** may result in right and left heart failure; tricuspid regurgitation	Senile or primary amyloidosis, sarcoidosis, hemochromatosis (associated with systemic diseases)	Peripheral **edema,** ascites, jugular venous distention	Differentiate from hypertrophic cardiomyopathy
Hypertrophic (diastolic dysfunction or loss of compliance)	Ventricular and ventricular septal hypertrophy, mitral regurgitation	Usually **autosomal dominant** (the most common gene affected is β-myosin); young **athletes**	Dyspnea, syncope, **S4,** systolic murmur, cardiomegaly on chest radiograph	Relieved by **squatting, worsened by Valsalva,** exacerbated by physical exertion, sudden death

JVP, jugular venous pressure.

QUICK HIT

Mitral valve prolapse (MVP) is the most frequently occurring valvular lesion, often found in young women and in patients with Marfan syndrome and related to tissue laxity. Characteristics of the heart sound in MVP include midsystolic click, followed by late systolic murmur.

V. Valvular heart diseases *(Table 3-11)*

TABLE 3-11 **Valvular Heart Disease and Murmurs**

Valvular Disease	Etiology	Physical Examination	Clinical Manifestations
Systolic murmurs			
Aortic stenosis	**Bicuspid aortic valves, degenerative calcification,** RHD, unicuspid aortic valve, syphilis	Delayed pulses, carotid thrill, **crescendo-decrescendo systolic ejection murmur** at right upper sternal border, decreased intensity with Valsalva	Syncope, angina, dyspnea/CHF, death, treat symptomatic patients with valve replacement
Mitral regurgitation	**RHD** (50% of cases), LV dilation, ischemic heart disease, endocarditis, MVP, papillary muscle dysfunction (secondary to myocardial infarction)	Splitting of S2; S3; **holosystolic** murmur at apex, radiating to the left axilla, increased intensity with squatting or handgrip	Arrhythmias, dilated left atrium, holosystolic murmur
Mitral valve prolapse (MVP)	Myxomatous degeneration of mitral valve leaflets, such that leaflets billow into the left atrium during systole	**Midsystolic click**, often followed by a late systolic murmur; decreased intensity with squatting	Can be associated with chest pain, palpitations, lightheadedness, panic attacks
Ventricular septal defect	Congenital defect	Harsh, holosystolic murmur	
Diastolic murmurs			
Aortic regurgitation	Rheumatic heart disease, syphilitic aortitis, nondissecting aortic aneurysm, Marfan syndrome	Wide pulse pressure, water-hammer-pulse, **S3, blowing, decrescendo diastolic murmur**	Left ventricular enlargement, dyspnea, early diastolic murmur
Mitral stenosis	Usually **rheumatic heart disease**	Cyanosis, **opening snap,** diastolic rumbling murmur	Dyspnea, orthopnea, left atrial enlargement, mid to late diastolic murmur

CHF, congestive heart failure; LV, left ventricular; RHD, rheumatic heart disease.

VI. **Peripheral vascular diseases** *(Table 3-12)*

TABLE 3-12 **Peripheral Vascular Diseases**

Disease	Pathology	Vessels Affected	Clinical Manifestations	Notes
Churg–Strauss	Eosinophils, vasculitis, perinuclear antineutrophil cytoplasmic antibody (p-ANCA)	Small and medium-sized arteries	**Asthma, elevated plasma eosinophils,** heart disease	May be associated with p-ANCA
Henoch–Schönlein purpura	**IgA** immune complex–mediated acute vasculitis, renal deposits in mesangium	Arterioles, capillaries, venules	Hemorrhagic urticaria, palpable purpura, fever, red blood cell casts in urine, **atopic** patient	Often associated with an **upper respiratory infection;** affects **children**
Kaposi sarcoma	Viral origin, common malignancy in patients with AIDS	Cutaneous and visceral vasculature	Malignant vascular tumor, especially in **homosexual** men	Probably results from reactivation of latent human herpesvirus 8 (HHV-8) infection
Kawasaki disease	Acute necrotizing inflammation	Large, medium, and small vessels	Fever, conjunctival lesions, lymphadenitis, coronary artery aneurysms	Affects **young children**
Rendu–Osler–Weber syndrome	**Autosomal dominant;** hereditary hemorrhagic telangiectasia	Dilation of venules and capillaries	Epistaxis, gastrointestinal (GI) bleeding	Increased occurrence in **Mormon** population
Polyarteritis nodosa (PAN)	Necrotizing degeneration of tunica media, aneurysms	Small and medium-sized arteries	Fever, weight loss, abdominal pain (GI), hypertension (renal)	Associated with **hepatitis B infection**
Takayasu arteritis (pulseless disease)	Inflammation leading to stenosis; **aortic arch** and the origins of great vessels	Medium and large arteries	**Loss of carotid, radial, and ulnar pulses;** fever; night sweats; deficits arthritis; visual; low blood pressure in upper extremities; claudication caused by lack of blood reaching extremities	Pathology referred to as "aortic arch syndrome"; young **Asian females;** corkscrew, widened aorta on angiogram
Temporal arteritis (giant cell arteritis)	Nodular inflammation of branches of carotid (especially **temporal**)	Medium and large arteries	**Headache,** absence of pulse in affected vessels, **visual deficits,** polymyalgia rheumatica	Significant elevation of **sedimentation rate;** affects the **elderly**
Thromboangiitis obliterans (Buerger disease)	Acute, full-thickness inflammation of vessels; may extend to nerves; occlusive lesions in extremities	Small and medium arteries and veins	Cold, pale limb; pain; **Raynaud phenomenon;** gangrene	Typical patient is a young **Jewish** man who **smokes heavily**
Wegener granulomatosis	Antineutrophil antibodies (cytoplasmic antineutrophil cytoplasmic antibody **[c-ANCA]**) causes necrotizing, **granulomatous lesions** in **kidney, lung,** and upper respiratory tract	Small arteries, small veins of kidneys and respiratory tract	Cough, ulcers of sinuses and **nasal septum,** red blood cell casts in urine, classic triad: (a) necrotizing vasculitis (b) necrotizing granulomas of respiratory tract (c) necrotizing glomerulitis	More common in males

CARDIAC NEOPLASMS

I. Metastatic tumors to the heart are more common than primary tumors

II. Primary tumors

A. Myxomas
   1. 90% found in atria
   2. Left atrium > right atrium
   3. Cause **ball-valve obstruction**, embolism, and fever

B. Rhabdomyoma
   1. Most common primary cardiac tumor found in children
   2. Often seen with tuberous sclerosis
   3. Composed of "spider cells" and glycogen vacuoles

DISEASES OF THE PERICARDIUM

I. Cardiac tamponade

A. This is an accumulation of fluid in the pericardial sac, which causes cardiac filling defects because of compression of the heart.
   1. Blood is usually indicative of a traumatic perforation of the heart or aorta or rupture as a consequence of an MI.
   2. Serous transudate may accumulate as a result of edema or CHF.

B. The most common causes are neoplasms, idiopathic pericarditis, and uremia.

C. Principal features of cardiac tamponade include:
   1. Intracardiac pressure is elevated.
   2. Ventricular filling is limited.
   3. Cardiac output is reduced.
   4. Decreased or absent heart sounds on auscultation

D. Pulsus paradoxus is a greater than normal (10 mm Hg) decline in systolic arterial pressure on inspiration.

E. Treatment involves pericardiocentesis (removal of fluid from the pericardial cavity).

II. Pericarditis

A. Pericarditis is defined as an inflammation of the pericardium (fibroserous membrane) covering the heart.

B. Causes
   1. Usually idiopathic
   2. Coxsackievirus A or B (serous pericarditis)
   3. Tuberculosis (hemorrhagic pericarditis)
   4. Uremia (serofibrinous pericarditis)
   5. SLE (serous pericarditis)
   6. Scleroderma (serous pericarditis)
   7. Post-MI (Dressler syndrome; fibrinous pericarditis)

C. Physical examination
   1. Jugular venous distention (JVD)
   2. Increase of JVP with inspiration (Kussmaul sign)
   3. Pericardial friction rub
   4. Distant heart sounds

D. Characteristics
   1. Pain exacerbated by inspiration
   2. Pain relieved by sitting
   3. Cardiomegaly
   4. Hypotension
   5. Diffuse ST elevation on ECG

E. Persistent, acute pericarditis leads to chronic, constrictive pericarditis.
   1. Both acute and chronic pericarditis mimic right-sided heart failure.
   2. Both acute and chronic pericarditis lead to obliteration of pericardial cavity.
   3. Fibrous tissue proliferation and calcification result.

QUICK HIT

Temporal arteritis is the most common vasculitis in the United States.

QUICK HIT

Primary tumors of the heart are very rare. Metastatic (secondary) tumors are more common. Atrial myxomas are the most frequently occurring primary tumors.

QUICK HIT

The needle for a pericardiocentesis passes through the skin, superficial fascia, pectoralis major muscle, external intercostal membrane, internal intercostal membrane, fibrous pericardium, and parietal layer of serous pericardium.

QUICK HIT

An MI also produces ST elevation. However, in an MI, ST elevation is limited to certain leads (corresponding to anatomical regions) and associated with possible QRS changes.

QUICK HIT

Autoregulation of blood flow in the heart is altered to meet the demands of tissue metabolism via nitric oxide and adenosine. Autoregulation also occurs in the kidney and brain.

QUICK HIT

Septic shock is associated with vasodilation, hypotension, and warm extremities.

SHOCK

I. Shock is defined as a metabolic state in which oxygen delivery is inadequate to meet the oxygen demand.

II. Signs and symptoms

A. Tachycardia
B. Hypotension
C. Oliguria
D. Mental status changes
E. Weak pulses
F. Cool extremities

III. Types of shock *(Table 3-13)*

TABLE 3-13 Shock

Type of Shock	SVR	HR	PCWP	PCWP After Fluid Challenge	Mechanism	Clinical Causes
Cardiogenic	High	Varies	High	Very high	Pump failure	Arrhythmias, heart failure, myocardial infarction
Hypovolemic	High	High	Low	Unchanged or high	Volume loss	Blood/fluid/plasma loss, burns, severe vomiting or diarrhea
Obstructive (tension pneumothorax, massive hemothorax)	High	High	Low or normal	Unchanged or increased	Extracardiac obstruction of blood flow	Tension pneumothorax, massive hemothorax
Obstructive (cardiac tamponade)	High	High	High	High or very high	Extracardiac obstruction of blood flow	Cardiac tamponade
Septic	Low	Low	Low or normal	High	Increased venous capacitance	Gram-negative endotoxemia, direct toxic injury
Neurogenic	Low	Low	Low or normal	high	Massive peripheral vasodilation	Severe cerebral, brain stem, or spinal cord injury
Anaphylactic	Low	High	Low	High	Increased venous capacitance due to histamine release	Type I hypersensitivity reaction to allergen

HR, heart rate; PCWP, pulmonary wedge capillary pressure; SVR, systemic vascular resistance.

IV. Clinical manifestations of shock
A. Acute tubular necrosis
B. Necrosis in the brain
C. Fatty change in the heart and liver
D. Patchy hemorrhages in the colon
E. Pulmonary edema due to acute lung injury

QUICK HIT

Doxorubicin, daunorubicin, and anthracyclines used to treat sarcomas, breast cancer, lung cancer, and acute lymphocytic leukemia result in dose-dependent, irreversible cardiotoxicity.

DRUGS THAT CAUSE ADVERSE EFFECTS TO THE CARDIOVASCULAR SYSTEM

I. Thrombotic complications: oral contraceptives (estrogen and progestins)

II. Cardiac toxicity: doxorubicin (antineoplastic), daunorubicin (antineoplastic), anthracyclines, tricyclic antidepressants, and lithium

III. Torsades de pointes: class IA (quinidine), class III (sotalol) antiarrhythmics, and tricyclic antidepressants

4 The Respiratory System

DEVELOPMENT

I. The lung bud forms from the foregut during week 4 of embryologic development.

II. The lining of the lower respiratory tract is derived from endoderm, whereas the connective tissue cartilage and muscle are derived from mesoderm.

III. Normal development causes the lung bud to completely separate from the esophagus at the level of the larynx.

IV. Incomplete separation causes a tracheoesophageal (TE) fistula *(Figure 4-1)*.

A. In the most common form of TE fistula, the esophagus ends in a blind pouch (esophageal atresia) and air enters the stomach (gastric bubble on radiograph).

B. Signs and symptoms of esophageal atresia with a TE fistula

1. Feeding difficulties within the first few days of life
2. Possible aspiration pneumonia with respiratory distress
3. Inability to pass nasogastric tube
4. Copious secretions

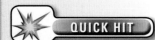

> **QUICK HIT**
> TE fistula is the most common anomaly of the lower respiratory tract.

> **QUICK HIT**
> Polyhydramnios is often associated with TE fistula due to the inability of excess amniotic fluid to pass through the stomach and intestine for absorption by the placenta into the mother's circulation.

FIGURE 4-1 **Tracheoesophageal fistula**

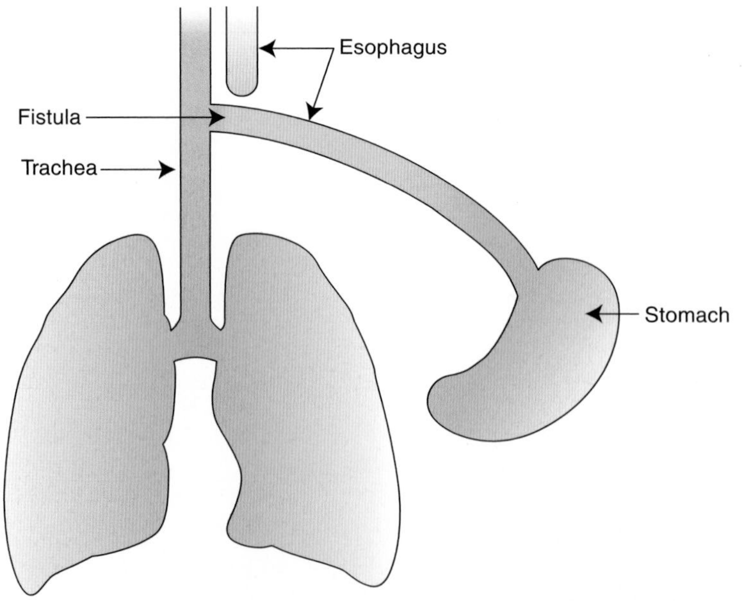
Esophagus
Fistula
Trachea
Stomach

V. Diaphragm muscle

A. This is the primary muscle used for breathing.
B. The diaphragm muscle separates the pleural and peritoneal cavities.
C. It is formed from fusion of the following structures:
   1. **Septum transversum**
   2. Paired **pleuroperitoneal membranes**
   3. **Dorsal mesentery** of the **esophagus**
   4. **Body wall**
D. It is innervated by the phrenic nerves (C3, C4, and C5).
E. Improper formation of the pleuroperitoneal membrane or its failure to fuse with the other three parts of the diaphragm can lead to a **congenital diaphragmatic hernia (CDH)**, a condition with serious complications.
   1. Abdominal contents are forced into the pleural cavity.
   2. Lung hypoplasia results from compression by abdominal viscera.
   3. Hernias appear most often on the **left side** (posterolateral).
   4. Diaphragmatic hernia is associated with polyhydramnios.
   5. Diaphragmatic hernia presents at birth as a flattened abdomen, cyanosis, and inability to breathe.

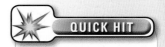

QUICK HIT

The defect of CDH is also known as the foramen of Bochdalek and occurs on the left side in nearly 90% of cases due to the earlier closure of the right pleuroperitoneal opening.

MNEMONIC

C3, C4, and C5 keep the diaphragm phrenically alive.

PHYSICS AND FUNCTION OF THE LUNG

I. Lung volumes

A. **Capacities and volumes in the normal lung** (Figure 4-2)
B. Volumes and pressure during the breathing cycle (Figure 4-3)
C. Spirometry tracing—normal versus diseased (Figure 4-4)
D. Pulmonary function tests—obstructive versus restrictive (Figure 4-5)

II. Compliance

A. Defined as $\Delta V/\Delta P$, where V is volume and P is pressure, compliance describes the ability of the chest wall and lung to expand when stretched.
   1. At functional residual capacity (FRC), the lungs have a tendency to collapse.
   2. This force is exactly balanced by the chest wall, which has a tendency to expand.
   3. Because these forces are in balance at FRC, the airway pressure is 0 mm Hg. Lung volumes above FRC create a positive airway pressure, whereas volumes below FRC create a negative airway pressure.

QUICK HIT

The sternocleidomastoid and the internal and external intercostals are accessory muscles of respiration. They are used when there is an increased demand for oxygen (such as in exercise) or in disease states.

QUICK HIT

Compliance is given by the slope of pressure versus volume curve.

QUICK HIT

Residual volume (RV) or volumes containing RV cannot be directly measured by plethysmography or spirometry but are derived from helium dilution techniques.

FIGURE 4-2 Lung volumes

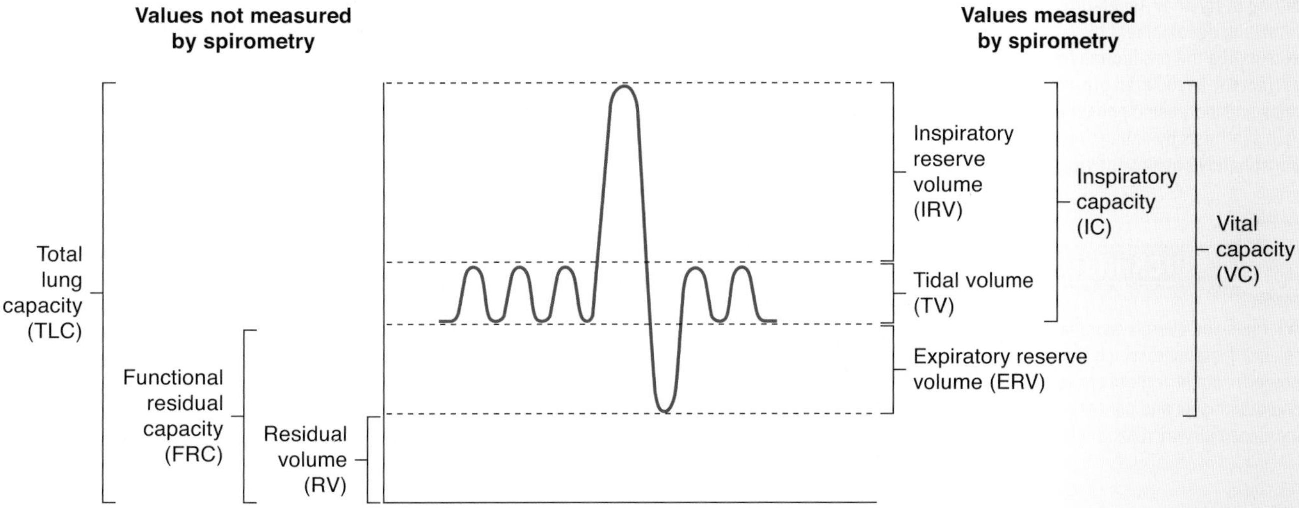
Values not measured by spirometry
Values measured by spirometry
Total lung capacity (TLC)
Functional residual capacity (FRC)
Residual volume (RV)
Inspiratory reserve volume (IRV)
Tidal volume (TV)
Expiratory reserve volume (ERV)
Inspiratory capacity (IC)
Vital capacity (VC)

QUICK HIT

SRS-A is a combination of the leukotrienes C_4 and D_4 (LTC_4 and LTD_4). In the treatment of asthma, zileuton blocks production of leukotrienes by inhibiting the lipoxygenase enzyme, whereas zafirlukast blocks leukotriene receptors. Leukotriene A_4 (LTA_4) is a precursor to leukotriene B_4 (LTB_4, LTC_4, and LTD_4). LTB_4 is responsible for chemotaxis of neutrophils and adhesion of white blood cells.

QUICK HIT

The primary molecule of surfactant is dipalmitoylphosphatidylcholine (lecithin). A lecithin-to-sphingomyelin ratio of 2:1 is the normal ratio of surfactant molecules in a newborn. A ratio below 2:1 can result in neonatal respiratory distress, especially in cesarean section delivery.

QUICK HIT

Type II pneumocytes are cuboidal cells with round nuclei, foamy cytoplasm (because of lipid content), and lamellar bodies (secreting granules) containing the surfactant.

QUICK HIT

Glucocorticoids administered during pregnancy accelerate fetal lung development by stimulating the production of surfactant-associated proteins and increasing phospholipid synthesis by enhancing phosphatidylcholine activity.

QUICK HIT

Allergies and allergic asthma release histamine, which is a powerful constrictor of airway smooth muscle and causes increased airway resistance.

FIGURE 4-3 **Breathing cycle**

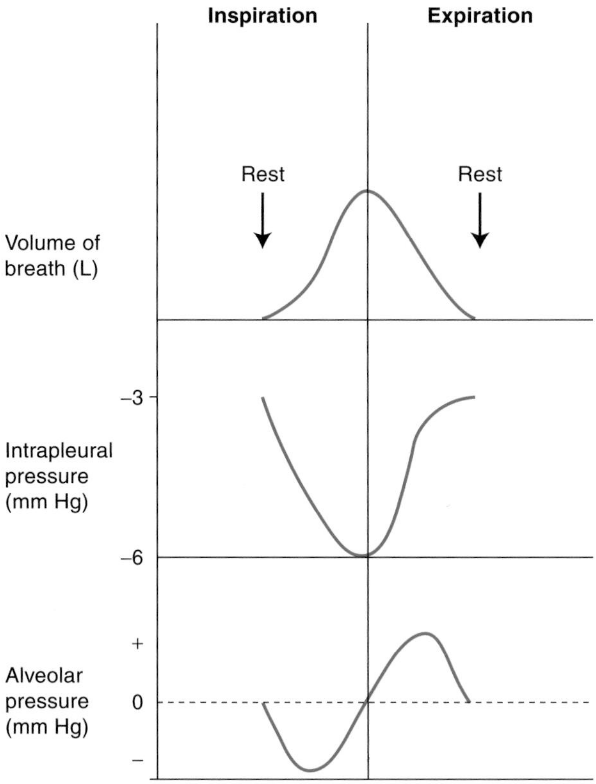

Inspiration
Expiration
Rest
Rest
Volume of breath (L)
–3
Intrapleural pressure (mm Hg)
–6
+
Alveolar pressure (mm Hg)
0
–

4. Low compliance implies a stiff chest wall or lung as seen in:
   a. **Pulmonary fibrosis due to asbestosis, sarcoidosis, and adult respiratory distress syndrome (ARDS)**
   b. **Pulmonary edema**
   c. **Paralysis of the respiratory muscles**
5. High compliance implies a flaccid lung as a result of:
   a. Decreased elastic recoil as seen in **emphysema** and **old age**
   b. **Bronchospasm** as in **asthma** (Figure 4-4)

B. **Surfactant** plays an important role in lung compliance.
1. Alveoli have a tendency to collapse.
2. An alveolus with a small radius has more collapsing pressure than an alveolus with a large radius, according to **Laplace law:**

   $$P \propto T/r$$

   where P is pressure required to prevent alveolar collapse, T is surface tension, and r is alveolar radius.
3. Surfactant reduces the pressure and prevents collapse by reducing the intermolecular forces between water molecules lining the alveoli.
4. Surfactant increases compliance and allows the alveoli to expand more easily.
5. **Neonatal respiratory distress syndrome** (NRDS) occurs in premature infants (<37 weeks' gestation) because **type II** (surfactant-producing) **pneumocytes** are not yet fully developed and fail to produce sufficient surfactant.
6. Atelectasis (collapsed alveoli) can result from NRDS.

III. Airway resistance

A. Airway resistance (R) is inversely proportional to the fourth power of the radius (r) (formula: $R \propto 1/r^4$); thus, any mechanism that decreases the radius of the bronchi will greatly affect the airway resistance.

FIGURE 4-4 **Spirometry tracings: normal versus diseased**

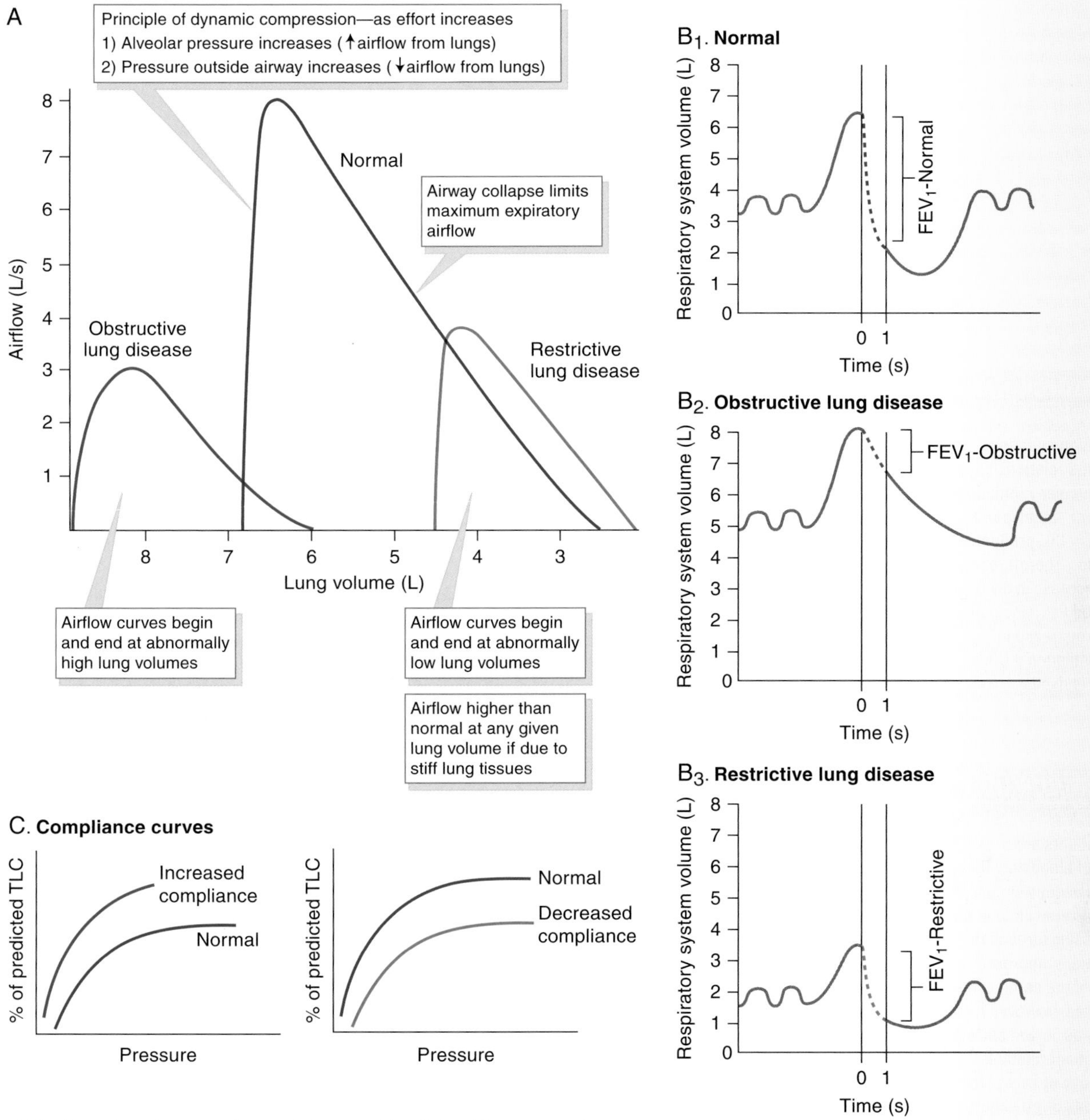
A
Principle of dynamic compression—as effort increases
1) Alveolar pressure increases (↑airflow from lungs)
2) Pressure outside airway increases (↓airflow from lungs)
Airflow (L/s)
8
7
6
5
4
3
2
1
Normal
Airway collapse limits maximum expiratory airflow
Obstructive lung disease
Restrictive lung disease
8
7
6
5
4
3
Lung volume (L)
Airflow curves begin and end at abnormally high lung volumes
Airflow curves begin and end at abnormally low lung volumes
Airflow higher than normal at any given lung volume if due to stiff lung tissues
B1. Normal
Respiratory system volume (L)
FEV1-Normal
Time (s)
B2. Obstructive lung disease
FEV1-Obstructive
B3. Restrictive lung disease
FEV1-Restrictive
C. Compliance curves
% of predicted TLC
Increased compliance
Normal
Decreased compliance
Pressure

FEV_1, forced expiratory volume at 1 second; TLC, total lung capacity.

B. The **airway radius** is under the control of the parasympathetic and sympathetic nervous systems.

1. **Parasympathetic nervous system**
   a. Causes **constriction** of the airways
   b. Mediated by direct stimulation, airway irritation, and slow-reacting substance of anaphylaxis (SRS-A)
   c. Stimulates mucus secretion
2. **Sympathetic nervous system**
   a. Causes **dilation** of airways
   b. Used as treatment for allergy and asthma (β_2-agonists)
   c. Functions in fight-or-flight autonomic reflexes; dilates airways to help provide oxygen in times of stress

FIGURE 4-5 Interpreting pulmonary function tests: obstructive versus restrictive

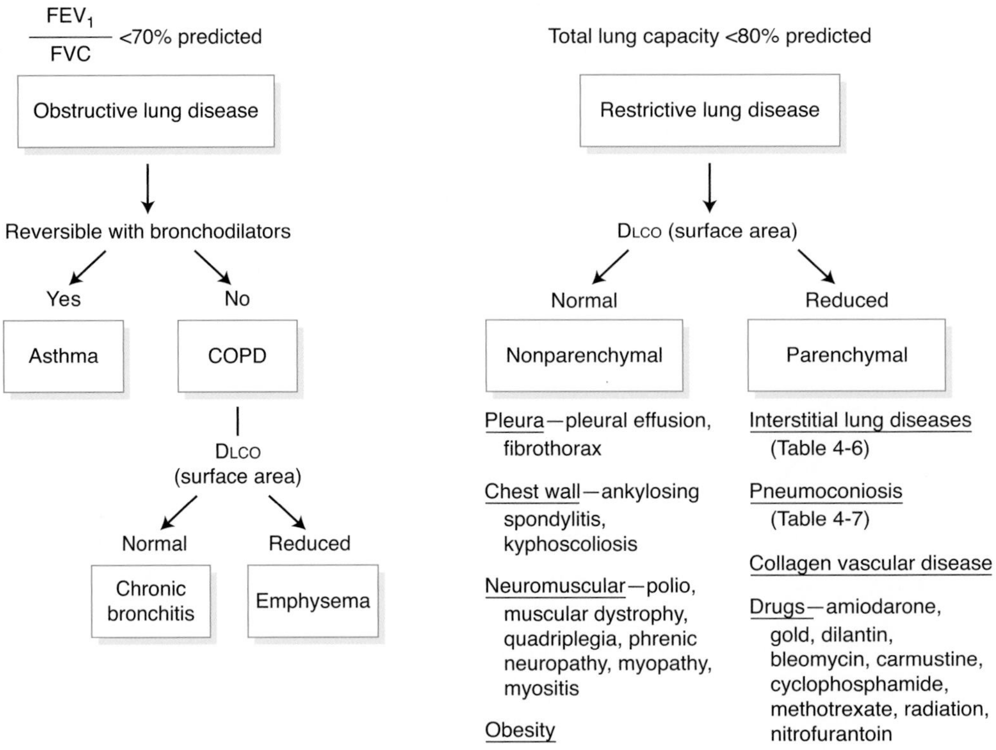
FEV1/FVC <70% predicted
Obstructive lung disease
Reversible with bronchodilators
Yes
No
Asthma
COPD
DLCO (surface area)
Normal
Reduced
Chronic bronchitis
Emphysema
Total lung capacity <80% predicted
Restrictive lung disease
DLCO (surface area)
Normal
Reduced
Nonparenchymal
Parenchymal
Pleura—pleural effusion, fibrothorax
Chest wall—ankylosing spondylitis, kyphoscoliosis
Neuromuscular—polio, muscular dystrophy, quadriplegia, phrenic neuropathy, myopathy, myositis
Obesity
Interstitial lung diseases (Table 4-6)
Pneumoconiosis (Table 4-7)
Collagen vascular disease
Drugs—amiodarone, gold, dilantin, bleomycin, carmustine, cyclophosphamide, methotrexate, radiation, nitrofurantoin

COPD, chronic obstructive pulmonary disease; DLCO, diffusing capacity of lung for carbon monoxide; FEV_1, forced expiratory volume at 1 second; FVC, forced vital capacity.

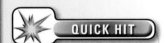

QUICK HIT

The ventilation equation quantifies the relationship between alveolar ventilation and alveolar PCO_2: **alveolar ventilation = CO_2 production/alveolar PCO_2**. Therefore, a threefold increase in alveolar PCO_2 (expired PCO_2) indicates a threefold decrease in alveolar ventilation if CO_2 production is fixed.

QUICK HIT

Anatomic shunts are passageways of blood flow that go from the venous circulation to the arterial circulation without passing through the lungs. Normally, approximately 2% of the cardiac output is shunted; however, it can be as much as 50% in certain congenital malformations (e.g., tetralogy of Fallot produces a right-to-left shunt).

QUICK HIT

There are two types of dead space:
(1) **Anatomic dead space**, measured by the **Fowler method**, is usually about 150 mL.
(2) **Physiologic dead space**, measured by the Bohr method, is considered to be the volume of the lung that does not eliminate CO_2.

3. Airway radius is also affected by the lung parenchyma, which is bound to the airway and exerts radial traction on it.
   a. In restrictive disorders such as interstitial fibrosis, radial traction of the airway increases → increasing airway diameter → decreasing airway resistance → increasing expiratory airflow. Despite the increased expiratory airflow, the reduced lung compliance will decrease both forced vital capacity (FVC) and forced expiratory volume at 1 second (FEV_1). Therefore, the FEV_1/FVC ratio is normal or increased.
   b. In obstructive disorders such as emphysema, destruction of elastic fibers → decreases radial traction → decreasing airway diameter → increasing resistance → decreasing expiratory airflow and FEV_1/FVC ratios.

IV. Ventilation and perfusion

A. **Ventilation/perfusion (V/Q) ratio**: the ratio of the rate of alveolar ventilation to the rate of pulmonary blood flow

B. Varies over the entire lung (higher in the apices, lower in the bases in an upright patient), but is 0.8 on average

C. Dead space
   1. Anatomic dead space is regions of the lung, such as the conducting airways, which are incapable of exchanging oxygen (O_2) and carbon dioxide (CO_2).
   2. Physiologic dead space is the volume of the lungs which does not participate in the elimination of CO_2.

$$V_D = V_T \times [(PaCO_2 - PECO_2)/PaCO_2]$$

V_D, physiologic dead space (mL); V_T, tidal volume (mL); Pa_{CO_2}, partial pressure of carbon dioxide, arterial blood (mm Hg); PE_{CO_2}, partial pressure of carbon dioxide in expired air (mm Hg).

3. It causes a reduction in ventilation.
4. V/Q is reduced to 0 in complete airway occlusion.
5. A V/Q of 0 is considered a shunt and no gas exchange will occur (areas are perfused but not ventilated).

D. Blood flow obstruction
  1. Blockage of a pulmonary artery or smaller vessel causes a reduction in perfusion.
  2. A perfusion value of 0 yields an infinite V/Q ratio.
  3. A V/Q of infinity is considered **physiologic dead space**.

E. Pulmonary embolism results in increased V/Q ratio (Table 4-1).

F. Blood flow and ventilation vary over the regions of the lung (Figure 4-6) due primarily to gravity.

TABLE 4-1 **Causes of Hypoxemia**

Cause	Associated Conditions	A–a Gradient	Lab Values	Notes
Right-to-left shunt	Congenital anomaly	Increased		Does not respond to oxygen
Ventilation/perfusion mismatch	Pneumonia, COPD, atelectasis, pulmonary infarction, tumors, granulomatous disease		Increased	Responds to oxygen (A–a gradient corrects)
Decreased diffusion capacity	Thick blood–air barrier (diffuse interstitial fibrosis, sarcoidosis, asbestosis, respiratory distress syndrome), decreased surface area (pneumonectomy, emphysema), decreased hemoglobin (anemia, PE)	Increased	DLCO decreased	Responds to oxygen but A–a gradient remains same
Decreased P_{O_2} in inspired air	High altitudes, erroneous setting on ventilator	Normal		Responds to oxygen
Hypoventilation of central origin	Opioid or barbiturate overdose	Normal	Elevated P_{CO_2}	Responds to oxygen
Hypoventilation of peripheral origin	Polio, chest trauma (multiple rib fractures → pain with breathing), tetanus, obesity (Pickwickian syndrome), suffocation, drowning, skeletal disease, phrenic nerve paralysis	Normal	Elevated P_{CO_2}	Responds to oxygen

A–a gradient, alveolar–arterial gradient; COPD, chronic obstructive pulmonary disease; DLCO, diffusing capacity of lung for carbon monoxide; PE, pulmonary embolus.

In determining the cause of hypoxemia in a patient, use a three-tier approach: (1) Check whether the A–a gradient is elevated; (2) check whether O_2 administration improved the condition and if the A–a gradient was corrected; and (3) look for other lab findings or associated conditions.

QUICK HIT

During exercise, pulmonary vascular resistance decreases as a result of dilation of the lung arterioles by metabolic products. The V/Q ratio becomes uniform over the entire lung. Conversely, during hypoxia, lack of oxygen constricts local lung vasculature, thus increasing pulmonary vascular resistance; this is the opposite of what takes place in the systemic circulation, wherein lack of oxygen results in vasodilation.

FIGURE 4-6 Pulmonary circulation

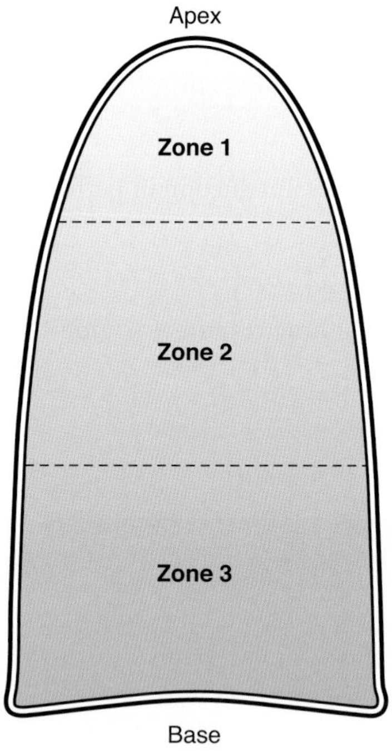
Apex
Zone 1
Zone 2
Zone 3
Base

Zone 1
- Lowest blood flow
- Alveolar pressure > arterial pressure > venous pressure
- Capillaries collapse due to high alveolar pressure
- Ventilation ($\dot{V}$) is decreased less than blood flow [also called perfusion ($\dot{Q}$)]

so: $\frac{\dot{V}}{\dot{Q}} = \frac{\downarrow}{\downarrow\downarrow} = \uparrow$ (Ventilation in excess of perfusion)

Zone 2
- Blood flow is higher than Zone 1 but lower than Zone 3
- Arterial pressure > alveolar pressure > venous pressure
- Capillaries remain open because arterial pressure is greater than alveolar pressure
- Ventilation ($\dot{V}$) is approximately equivalent to perfusion ($\dot{Q}$)

so: $\frac{\dot{V}}{\dot{Q}} \approx 1$

Zone 3
- Highest blood flow
- Arterial pressure > venous pressure > alveolar pressure
- Capillaries remain open because arterial pressure is higher than both alveolar and venous pressure
- Ventilation ($\dot{V}$) is increased less than perfusion ($\dot{Q}$)

so: $\frac{\dot{V}}{\dot{Q}} = \frac{\uparrow}{\uparrow\uparrow} = \downarrow$ (Perfusion in excess of ventilation)

CONTROL OF BREATHING

I. Medulla

A. Mediates inspiration and expiration
B. Generates the basic breathing rhythm
C. Receives input via the vagus and glossopharyngeal nerves
D. Sends output via the phrenic nerve to the diaphragm and via the spinal nerve to the intercostals and abdominal wall
E. The cerebral cortex can override the medulla and provide voluntary control of breathing if desired

II. The central nervous system (CNS) seeks to keep $Pa{CO_2}$ within a narrow range. On the other hand, in the case of oxygen, the nervous system responds only to very low levels of $Pa{O_2}$.

III. Depth and rate of respiration control these variables.

A. **Central control**
1. Chemoreceptors in the **medulla** sense the pH of the cerebrospinal fluid (CSF).
2. CO_2 crosses the blood–brain barrier, where it binds with H_2O to form carbonic acid (H_2CO_3). H_2CO_3 dissociates to hydrogen ion (H^+) and bicarbonate (HCO_3), causing an increase in H^+ (decreasing the pH of the CSF).
3. Increases in [H^+] (hydrogen ion concentration) directly stimulate the central chemoreceptors, which stimulate breathing.
4. Decreases in [H^+] reduce stimulation of the receptors and slow respiration.

B. **Peripheral control**
1. Chemoreceptors in the **carotid bodies** and at the aortic arch bifurcation sense changes in $Pa{O_2}$, $Pa{CO_2}$, and [H^+].
2. Decreases in **$Pa{O_2}$** below 60 mm Hg stimulate the peripheral chemoreceptors to increase rate and depth of breathing (in the absence of lung disease, decreased $Pa{O_2}$ is rarely the driving force for respiration).
3. Increases in **$Pa{CO_2}$** potentiate peripheral chemoreceptor response to $Pa{O_2}$ (major direct effect of changes in $Pa{CO_2}$ is on the central chemoreceptors).

QUICK HIT

Administering high fraction of inspired oxygen ($F{IO_2}$) to patients with chronic hypercapnia (e.g., COPD patients) can lead to respiratory failure because hypoxia is the only stimulus for respiration.

QUICK HIT

Hyperventilation associated with states of anxiety leads to decreased arterial $P{CO_2}$, which causes constriction of cerebral vasculature, decreasing blood flow to the brain and producing feelings of faintness, suffocation, blurred vision, and chest tightness.

4. Increases in arterial [H^+] directly stimulate the chemoreceptors, independent of the Pa_{CO_2} (causes increased respiration in metabolic acidosis).
5. Stimulation of irritant receptors in large airways and stretch receptors in small airways inhibits inspiration.

C. **Abnormal breathing**

1. **Cheyne–Stokes breathing**
   a. Tidal volumes variably increase and decrease and are separated by a period of apnea.
   b. This breathing abnormality is a result of pontine dysfunction and is associated with drug overdose, hypoxia, CNS depression, congestive heart failure (CHF), and increased intracerebral pressure.
2. **Kussmaul breathing**
   a. Deep, labored breathing pattern associated with severe metabolic acidosis (e.g., diabetic ketoacidosis)
   b. Can be either fast or slow
3. **Sleep apnea**
   a. **Obstructive sleep apnea**
      - Risk factors: middle age, male sex, obesity, smoking, hypertension, pharyngeal malformations, use of alcohol and other drugs
      - **Characteristics**
        (1) Ventilatory effort exists.
        (2) Airway is obstructed.
        (3) Apnea is terminated by self-arousal.
        (4) Apnea usually occurs in the nasopharynx or oropharynx when muscles relax during rapid eye movement (REM) sleep.
   b. **Central sleep apnea**
      - Ventilatory effort does not exist.
      - Airway is not obstructed.
      - Patient does not arouse self.
      - Central sleep apnea, like obstructive sleep apnea, occurs in the REM stage of sleep.
      - It is CO_2 threshold–dependent; that is, there is decreased chemoreceptor sensitivity to O_2 and CO_2 concentrations.
   c. **Therapy** includes weight loss (for obstructive sleep apnea) and continuous positive airway pressure (CPAP); multiple drugs have been used in treatment, but none is as effective as CPAP.

QUICK HIT

Obstructive sleep apnea causes CO_2 retention, leading to respiratory acidosis and hypoxemia.

QUICK HIT

Patients with unexplained daytime sleepiness, arrhythmias, and mood changes should be evaluated for sleep apnea.

QUICK HIT

Remember that air contains higher oxygen levels (P_{O_2} = 160 mm Hg) and virtually no CO_2 (P_{CO_2} = 0 mm Hg) as compared to arterial gas levels (P_{O_2} = 100 mm Hg, P_{CO_2} = 40 mm Hg).

IV. Gas exchange

A. Diffusion of gas depends on the **partial pressure difference** between the gas in the alveolus and the gas in the blood (i.e., the difference in pressure across the blood–air barrier).

B. Partial pressure

1. The alveolar partial pressure of oxygen (P_AO_2) can be calculated as follows:

$$\mathbf{P_AO_2 = (760 - 47\ mm\ Hg)\ F_iO_2 - (P_ACO_2/0.8)}$$

where 760 mm Hg = total atmospheric pressure (at sea level);
47 mm Hg = partial pressure of completely humidified air as found in the alveoli;
F_iO_2 = percent of air that is oxygen (normally 0.21);
P_ACO_2 = partial pressure of CO_2 in the alveoli (normally 40);
and 0.8 = the ratio of volume of CO_2 produced to the volume of O_2 consumed (respiratory quotient).

2. For O_2, higher pressures will force more oxygen into the blood and allow it to equilibrate more readily.
3. For CO_2, higher partial pressures in the blood (or lower in the alveoli) will force more CO_2 out of the blood and into the lungs, where it can be expired.
4. The amount of O_2 delivered to the tissues is also determined by hemoglobin concentration and red blood cell number (hematocrit) (see Chapter 10).

QUICK HIT

The blood–air barrier is made up of:
(1) Membrane and cytoplasm of type I pneumocytes
(2) Fused basement membrane of type I pneumocytes and endothelial cells
(3) Membrane and cytoplasm of endothelial cells

QUICK HIT

The **right main bronchus** is more vertically oriented than the **left main bronchus** and is therefore the path commonly taken by aspirated particles. If a patient is supine, the object is most likely to enter the **lower lobe.**

C. Disease affects diffusion capacity of the lung.
   1. Fibrosis causes a thickening of the interstitium, which hinders diffusion across the blood–air barrier.
   2. Emphysema destroys the alveolar walls and decreases the area available for gas exchange.

QUICK HIT

Slow, deep breaths increase the deposition of dust by sedimentation and diffusion, whereas exercise results in higher rates of airflow and increased deposition by impaction.

LUNG DEFENSES

I. Anatomic barriers

A. Impaction
   1. Large particles (**greater than 10 μm in diameter**) fail to turn the corners of the respiratory tract.
   2. Common site: **nasopharynx**

B. Sedimentation
   1. Medium particles (**between 2 and 10 μm in diameter**) settle as a result of weight.
   2. Common site: **small airways**

C. Diffusion
   1. Small particles (**between 0.5 and 2 μm in diameter**) are engulfed by alveolar macrophages (dust cells).
   2. Common site: **alveoli**

D. Suspension: particles **less than 0.5 μm in diameter** remain suspended in air.

QUICK HIT

Kartagener syndrome is an autosomal recessive disorder causing a defect in the dynein arms of cilia, resulting in infertility, situs inversus, chronic sinusitis, and bronchiectasis.

II. Nonspecific

A. **Mucociliary escalator**
   1. Particles are trapped in the gel layer of the upper airway.
   2. Ciliary motion removes particles.

B. **Cough**
   1. Cough is a bronchoconstriction that occurs to prevent penetration of particles.
   2. It is also defined as deep inspiration followed by forced expiration.
   3. The cough reflex can be suppressed by antitussive agents such as opioids (see Chapter 9).
   4. Specific mechanisms include secretory immunoglobulin A (IgA) and complement.

QUICK HIT

Hyaline membrane refers to eosinophilic membranous structures lining the alveolar wall.

QUICK HIT

Hyaline membrane disease is associated with diabetes of the mother.

ADULT RESPIRATORY DISTRESS SYNDROME AND NEONATAL RESPIRATORY DISTRESS SYNDROME

This group of diseases often leads to respiratory failure and death (Table 4-2).

QUICK HIT

Hyaline membranes are characteristic of both ARDS and NRDS but are caused by distinctly different pathologic mechanisms.

QUICK HIT

Neutrophils are implicated in the pathogenesis of ARDS. Essentially, injury promotes neutrophil recruitment. Neutrophils release chemokines, ultimately leading to production of oxygen radicals, prostaglandins, and proteases and resulting in damage to the alveolar epithelium.

TABLE 4-2 Adult Respiratory Distress Syndrome (ARDS) and Neonatal Respiratory Distress Syndrome (NRDS)

	ARDS (Diffuse Alveolar Damage)	NRDS (Hyaline Membrane Disease)
Age group	Adults	Premature infants
Causes	**Shock, infection, trauma, or aspiration** resulting in **neutrophil** recruitment and free radical production (oxygen toxicity)	**Lack of surfactant** production
Pathophysiology	Impaired gas exchange caused by pulmonary hemorrhage, pulmonary edema, or atelectasis	Increased work to expand lungs; infant can clear lungs of fluids but cannot fill lungs with air; atelectasis
Features	Respiratory insufficiency; cyanosis; hypoxemia; heavy, wet lungs; diffuse pulmonary infiltrates on radiograph; hyaline membranes in alveoli; pneumothorax may result—may be rapid and fatal	Respiratory insufficiency; cyanosis; hypoxemia; heavy, wet lungs; diffuse pulmonary infiltrates on radiograph; hyaline membranes in alveoli

PNEUMOTHORAX

I. Simple pneumothorax

A. May be caused by **spontaneous** rupture of a bleb (congenital or secondary to paraseptal emphysema) or penetrating trauma causing a loss of negative intrathoracic pressure

B. Is most commonly seen in tall, slender **men 20 to 40 years of age**

C. Presents as sudden chest pain, shortness of breath (SOB), **cough, hyperresonance**, and **decreased breath sounds** over affected lung; chest radiograph shows **radiolucency** and in the case of a **tension pneumothorax**, the **trachea deviates to the side of the pneumothorax**

D. Has a 50% recurrence rate

E. Treatment includes the insertion of a chest tube with suction to create a vacuum for larger defects as well as monitoring for small defects such as air leaks.

II. Tension pneumothorax

A. A flap of tissue allows air to enter pleural space but not to escape, causing an increase in pleural cavity pressure.

B. Pressure builds, the mediastinum is displaced, the **trachea deviates away from the lesion**, jugular venous distention (JVD) occurs, and breath sounds are uneven.

C. Cardiovascular and respiratory compromise may be rapidly fatal.

III. Open sucking chest wound

A. Penetrating trauma to the chest wall and pleura can cause this condition.

B. If the diameter of the lesion approaches the diameter of the trachea, air will preferentially enter through the defect.

PULMONARY VASCULAR DISEASES

A variety of diseases primarily affect the vasculature of the lungs (Table 4-3).

TABLE 4-3 Pulmonary Vascular Diseases

Disease	Etiology	Features	Complications
Pulmonary hypertension	Primary—may be associated with proliferation of vascular smooth muscle Secondary—owing to COPD or increased pulmonary blood flow (as seen with a left-to-right shunt)	Loud S2 **Left parasternal heave due to right ventricular hypertrophy** Heart failure cells	Leads to cor **pulmonale**
Pulmonary embolism	Commonly from proximal **deep vein thrombosis** (usually lower limb such as femoral veins) as a result of **Virchow triad:** blood stasis, endothelial damage (fat, infection, trauma), and hypercoagulable states	**Respiratory alkalosis; increased A–a gradient; hemorrhagic,** red, wedge-shaped infarct Acute-onset dyspnea, chest pain, tachycardia, hypotension *V/Q* ratio approaches infinity saddle embolus—an embolus lodged at the pulmonary artery bifurcation, often fatal	Can lead to cardiovascular collapse and sudden death

(continued)

QUICK HIT

Decreased breath sounds and hyporesonance indicate pleural effusion.

QUICK HIT

Lab values expected in a pneumothorax include increased P_{CO_2}, depressed P_{O_2}, acidotic pH, and compensatory increase in bicarbonate.

QUICK HIT

Bronchial obstruction can also lead to tracheal deviation with decreased breath sounds; however, in this case, the tracheal deviation is toward the side of the lesion because of the loss of volume. Decreased ventilation to the affected lung also leads to loss of tactile fremitus and hyporesonance.

QUICK HIT

Flail chest is caused by multiple fractures of consecutive ribs (each fractured in at least two places), leading to paradoxical movement of the injured area of the chest wall with respiration.

QUICK HIT

The clinical settings in which a pulmonary embolus can occur include cancer, multiple fractures, oral contraceptive use, prolonged bed rest, or CHF.

QUICK HIT

Fat emboli are often caused by crush injury with fracture of the long bones and orthopedic surgery.

QUICK HIT

Pulmonary edema caused by heart failure is characterized histologically by hemosiderin-laden macrophages ("heart failure cells") and congested alveolar capillaries.

QUICK HIT

Chronic obstructive pulmonary disease (COPD) is characterized by airflow obstruction. This is in contrast to restrictive pulmonary diseases, which demonstrate defective lung expansion. Obstructive disorders have increased TLC, decreased FEV_1, and decreased FEV_1/FVC. Restrictive disorders show reduced lung volumes and normal or increased FEV_1/FVC. Normal FEV_1/FVC ratio is approximately 80%.

QUICK HIT

Status asthmaticus is a prolonged asthmatic attack that does not respond to therapy and can be fatal.

QUICK HIT

There are many types of asthma, including extrinsic (children), intrinsic (adults), exercise induced, and cold air induced.

QUICK HIT

Reid index: Ratio (normally > 0.4) between the thickness of the submucosal mucus-secreting glands and the thickness between the epithelium and cartilage overlying the bronchus.

QUICK HIT

"Blue bloater": Blue refers to cyanosis; bloater refers to the peripheral edema in these patients from pulmonary hypertension and right ventricular overload.

TABLE 4-3 **Pulmonary Vascular Diseases** *(Continued)*

Disease	Etiology	Features	Complications
Pulmonary edema	Obliteration of alveoli as a result of intra-alveolar accumulation of fluid	Heart failure or overload leads to **increased hydrostatic pressure** Inflammatory alveolar reactions (caused by drugs, pneumonia, sepsis, and uremia) leads to **increased capillary permeability**	Hypoxia
Wegener granulomatosis	Etiology is unknown but thought to be autoimmune in nature	Focal necrotizing **vasculitis** affecting small-sized to medium-sized vessels Acute necrotizing **granulomas of upper and lower respiratory tract** Bilateral nodular and cavitary infiltrates seen on chest radiograph Mucosal ulceration of nasopharynx seen on examination Associated with c-ANCA	Untreated disease is fatal within several years

A–a gradient, Alveolar–arterial gradient; c-ANCA, cytoplasmic antineutrophil cytoplasmic antibody; COPD, chronic obstructive pulmonary disease; V/Q, ventilation/perfusion.

CHRONIC OBSTRUCTIVE PULMONARY DISEASE

I. Types of chronic obstructive pulmonary disease (COPD) *(Table 4-4)*

TABLE 4-4 **Types of Chronic Obstructive Pulmonary Disease**

Disease	Pathophysiology	Clinical Features and Management
Asthma	**Increased sensitivity** of bronchioles causes bronchoconstriction, muscle hypertrophy, **Curschmann spirals** (twisted, mucus casts of small airways), and **Charcot–Leyden crystals** (enzymes present within eosinophils)	**Cough, wheezing,** dyspnea; common treatment options include inhaled steroids and β_2-agonists
Chronic bronchitis	Caused by persistent irritants and infections; most common cause is smoking; hyperplasia of goblet cells and submucosal glands **(increased Reid index); excess mucus;** possible cor pulmonale	**Productive cough** for at least 3 consecutive months over 2 consecutive years; cyanosis due to decreased O_2 saturation, wheezing; "blue bloater"; chronic respiratory acidosis as mucus plugs block the exhalation of CO_2; **smoking cessation**

(continued)

TABLE 4-4 **Types of Chronic Obstructive Pulmonary Disease** *(Continued)*

Disease	Pathophysiology	Clinical Features and Management
Emphysema	Dilated alveoli; damaged alveolar walls; **damaged alveolar septae** leads to **enlarged alveolar airspaces;** destruction of structural support to lymphatic vessels leads to heavy pigment deposition; **decreased elastic recoil;** centrilobular (associated with smoking), panacinar (α_1-antitrypsin deficiency), paraseptal (associated with scarred tissue, may lead to spontaneous pneumothorax in young patients), and irregular forms	"Pink puffer"; paraseptal type may lead to pneumothorax; anteroposterior diameter increased ("barrel chested"); hypertrophy of accessory respiratory muscles; episodes of nonproductive cough; **smoking cessation**
Bronchiectasis	**Chronic infection leads to irreversible bronchial dilation;** destruction of bronchial wall; commonly caused by bronchial **obstruction** (e.g., tumor)	Copious amounts of purulent sputum; hemoptysis; possible lung abscess; associated with CF and Kartagener syndrome

CF, cystic fibrosis; CO_2, carbon dioxide; COPD, chronic obstructive pulmonary disease.

II. Therapeutic agents used in asthma and COPD *(Table 4-5)*

A. Inhaled agents

1. β_2-Agonists
   a. β_2-Agonists are useful for treatment of an acute asthma attack characterized by SOB, chest tightness, wheezing, and cough as a result of bronchoconstriction.
   - The β_2-agonists stimulate adenylyl cyclase, resulting in the conversion of adenosine triphosphate (ATP) to cyclic adenosine monophosphate (cAMP); the increased levels of cAMP result in myriad effects, depending on the cell type in question.
   - β_2-Agonists are potent dilators of the bronchi. They act by relaxing smooth muscle in the airways.
   - Systemic activation of β_2-specific receptors (which is minimal with inhaled β_2-agonists) may result in vasodilation, a slight decrease in peripheral resistance, bronchodilation, increased glycogenolysis in muscle and in the liver, increased release of glucagons, and relaxation of uterine smooth muscle.

   b. Side effects include tachycardia, hyperglycemia, hypokalemia, and hypomagnesemia.
   c. β_2-Agonists have no effect on the inflammation associated with asthma.
   d. Selected β_2-agonists:
   - **Albuterol** or **terbutaline** provides immediate relief of acute attacks without β_1-adrenoceptor stimulation.
   - **Salmeterol** has a longer duration of action and a slower onset of action.

2. Corticosteroids
   a. In cases of moderate asthma, corticosteroids (inhaled or systemic) can be used to decrease the associated inflammation.
   b. Inhaled corticosteroids such as beclomethasone, triamcinolone, and flunisolide decrease the effect that inflammatory cells (mast cells, eosinophils, macrophages) have on the airway.

QUICK HIT

Emphysema and bronchitis often coexist in the same patient.

QUICK HIT

Two types of emphysema: Centriacinar primarily affects the respiratory bronchioles, is associated with smoking, and predominantly involves the upper lobes; panacinar is dilation of the entire alveolus, predominantly involves the lower segments, and involves α_1-antitrypsin deficiency.

QUICK HIT

In emphysema, smoking attracts neutrophils, which release elastase. α_1-Antitrypsin normally inhibits elastase; however, free radicals caused by smoking inhibit α_1-antitrypsin, allowing elastase to damage the alveolar walls, causing dilation.

QUICK HIT

"Pink puffer": Pink refers to the lack of cyanosis from the nearly normal arterial oxygen pressures; puffer refers to the severe dyspnea seen in these patients.

QUICK HIT

Order of β-agonist potency (most potent to least potent): isoproterenol, epinephrine, and norepinephrine. Order of α-agonist potency (most potent to least potent): epinephrine, norepinephrine, and isoproterenol.

QUICK HIT

β_2-Selective agents such as terbutaline can be used in premature labor to prevent contractions.

TABLE 4-5 Therapeutic Agents for Asthma and Chronic Obstructive Pulmonary Disease

Therapeutic Agent (common name, if relevant) [trade name, where appropriate]	Class–Pharmacology and Pharmacokinetics	Indications	Side Effects or Adverse Effects	Contraindications or Precautions to Consider; Notes
Epinephrine [Primatene Mist]	Adrenergic agonist (nonselective)—relaxes bronchial smooth muscle through β_2-receptor activity	Asthma	Tachycardia (β_1-receptor activity)	
Isoproterenol [Isuprel]	β-agonist (nonselective)—relaxes bronchial smooth muscle through β_2-receptor activity	Asthma	Tachycardia (β_1-receptor activity)	
Albuterol [Proventil, Ventolin], **levalbuterol** [Xopenex]	**β_2-agonist—leads to relaxation of smooth muscle**	Asthma, **COPD,** bronchitis	**Tremor, tachycardia, arrhythmia,** headache, nausea, vomiting	
Salmeterol [Serevent]	**Long-acting β_2-agonist—leads to relaxation of smooth muscle**	Asthma prophylaxis	**Hand tremor,** headache, nervousness, dizziness, cough, stuffed nose, runny nose, muscle pain/cramps, sore throat	Not for acute asthmatic attacks
Theophylline [Aerolate, Theo-24, Theo-Dur, Theolair, Uniphyl]	Methylxanthines—unknown mechanism; may inhibit phosphodiesterase → decreases cAMP hydrolysis → promotes bronchodilation; stimulates CNS, cardiac muscle; relaxes smooth muscle; produces diuresis; increases cerebral vascular resistance	Asthma	Cardiotoxicity, neurotoxicity	Metabolized by cytochrome P450. Narrow therapeutic window
Ipratropium [Atrovent]	Muscarinic antagonist—competitively blocks muscarinic receptors → prevents bronchoconstriction	Asthma, COPD		
Beclomethasone, dexamethasone, prednisone	Corticosteroids—inhibits leukotriene synthesis → reduces inflammation and leads to bronchodilation	Asthma, COPD	**Osteoporosis, Cushingoid reaction, psychosis, glucose intolerance, infection, hypertension, cataracts, acne**	
Zileuton	Antileukotriene—**5-lipoxygenase inhibitor** → inhibits conversion of arachidonic acid to leukotriene → prevents bronchoconstriction and inflammatory cell infiltration	Asthma		
Zafirlukast [Accolate], **montelukast** [Singulair]	Antileukotriene—**blocks leukotriene receptors (LTD_4)** → prevents bronchoconstriction and inflammatory cell infiltration	Asthma (especially Aspirin-induced asthma)		
Cromolyn	Prevents release of mediators from mast cells → prevents bronchoconstriction and inflammation	Asthma prophylaxis		Not for acute asthmatic attacks
Nedocromil [Tilade]	Stabilizes membranes of mast cells and prevents mediator release	Asthma	Unpleasant taste	Not for acute asthmatic attacks

cAMP, cyclic adenosine monophosphate; CNS, central nervous system; COPD, chronic obstructive pulmonary disease; LTD_4, leukotriene D_4.

Clinical Vignette 4-1

CLINICAL PRESENTATION: A 59-year-old woman presents with a chief complaint of **shortness of breath (SOB).** Patient states she has been experiencing worsening SOB with minimal physical exertion. She has been experiencing bouts of **productive cough** every morning for the past 2 years. She has smoked two packs of cigarettes a day for the past 35 years. Patient denies any fevers or bloody sputum. Physical exam reveals an **increased anteroposterior diameter of the chest wall** and **wheezes** and **rhonchi** on inspiration. Temperature = 98.3° F; blood pressure = 142/92 mm Hg; heart rate = 93 bpm; respiration rate = 23 breaths/min.
DIFFERENTIALS: COPD, asthma, CHF. Given the patient's presentation and long-standing history of smoking, this patient most likely has COPD.
LABORATORY STUDIES: Proper follow-up management would include an **arterial blood gas** to provide information regarding the patient's O_2 status because hypoxemia and hypercapnia may be present. **Spirometry** is the next best step in the evaluation process. **Flow volume loops** will assist in identifying restrictive from obstructive pulmonary disease. A forced expiratory volume at 1 second/forced vital capacity ratio in obstructive pulmonary diseases will be below the normal ratio of 0.8.
MANAGEMENT: Initial step in management is smoking cessation. **β-Agonists and anticholinergic agents** provide bronchodilation via nebulizers. Administration of **oxygen** is necessary to correct hypoxemia. **Corticosteroids** can be used in acute exacerbations along with **antibiotics** if there is suspicion of an underlying infection.

c. In cases of severe asthma, intravenous methylprednisolone or oral prednisone may be necessary for a short period.
d. The side effects of inhaled steroids are minimal when compared with systemic steroid use. However, adverse reactions can occur and include oral candidiasis, and, with long-term use, osteoporosis.

B. Other asthma medications
1. **Cromolyn**, a prophylactic anti-inflammatory agent
2. **Ipratropium**, a derivative of atropine that blocks the vagal aspect of airway smooth muscle contraction and mucus secretion
3. **Theophylline**, a bronchodilator, which may result in seizures and arrhythmias
4. Newer agents
a. **Zileuton**, a 5-lipoxygenase inhibitor, blocks the conversion of arachidonic acid into leukotrienes, which are responsible for chemotaxis, increased secretion, and bronchospasm.
b. **Zafirlukast** prevents the chemotactic and bronchospastic effects of leukotriene D_4 (LTD_4) by blocking its receptor.

QUICK HIT

Agents useful in the treatment of an acute COPD exacerbation include albuterol, ipratropium, systemic corticosteroids, and doxycycline. Even in the absence of a respiratory infection, doxycycline has anti-inflammatory properties, which are useful in an acute exacerbation.

QUICK HIT

Agents useful in treating acute asthmatic exacerbation include albuterol, ipratropium, systemic corticosteroids, and magnesium. The use of leukotriene receptor antagonists may also be helpful in the acute setting, although this is controversial.

QUICK HIT

Agents useful in the long-term management of chronic asthma include inhaled β-agonists (both short acting and long acting), inhaled corticosteroids, cromolyn, theophylline, and antileukotrienes.

INTERSTITIAL LUNG DISEASE *(Table 4-6)*

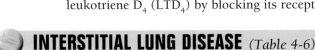

Insterstitial lung disease (ILD) is a noninfectious, nonmalignant condition characterized by inflammation and pathologic changes of the alveolar wall. Differentiation and diagnosis often require histologic evaluation of the lung. It is characterized as having decreased lung volumes and a normal to increased FEV_1/FVC ratio.

QUICK HIT

Interstitial lung disease (ILD) can be a side effect of bleomycin, methotrexate, and amiodarone.

QUICK HIT

Interstitial lung diseases demonstrate alveolar wall fibrosis.

TABLE 4-6 **Interstitial Lung Disease**

Disease	Pathophysiology	Population Most at Risk	Clinical Features
Eosinophilic granuloma	Presence of Langerhans-like cells and **Birbeck granules;** subset of histiocytosis X	Former **smokers**	Lesions in lung or ribs, pneumothorax
Goodpasture syndrome	Pulmonary hemorrhage, anemia, glomerulonephritis, **antibasement membrane antibodies**	Men, middle-aged people	Hemoptysis, hematuria

(continued)

QUICK HIT

Patients with sarcoidosis often demonstrate **anergy** when challenged with the tuberculin skin test despite a polyclonal hyperglobulinemia.

QUICK HIT

The three most common causes of hemoptysis are tuberculosis (TB), malignancy, and Goodpasture syndrome.

QUICK HIT

Bloody pleural effusions are most commonly from TB, malignancy, or trauma.

QUICK HIT

Anthracotic, blackened lungs are endemic to urban environments.

QUICK HIT

Silicosis is an occupational disease seen in individuals involved in mining, stonecutting, and glass production.

QUICK HIT

Malignant mesothelioma is most specific but not most commonly associated with asbestos exposure. Bronchogenic carcinoma is most commonly associated with asbestosis.

TABLE 4-6 Interstitial Lung Disease *(Continued)*

Disease	Pathophysiology	Population Most at Risk	Clinical Features
Idiopathic pulmonary fibrosis	Chronic **inflammation of alveolar wall;** leukocytes release cytokines that lead to fibrosis; cystic spaces	Sixth decade of life	**Honeycomb lung;** fatal within years
Sarcoidosis	Interstitial fibrosis; diagnosis by exclusion of other causes and biopsy showing **non-caseating granulomatous lesions;** asteroid and Schaumann bodies; increased angiotensin-converting enzyme levels; uveitis; polyarthritis; hypercalcemia; erythema nodosum; cardiomyopathy; central and peripheral neuropathies	**Young Black females**	Dyspnea on exertion, dry cough, fever, fatigue, bilateral hilar lymphadenopathy visible on chest x-ray, increased levels of angiotensin-converting enzyme, hypercalcemia
Hypersensitivity pneumonitis (farmer's lung, pigeon breeder's lung)	Prolonged exposure to organic antigens in atopic individuals; interstitial inflammation; alveolar damage leads to chronic, fibrotic lung	People with an occupational history of farming or bird-keeping	**Dry cough, chest tightness,** general malaise, and fever

ENVIRONMENTAL LUNG DISEASES (PNEUMOCONIOSIS) *(Table 4-7)*

This group of diseases is often caused by workplace exposure to various organic and chemical irritants. A careful history and pulmonary function testing are often important for diagnosis.

Approximately 70% to 80% of newly diagnosed pulmonary tuberculosis (TB) cases in adults are actually a result of reactivation of a clinically unsuspected infection acquired years to decades previously.

TABLE 4-7 Environmental Lung Diseases (Pneumoconiosis)

Disease	Pathophysiology	Clinical Features
Anthracosis	Carbon dust ingested by alveolar macrophages, visible **black deposits seen on gross lung tissue samples**	Usually asymptomatic
Asbestosis	Asbestos fibers ingested by alveolar macrophages, fibroblast proliferation, interstitial fibrosis (lower lobes), **asbestos bodies and ferruginous bodies (hemosiderin laden asbestos fibers),** pleural plaques and effusions	Increased risk of bronchogenic carcinoma and **malignant mesothelioma,** synergistic effect of asbestos and tobacco in causing bronchogenic carcinoma
Coal worker's pneumoconiosis	Carbon dust ingested by alveolar macrophages forms bronchiolar **macules;** may progress to fibrosis	Plaques are asymptomatic; often benign, may progress to fibrosis; may be fatal owing to pulmonary hypertension and **cor pulmonale; no evidence of increased risk for TB or lung cancer**
Silicosis	Silica dust ingested by alveolar macrophages causing release of harmful enzymes; **silicotic nodules** (of collagen that may calcify) and thick pleural scars	Nodules may obstruct air or blood flow; concurrent TB common **(silicotuberculosis)**
Berylliosis	Induction of cell-mediated immunity leads to non-caseating granulomas, several organ systems affected; histologically identical to sarcoidosis	Increases lung cancer

TB, tuberculosis.

RESPIRATORY INFECTIONS

I. Pneumonia

A. Pathogenesis

1. Most commonly, pneumonia is caused by **microaspiration** from the oropharynx or **inhalation of infectious droplets or particles**.
2. Alcoholism, nasogastric tubes, and obtunded states increase risk of contracting pneumonia.
3. Normal oral flora consists of gram-positive cocci.
4. Hospitalized patients may be colonized by gram-negative rods (nosocomial infections).
5. Other portals of entry include respiratory droplets, hematogenous spread, contiguous spread, and traumatic inoculation.

B. **Clinical manifestations**

1. **Typical pneumonia** presents with acute fever, purulent sputum, pleuritic pain, and lobar "whited out" infiltrate on chest radiograph (e.g., *Streptococcus pneumoniae*).
2. **Atypical pneumonia** is characterized by slow onset of nonproductive cough, headache, gastrointestinal (GI) symptoms, and diffuse patchy infiltrate on chest radiograph (e.g., *Mycoplasma pneumoniae*).
3. **Nosocomial pneumonia** commonly occurs in the setting of an underlying disease, immunosuppression, or use of a ventilator (e.g., *Pseudomonas aeruginosa, Escherichia coli*).

C. Location of pathology and typical organisms

1. **Lobar** (intra-alveolar infiltrate): *Streptococcus pneumoniae*
2. **Bronchopneumonia** (bronchiolar infiltrate): *Staphylococcus aureus, Haemophilus influenzae, Streptococcus pneumoniae*, viral
3. **Interstitial** (diffuse infiltrate in alveolar wall): *M. pneumoniae, Legionella, Pneumocystis jirovecii*, viral

D. Etiology

1. Bacterial and mycoplasmal pneumonias (Table 4-8)
2. Viral pneumonia (Table 4-9)
3. Fungal pneumonia (Table 4-10)
4. Clinical diagnosis of pneumonia (Tables 4-11 and 4-12)

QUICK HIT

The most likely cause for lung abscess formation in a comatose patient is aspiration pneumonia as a consequence of a depressed cough reflex. Other causes of lung abscess formation are septic emboli (from infective endocarditis), spread from adjacent organs, and malignant tumors.

QUICK HIT

Typical pneumonia is characterized histopathologically by intra-alveolar exudation of neutrophils, fibrin, erythrocytes, and bacteria. Sputum is essentially pus consisting of bacteria and neutrophils. However, because organisms causing atypical pneumonia are generally intracellular pathogens, we see the alveolar septae swollen with T cells and macrophages and therefore no sputum production (hence nonproductive cough).

TABLE 4-8 Bacterial and Mycoplasmal Pneumonia

Bacteria	Presentation	Population Most at Risk	Clinical Features
Streptococcus pneumoniae	Typical	**Adults**	Most common cause of community-acquired pneumonia
Haemophilus influenzae	Typical	Elderly	Complicates viral infection, chronic respiratory disease
Staphylococcus aureus	Typical	Can cause typical community-acquired pneumonia but also infects immunocompromised and hospitalized patients	Abscesses, complicates viral infection, especially influenza
Streptococcus agalactiae	Typical	**Neonates**	Similar to *Streptococcus pneumoniae*
Mycoplasma pneumoniae	Atypical	**Young adults**	Most common cause of atypical pneumonia; positive cold agglutinin test
Legionella pneumophila	Atypical	Immunocompromised patients	Found in drinking water and air conditioners
Klebsiella pneumoniae	Atypical	Patients with alcoholism	Aspiration of gastric contents
Chlamydophila psittaci	Atypical	**Pet bird** owners	Bradycardia, splenomegaly
Chlamydia trachomatis (trachoma)	Atypical	**Neonates**	Most common cause of *trachoma*, preventable blindness
Chlamydophila pneumoniae	Atypical	**Young adults**	Upper and lower pulmonary tract infection
Coxiella burnetii	Atypical	Dairy workers (via inhalation)	Fever
Francisella tularensis	Atypical	Hunters, veterinarians, livestock workers	Granulomatous nodules

QUICK HIT

Consolidation of lungs in bacterial pneumonia leads to increased fremitus because sounds are better transmitted through consolidation. Bronchial breath sounds may also be appreciated. Conversely, viral pneumonia should not cause lung consolidation, and therefore fremitus should be decreased.

QUICK HIT

Aspirin therapy for the fever of influenza and varicella zoster infections in children is contraindicated because it may cause Reye syndrome. Clinical manifestations of Reye syndrome include encephalopathy and potentially fatal liver damage.

QUICK HIT

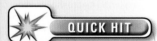

Other less common sources of fungal lung infection include *Cryptococcus neoformans* and *Aspergillus* in immunocompromised individuals.

QUICK HIT

Pneumocystis jirovecii is now classified as a fungus but was previously classified as a protozoa.

TABLE 4-9 Viral Pneumonia

Virus	Pathophysiology	Clinical Features
Respiratory syncytial virus (types 1 and 2)	Atypical	Also causes bronchiolitis; more common in winter months; can cause serious respiratory distress in infants
Influenza	Atypical	**Often complicated by secondary bacterial infection**

TABLE 4-10 Fungal Pneumonia

Etiology	Pathophysiology	Clinical Features
Histoplasma capsulatum	Atypical	Most infections are subclinical; tiny yeast forms in macrophages; found in Ohio, Mississippi, and Missouri River Valleys; yeast with a thin cell wall but no true capsule
Coccidioides immitis	Atypical	Most infections are subclinical; nonbudding spherules filled with endospores; "valley fever" found in southwestern deserts of United States
Pneumocystis jirovecii	Atypical	Often fatal common opportunistic infection in immunocompromised patients (such as patients with HIV)
Paracoccidioides brasiliensis	Atypical	Budding yeast resemble spokes of a "captain's wheel"; found in Central and South Americas; yeast with multiple budding
Sporotrichosis	Atypical	Skin nodules that occur along lymphatics in the arms of rose gardeners
Aspergillus	Atypical	Fungal ball of hyphae (aspergilloma) in preexisting lung cavities or invasive pulmonary disease in immunocompromised patients
Blastomyces dermatitidis	Atypical	Yeast forms in body; 5–25-mm yeast with thick refractile wall and broad-based budding; found in Mississippi–Ohio River basins and around the Great Lakes
Candida albicans	Atypical	Yeast and hyphae
Cryptococcus neoformans	Atypical	Yeast with broad capsule

TABLE 4-11 Clinical Diagnosis of Pneumonia

	Bacterial	Viral	Mycoplasma
Age	Any; often younger than 2 years old	Any	Young adults (teenagers)
Fever	>102.28° F	<102.28° F	<102.28° F
Onset	Abrupt	Gradual	Gradual fever, gradual cough
Relatives	Healthy	Sick (concurrent)	Sick (2–3 weeks previous)
Cough	Productive	Dry	Paroxysmal
Pleuritic chest pain	Yes (splinting)	No	No
Physical examination	Tubular breath sounds; dull to percussion	Bilateral, diffuse rales	Rales in one or two segments
Radiographic findings	Consolidated "whited out" lobe	Diffuse, patchy, bilateral	Patchy; one or two lobes; no consolidation

TABLE 4-12 Most Common Causative Agents of Pneumonia by Age

Neonates (Birth–4 weeks)	Children (1 month–20 years)	Young Adults (20–40 years)	Adults (40–60 years)	Elderly (≥60 years)
Group B streptococcus	Viral: RSV, parainfluenza, influenza	*Mycoplasma pneumoniae*	*Streptococcus pneumoniae*	*S. pneumoniae*
Escherichia coli	*S. pneumoniae*	*S. pneumoniae*	*M. pneumoniae*	Anaerobes
	M. pneumoniae	*Chlamydophila pneumoniae*	*Haemophilus influenzae*	*H. influenzae*
	C. pneumoniae		Viruses	Gram-negative rods
			Anaerobes	

RSV, respiratory syncytial virus.

QUICK HIT

Primary TB occurs in the upper part of the lower lobe or lower part of the upper lobe. However, secondary TB occurs in the apical area.

MNEMONIC

Miliary TB—think millet seed to remember multiple seedlike, white-gray lesions.

II. Tuberculosis and its treatment *(Figure 4-7)*

A. Multiple drug therapy is used for the treatment of TB in an effort to combat drug resistance.

B. A common therapeutic regimen includes **isoniazid** (INH), **rifampin**, **ethambutol**, and **pyrazinamide** for a period of 2 months, followed by INH and rifampin for a period of 4 to 7 months.

1. INH
   a. INH, which diffuses into all body fluids, including breast milk, targets the outer layer of the mycobacteria.
   b. A common side effect of INH therapy is paresthesia, which can be corrected by the administration of **pyridoxine** (vitamin B_6).
2. Rifampin
   a. Rifampin inhibits RNA synthesis by blocking the β subunit of bacterial DNA-dependent RNA polymerase.
   b. Rifampin also induces **cytochrome P450 enzymes** in the liver and can decrease the half-lives of other agents in this way.
   c. One side effect of rifampin is the **orange-red color** of bodily fluids.

QUICK HIT

Mycobacterium tuberculosis are acid-fast bacteria because they have an envelope that contains large amounts of lipid and even true waxes that prevent the acid-fast stain (carbolfuchsin) from leaking out.

QUICK HIT

Rifampin decreases the half-lives of oral contraceptives as well as warfarin, digitoxin, ketoconazole, propranolol, and prednisone. Consequently, higher doses of these medications may be required to achieve the same therapeutic effect.

FIGURE 4-7 Tuberculosis

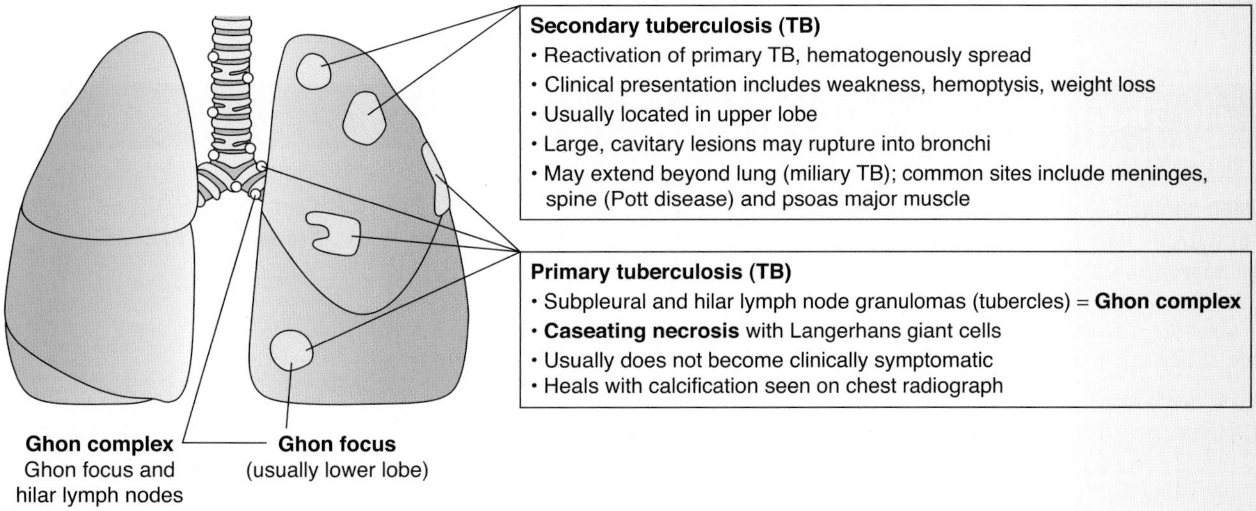
Secondary tuberculosis (TB)
• Reactivation of primary TB, hematogenously spread
• Clinical presentation includes weakness, hemoptysis, weight loss
• Usually located in upper lobe
• Large, cavitary lesions may rupture into bronchi
• May extend beyond lung (miliary TB); common sites include meninges, spine (Pott disease) and psoas major muscle
Primary tuberculosis (TB)
• Subpleural and hilar lymph node granulomas (tubercles) = Ghon complex
• Caseating necrosis with Langerhans giant cells
• Usually does not become clinically symptomatic
• Heals with calcification seen on chest radiograph
Ghon complex
Ghon focus and hilar lymph nodes
Ghon focus
(usually lower lobe)

III. Upper respiratory infections

A. Otitis externa—most common cause is *P. aeruginosa*

B. Otitis media—most pathogens involved are *S. pneumoniae* and nontypable *H. influenzae*

C. Sinusitis
   1. Results from obstructed drainage outlets of the sinuses
   2. Caused by *S. pneumoniae, H. influenzae,* and *Moraxella*

D. Rhinitis
   1. Viral rhinitis
      a. Most commonly caused by rhinoviruses and coronaviruses, also by adenoviruses and parainfluenza viruses
      b. Common cold
   2. Bacterial rhinitis
      a. Often secondary to viral infection
      b. Commonly caused by *Streptococcus, Staphylococcus,* and *H. influenzae*
   3. Allergic rhinitis
      a. Type I hypersensitivity reactions
      b. Characterized by eosinophilia

E. Laryngitis
   1. Characterized by edema and inflammation of the vocal cords
   2. Caused by infection (*M. pneumoniae,* parainfluenza virus) or overuse

F. Croup versus epiglottitis (Table 4-13)

IV. Therapeutic agents *(Table 4-14)*

QUICK HIT

Parainfluenza virus causes a disease resembling the common cold in adults and is transmitted via respiratory droplets.

QUICK HIT

The incidence of epiglottitis caused by *Haemophilus influenzae* has decreased dramatically with the introduction of the *H. influenzae* type B vaccine. *H. influenzae* can also cause meningitis in unvaccinated children.

TABLE 4-13 **Croup versus Epiglottitis**

	Croup	Epiglottitis
Organism	Parainfluenza virus (type 1 or 2)	*Haemophilus influenzae* type B
Pathology	Inflammation of subglottic trachea	Inflamed epiglottis
Age	6 months to 2 years	1–5 years
Fever	<102° F	>102° F
Onset	**Gradual** (barking cough to **stridor**)	**Abrupt; stridor**
Associated symptoms	Rhinorrhea, hoarseness, conjunctivitis	None
Degree of illness	Not toxic, degree of symptoms greater than degree of illness	Toxic
Physical examination	Writhing, anxious, **subglottic edema and "steeple sign"** on radiograph	Quiet, **"sniffing position,"** drooling, **"thumbprint"** epiglottis on radiograph
Outcome	Self-limiting	Medical emergency; 90% of patients require surgery to reestablish airway

TABLE 4-14 **Therapeutic Agents for Allergy, Cough, and Cold**

Therapeutic Agent (common name, if relevant) [trade name, where appropriate]	Class–Pharmacology and Pharmacokinetics	Indications	Side Effects or Adverse Effects	Contraindications or Precautions to Consider; Notes
Diphenhydramine, dimenhydrinate, chlorpheniramine	H_1 blocker (first generation)	Allergy, motion sickness, insomnia	Sedation, anti-muscarinic, anti-α adrenergic	
Loratadine, fexofenadine, desloratadine, cetirizine	H_1 blocker (second generation)	Allergy	Sedating	Less sedating than first-generation H_1 blocker due to decreased CNS entry

(continued)

TABLE 4-14 **Therapeutic Agents for Allergy, Cough, and Cold** *(Continued)*

Therapeutic Agent (common name, if relevant) [trade name, where appropriate]	Class–Pharmacology and Pharmacokinetics	Indications	Side Effects or Adverse Effects	Contraindications or Precautions to Consider; Notes
Fluticasone [Flonase], beclomethasone, flunisolide [Nasarel], budesonide [Rhinocort], mometasone furoate	Intranasal glucocorticoids—decrease cytokine synthesis, downregulate inflammatory response in the nasal mucosa	Nasal congestion, allergic rhinitis	Local irritation of nasal mucosa, epistaxis	
Guaifenesin [Robitussin]	Expectorant—thins mucus and lubricates irritated respiratory tract	Cough associated with common cold and minor upper respiratory tract infections		Does not suppress cough reflex
N-acetylcysteine	Mucolytic—loosens mucus plugs	Cough (especially in patients with CF), acetaminophen overdose		

CF, cystic fibrosis; CNS, central nervous system.

CYSTIC FIBROSIS

I. Cystic fibrosis (CF) is the most common lethal genetic disease in Caucasians.

II. Autosomal recessive mutation occurs on chromosome 7, the CF transmembrane conductance regulator (CFTR) gene. This leads to:

A. Deletion of phenylalanine at position 508 in 90% of patients with CF in the United States

B. Altered chloride and water transport in epithelial cells

C. High sodium and chloride concentrations on sweat test

D. Increased mucosal viscosity obstructs exocrine glands, which leads to organ failure

E. An abnormally high rate of sodium absorption from luminal secretions and a decreased rate of chloride secretion into luminal secretions reduce the salt and water content of bronchiolar secretions.

III. Chronic pulmonary disease

A. Most serious complication and leading cause of death in patients with CF

B. *P. aeruginosa* infections are the most common in adults, followed by *S. aureus* and *H. influenzae*. In children, *S. aureus* is the most common infection.

C. Increased residual volume (RV) and increased total lung capacity (TLC) are characteristics of COPD.

D. Atelectasis

E. Bronchiectasis

IV. Pancreatic insufficiency

A. Nutritional deficiencies (especially of fat-soluble vitamins A, D, E, and K)

B. Steatorrhea

C. β-Cells are initially spared but become functionally inactive with age, leading to an increased need for insulin.

V. Meconium ileus

A. Usually presents in infant with abdominal distention, small bowel obstruction, and emesis

QUICK HIT

N-acetylcysteine is indicated for the treatment of acetaminophen overdose, as a mucolytic in CF, and is used off-label as prophylaxis against radiocontrast-induced nephropathy.

QUICK HIT

Superior sulcus tumors (**Pancoast tumors**) involve the apex of the lung and result in **Horner syndrome** (ptosis, miosis, anhydrosis). **Superior vena cava (SVC) syndrome** occurs when the SVC is obstructed, resulting in facial cyanosis and swelling.

VI. Treatment of CF includes symptomatic treatment and gene therapy.

A. Mucolytics: *N*-acetylcysteine lyses the disulfide linkages between mucoproteins, resulting in decreased mucus viscosity.

B. **Inhaled bronchodilators**

C. Corticosteroids: Prednisone has been shown to increase pulmonary function and body weight in patients with CF.

D. **Antibiotics as needed to manage infections**

LUNG NEOPLASMS *(Tables 4-15 to 4-17)*

I. Lung neoplasms are the leading cause of cancer death for both men and women in the United States.

II. Lung is the second most common type of cancer (with the first being prostate cancer in men and breast cancer in women).

III. Lung cancer deaths among women are rising rapidly as a result of increased smoking in this population.

IV. Symptoms include cough, hemoptysis, airway obstruction, weight loss, and paraneoplastic syndromes.

TABLE 4-15 **Lung Neoplasms**

Tumor	Location and Histology	Clinical Features
Adenocarcinoma	**Peripheral;** subpleural; usually on preexisting parenchymal **scars;** glandular	**Most common type;** may be related to smoking; CEA-positive; K-*ras* oncogenes
Bronchioalveolar	**Peripheral;** subtype of adenocarcinoma; tumor cells line alveolar walls	**Less strongly associated with smoking;** autoantibodies to surfactant may exist
Carcinoid	Major bronchi; spread by direct extension	Increased secretion of **5-HT,** flushing, wheezing, recurrent diarrhea, heart disease, low malignancy
Large cell	**Peripheral;** undifferentiated; giant cells with pleomorphism	Poor prognosis; metastasis to the brain; smoking
Metastasis	**Cannonball** lesions	**Higher incidence than primary lung cancer**
Small cell (oat cell)	**Central;** undifferentiated; **most aggressive;** small, dark blue cells; arise from neuroendocrine (Kulchitsky) cells	Poor prognosis; strongly associated with smoking; ectopic ACTH; ADH secretion
Squamous cell	**Central;** mass from bronchus; keratin pearls; cavitation	Strongly associated with smoking; secretion of **PTH-like peptide**

5-HT, serotonin; ACTH, adrenocorticotropic hormone; ADH, antidiuretic hormone; CEA, carcinoembryonic antigen; PTH, parathyroid hormone.

QUICK HIT

Nasopharyngeal carcinoma, common in Southeast Asia and East Africa, is caused by the Epstein–Barr virus.

TABLE 4-16 **Other Respiratory Carcinomas**

Tumor	Histology	Risk Factors
Nasopharyngeal carcinoma	Lymphoepithelioma (rich in lymphocytes)	Epstein–Barr virus infection; common in Southeast Asia (adult) and East Africa (childhood)
Laryngeal carcinoma	Squamous cell carcinoma	Smoking

TABLE 4-17 **Paraneoplastic Syndromes of Lung Cancer**

Disorder	Causes and Clinical Presentation
Horner syndrome	Superior sulcus tumors (Pancoast tumors); ptosis, miosis, anhidrosis
Superior vena cava (SVC) syndrome	Insidious compression or obstruction of the SVC; facial cyanosis, facial swelling, headache, venous distention of the neck, upper chest, and arms
Cushing syndrome	**ACTH** secretion; associated with small cell carcinoma; fat deposition of the face (moon faces), upper back (buffalo hump), truncal obesity, muscle weakness, purple striae
Hypercalcemia	Secretion of **PTH-related protein** (PTHrP); associated with **squamous cell lung cancer**
SIADH	Ectopic **antidiuretic hormone (ADH)** production; hyponatremia (Na^+ below 120 mEq/L)
Lambert–Eaton myasthenic syndrome	Proximal muscle weakness with autonomic dysfunction; antibodies produced against presynaptic calcium channels of the neuromuscular junction, no improvement with administration of anticholinesterase agents

ACTH, adrenocorticotropic hormone; PTH, parathyroid hormone; SIADH, syndrome of inappropriate antidiuretic hormone.

QUICK HIT

Paraneoplastic syndrome is a clinical and biochemical disturbance caused by a neoplasm that is not directly related to the primary tumor or metastases. Secretion of parathyroid hormone (PTH)–like hormone results in hypercalcemia. Ectopic antidiuretic hormone (ADH) production leads to syndrome of inappropriate antidiuretic hormone (SIADH) secretion with urinary retention and high urine osmolality. Adrenocorticotropic hormone (ACTH)–producing tumors lead to Cushing syndrome.

MNEMONIC

To remember the symptoms of Horner syndrome, think "PAM is Horny." P is ptosis, A is anhydrosis, M is miosis.

MNEMONIC

To remember the location, risk factors, and hormone-producing properties for small cell and squamous cell carcinoma, think **s** with **c**entral, **s**moking, and **s**ecretions.

Clinical Vignette 4-2

CLINICAL PRESENTATION: A 74-year-old man presents with shortness of breath, a chronic **bloody cough, increased fatigue, and a weight loss of 20 lb over a 3-month period.** Past medical history is significant for **hypertension, emphysema, coronary artery disease**, and a 26-pack-year history of **smoking.** Physical examination reveals wheezing in the right upper lobe. Temperature = 98.7° F; blood pressure = 140/92 mm Hg; heart rate = 80 bpm; and respiration rate = 25 breaths/min.

DIFFERENTIALS: Lung cancer, TB, pneumonia, left heart failure. Given the patient's presentation and long-standing history of smoking, this patient most likely has lung cancer. The two most common causes of hemoptysis in the United States are bronchitis and lung cancer.

LABORATORY STUDIES: Proper follow-up for this patient would include imaging, such as a chest **CT scan** or a **chest x-ray.** If imaging reveals a mass, **bronchoscopy** can be performed to obtain cells via brushings, bronchoalveolar lavage, or biopsy. **CT-guided fine needle biopsy** can also be performed to gather cells.

MANAGEMENT: Treatments include **surgical resection** and **chemotherapy** independently or in combination with **radiation.** Non–small cell lung cancer should be staged using the TNM (tumor, node, metastasis) system. Patients with stage I or II non–small cell lung cancers can be cured with surgical resection and radiotherapy. Small cell lung cancer often has metastasized at the time of diagnosis, making surgical resection futile and limiting radiotherapy and chemotherapy as the only treatment options.

DRUGS THAT CAUSE ADVERSE EFFECTS TO THE RESPIRATORY SYSTEM

I. Pulmonary fibrosis: bleomycin (antineoplastic), amiodarone (antiarrhythmic), busulfan (antineoplastic)

II. Cough: angiotensin-converting enzyme inhibitors (versus angiotensin II receptor blockers = no cough)

5 The Gastrointestinal System

INNERVATION AND BLOOD SUPPLY OF THE GASTROINTESTINAL TRACT *(Figure 5-1)*

FIGURE 5-1 **Innervation and blood supply of the gastrointestinal tract**

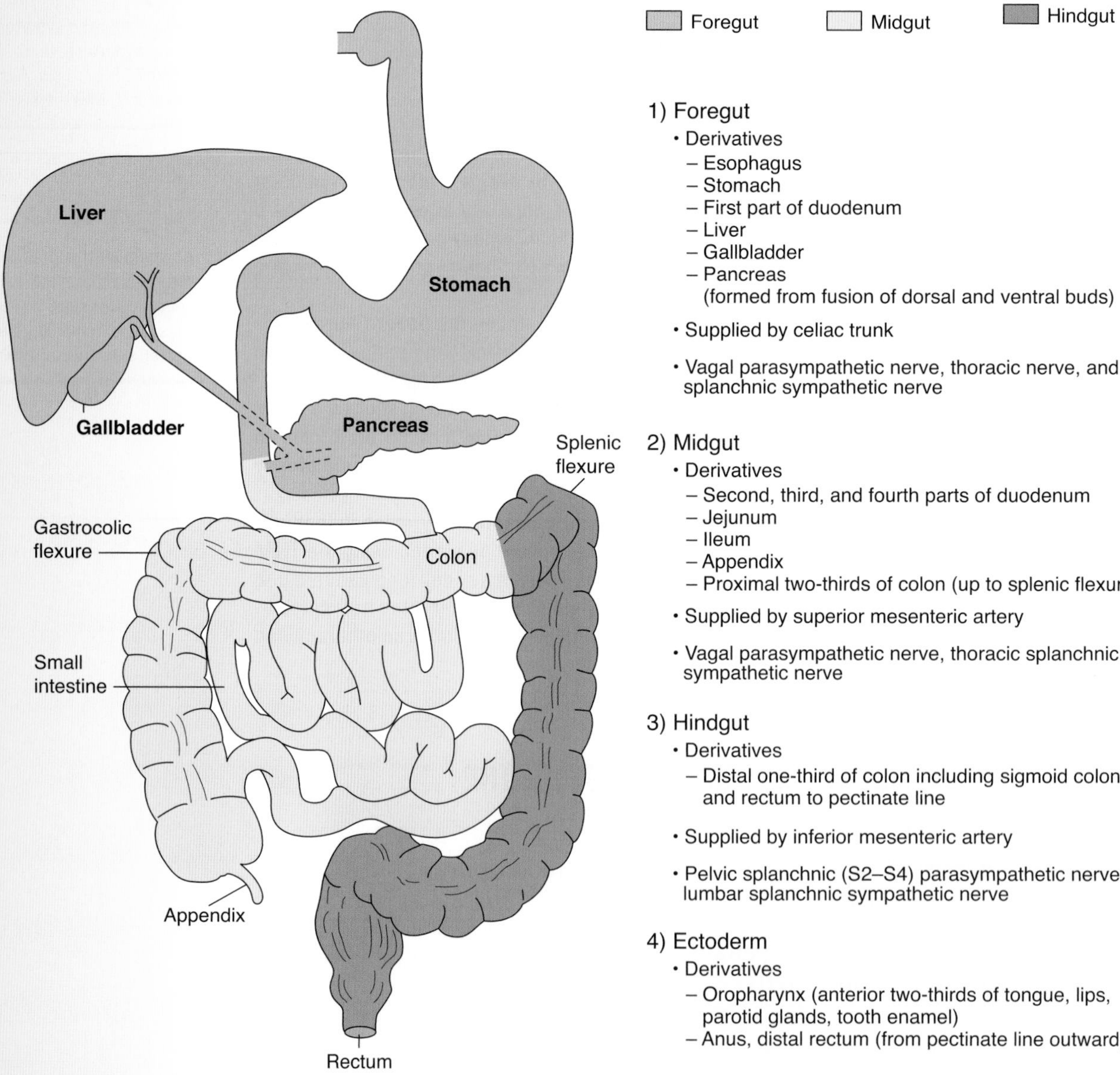

Liver
Stomach
Gallbladder
Pancreas
Splenic flexure
Gastrocolic flexure
Colon
Small intestine
Appendix
Rectum
Foregut
Midgut
Hindgut

1) Foregut
   - Derivatives
     - Esophagus
     - Stomach
     - First part of duodenum
     - Liver
     - Gallbladder
     - Pancreas (formed from fusion of dorsal and ventral buds)
   - Supplied by celiac trunk
   - Vagal parasympathetic nerve, thoracic nerve, and splanchnic sympathetic nerve

2) Midgut
   - Derivatives
     - Second, third, and fourth parts of duodenum
     - Jejunum
     - Ileum
     - Appendix
     - Proximal two-thirds of colon (up to splenic flexure)
   - Supplied by superior mesenteric artery
   - Vagal parasympathetic nerve, thoracic splanchnic sympathetic nerve

3) Hindgut
   - Derivatives
     - Distal one-third of colon including sigmoid colon and rectum to pectinate line
   - Supplied by inferior mesenteric artery
   - Pelvic splanchnic (S2–S4) parasympathetic nerve and lumbar splanchnic sympathetic nerve

4) Ectoderm
   - Derivatives
     - Oropharynx (anterior two-thirds of tongue, lips, parotid glands, tooth enamel)
     - Anus, distal rectum (from pectinate line outward)

HORMONES OF THE GASTROINTESTINAL SYSTEM *(Figure 5-2)*

FIGURE 5-2 **Hormones of the gastrointestinal system**

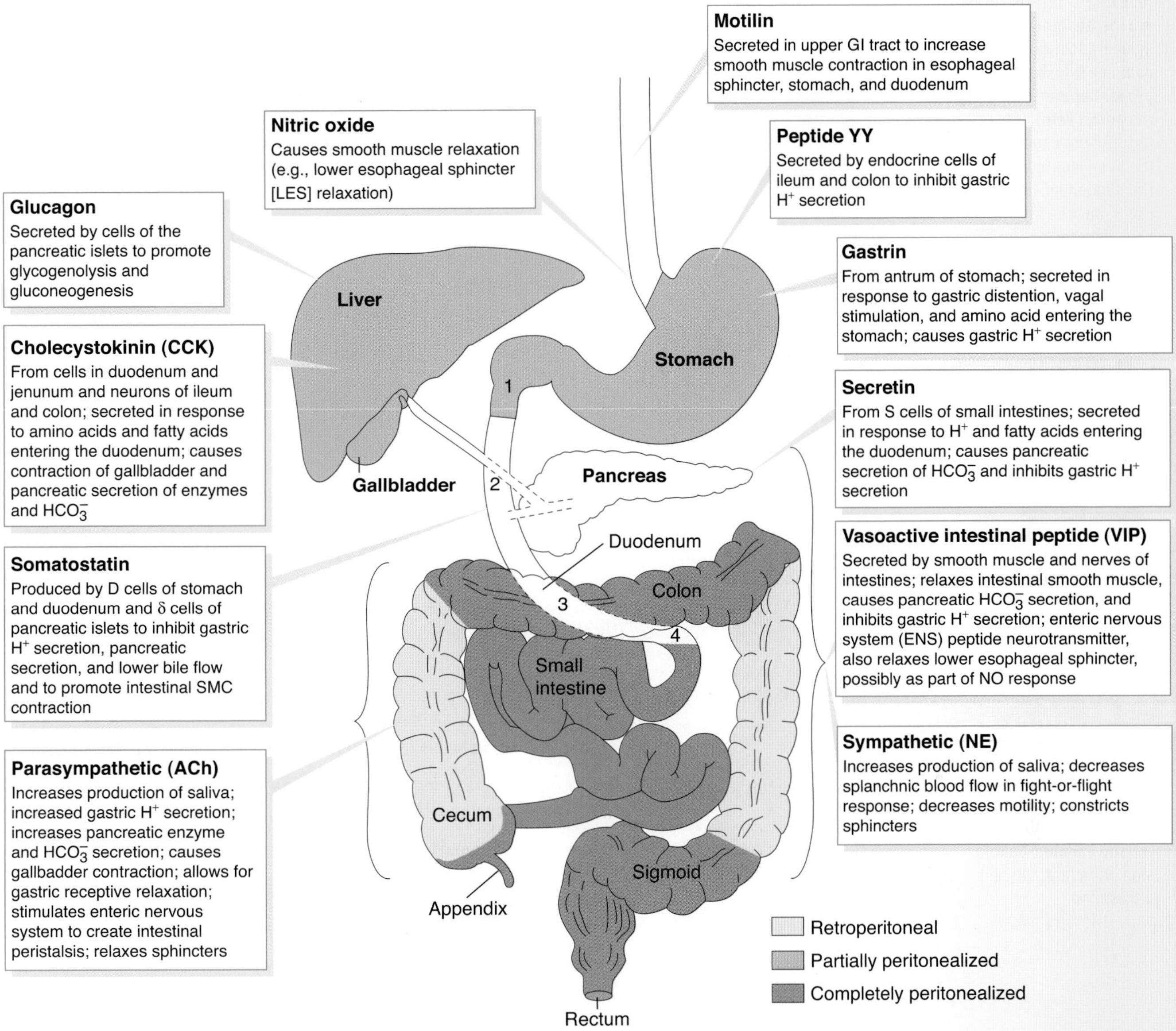
Motilin
Secreted in upper GI tract to increase smooth muscle contraction in esophageal sphincter, stomach, and duodenum
Nitric oxide
Causes smooth muscle relaxation (e.g., lower esophageal sphincter [LES] relaxation)
Peptide YY
Secreted by endocrine cells of ileum and colon to inhibit gastric H^+ secretion
Glucagon
Secreted by cells of the pancreatic islets to promote glycogenolysis and gluconeogenesis
Gastrin
From antrum of stomach; secreted in response to gastric distention, vagal stimulation, and amino acid entering the stomach; causes gastric H^+ secretion
Cholecystokinin (CCK)
From cells in duodenum and jenunum and neurons of ileum and colon; secreted in response to amino acids and fatty acids entering the duodenum; causes contraction of gallbladder and pancreatic secretion of enzymes and HCO_3^-
Secretin
From S cells of small intestines; secreted in response to H^+ and fatty acids entering the duodenum; causes pancreatic secretion of HCO_3^- and inhibits gastric H^+ secretion
Somatostatin
Produced by D cells of stomach and duodenum and δ cells of pancreatic islets to inhibit gastric H^+ secretion, pancreatic secretion, and lower bile flow and to promote intestinal SMC contraction
Vasoactive intestinal peptide (VIP)
Secreted by smooth muscle and nerves of intestines; relaxes intestinal smooth muscle, causes pancreatic HCO_3^- secretion, and inhibits gastric H^+ secretion; enteric nervous system (ENS) peptide neurotransmitter, also relaxes lower esophageal sphincter, possibly as part of NO response
Parasympathetic (ACh)
Increases production of saliva; increased gastric H^+ secretion; increases pancreatic enzyme and HCO_3^- secretion; causes gallbadder contraction; allows for gastric receptive relaxation; stimulates enteric nervous system to create intestinal peristalsis; relaxes sphincters
Sympathetic (NE)
Increases production of saliva; decreases splanchnic blood flow in fight-or-flight response; decreases motility; constricts sphincters
Liver
Stomach
1
Gallbladder
2
Pancreas
Duodenum
3
Colon
4
Small intestine
Cecum
Sigmoid
Appendix
Rectum
Retroperitoneal
Partially peritonealized
Completely peritonealized

ACh, acetylcholine; GI, gastrointestinal; HCO_3^-, bicarbonate; NE, norepinephrine; NO, nitric oxide; SMC, smooth muscle cells.

QUICK HIT

The boundaries of the epiploic foramen of Winslow (opening of the lesser sac) are the hepatoduodenal ligament (containing **the common bile duct [CBD], the proper hepatic artery, and the portal vein**), located anteriorly; the caudate lobe of the liver, located superiorly; the duodenum, located inferiorly; and the inferior vena cava, located posteriorly.

MNEMONIC

Rule of 2s for Meckel diverticulum: 2 feet from ileocecal junction; 2 inches long; 2% of the population affected; 2 times more common in men; and 2 types of ectopic tissue involved (gastric or pancreatic). Remember Meckel diverticulum as the disease associated with 2 because **"di-"** means **"2."**

QUICK HIT

Duodenal atresia is associated with Down syndrome and demonstrates a characteristic **"double-bubble"** sign on radiograph and ultrasound.

QUICK HIT

Many GI disorders present with abdominal pain—use the quality of pain to help you: **sharp, stabbing epigastric pain** that radiates to the back suggests pancreatitis; **burning epigastric pain** suggests a gastric or duodenal ulcer; and **pain that shifts** from the epigastrium to the right lower quadrant suggests appendicitis.

IMPORTANT CONGENITAL MALFORMATIONS OF THE GASTROINTESTINAL SYSTEM *(Table 5-1)*

With the exception of a Meckel diverticulum, which can remain asymptomatic throughout the lifespan, congenital malformations of the gastrointestinal (GI) tract will manifest themselves during the neonatal period.

TABLE 5-1 Important Congenital Malformations of the Gastrointestinal System

Malformation	Clinical Features
Hypertrophic pyloric stenosis	Thickening of the pylorus musculature **Projectile vomiting** Palpable knot "olive" in the pyloric region
Extrahepatic biliary atresia	Incomplete recanalization of the bile duct during development Presents shortly after birth Dark urine Clay-colored stool Jaundice
Annular pancreas	Abnormal fusion of ventral and dorsal pancreatic buds, forming a constricting ring around the duodenum Duodenal obstruction (bilious vomiting); presents shortly after birth
Meckel diverticulum	Persistent remnant of the vitelline duct Forms an outpouching (true diverticulum) in the ileum Ulceration and bleeding Fifty percent contain either gastric or pancreatic tissue when symptomatic
Malrotation of the midgut	Normal 270-degree rotation is not completed Cecum and appendix lie in upper abdomen Associated with **volvulus** (twisting of intestine), causing an obstruction
Intestinal stenosis or atresia	Results from failure of the normal recanalization of the lumen May produce failure to thrive
Hirschsprung disease (congenital or toxic megacolon)	Failure of **neural crest cells** to migrate to colon No peristalsis Constipation and abdominal distention in newborn **Bowel movement precipitated by digital rectal examination**
Anal agenesis	Lack of anal opening as a result of improper formation of the urorectal septum May cause rectovesical (anus to bladder), rectovaginal, or rectourethral fistula

THE OROPHARYNX, ESOPHAGUS, AND STOMACH

I. The digestion of food begins in the oral cavity with salivary enzymes.

II. The esophagus transports food to the stomach.

A. The upper third of the esophagus is skeletal muscle.
B. The middle third is both skeletal and smooth muscle.
C. The lower third is smooth muscle.
D. The lower esophageal sphincter (LES) relaxes in preparation for the passage of food into the stomach.

III. The stomach receives and stores food.

A. Receptive relaxation—the stomach relaxes to accommodate the entering food (a vagovagal reflex).

B. Three phases of gastric secretion
  1. **Cephalic phase**—the sight, smell, taste, or thought of food stimulates secretion.
  2. **Gastric phase**—secretion is caused by the entry of food into the stomach.
  3. **Intestinal phase**—food entering the intestine causes a feedback stimulation of gastric secretion.

C. Important gastric secretions
  1. **Hydrochloric acid (HCl)** is secreted by parietal cells of the fundus.
     a. Stimulated by gastrin, histamine, and vagal stimulation
     b. Inhibited by **omeprazole** (proton pump inhibitor), **cimetidine** (H_2 blocker), chyme in small intestine via gastric inhibitory peptide (GIP), and secretin
  2. **Intrinsic factor** is secreted by parietal cells of the fundus.
     a. Binds to vitamin B_{12} (extrinsic factor)
     b. **Vitamin B_{12}–intrinsic factor complex** absorbed in **terminal ileum**
  3. **Pepsinogen** is secreted by chief cells.
     a. Pepsinogen is converted to pepsin by the low pH of the stomach.
     b. Pepsin begins the digestion of protein.
  4. **Gastrin** secreted by the G cells of the antrum and pylorus stimulates the release of HCl from parietal cells.
  5. **Somatostatin is secreted by a variety of cells throughout the GI tract and has a global inhibitory effect.**

D. The stomach grinds food into small particles and forces it into the duodenum.
  1. Grinding (trituration) takes place in peristaltic waves occurring at a rate of three to five waves per minute.
  2. **Migrating motor complexes (MMCs)**, stimulated by motilin, occur in the interdigestive period and serve to flush undigested food through the GI system.

IV. Nonneoplastic disorders of the oropharynx, esophagus, and stomach *(Table 5-2)*

TABLE 5-2 Nonneoplastic Disorders of the Oropharynx, Esophagus, and Stomach

Disorder	Etiology and Pathology	Clinical Features	Notes
Sialolithiasis	Blockage of salivary gland duct preventing release of saliva; follows chronic sialadenitis (inflammation of the salivary glands)	Acute pain; usually in submandibular gland or Stensen duct of the parotid gland	Passage of stone can be induced by stimulating the secretion of saliva (e.g., by sucking on a lemon)
Pleomorphic adenoma	Increased risk with radiation exposure	Benign, recurring, mixed cell tumor of the parotid; may lead to facial nerve injury	Most frequent salivary gland tumor; more common in women 20–40 years of age
Esophageal variceal bleeding	Bleeding from esophageal varices owing to portal HTN	Hematemesis, signs of portal HTN (i.e., caput medusae, ascites)	Usually treated with vasoconstrictors (vasopressin); endoscopy required for diagnosis (to rule out bleeding ulcers)
Boerhaave syndrome	Complete rupture of the esophagus (all layers); caused by severe retching	Often presents as left pneumothorax; surgical correction necessary	Esophageal reflux disease predisposes to this condition
Mallory–Weiss tear	Laceration of the gastroesophageal junction; usually caused by severe retching	Poststretching hematemesis	Alcoholics and bulimics are at an increased risk

(continued)

QUICK HIT

Gastroesophageal reflux disease (GERD), a common gastroesophageal disorder, is usually treated with H_2 blockers such as cimetidine or ranitidine or, in more severe cases, with proton pump inhibitors such as omeprazole or lansoprazole.

QUICK HIT

Cyclooxygenase-2 (COX-2) inhibitors such as celecoxib and rofecoxib not only reduce the adverse GI side effects and ulcers of normal nonsteroidal anti-inflammatory drugs (NSAIDs) but also do not inhibit platelet function.

QUICK HIT

Helicobacter pylori infection is pharmacologically treated with **"triple therapy."** The therapeutic regimen typically includes a proton pump inhibitor (omeprazole) and clarithromycin plus either amoxicillin or metronidazole.

TABLE 5-2 Nonneoplastic Disorders of the Oropharynx, Esophagus, and Stomach *(Continued)*

Disorder	Etiology and Pathology	Clinical Features	Notes
Acute gastritis	NSAIDs, smoking, alcohol, aspirin, steroids, burn injury (Curling ulcer), brain injury (Cushing ulcer)	Erosive; acute inflammation; necrosis; hemorrhage; **"coffee-ground" vomitus**	Blood in the nasogastric tube
Chronic gastritis	Type A (fundal): autoimmune pernicious anemia, aging Type B (antral): *Helicobacter pylori*	Nonerosive; mucosal inflammation and atrophy of mucosa	Risk factor for gastric carcinoma
Gastric ulcers	***H. pylori*** (70% of cases); bile-induced gastritis; increased permeability of gastric mucosa; associated with the use of aspirin and NSAIDs	Postprandial pain, bleeding, perforation, obstruction	Usually near the lesser curvature; not dependent on increased gastric acid secretion; not precancerous
Dumping syndrome	Postvagotomy; unimpeded passage of hypertonic food to the small intestine, causing distention as a result of osmotic flow of water into the lumen	Nausea, diarrhea, palpitations, sweating, lightheadedness, reactive hypoglycemia	Can be prevented by eating only small meals and ingesting solids and liquids separately

HTN, hypertension; NSAIDs, nonsteroidal anti-inflammatory drugs.

QUICK HIT

Leiomyoma is the most common benign tumor of the stomach.

V. Neoplastic disorders of the oropharynx, esophagus, and stomach *(Table 5-3 and Figure 5-3)*

Nonneoplastic and neoplastic disorders originating proximal to the pyloric sphincter often present with hematemesis and dysphagia as a result of alcohol and tobacco abuse.

TABLE 5-3 Neoplastic Disorders of the Oropharynx, Esophagus, and Stomach

Disorder	Etiology and Pathology	Clinical Features	Notes
Oral cancer	**Smoking,** chewing tobacco, alcohol	Squamous cell carcinoma; may involve tongue	Leukoplakia (white patch on the mucus membrane that cannot be wiped off) is a common precursor lesion
Esophageal adenocarcinoma	**Barrett esophagus;** complication of GERD	**Columnar metaplasia of esophageal squamous epithelium;** distal third of the esophagus	More common in Whites
Esophageal squamous cell carcinoma	Alcohol and tobacco use; esophagitis	Dysphagia, anorexia, pain	More common in Blacks
Gastric carcinoma	***Helicobacter pylori;*** gastritis; low-fiber diet, nitrosamines; blood group A; high-salt diet; increased incidence in Japan owing to greater consumption of smoked foods	Aggressive spread from antrum to nodes and liver; **Virchow node** (enlarged left-sided supraclavicular lymph node); **Krukenberg tumor** (metastatic disease to the ovaries from the stomach characterized by mucinous, signet ring cells)	More common in men older than 50 years; infiltration of stomach walls with tumor cells and subsequent fibrosis leads to linitis plastica (leather-bottle stomach)

GERD, gastroesophageal reflux disease.

FIGURE 5-3 **Barium-swallow radiograph of achalasia**

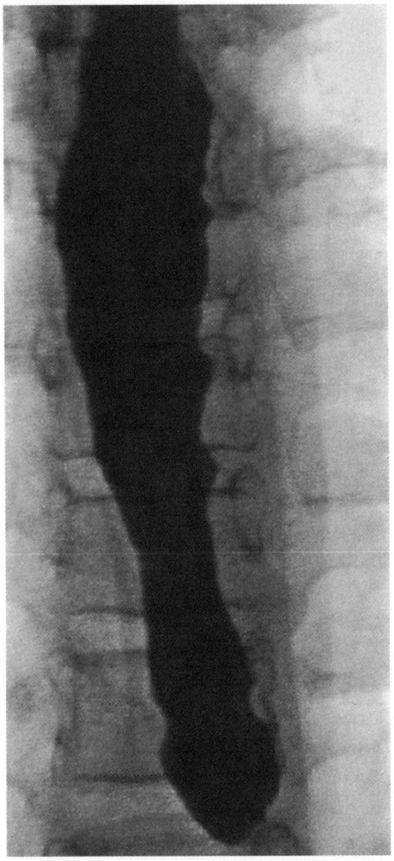

(Reproduced with permission from Humes DH, Dupont HL, Gardner LB, et al. *Kelley's Textbook of Internal Medicine.* 4th ed. Philadelphia, PA: Lippincott Williams & Wilkins; 2000:821.)

Clinical Vignette 5-1

CLINICAL PRESENTATION: During a visit to her primary care physician, a 39-year-old woman complains of **difficulty swallowing.** She also reports some heartburn and weight loss but denies pain on swallowing. She is an otherwise healthy female with no medical problems. Physical examination shows intact cranial nerves, swallowing mechanisms, and motor function of extremities. Vital signs are stable. Barium-swallow radiograph is shown previously.

DIFFERENTIALS: Mechanical obstruction—cancer, strictures, and rings; **oropharyngeal motility disorders**—multiple sclerosis, stroke, poliomyelitis, Parkinson disease, and myasthenia gravis; **esophageal motility disorders**—achalasia, scleroderma, and diffuse esophageal spasm. To remember the differentials for dysphagia, group them according to the phase of swallowing that has been disturbed and the type of pathology present (obstruction or motility disorder). To sort through the differentials, look for three symptoms specific to esophageal pathology: dysphagia (difficulty swallowing), odynophagia (pain on swallowing), and heartburn. Odynophagia would suggest diffuse esophageal spasm, whereas heartburn would suggest gastroesophageal reflux disease (GERD). Determine the type of dysphagia: difficulty with solids indicates mechanical obstruction; trouble with both solids and liquids suggests esophageal motility disorders; and problems in transferring food from the oral cavity suggest oropharyngeal disorders. For oropharyngeal disorders, look for details in the history and physical examination such as aspiration pneumonia, nasal regurgitation, and cranial nerve pathology.

LABORATORY STUDIES: In this case, the **barium-swallow chest radiograph** shows dilation of the esophagus with narrowing at the LES confirming a diagnosis of achalasia. Other significant findings on chest radiograph include pneumonia, thickened esophageal folds, ulcerations, and strictures. **Manometry** is also helpful in esophageal motility disorders, and, in achalasia,

(continued)

MNEM...

Various emetic su... blood stimulate the... trigger zone and area... to produce feelings of na... and vomiting. Remember the... extraintestinal causes of vomiti... as part of your differential:

- **V**estibular disturbance/**V**agal
- **O**piates
- **M**igraine/**M**etabolic (diabetic ketoacidosis, gastroparesis, hypercalcemia)
- **I**nfections
- **T**oxicity
- **I**ncreased intracranial pressure (ICP)/**I**ngested alcohol
- **N**eurogenic, psychogenic
- **G**estation

MNEMONIC

To remember one cause and treatment of a**CHA**lasia, think **CHA**gas disease and calcium-**CHA**nnel blocker.

Clinical Vignette 5-1 (Continued)

it would classically show a lack of ordered peristalsis, increased LES pressures, and failure of LES relaxation after swallowing. **Esophagoscopy** is helpful in visualizing and qualifying obstruction and mucosal wall integrity and is important to rule out cancer. **Esophageal pH monitoring** would also be done in this case to rule out GERD. If an oropharyngeal disorder is suspected, a **swallowing electromyography** is indicated and electromyelograms would be abnormal.

MANAGEMENT: Achalasia is treated by calcium channel blockers and nitrates to decrease LES pressure. Patients refractory to medical treatment can undergo endoscopic injection of botulinum toxin at the LES to block the release of acetylcholine locally. Surgical management options include myotomy of the gastroesophageal junction to relieve LES pressure with partial fundoplication to prevent reflux.

THE SMALL INTESTINE, LARGE INTESTINE, AND RECTUM

I. Muscular layers of the GI tract is shown in Figure 5-4.

FIGURE 5-4 **Picture of muscular layer of the gastrointestinal tract**

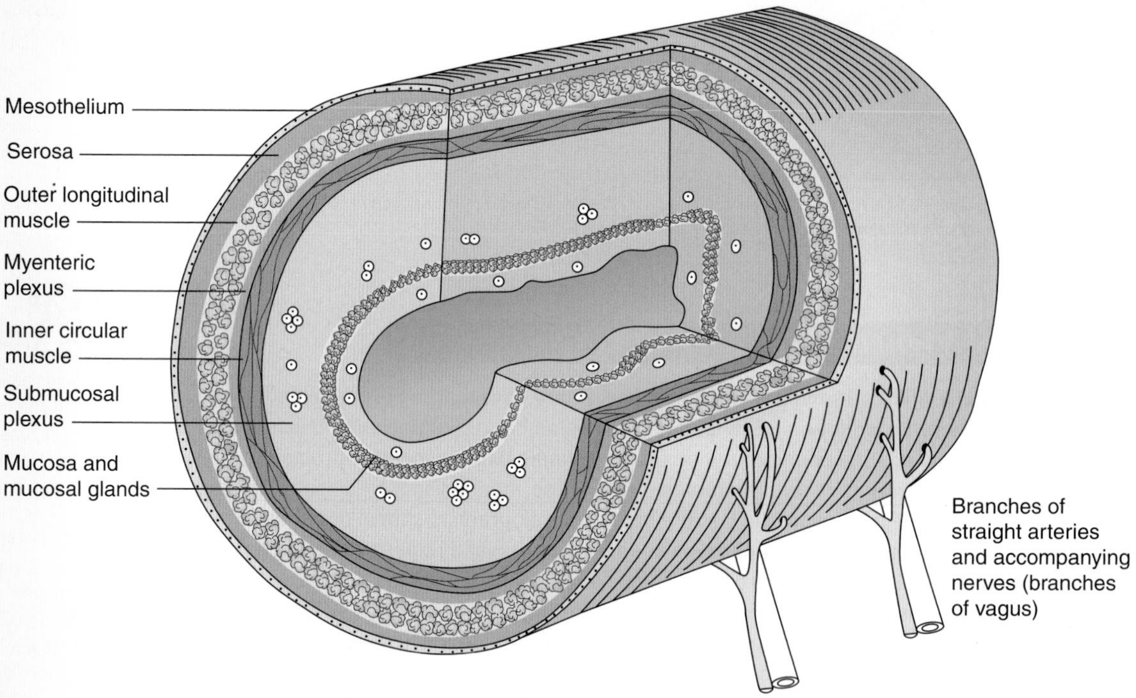
Mesothelium
Serosa
Outer longitudinal muscle
Myenteric plexus
Inner circular muscle
Submucosal plexus
Mucosa and mucosal glands
Branches of straight arteries and accompanying nerves (branches of vagus)

II. The small intestine digests and absorbs the food.

A. Digestion is mediated by a variety of GI hormones, including cholecystokinin (CCK), secretin, somatostatin, and others (Figure 5-2).

B. Carbohydrates

1. Pancreatic amylase hydrolyzes glycogen, starch, and most other complex carbohydrates to disaccharides.
2. Disaccharides are broken down to monosaccharides by intestinal brush border enzymes and absorbed.
3. Monosaccharides are absorbed by a variety of mechanisms:
   a. Glucose and galactose are absorbed by sodium (Na^+)-dependent transport.
   b. Fructose is absorbed by facilitated diffusion.

QUICK HIT

Lactose intolerance is caused by a genetic absence or decrease in lactase. Lactose cannot be broken down; it remains in the lumen of the gut and causes **osmotic** diarrhea.

C. **Protein**
   1. It is degraded to amino acids, dipeptides, and tripeptides by proteases produced by the pancreas.
      a. Activation of **trypsinogen to trypsin**
         - Autoactivated
         - Activated by intestinal brush border enterokinases
      b. Trypsin degrades the peptide bonds of arginine or lysine.
      c. Trypsin also **activates the other proteolytic pancreatic enzymes**.
   2. Proteins are absorbed by an Na^+-dependent transport.
      a. There are separate carriers for acidic, basic, and neutral amino acids.
      b. Dipeptides and tripeptides are absorbed faster than single amino acids.

D. Fats
   1. Lipids are broken into droplets by the mixing action of the stomach.
   2. **Pancreatic lipase** (and to a lesser extent salivary lipase) **hydrolyzes triacylglycerol to fatty acids and 2-monoacylglycerol. Chronic pancreatitis** decreases fat digestion and absorption due to decreased lipase release from the exocrine pancreas.
   3. Bile salts (amphipathic molecules) emulsify the hydrolyzed products and form micelles.
   4. Micelles allow for fat absorption (Figure 5-5).
   5. A variety of familial and acquired disorders may disrupt lipid metabolism, resulting in **hyperlipidemia**.
      a. Hyperlipidemia, especially high levels of low-density lipoproteins (LDLs), is associated with coronary artery disease (CAD).
      b. Typically, treatment first involves dietary intervention and then drug therapy, regardless of the cause of the hyperlipidemia.
         - **3-Hydroxy-3-methylglutaryl coenzyme A (HMG-CoA) reductase inhibitors**, also known as "**statins**," such as atorvastatin, lovastatin, and pravastatin, are an effective and widely used means of lowering LDL.

QUICK HIT

Often, the amino acid transporter found in the intestines is identical to the amino acid transporter found in the renal tubules. As such, diseases that affect these transporters have multiorgan system effects. One of these diseases is Hartnup disease, which is a defect in the intestinal and renal tubular absorption of neutral amino acids leading to excretion of tryptophan derivatives and causing pellagra-like symptoms.

QUICK HIT

Although the statins work well as cholesterol-lowering agents, they can be **hepatotoxic**. Consequently, patients who take them should undergo routine liver function tests.

The Gastrointestinal System

FIGURE 5-5 **Absorption and digestion of fats (lipid metabolism)**

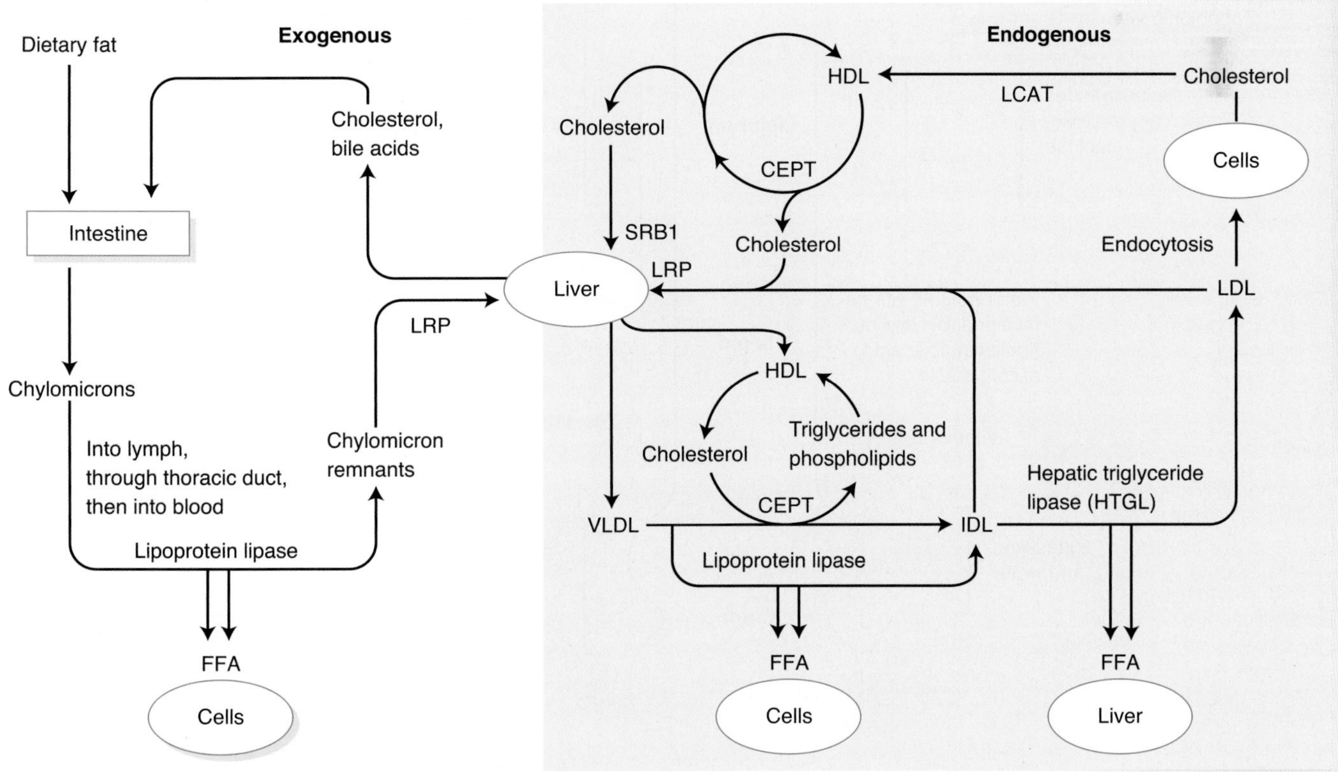

Exogenous
Endogenous
Dietary fat
Intestine
Cholesterol, bile acids
Chylomicrons
Into lymph, through thoracic duct, then into blood
Lipoprotein lipase
Chylomicron remnants
LRP
FFA
Cells
Liver
Cholesterol
SRB1
LRP
HDL
CEPT
Cholesterol
LCAT
Cholesterol
Cells
Endocytosis
LDL
HDL
Cholesterol
Triglycerides and phospholipids
CEPT
VLDL
IDL
Lipoprotein lipase
Hepatic triglyceride lipase (HTGL)
FFA
Cells
FFA
Liver

CEPT, cholesterol ester transfer protein; FFA, free fatty acid; HDL, high-density lipoprotein; IDL, intermediate-density lipoprotein; LCAT, lecithin-cholesterol acyltransferase; LDL, low-density lipoprotein; LRP, lipoprotein-related receptor protein; SRB1, scavenger receptor class B1; VLDL, very low-density lipoprotein.

- **Bile acid-binding resins** such as cholestyramine and colestipol work by binding bile acids in the intestine and promoting their subsequent loss in the stool, which ultimately lowers LDL levels.
- **Nicotinic acid (niacin)** inhibits the release of lipoproteins from the liver, lowering very low-density lipoproteins (VLDLs) and LDL.

III. The large intestine stores and excretes nondigestible material.

A. Absorbs 2 to 3 L per day of water
B. **Secretes potassium (K^+)**
C. Mediates defecation of undigested material through both voluntary and involuntary (rectosphincteric reflex) mechanisms

> **QUICK HIT**
> The sweetener sucralose, a chloride derivative of sucrose, is absorbed at a level only 11% to 27% of intake, and most of it is excreted, unmetabolized, in feces.

LOCATION OF ABSORPTION OF VITAMINS, MINERALS, AND NUTRIENTS *(Figure 5-6)*

FIGURE 5-6 Location of absorption of vitamins, minerals, and nutrients

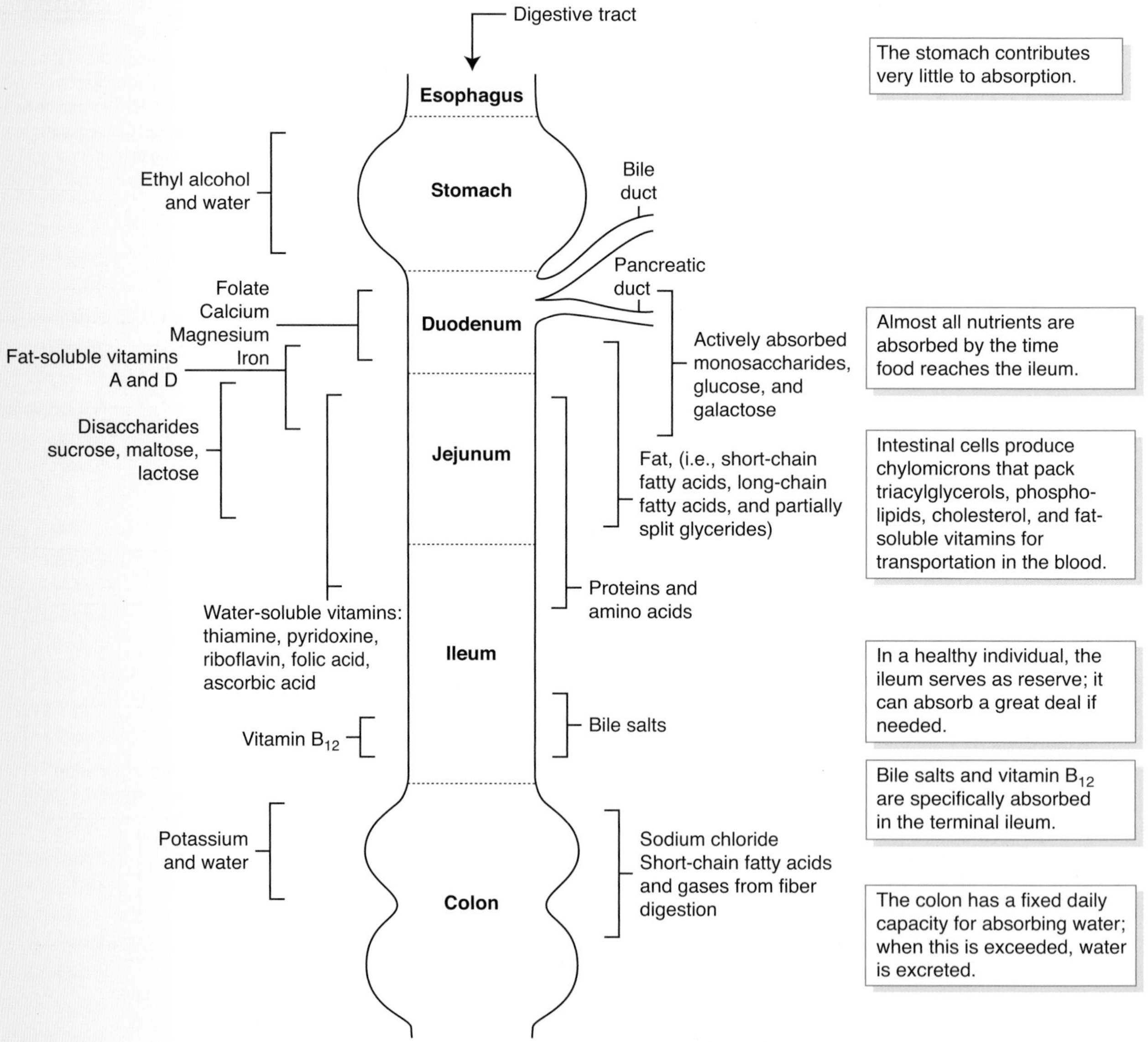

Digestive tract
Esophagus
Stomach
Duodenum
Jejunum
Ileum
Colon
Bile duct
Pancreatic duct
Ethyl alcohol and water
Folate
Calcium
Magnesium
Iron
Fat-soluble vitamins A and D
Disaccharides sucrose, maltose, lactose
Water-soluble vitamins: thiamine, pyridoxine, riboflavin, folic acid, ascorbic acid
Vitamin B12
Potassium and water
Actively absorbed monosaccharides, glucose, and galactose
Fat, (i.e., short-chain fatty acids, long-chain fatty acids, and partially split glycerides)
Proteins and amino acids
Bile salts
Sodium chloride
Short-chain fatty acids and gases from fiber digestion
The stomach contributes very little to absorption.
Almost all nutrients are absorbed by the time food reaches the ileum.
Intestinal cells produce chylomicrons that pack triacylglycerols, phospholipids, cholesterol, and fat-soluble vitamins for transportation in the blood.
In a healthy individual, the ileum serves as reserve; it can absorb a great deal if needed.
Bile salts and vitamin B12 are specifically absorbed in the terminal ileum.
The colon has a fixed daily capacity for absorbing water; when this is exceeded, water is excreted.

COMMON CLINICAL DISORDERS OF THE SMALL INTESTINE, LARGE INTESTINE, AND RECTUM *(Table 5-4)*

Common clinical disorders of the GI tract, distal to the pyloric sphincter, will usually present as vague abdominal pain as a result of stimulation of the visceral afferent nerves. If the parietal peritoneum (the abdominal wall), innervated by the somatic afferent nerves, is irritated by the lesion, the pain will become more localized (as is seen in acute appendicitis).

TABLE 5-4 **Common Clinical Disorders of the Small Intestine, Large Intestine, and Rectum**

Disorder	Etiology and Pathology	Clinical Features	Notes
Hiatal hernia	Saclike herniation of stomach through diaphragm; smoking; obesity	Retrosternal pain (worse in supine position); can lead to **GERD**	Usually occurs in the sliding (versus rolling) form
Duodenal ulcers	***Helicobacter pylori*** (in 90% of cases); hypersecretion of acid; smokers; Zollinger–Ellison syndrome; blood group O; associated with NSAID use	Coffee-ground vomitus; **smooth border;** clean base; black stools; pain at night or 2 h postprandial; perforation may result in acute pancreatitis	Not precancerous
Ischemic bowel disease	Atherosclerosis of celiac artery or mesenteric artery	Abdominal pain, nausea, vomiting, stool positive for blood test	Usually affects watershed areas (splenic flexure or rectosigmoid junction)
Diverticulitis	Outpouchings of the colon obstructed with fecalith leading to inflammation or infection; low-fiber diet	Usually involves the **sigmoid colon;** fever; leukocytosis; colicky pain; usually multiple in number and causes increased risk of perforation	False diverticula: pockets of mucosa and submucosa herniated through muscular layer (not all layers)
Appendicitis	Obstruction (usually fecalith or lymphoid hyperplasia); bacterial proliferation and mucosal invasion	Nausea, vomiting, anorexia, abdominal pain that migrates from epigastrium to right lower quadrant, pain at **McBurney point,** psoas sign or obturator sign, increased WBCs in blood	Differential diagnosis in females includes ectopic pregnancy, ovarian torsion, ruptured ovarian cyst, and pelvic inflammatory disease
Adenocarcinoma	Chronic IBD, low-fiber diet, older age, hereditary polyposis or adenomatous disorders	**Increased CEA** (not diagnostic, used to assess treatment); rectosigmoid tumors present in an **annular manner** producing early obstruction and constipation; **left-sided tumors present with blood in the stool, whereas right-sided tumors typically present with anemia as a result of occult blood loss**	Screen for occult blood in stool and flexible sigmoidoscopy; screening colonoscopy with a positive family history; third most common cause of cancer death (after lung and prostate/breast)
Carcinoid tumor	Arises from **neuroendocrine cells** (Kulchitsky cells); releases vasoactive peptides such as histamine, serotonin, and prostaglandins	**Increased 5-HIAA in urine,** diarrhea, **flushing,** right-sided heart valve lesions, hypotension, bronchospasm	Most common tumor of the appendix but also found in the ileum, rectum, and bronchus

5-HIAA, 5-hydroxyindoleacetic acid; CEA, carcinoembryonic antigen; GERD, gastroesophageal reflux disease; IBD, inflammatory bowel disease; NSAID, nonsteroidal anti-inflammatory drug; WBC, white blood cell.

QUICK HIT

Posterior duodenal ulcers are associated with erosion of the gastroduodenal artery and subsequent hemorrhage.

QUICK HIT

Duodenal versus gastric ulcer: In **d**uodenal ulcers, pain ***d**ecreases after meals/antacids* whereas in gastric ulcers, *pain persists after meals/antacids.* Also, duodenal ulcers are associated with *increased acid production,* whereas patients with gastric ulcers have *decreased to normal acid production.* Finally, although all gastric ulcers should be biopsied to rule out gastric *carcinoma,* duodenal ulcers require no such intervention.

QUICK HIT

Diverticulosis, the most common cause of bleeding from the lower GI tract, can be differentiated from diverticulitis because diverticulitis typically does not cause bleeding but is painful, whereas diverticulosis does cause bleeding but is typically painless.

QUICK HIT

Small-bowel obstructions are usually caused by adhesions, whereas large-bowel obstructions are most commonly a result of neoplasms. Ileus, a common cause of temporary small-bowel paralysis, commonly occurs postoperatively.

MNEMONIC

Left-sided valvular lesions are not observed in carcinoid syndrome because the lung metabolizes serotonin (5-HT). Remember the symptoms of carcinoid syndrome as "**Be FDR**": **B**ronchospasm, **F**lushing, **D**iarrhea, and **R**ight-sided valvular lesions.

QUICK HIT

The shift of pain that is observed classically in appendicitis occurs because the visceral peritoneum is irritated first, which produces a diffuse sensation of pain. As the appendicitis progresses, the parietal peritoneum becomes inflamed, resulting in a more localized sensation of pain in the right lower quadrant.

QUICK HIT

A **positive psoas sign** elicited by pain on extension of the leg indicates retroperitoneal inflammation and suggests the appendix is located behind the cecum retroperitoneally. A **positive obturator sign** elicited by pain on abduction/adduction at the hip joint of a leg flexed at the knee suggests the appendix is located in the pelvic region; a pelvic appendix can also be palpated on rectal examination.

MNEMONIC

To quickly remember the pH changes associated with GI losses, think: With vomiting, both the pH and food come up. With diarrhea, both the pH and food go down.

Clinical Vignette 5-2

CLINICAL PRESENTATION: A 21-year-old woman presents to the emergency department with **right lower quadrant pain** of several hours' duration. She reports that the **pain began in the epigastrium** and has since moved to the right lower quadrant. Since the onset of the pain, she reports **no appetite and nausea.** She is otherwise a healthy young female. Physical examination reveals **tenderness at McBurney point.** No peritoneal signs, psoas sign, or obturator sign. Rectal examination gives a negative result. Temperature = 100.3° F; blood pressure = 120/80 mm Hg; heart rate = 95 bpm; and respiration = 20 breaths/min.

DIFFERENTIALS: Appendicitis, mittelschmerz, ovarian cyst rupture, pelvic inflammatory disease, ectopic pregnancy, kidney stones, and Meckel diverticulum. The shift in pain described previously is classic for appendicitis. Also, anorexia, nausea, and vomiting beginning after the onset of pain are typical for appendicitis. Further, gynecologic history is needed on this patient to determine if midcycle pain associated with ovulation (mittelschmerz) was occurring. Also, a pelvic examination is indicated in this patient to further determine the pelvic pathology.

LABORATORY STUDIES: If this were a young man, the history and physical examination would be sufficient to indicate surgery for appendicitis. In a young woman, however, there is a longer differential list and a **computerized tomography (CT) scan** would be helpful in determining the cause of the pain. A **complete blood count (CBC)** often shows a mildly elevated white blood cell (WBC) count, but this is not a consistent finding. A **human chorionic gonadotropin (hCG) pregnancy test** and **pelvic ultrasound** should also be performed on this patient to rule out pelvic pathology.

MANAGEMENT: Laparoscopic or open appendectomy should be performed emergently because of the risk of rupture.

Diarrhea, the passage of abnormal amounts of fluid or semisolid fecal matter, can be mediated by a number of mechanisms. Osmotic diarrhea results when unabsorbed solutes increase intraluminal oncotic pressure, causing an outpouring of water. Surgical resection can lead to an inadequate surface for absorption of nutrients, resulting in a form of **osmotic diarrhea**. Active ion secretion causing obligatory water loss is termed **secretory diarrhea**. Altered intestinal motility, in which there is an alteration of the normally

Clinical Vignette 5-3

CLINICAL PRESENTATION: A 54-year-old woman presents to the emergency department with **severe abdominal pain** of 36 hours' duration. Her past medical history is significant for **CAD, hypertension (HTN),** and **diabetes.** Physical examination reveals a **soft, nondistended, nontender abdomen** with **normal bowel sounds** and no palpable masses. Temperature = 98.9° F; blood pressure = 140/90 mm Hg; heart rate = 99 bpm; and respiration rate = 21 breaths/min.

DIFFERENTIALS: Acute mesenteric ischemia, appendicitis, diverticulitis, colon adenocarcinoma, IBD, and pseudomembranous colitis. Pain disproportionate to the physical findings is strongly suggestive of mesenteric ischemia. As the ischemia progresses, peritonitis, sepsis, and shock may occur.

LABORATORY STUDIES: Mesenteric angiogram is the definitive diagnostic test for mesenteric ischemia. **Plain abdominal radiographs** are obtained to rule out other causes of acute abdominal pain. **Abdominal radiographs with barium enema** often show "thumbprinting" as a result of thickened edematous mucosal folds.

MANAGEMENT: Supportive therapy with intravenous (IV) fluids and broad-spectrum antibiotics should be started. Further treatment depends on the cause of the ischemia. Given the history of CAD in this patient, this is most likely **thrombotic** in nature, and direct **intra-arterial injection of papaverine** (a vasodilator) into the superior mesenteric system during arteriography will relieve the occlusion and vasospasm. An **embolic** occlusion indicates direct **intra-arterial infusion of thrombolytics or embolectomy.** If it is a **venous thrombosis, heparin anticoagulation** should be started. If signs of peritonitis develop, the **nonviable bowel should be resected.**

coordinated control of intestinal propulsion, may also result in diarrhea (often alternating with constipation). Finally, sloughing of colonic mucosa, caused by inflammation and necrosis, often as a result of infection, causes an **exudative form of diarrhea**.

- **Bacterial Causes of Diarrhea** (Table 5-5)
- **Viral Causes of Diarrhea** (Table 5-6)
- **Protozoal Causes of Diarrhea** (Table 5-7)

TABLE 5-5 **Bacterial Causes of Diarrhea**

Infectious Agent	Clinical Features	Treatment	Notes
Shigella	**Shiga toxin** causes **bloody** diarrhea, mild to severe, 1–2 weeks in duration; fever for 3–4 days; lactose (–)	Bismuth, ampicillin, ciprofloxacin, or trimethoprim-sulfamethoxazole	Fecal leukocytes and stool culture necessary for diagnosis
Salmonella	**Bloody** diarrhea, fever, cramps, nausea, motile, lactose (–)	Supportive therapy only; no opiates; tetracycline may be used if needed, symptoms may be prolonged with antibiotics	Commonly acquired from **eggs, poultry, or turtles;** diagnosis based on stool culture; increased susceptibility in immunocompromised patients
Campylobacter jejuni	**Bloody** diarrhea, fever, crampy abdominal pain, self-limited but may persist for 3–4 weeks	Supportive therapy or possibly erythromycin	**Leading cause of foodborne diarrhea** in United States, spiral (S-shaped), oxidase (+)
Vibrio cholerae	**Watery** diarrhea **(rice-water stools),** vomiting, and dehydration occur after 12–48 h of incubation	Supportive therapy only; no opiates	Caused by **toxin;** most often occurs in underdeveloped nations; commonly associated with consumption of raw oysters; comma-shaped with flagellum
Clostridium difficile	**Watery** diarrhea caused by antibiotic-induced suppression of normal colonic flora and *C. difficile* overgrowth; **pseudomembranes** on the colonic mucosa	Metronidazole, oral vancomycin	Exotoxin mediated; termed *pseudomembranous colitis* because of the false membranes created on the colon by the bacterial infection
Enterotoxigenic *Escherichia coli* (traveler's diarrhea)	**Watery** diarrhea; 3–6 days' duration; occasional fever and vomiting	Bismuth, trimethoprim-sulfamethoxazole, doxycycline, and ciprofloxacin	Antibiotics reduce duration of infection to 1–2 days
Enterohemorrhagic *E. coli* (0157:H7)	**Shiga-like toxin** causes **bloody** diarrhea	Supportive therapy	Typically, food-borne transmission (e.g., **undercooked hamburger**); diagnosis made by stool culture
Yersinia enterocolitica	**Bloody** diarrhea, fever, cramps, nausea	Supportive therapy only; no opiates	Transmitted by food or contaminated domestic animal feces; clinically indistinguishable from *Salmonella* and *Shigella*

QUICK HIT

Salmonella requires at least 100,000 organisms to be infectious; *Shigella,* however, requires only 100.

QUICK HIT

Vibrio cholerae produces an exotoxin that activates adenylate cyclase in the crypt cells. The increase in cyclic adenosine monophosphate (cAMP) activates chloride secretory channels. Consequently, sodium and water accompany chloride into the lumen, which results in an osmotic diarrhea.

QUICK HIT

Norwalk virus, in contrast to most viruses transmitted via the fecal-oral route, is uncommon in children.

TABLE 5-6 Viral Causes of Diarrhea

Infectious Agent	Clinical Features	Treatment	Notes
Rotavirus	Severe, dehydrating diarrhea; vomiting; low-grade fever	Supportive therapy only	**Most common cause of diarrhea in infants;** usually occurs during **winter** months
Norwalk virus	Mild diarrhea and vomiting	Supportive therapy only	Epidemics in underdeveloped countries; **affects older children and adults**
Adenovirus (serotypes 40 and 41)	Diarrhea and moderate omiting	Supportive therapy only	Second to rotavirus as the cause of gastroenteritis in children

QUICK HIT

The *Giardia* trophozoite has a very characteristic appearance. It is pear shaped, with four pairs of flagella and two nuclei that resemble eyes.

TABLE 5-7 Protozoal Causes of Diarrhea

Infectious Agent	Clinical Features	Treatment	Notes
Entamoeba histolytica	**Bloody** diarrhea, lower abdominal pain, may lead to dysentery with 10–12 bloody and mucous stools per day	Metronidazole	Caused by ingestion of viable cysts via fecal-oral route
Giardia lamblia	**Watery,** foul-smelling diarrhea; nausea; anorexia; cramps lasting weeks to months	Metronidazole	Fecal-oral transmission; often contracted while **camping**
Cryptosporidium	**Watery** diarrhea with large fluid loss; symptoms persist in immunocompromised patients; self-limited in healthy individuals	Supportive therapy	Immunocompromised patients (especially **patients with AIDS);** fecal-oral transmission of oocysts

- **Comparison of Inflammatory Bowel Conditions** (Table 5-8)

It is speculated that the pathogenesis of inflammatory bowel disease (IBD) is related to the activation of the immune system and the consequent release of cytokines and inflammatory mediators. The cause of IBD has yet to be discovered; however, there is some suggestion of a genetic component.

TABLE 5-8 Comparison of Inflammatory Bowel Conditions

	Crohn Disease	Ulcerative Colitis
Typical patient	• Young person of Jewish descent • Bimodal age distribution: 25–40 years of age and 50–65 years of age • Female > male	• Person of Jewish descent • Recently quit smoking • Bimodal age distribution: 20–35 years of age and 65+ years of age • Male > female
Clinical findings	• Diarrhea • Abdominal pain • Fever • Malabsorption • Obstruction	• Bloody, mucous diarrhea • Abdominal pain • Fever • Weight loss • Toxic megacolon

(continued)

TABLE 5-8 **Comparison of Inflammatory Bowel Conditions** *(Continued)*

	Crohn Disease	Ulcerative Colitis
Location	• Small intestine • Colon • "Mouth to anus"	• Colon • Rectum
Histologic findings	• Full-thickness inflammation • **Granulomas**	• Mucosal inflammation • **Crypt abscesses**
Gross findings	• **Cobblestone appearance** • Wall thickening with narrowed lumen • **Skipped areas** • **Fistulas**	• Pseudopolyps • Widened lumen • Toxic megacolon
Diagnostic evaluation	• Colonoscopy • Barium enema • Upper GI series with small-bowel follow-through	• Colonoscopy • Barium enema • Upper GI series with small-bowel follow-through
Risk of malignancy	• Small increase	• Large increase
Associated systemic manifestations	• Arthritis • Eye lesions • Erythema nodosum • Pyoderma gangrenosum • Aphthous ulcers (chancre sores)	• Arthritis • Eye lesions • Erythema nodosum • Pyoderma gangrenosum • Sclerosing cholangitis
Medical treatment	• Sulfasalazine • Steroids • Metronidazole	• Sulfasalazine • Steroids • Metronidazole
Indications for surgery	• Obstruction • Massive bleeding • Perforation • Refractory to medical treatment • Cancer • Toxic megacolon	• Toxic megacolon • Cancer • Massive bleeding • Failure to mature • Refractory to medical treatment

GI, gastrointestinal.

MALABSORPTION SYNDROMES OF THE SMALL INTESTINE

(Table 5-9)

Malabsorption may produce a variety of symptoms ranging from diarrhea to steatorrhea to specific nutrient deficiencies. For example, iron, vitamin B_{12}, fat-soluble vitamins (A, D, E, and K), or protein may be poorly absorbed and lead to systemic manifestations.

QUICK HIT

Celiac disease (nontropical sprue) causes decreased absorption of fat and fat-soluble vitamins, leading to skeletal and hematologic conditions due to decreased vitamin D and K.

TABLE 5-9 **Malabsorption Syndromes of the Small Intestine**

Syndrome	Pathology	Clinical Features	Notes
Abetalipoproteinemia	Lack of apolipoprotein B; defective chylomicron assembly; enterocytes congested with lipid	Acanthocytes ("burr" cells) in blood; **no chylomicrons, VLDL, or LDL in blood**; retinitis pigmentosa; peripheral neuropathy; mental retardation; ataxia	Autosomal recessive; vitamin E supplements may improve the retinopathy and neuropathy

(continued)

TABLE 5-9 **Malabsorption Syndromes of the Small Intestine** *(Continued)*

Syndrome	Pathology	Clinical Features	Notes
Celiac disease (non-tropical sprue)	Gluten sensitivity	Foul-smelling, pale stool; **villi of small intestine blunted;** stunted growth; symptoms disappear when gluten is removed from diet	Associated with HLA-B8 and HLA-DQW2; predisposes to T-cell lymphoma and GI and breast cancer; if unmanaged, causes vitamin deficiency resulting in skeletal, hematologic, and neurologic symptoms
Disaccharidase deficiency	Enzyme deficiency; bacterial digestion of unabsorbed disaccharide	Diarrhea, bloating	Most commonly lactase deficiency
Tropical sprue	Etiology unclear	Affects small intestine; may cause vitamin deficiencies and megaloblastic anemia	Possible infectious cause; does not improve with gluten removal
Whipple disease	Systemic disease caused by *Tropheryma whippelii*	Diarrhea, weight loss, lymphadenopathy; hyperpigmentation, **macrophages laden with *T. whippelii***	Older white males
Bacterial overgrowth	Bacterial overpopulation of small intestine owing to stasis, raised pH, impaired immunity, or **clindamycin** or **ampicillin** therapy	Inflammatory infiltrate in bowel wall	Treat with antibiotics, metronidazole, or oral vancomycin

GI, gastrointestinal; HLA-B8, human leukocyte antigen-B8; LDL, low-density lipoprotein; VLDL, very low-density lipoprotein.

NEOPLASTIC POLYPS *(Table 5-10)*

GI polyps can be very diverse in their presentation. Individuals can be asymptomatic, as is usually the case with tubular adenomas, or can present with serious systemic manifestations such as anemia secondary to invasive cancer.

- **Comparison of Polyposis Conditions** (Table 5-11)

TABLE 5-10 **Neoplastic Polyps**

Tubular Adenoma	Tubulovillous Adenoma	Villous Adenoma
Usually **benign**	Greater potential of malignancy than tubular adenoma	Highly **malignant**
Multiple	Morphologically, shares features of both tubular and villous adenomas	**Sessile** tumors Fingerlike projections
Pedunculated tumors Greater chance of malignancy if genetically predisposed Most common polyp		

TABLE 5-11 **Comparison of Polyposis Conditions**

Disease	Inheritance	Clinical Features
Familial adenomatous polyposis	Autosomal dominant	Colon lined with hundreds of polyps; potential for malignancy approaches 100%
Turcot syndrome	Autosomal dominant	Colonic polyps and **central nervous system (CNS) tumors;** potential for malignancy approaches 100%
Gardner syndrome	Autosomal dominant	Colonic polyps; soft-tissue and **bone tumors;** potential for malignancy approaches 100%
Peutz–Jeghers syndrome	Autosomal dominant	Benign hamartomatous polyps of the gastrointestinal tract (especially the small intestine); **hyperpigmented mouth, hands, and genitalia;** increased incidence of tumors of the uterus, breast, ovaries, lung, stomach, and pancreas; no malignant potential
Familial nonpolyposis syndrome	Autosomal dominant	**Defect in DNA repair** causing large number of colonic lesions (especially proximal); potential for malignancy approaches 50%

THE HEPATOBILIARY SYSTEM

MNEMONIC

Remember the drugs that cause hepatic necrosis by the phrase "**V**ery **A**ngry **H**epatocytes": **V**alproic acid, **A**cetaminophen, and **H**alothane.

I. **Microscopic organization of the liver** *(Figure 5-7)*

II. **Enterohepatic cycling and the excretion of bilirubin** *(Figure 5-8)*

III. **Important biochemical pathways of the liver and digestion** *(Figure 5-9)*

FIGURE 5-7 **Microscopic organization of the liver**

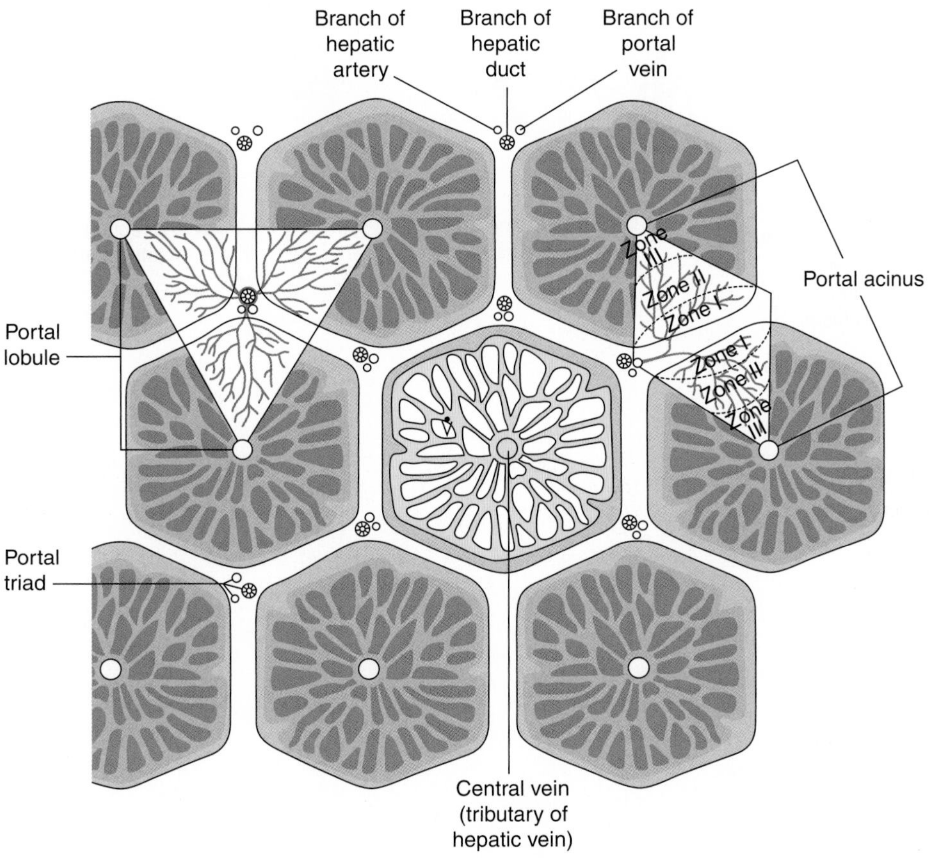
Branch of hepatic artery
Branch of hepatic duct
Branch of portal vein
Portal acinus
Zone III
Zone II
Zone I
Zone I
Zone II
Zone III
Portal lobule
Portal triad
Central vein (tributary of hepatic vein)

FIGURE 5-8 Enterohepatic cycling and the excretion of bilirubin

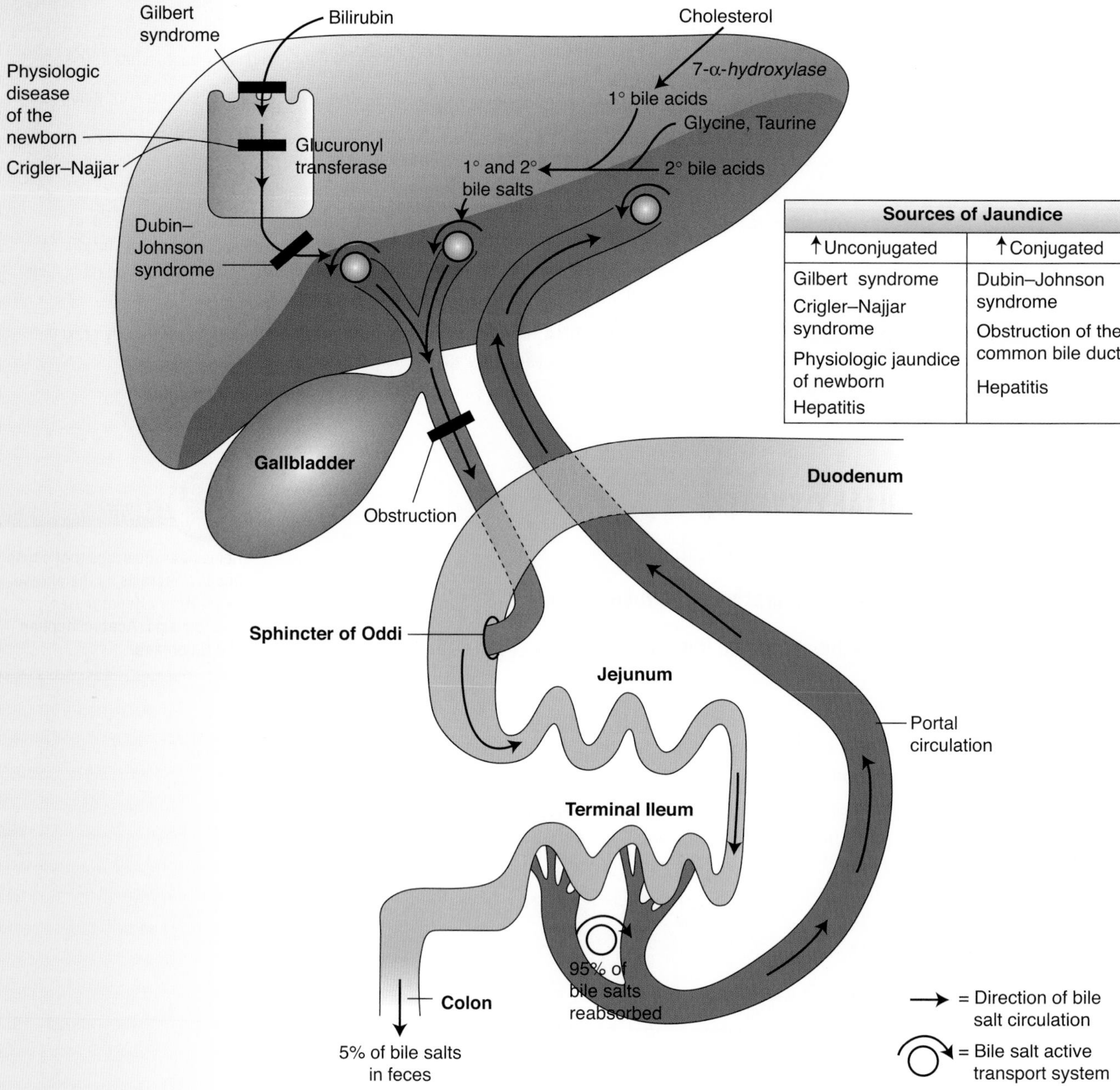
Gilbert syndrome
Bilirubin
Cholesterol
7-α-hydroxylase
1° bile acids
Glycine, Taurine
Physiologic disease of the newborn
Crigler–Najjar
Glucuronyl transferase
1° and 2° bile salts
2° bile acids
Dubin–Johnson syndrome
Gallbladder
Obstruction
Duodenum
Sphincter of Oddi
Jejunum
Portal circulation
Terminal Ileum
95% of bile salts reabsorbed
Colon
5% of bile salts in feces
= Direction of bile salt circulation
= Bile salt active transport system

Sources of Jaundice	
↑Unconjugated	↑Conjugated
Gilbert syndrome Crigler–Najjar syndrome Physiologic jaundice of newborn Hepatitis	Dubin–Johnson syndrome Obstruction of the common bile duct Hepatitis

FIGURE 5-9 **Important biochemical pathways of the liver and digestion**

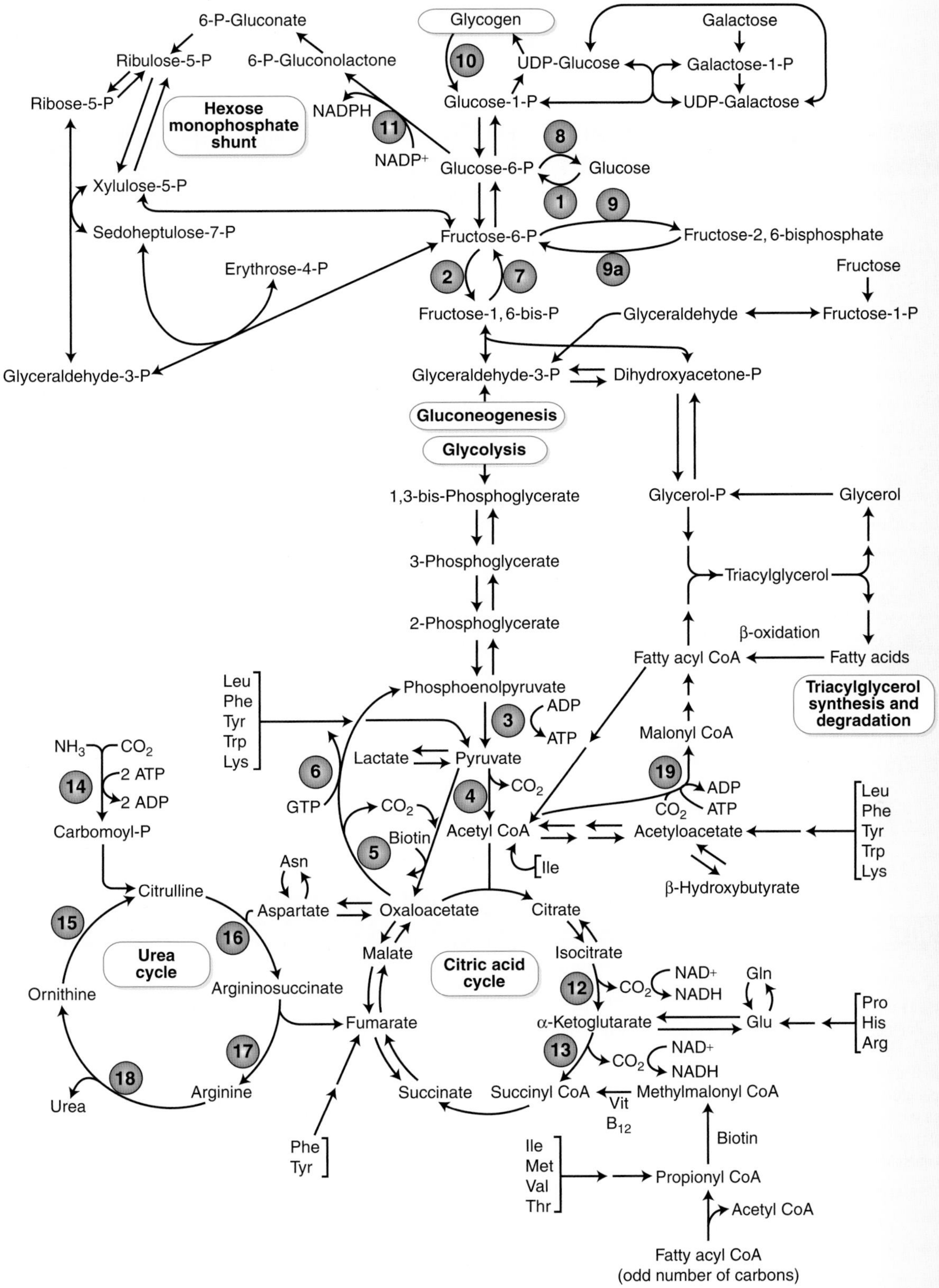
6-P-Gluconate
Ribulose-5-P
6-P-Gluconolactone
Ribose-5-P
Hexose monophosphate shunt
NADPH
NADP+
Xylulose-5-P
Sedoheptulose-7-P
Erythrose-4-P
Glyceraldehyde-3-P
Glycogen
UDP-Glucose
Glucose-1-P
Galactose
Galactose-1-P
UDP-Galactose
Glucose-6-P
Glucose
Fructose-6-P
Fructose-2, 6-bisphosphate
Fructose-1, 6-bis-P
Fructose
Glyceraldehyde
Fructose-1-P
Glyceraldehyde-3-P
Dihydroxyacetone-P
Gluconeogenesis
Glycolysis
1,3-bis-Phosphoglycerate
3-Phosphoglycerate
2-Phosphoglycerate
Phosphoenolpyruvate
ADP
ATP
Lactate
Pyruvate
Leu
Phe
Tyr
Trp
Lys
GTP
CO_2
Biotin
Acetyl CoA
Ile
Glycerol-P
Glycerol
Triacylglycerol
β-oxidation
Fatty acyl CoA
Fatty acids
Triacylglycerol synthesis and degradation
Malonyl CoA
Acetyloacetate
β-Hydroxybutyrate
NH_3
2 ATP
2 ADP
Carbomoyl-P
Citrulline
Asn
Aspartate
Oxaloacetate
Citrate
Isocitrate
Malate
Citric acid cycle
Urea cycle
Ornithine
Argininosuccinate
Fumarate
NAD+
NADH
Gln
Glu
α-Ketoglutarate
Pro
His
Arg
Arginine
Urea
Succinate
Succinyl CoA
Methylmalonyl CoA
Vit B_{12}
Biotin
Phe
Tyr
Ile
Met
Val
Thr
Propionyl CoA
Acetyl CoA
Fatty acyl CoA (odd number of carbons)
1
2
3
4
5
6
7
8
9
9a
10
11
12
13
14
15
16
17
18
19

ADP, adenosine diphosphate; Arg, arginine; Asn, asparagine; ATP, adenosine triphosphate; CoA, coenzyme A; CO_2, carbon dioxide; Gln, glutamine; Glu, glutamic acid; GTP, guanosine triphosphate; His, histidine; Ile, isoleucine; Leu, leucine; Lys, lysine; Met, methionine; $NADP^+$, nicotinamide adenide dinucleotide phosphate; NADPH, reduced nicotinamide adenide dinucleotide phosphate; NH_3, ammonia; Phe, phenylalanine; Pro, proline; Thr, threonine; Trp, tryptophan; Tyr, tyrosine; UDP, urine diphosphate; Val, valine.

IV. Glycolysis versus gluconeogenesis versus glycogenolysis *(Table 5-12)*

As food is absorbed, the glycolysis pathway is activated and energy is stored as glycogen in the liver. **Glycogenolysis** provides food for the periods between regular meals. After 30 hours of fasting, glycogen is completely depleted and **gluconeogenesis** becomes the only source of blood glucose.

TABLE 5-12 Glycolysis versus Gluconeogenesis versus Glycogenolysis

	Glycolysis	Gluconeogenesis	Glycogenolysis
Description of the process	Glucose is broken down to form pyruvate and energy is released	Glucose is formed after 4–6 h of fasting	**Glucose** is produced from glycogen stores after **2–3 hours of fasting**
Key enzymes and their regulation	Glucokinase (in liver), hexokinase (all tissues); requires ATP; (–) glucose-6-P; see enzyme 1, Figure 5-9 Phosphofructokinase-1 (PFK-1); requires ATP; **rate-limiting step in glycolysis;** (+) AMP, fructose-2-6-bis-P; (–) ATP, citrate; see enzyme 2, Figure 5-9 Pyruvate kinase; produces ATP; (+) fructose-1-6-bis-P; (–) alanine, phosphorylation, ATP; see enzyme 3, Figure 5-9 Pyruvate dehydrogenase; (+) pyruvate, insulin, ADP; (–) NADH, acetyl CoA, phosphorylation; see enzyme 4, Figure 5-9	Pyruvate carboxylase; requires **biotin, CO_2,** and **ATP;** (+) acetyl CoA; see enzyme 5, Figure 5-9 Phosphoenolpyruvate carboxykinase (PEPCK); requires GTP; (+) cortisol, glucagon; see enzyme 6, Figure 5-9 Fructose-1-6-bisphosphatase; (+) glucagon; (–) AMP, fructose-2-6-bis-P; see enzyme 7, Figure 5-9 Glucose-6-phosphatase; (+) glucagon; see enzyme 8, Figure 5-9	Glycogen phosphorylase; (+) AMP, phosphorylation; see enzyme 10, Figure 5-9 Phosphoglucomutase converts glucose-1-P to glucose-6-P

ADP, adenosine diphosphate; AMP, adenosine monophosphate; ATP, adenosine triphosphate; CoA, coenzyme A; CO_2, carbon dioxide; GTP, guanosine triphosphate; NADH, reduced nicotinamide adenine dinucleotide; P, phosphate.

V. Defective enzyme diseases *(Table 5-13)*

With a few exceptions, most defective enzyme diseases are autosomal recessive. Since the liver contains a high proportion of metabolic enzymes, it is often affected by these diseases.

QUICK HIT

McArdle disease is a glycogen-storage disease similar to von Gierke, Pompe, and Cori diseases, but it has no GI manifestations. It is a deficiency of muscle glycogen phosphorylase with consequent accumulation of glycogen in skeletal muscle.

TABLE 5-13 Defective Enzyme Diseases

Disease	Defective Enzyme	Clinical Features
Gaucher disease	Glucocerebrosidase	• Accumulation of **glucocerebroside** • Hepatosplenomegaly • Erosion of the head of the long bones (e.g., femur) • Gaucher cells (distinctive, **wrinkled paper** appearance) found in liver, spleen, and bone marrow
Niemann–Pick disease	Sphingomyelinase	• **Foamy histiocytes** in liver, spleen, lymph nodes, and skin • Hepatosplenomegaly • Anemia • Neurologic deterioration
von Gierke disease	Glucose-6-phosphatase	• Accumulation of glycogen in liver and kidney • Hepatomegaly • Hypoglycemia
Cori disease	Debranching enzyme	• Accumulation of glycogen in liver and striated muscle • Hepatomegaly • Hypoglycemia • Failure to grow

(continued)

TABLE 5-13 **Defective Enzyme Diseases** *(Continued)*

Disease	Defective Enzyme	Clinical Features
Pompe disease	α_1,4-Glucosidase (lysosomal enzyme)	• Accumulation of glycogen in liver and striated muscle • Cardiomegaly • Death caused by cardiac failure before 3 years of age
Galactosemia	Galactose-1-phosphate uridylyltransferase	• Accumulation of galactose-1-phosphate in many tissues • **Cataracts** • Cirrhosis • Mental retardation • Failure to thrive
Phenylketonuria	Phenylalanine hydroxylase	• Accumulation of phenylalanine • Cerebral myelin degeneration • **Mental retardation**
Maple syrup urine disease	Branched-chain α-ketoacid dehydrogenase	• Inability to metabolize leucine, isoleucine, and valine • Neurologic symptoms • High mortality

VI. Viral hepatitis *(Table 5-14 and Figure 5-10)*

Viral hepatitis can lead to **direct hyperbilirubinemia**, elevated serum transaminases, icterus, or hepatomegaly, but not ascites. Morphologically, changes range from multifocal hepatocellular necrosis (hepatitis A and hepatitis B) to ballooning degeneration (hepatitis B and hepatitis C) to piecemeal necrosis (hepatitis C).

MNEMONIC

To remember that hepatitis A and E are transmitted by the fecal-oral route, think of the phrase **"vowels are bowels."**

TABLE 5-14 **Viral Hepatitis**

	Hepatitis A	Hepatitis B	Hepatitis C	Hepatitis D	Hepatitis E
Virus family	Picornavirus	Hepadnavirus	Flavivirus	Delta agent	Calicivirus
Viral morphology	Single-stranded RNA	Circular, double-stranded DNA	Single-stranded RNA	Incomplete genome of single-stranded RNA	Single-stranded RNA
Mode of transmission	Fecal-oral	Sexual and parenteral, transplacental	Parenteral; limited sexual; transplacental	Sexual and parenteral, transplacental	Fecal-oral
Diagnostic test	IgM anti-HAV	HBsAg; anti-HBsAg; HBeAg; HBV DNA; IgM anti-HBcAg	Anti-HCV	Anti-sag	None
Severity	Mild	Moderate	Mild	Severe	Mild
Chronic infection	No	10% of adults, 80%–90% of infants, and immunocompromised patients	80%–90%	No increase over hepatitis B alone	No
Carrier state	No	Yes	Yes	Yes	No
Hepatocellular carcinoma	No	Yes	Yes	No	No
Prophylaxis and treatment	Immune globulin; vaccine	Hepatitis B immune globulin; vaccine Interferon and nucleoside analog inhibitors of viral DNA synthesis	Interferon and ribavirin	Hepatitis B immune globulin; vaccine	None
Notes	Incubation period of 14–15 days	**Dane particle:** viral DNA genome, DNA polymerase, HBcAg, HBeAg, HBsAg; has **reverse transcriptase;** incubation period 60–90 days	**Most frequent cause of transfusion-mediated hepatitis**	Defective in replication; **requires coinfection with hepatitis B**	Hepatitis infection in third-world nations; mortality in pregnant females

HAV, hepatitis A virus; HBcAg, hepatitis B core antigen; HBeAg, hepatitis B envelope antigen; HBsAg, hepatitis B surface antigen; HBV, hepatitis B virus; HCV, hepatitis C virus; IgM, immunoglobulin M.

QUICK HIT

Hepatitis B viral DNA, hepatitis B surface antigen (HBsAg), and hepatitis B envelope antigen (HBeAg) are indicators of virus replication. Antibody to hepatitis B surface antigen (HBsAb) is indicative of recovery and immunity. HBsAb is also positive following vaccination. Antibody to hepatitis B core antigen (HBcAb) is positive in early infection; in addition, HBcAb acts as a marker for hepatitis infection during the "window" period, which is the period during acute infection when HBsAg is undetectable and HBsAb has not yet appeared. During the window period, equivalent amounts of surface antigen and antibody neutralize each other and thus are not detectable by testing.

FIGURE 5-10 Hepatitis B serology and interpretation of hepatitis B panel

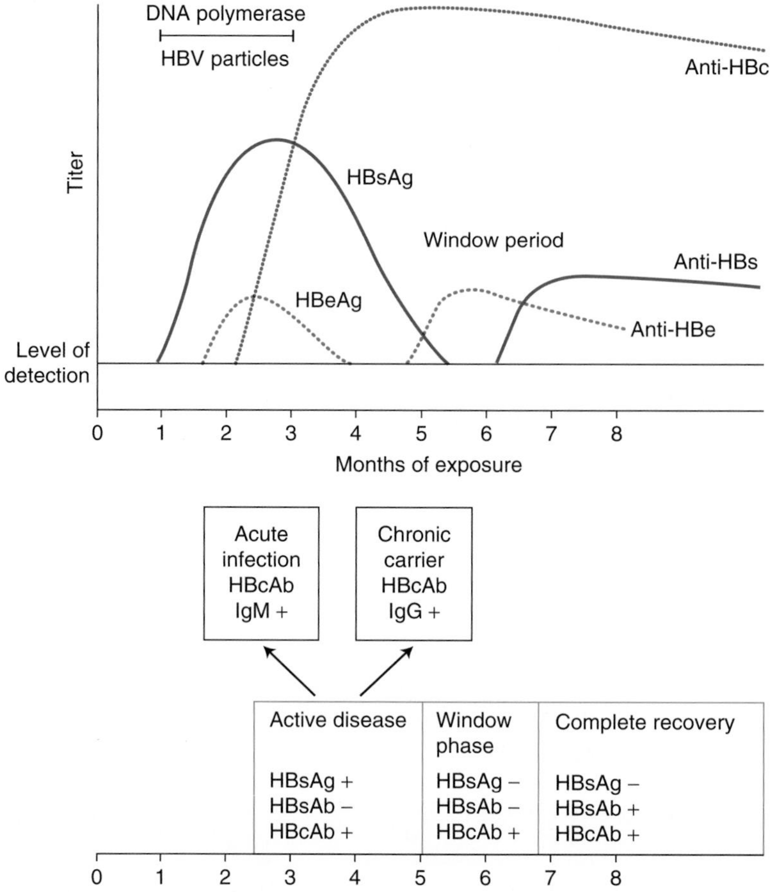
DNA polymerase
HBV particles
Anti-HBc
Titer
HBsAg
Window period
Anti-HBs
HBeAg
Anti-HBe
Level of detection
0 1 2 3 4 5 6 7 8
Months of exposure
Acute infection HBcAb IgM +
Chronic carrier HBcAb IgG +
Active disease
HBsAg +
HBsAb –
HBcAb +
Window phase
HBsAg –
HBsAb –
HBcAb +
Complete recovery
HBsAg –
HBsAb +
HBcAb +
0 1 2 3 4 5 6 7 8

HBcAb, hepatitis B core antibody; HBeAg, hepatitis B envelope antigen; HBsAb, antibody to hepatitis B surface antigen; HBsAg, hepatitis B surface antigen; HBV, hepatitis B virus; IgG, immunoglobulin G; IgM, immunoglobulin M.

VII. Cirrhosis *(Table 5-15)*

Cirrhosis is a disease of the liver characterized by fibrosis and disorganization of the lobular and vascular structure owing to the destruction and regeneration of hepatocytes.

QUICK HIT

Cirrhosis often leads to **portal hypertension.** There are three major collateral circulation pathways that allow blood to return to the heart: (a) left gastric to esophageal plexus to azygous to the superior vena cava (SVC) **(esophageal varices)**; (b) inferior mesenteric to superior rectal to inferior rectal to inferior vena cava (IVC) **(hemorrhoids)**; and (c) ligamentum teres to superficial abdominals to SVC or IVC **(caput medusae).**

TABLE 5-15 Cirrhosis

Etiology	Pathology	Clinical Manifestation	Notes
Chronic alcohol abuse	**Micronodular** fatty liver; decreased metabolism of estrogen; decreased synthesis of coagulation factors	**Jaundice,** bleeding, gynecomastia, testicular atrophy, edema, **asterixis,** portal HTN **(esophageal varices,** spider angiomata, and splenomegaly), encephalopathy	**Most common cause of cirrhosis in the United States**
Wilson disease	**Decreased ceruloplasmin**	Copper deposits in liver, basal ganglia (causing extrapyramidal signs), and Descemet membrane of cornea **(Kayser–Fleischer ring)**	Autosomal recessive
Hemochromatosis	Familial; increased total iron; decreased TIBC; increased ferritin; increased transferrin saturation	Iron deposits in liver, diabetes mellitus, increased skin pigmentation, cardiomyopathy	Bronze diabetes; increased risk of hepatocellular carcinoma

(continued)

TABLE 5-15 **Cirrhosis** *(Continued)*

Etiology	Pathology	Clinical Manifestation	Notes
Primary biliary cirrhosis	Autoimmune; **antimitochondrial antibodies**	Jaundice, pruritus, hypercholesterolemia, beading on ERCP	More common in women and middle-aged people
Posthepatic cirrhosis	Chronic active hepatitis caused by HBV and HCV infection	Jaundice, pruritus	**Most likely cause of cirrhosis to lead to hepatocellular carcinoma**
α_1-Antitrypsin deficiency	Autosomal recessive; defective α_1-antitrypsin accumulates in hepatocytes	Jaundice, **panacinar emphysema**, pancreatic manifestations	**More severe in homozygous form** (PI*ZZ alleles)
Congestive heart failure	Passive congestion	**Nutmeg liver**	Most often a result of right heart failure

ERCP, endoscopic retrograde cholangiopancreatography; HBV, hepatitis B virus; HCV, hepatitis C virus; HTN, hypertension; TIBC, total iron-binding capacity.

VIII. Common clinical disorders of the hepatobiliary system *(Table 5-16 and Figures 5-11, 5-12, and 5-13)*

TABLE 5-16 **Common Clinical Disorders of the Hepatobiliary System**

Disorder	Etiology and Pathology	Clinical Features	Notes
Cholelithiasis (gallstones)	Very common disease; women older than 40 years of age; obesity; multiparity	Steatorrhea, nausea, vomiting, bile duct obstruction, jaundice, may lead to cholangitis or cholecystitis, malignancy, positive Murphy sign	Cholesterol stones (large); pigment stones (seen in hemolytic anemia or excess bilirubin production); mixed stones (majority)
Primary biliary cirrhosis	**Autoimmune** disease leading to the destruction of intrahepatic bile ducts; middle-aged women	**Pruritus, jaundice, hypercholesterolemia,** RUQ discomfort, portal HTN	Positive **antimitochondrial antibodies;** associated with other autoimmune diseases
Primary sclerosing cholangitis	Fibrosis and stenosis of intrahepatic or extrahepatic bile ducts	Jaundice, pruritus, weight loss	Strong association with **ulcerative colitis;** increased incidence of cholangiocarcinoma
Adenocarcinoma of the gallbladder	Gallstones	Obstructive jaundice, enlarged gallbladder	**Courvoisier law:** obstruction of CBD enlarges the gallbladder, whereas obstructing stones do not; caused by scarring of the gallbladder
Hepatocellular adenoma (hepatoma)	Benign tumor; women 20–30 years of age taking **oral contraceptives**	Usually found incidentally; may cause pain or hemorrhage	10% may become malignant; oral contraceptive use should be stopped, lesion regresses with the cessation of contraceptive
Hepatocellular carcinoma	Cirrhosis, **hepatitis B, hepatitis C,** aflatoxin B (carcinogen in contaminated peanuts)	Increased α-fetoprotein, jaundice, abdominal distention, ascites	**Hematogenous spread**

CBD, common bile duct; HTN, hypertension; RUQ, right upper quadrant.

QUICK HIT

Pigment gallstones occurring in children or young adults with no history of pregnancy may be a result of a congenital hemoglobinopathy (e.g., sickle cell disease or thalassemia).

QUICK HIT

Murphy sign: Cessation of inspiration as a result of deep palpation of RUQ by examiner during inspiration; **Charcot triad:** Fever, RUQ pain, and jaundice; **Reynold pentad:** Charcot triad plus hypotension and mental status changes.

QUICK HIT

Metastatic disease is the most common source of malignancy in the liver.

FIGURE
5-11 Approach to liver studies

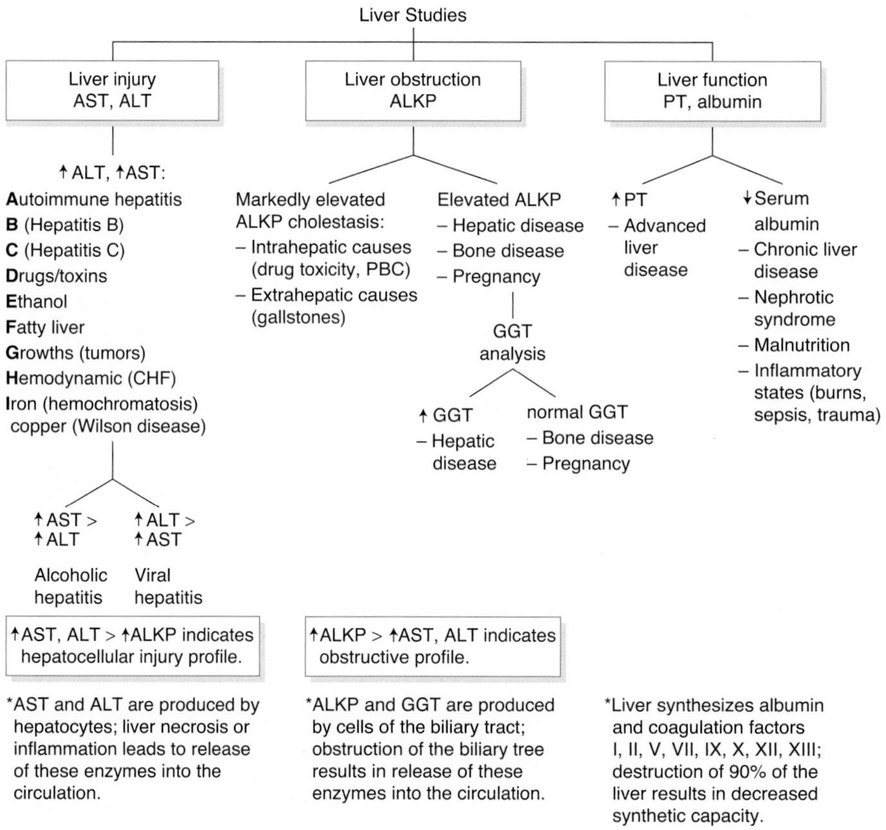
Liver Studies
Liver injury
AST, ALT
Liver obstruction
ALKP
Liver function
PT, albumin
↑ALT, ↑AST:
Autoimmune hepatitis
B (Hepatitis B)
C (Hepatitis C)
Drugs/toxins
Ethanol
Fatty liver
Growths (tumors)
Hemodynamic (CHF)
Iron (hemochromatosis)
copper (Wilson disease)
↑AST > ↑ALT
↑ALT > ↑AST
Alcoholic hepatitis
Viral hepatitis
Markedly elevated ALKP cholestasis:
– Intrahepatic causes (drug toxicity, PBC)
– Extrahepatic causes (gallstones)
Elevated ALKP
– Hepatic disease
– Bone disease
– Pregnancy
GGT analysis
↑GGT
– Hepatic disease
normal GGT
– Bone disease
– Pregnancy
↑PT
– Advanced liver disease
↓Serum albumin
– Chronic liver disease
– Nephrotic syndrome
– Malnutrition
– Inflammatory states (burns, sepsis, trauma)
↑AST, ALT > ↑ALKP indicates hepatocellular injury profile.
↑ALKP > ↑AST, ALT indicates obstructive profile.
*AST and ALT are produced by hepatocytes; liver necrosis or inflammation leads to release of these enzymes into the circulation.
*ALKP and GGT are produced by cells of the biliary tract; obstruction of the biliary tree results in release of these enzymes into the circulation.
*Liver synthesizes albumin and coagulation factors I, II, V, VII, IX, X, XII, XIII; destruction of 90% of the liver results in decreased synthetic capacity.

ALKP, alkaline phosphatase; ALT, alanine aminotransferase; AST, aspartate aminotransferase; CHF, congestive heart failure; GGT, gamma glutamyl transpeptidase; PBC, primary biliary cirrhosis; PT, prothrombin time.

FIGURE
5-12 Diseases of the gallbladder and biliary tract

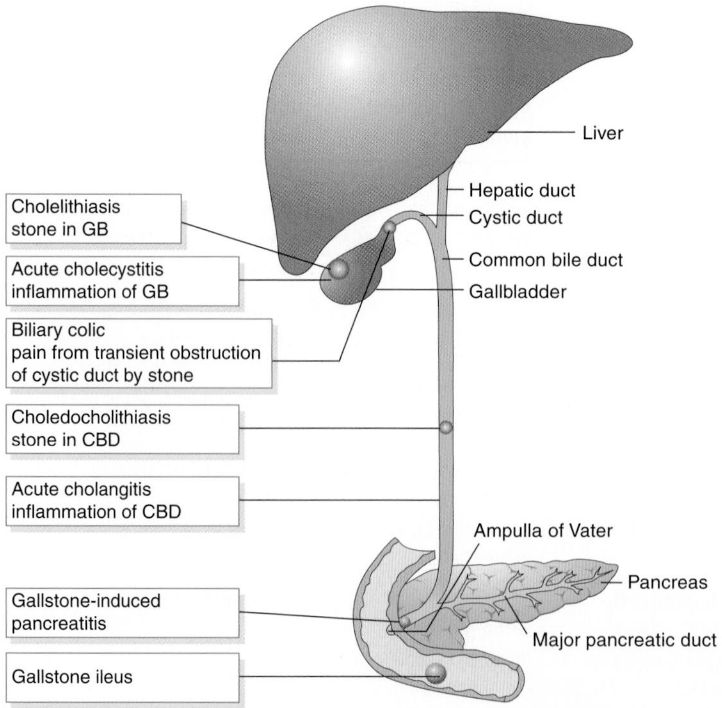
Liver
Hepatic duct
Cystic duct
Common bile duct
Gallbladder
Cholelithiasis
stone in GB
Acute cholecystitis
inflammation of GB
Biliary colic
pain from transient obstruction of cystic duct by stone
Choledocholithiasis
stone in CBD
Acute cholangitis
inflammation of CBD
Ampulla of Vater
Pancreas
Major pancreatic duct
Gallstone-induced pancreatitis
Gallstone ileus

CBD, common bile duct; GB, gallbladder.

The Gastrointestinal System

FIGURE 5-13 **Approach to fractionate bilirubin studies**

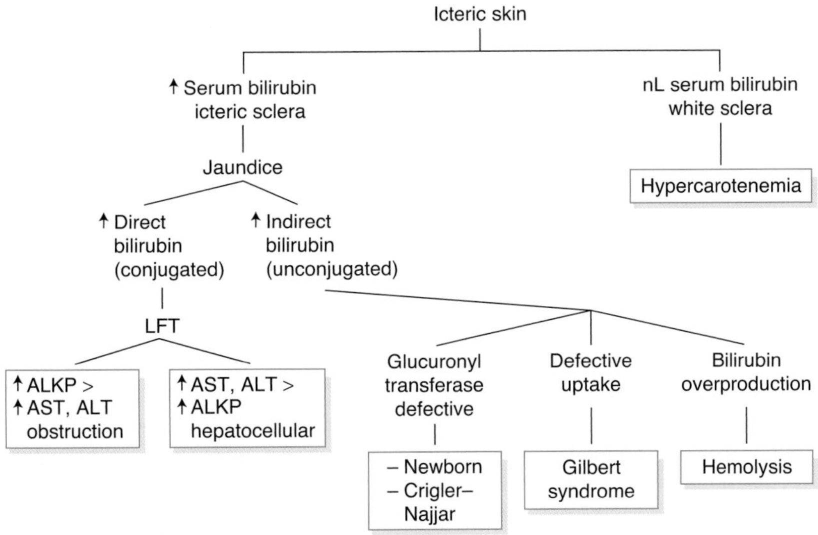
Icteric skin
↑ Serum bilirubin icteric sclera
nL serum bilirubin white sclera
Jaundice
Hypercarotenemia
↑ Direct bilirubin (conjugated)
↑ Indirect bilirubin (unconjugated)
LFT
↑ ALKP > ↑ AST, ALT obstruction
↑ AST, ALT > ↑ ALKP hepatocellular
Glucuronyl transferase defective
Defective uptake
Bilirubin overproduction
– Newborn – Crigler–Najjar
Gilbert syndrome
Hemolysis

ALKP, alkaline phosphatase; ALT, alanine aminotransferase; AST, aspartate aminotransferase; LFT, liver function test.

Clinical Vignette 5-4

CLINICAL PRESENTATION: A 6-year-old boy presents to the emergency department with multiple episodes of **nausea and vomiting** of 2 days' duration, and today his **"stomach hurts."** The worried mother reports finding the Tylenol bottle half empty this morning. On physical examination, the patient is **jaundiced** and diaphoretic, with **right upper quadrant (RUQ) tenderness.** Temperature = 98.6° F; blood pressure = 110/70 mm Hg; heart rate = 103 bpm; and respiration rate = 22 breaths/min.

DIFFERENTIALS: Acetaminophen-induced liver toxicity and gastroenteritis. The chemical structure of acetaminophen is *N*-acetyl-*p*-aminophenol (APAP). APAP itself is nontoxic but it is metabolized primarily in the liver by cytochrome P450 to a toxic metabolite, *N*-acetyl-*p*-benzoquinoneimine (NAPQI). Glutathione can bind NAPQI and lead to the excretion of nontoxic mercapturate conjugates in the urine. As the glutathione stores are diminished, NAPQI accumulates and covalently binds to the hepatocyte lipid bilayer, causing centrilobular necrosis. Inducers of cytochrome P450, such as ethanol, isoniazid, rifampin, phenytoin, barbiturates, and carbamazepine, can lead to an increased production of NAPQI.

LABORATORY STUDIES: Elevated **serum APAP levels** and **transaminase levels** greater than 1,000 U/L support the diagnosis of APAP hepatotoxicity. **Coagulation studies** should also be obtained to monitor the liver function.

MANAGEMENT: Glutathione stores can be replaced orally or intravenously by sulfhydryl-containing compounds like ***N*-acetylcysteine.** *N*-acetylcysteine also directly detoxifies NAPQI to nontoxic metabolites by acting as a substrate for sulfation. In addition to *N*-acetylcysteine, if the patient presents within hours of the incident, **gastric lavage** and **oral charcoal** could also be performed.

The Gastrointestinal System

Clinical Vignette 5-5

CLINICAL PRESENTATION: During a visit to her primary care physician, a 42-year-old woman complains of intermittent **right upper quadrant (RUQ) pain** of several months' duration that is worse after **large and fatty meals.** Pain is **steady** and **lasts 1 to 4 hours** and is sometimes associated with nausea and vomiting. Physical exam reveals a soft, nondistended abdomen with mild tenderness in the RUQ, normal bowel sounds, and no palpable masses. No cough tenderness, rebound tenderness, or tenderness to percussion. Temperature = 98.7° F; blood pressure = 130/80 mm Hg; heart rate = 85 bpm; and respiration rate = 20 breaths/min.
DIFFERENTIALS: Biliary colic/cholelithiasis, acute cholecystitis, choledocholithiasis, and acute cholangitis. When differentiating between the various causes of RUQ pain, use these findings to guide your approach: (a) when **obstructive symptoms (jaundice, pruritus, light-colored stools, tea-colored urine, etc.)** are present, consider a stone in the common bile duct (CBD) (e.g., choledocholithiasis or acute cholangitis); (b) **inflammation of the parietal peritoneum** elicited by **cough tenderness, rebound tenderness, tenderness to percussion,** and **still posture** indicates an inflammatory condition (e.g., acute cholecystitis or acute cholangitis); and (c) look for specific signs: **Murphy sign** (acute cholecystitis), **Charcot triad** (acute cholangitis), and **Reynold pentad** (acute suppurative cholangitis).
LABORATORY STUDIES: **Ultrasound** is the most effective imaging study for diagnosing cholelithiasis and is superior to CT and radiography. Relevant findings include stones, a thickened gallbladder wall, and pericholecystic fluid. Dilation of the CBD suggests obstruction. To sort through the differentials, look for an obstructive pattern on **fractionate bilirubin** and **liver enzyme studies** to support choledocholithiasis and acute cholangitis: elevated direct bilirubin and marked increases in alkaline phosphatase in comparison to mild increases in aspartate aminotransferase (AST) and alanine aminotransferase (ALT). **Complete blood count studies** showing an increase in white blood cells with a left shift would support an inflammatory condition (acute cholecystitis or cholangitis).
MANAGEMENT: Uncomplicated cholelithiasis and acute cholecystis are treated surgically with a cholecystectomy. Choledocholithiasis and acute cholangitis are treated by endoscopic retrograde cholangiopancreatography (ERCP); if this fails, surgical exploration of the CBD is attempted. In acute cholecystitis and cholangitis, antibiotics are also given to resolve the underlying infection.

THE PANCREAS

- Common Clinical Disorders of the Pancreas (Table 5-17)

In the United States, alcohol is the most common cause of pancreatic pathology.

QUICK HIT

Multiple endocrine neoplasia type 1 (MEN 1) involves neoplasia or hyperplasia of the pancreas, the parathyroids, and the pituitary.

QUICK HIT

Use patient **history** to determine whether the cause of pancreatitis is gallstones or alcohol abuse. The **amylase/lipase levels** are markedly elevated in gallstone pancreatitis (thousands) in comparison to the increase seen in alcoholic pancreatitis (hundreds); chronic alcohol consumption may lead to less functioning pancreatic tissue.

TABLE 5-17 Common Clinical Disorders of the Pancreas

Disorder	Etiology and Pathology	Clinical Features	Notes
Acute pancreatitis	Gallstones (obstructing the ampulla of Vater); alcohol abuse	**Midepigastric pain radiating to the back; increased serum amylase** and lipase; hemorrhage may lead to Cullen or Grey Turner sign; hypocalcemia	Activation of pancreatic enzymes leads to autodigestion
Chronic pancreatitis	**Alcoholism** in adults; cystic fibrosis in children	**Increased serum amylase** and lipase, **pancreatic calcifications,** epigastric pain, steatorrhea	Irreversible; leads to organ atrophy; may lead to formation of pancreatic pseudocyst
Adenocarcinoma of the exocrine pancreas	More common in smokers	Invasive; **Trousseau syndrome** (migratory thrombophlebitis); radiating abdominal pain; obstructive jaundice; **increased carcinoembryonic antigen**	Poor prognosis; over 50% in the head of the pancreas; more common in Blacks, males, patients with diabetes, and people older than 60 years

(continued)

TABLE 5-17 Common Clinical Disorders of the Pancreas *(Continued)*

Disorder	Etiology and Pathology	Clinical Features	Notes
Insulinoma (endocrine pancreas)	Originates in β cells	**Whipple triad:** hypoglycemia, CNS dysfunction, and reversal of CNS abnormalities with glucose	Most common islet cell tumor
Gastrinoma (Zollinger–Ellison syndrome)	Gastrin-secreting tumor (most commonly, islet cell origin)	Recurrent peptic ulcers	Part of **multiple endocrine neoplasia type 1**

CNS, central nervous system.

QUICK HIT

The presence of **C-peptide** in the blood distinguishes endogenous insulin secretions (as in an insulinoma) from exogenous insulin administration (as seen in Munchausen syndrome).

PATHOGENS OF THE GASTROINTESTINAL TRACT

I. Bacterial

Enterobacteriaceae
Salmonella
Shigella
Escherichia coli
Vibrio cholerae
Staphylococcus aureus
Campylobacter jejuni
Helicobacter pylori
Clostridium botulinum
Clostridium difficile
Bacillus fragilis

II. Parasitic

Entamoeba histolytica
Giardia lamblia
Cryptosporidium
Trichuris trichiura
Ascaris lumbricoides
Strongyloides stercoralis

III. Viral

Adenovirus
Coronavirus
Echovirus
Rotavirus
Norwalk agent
Reovirus

THERAPEUTIC AGENTS FOR THE GASTROINTESTINAL SYSTEM

Various therapeutic agents have been designed to treat GI diseases such as heartburn (Table 5-18), diarrhea (Table 5-19), nausea (Table 5-20), and constipation (Table 5-21).

TABLE 5-18 Therapeutic Agents for Heartburn

Therapeutic Agent (common name, if relevant) [trade name, where appropriate]	Class—Pharmacology and Pharmacokinetics	Indications	Side Effects or Adverse Effects	Contraindications or Precautions to Consider; Notes
Cimetidine, ranitidine [Zantac]	**H_2 blocker—blocks histamine H_2 receptors; reversibly decreases proton secretion by parietal cells**	**Peptic ulcer disease, gastritis, esophageal reflux**	**Gynecomastia, impotence,** and decreased libido in males (cimetidine only); **dizziness and headaches**	**Crosses placenta; decreases renal excretion of creatinine; cytochrome P450 inhibitor**
Famotidine [Pepcid], **Nizatidine**	**H_2 blocker—blocks histamine H_2 receptors; reversibly decreases proton secretion by parietal cells**	**Peptic ulcer disease, gastritis, esophageal reflux**	**Gynecomastia** (rare); confusion, dizziness, and headaches	**Crosses placenta; milder side effect profile** than cimetidine and ranitidine

(continued)

TABLE 5-18 **Therapeutic Agents for Heartburn** *(Continued)*

Therapeutic Agent (common name, if relevant) [trade name, where appropriate]	Class—Pharmacology and Pharmacokinetics	Indications	Side Effects or Adverse Effects	Contraindications or Precautions to Consider; Notes
Omeprazole [Prilosec], **lansoprazole, esomeprazole**	**Proton pump inhibitor—irreversibly inhibits H^+/K^+-ATPase in gastric parietal cells → decreases proton secretion by parietal cells**	Peptic ulcer disease, gastritis, esophageal reflux, and **Zollinger–Ellison syndrome**		**Inhibits cytochrome P450;** given with clarithromycin and **amoxicillin** for ***Helicobacter pylori***
Bismuth [Pepto-Bismol], **sucralfate**	**Cytoprotectant—binds to ulcer base → protection; allows bicarbonate ion secretion to reestablish pH gradient in the mucous layer**	**Traveler's diarrhea,** peptic ulcer disease		
Misoprostol	**Cytoprotectant—PGE_1 analog → increased production and secretion of gastric mucosa barrier; decreased acid production**	**Prevents NSAID-induced peptic ulcers;** maintains patent ductus arteriosus	**Diarrhea**	**Abortion-inducing drug,** contraindicated in women of childbearing age
Pirenzepine, propantheline	**Muscarinic antagonist—blocks M_1 receptors on ECL cells → decreases histamine secretion; blocks M_3 receptors on parietal cells → decreases acid secretion**	Peptic ulcer	**Tachycardia, dry mouth, blurry vision** (difficulty accommodating)	
Aluminum hydroxide	**Antacid**—buffers gastric acid by raising pH	Peptic ulcer, gastritis, esophageal reflux, and diarrhea	**Constipation,** hypophosphatemia, muscle weakness, **osteodystrophy,** seizures, and **hypokalemia**	Can affect the **absorption, bioavailability,** or **urinary excretion** of drugs by changing the **gastric pH, urinary pH,** or **gastric emptying**
Magnesium hydroxide (milk of magnesia)	**Antacid**—buffers gastric acid by raising pH	Peptic ulcer, gastritis, esophageal reflux, and constipation	**Diarrhea, hyporeflexia, hypotension, cardiac arrest, hypokalemia**	Can affect the **absorption, bioavailability,** or **urinary excretion** of drugs by chang- ing **the gastric pH, urinary pH, or gastric emptying**
Calcium carbonate [TUMS, Caltrate]	**Antacid**—buffers gastric acid by raising pH	Peptic ulcer, gastritis, esophageal reflux, and calcium deficiency	**Hypercalcemia, rebound acid increase, and hypokalemia**	Can affect the **absorption, bioavailability,** or **urinary excretion** of drugs by changing **the gastric pH, urinary pH, or gastric emptying**

ATPase, adenosine triphosphatase; ECL, enterochromaffin-like; PGE_1, prostaglandin E_1.

TABLE 5-19 Therapeutic Agents for Diarrhea, Ulcerative Colitis, and Crohn Disease

Therapeutic Agent (common name, if relevant) [trade name, where appropriate]	Class—Pharmacology and Pharmacokinetics	Indications	Side Effects or Adverse Effects	Contraindications or Precautions to Consider; Notes
Loperamide [Imodium]	**Antidiarrheal—similar to opioid agonist**	**Oral antidiarrheal**		
Aluminum hydroxide	**Antidiarrheal—delays gastric emptying**	Peptic ulcer, gastritis, esophageal reflux, and diarrhea	**Constipation,** hypophosphatemia, muscle weakness, **osteodystrophy,** seizures, and **hypokalemia**	Can **affect the absorption, bioavailability, or urinary excretion of drugs** by changing the **gastric pH, urinary pH,** or **gastric emptying**
Sulfasalazine	**Anti-inflammatory—sulfapyridine (antibacterial)** and **mesalamine (anti-inflammatory)**	Ulcerative colitis, Crohn disease	Malaise, nausea, **sulfonamide toxicity,** reversible **oligospermia**	**Activated by colonic bacteria**
Infliximab	**Anti-inflammatory—monoclonal antibody** that binds TNF → **inhibits proinflammatory effects** of TNF	**Crohn disease,** rheumatoid arthritis	Respiratory infection, fever, and hypotension	

TNF, tumor necrosis factor.

TABLE 5-20 Therapeutic Agents for Nausea

Therapeutic Agent (common name, if relevant) [trade name, where appropriate]	Class—Pharmacology and Pharmacokinetics	Indications	Side Effects or Adverse Effects	Contraindications or Precautions to Consider; Notes
Scopolamine	**Anticholinergic**—M_1-muscarinic receptor antagonist	**Motion sickness;** prophylaxis	**Dry mouth,** drowsiness, and **vision disturbances**	**Delivered transdermally**
Promethazine [Phenergan]	**Antihistamine**—D_2-receptor antagonist; H_1 blocker	Counteracts nausea of **migraine;** allergies; **motion sickness**	Sedation, CNS depression, atropine-like effects, allergic dermatitis, blood dyscrasias, **teratogenicity,** acute antihistamine poisoning	
Prochlorperazine [Compazine]	**Dopamine antagonist**—D_2-receptor antagonist	**Nausea;** counteracts nausea of **migraine**	Teratogenic	
Metoclopramide [Reglan]	**Dopamine antagonist—central and peripheral D_2 antagonism at low doses and** weak 5-HT_3 antagonism at high doses; enhances acetylcholine release, prokinetic	**Nausea;** counteracts nausea of **migraine;** increases stomach motility	Sleepiness, fatigue, headache, insomnia, dizziness, nausea, akathisia, **dystonia,** and tardive dyskinesia	
Ondansetron [Zofran]	**Serotonin antagonist—5-HT_2 blocker**	**Nausea** (caused by **cancer therapy** or **postoperative state)**	Headache, constipation, and dizziness	

5-HT, serotonin; CNS, central nervous system.

The Gastrointestinal System

TABLE 5-21 Therapeutic Agents for Constipation

Therapeutic Agent (common name, if relevant) [trade name, where appropriate]	Class—Pharmacology and Pharmacokinetics	Indications	Side Effects or Adverse Effects	Contraindications or Precautions to Consider; Notes
Methylcellulose [Citrucel] **Psyllium** [Perdiem Fiber]	**Bulk-forming laxative**—dietary fiber	Constipation	Impaction above strictures, fluid overload, gas, and bloating	
Lactulose	**Osmotic laxative**	Decreases ammonia in hepatic encephalopathy; constipation	Abdominal bloating and flatulence	Lowers colon pH so that ammonia is trapped and then excreted
Magnesium hydroxide [Milk of Magnesia]	**Osmotic laxative**	Constipation, peptic ulcer, gastritis, and esophageal reflux	Diarrhea	
Magnesium sulfate, Magnesium citrate	**Osmotic laxative**		Magnesium toxicity (in renal insufficiency)	
Docusate	**Stool softener;** by emulsifying stool, it makes the passage of stool easier	Constipation	Skin rash	
Bisacodyl [Dulcolax]	**Stimulant laxative;** increases peristalsis	Constipation	Electrolyte imbalances (chronic use); gastric irritation	
Senna [Senokot]	**Stimulant laxative;** increases peristalsis	Constipation	Electrolyte imbalances (chronic use); melanosis coli	
Phenolphthalein [Ex-Lax]	**Stimulant laxative**—reduces the absorption of electrolytes and water from the gut	Constipation	Tumorigenic	
Anthraquinones	**Stimulant laxative**—reduces the absorption of electrolytes and water from the gut	Constipation		
Castor oil	**Stimulant laxative**—reduces the absorption of electrolytes and water from the gut; active component is ricinoleic acid	Constipation, labor induction		
Mineral oil [Fleet Mineral Oil Enema]	**Hyperosmolar agent**—draws water into the gut lumen → gut distension → promotes peristalsis and evacuation of bowel	**Preoperative patients;** short-term treatment of constipation		May interfere with the absorption of fat-soluble vitamins
Metoclopramide [Reglan]	**Prokinetic agent—D_2-receptor antagonist;** increases resting tone, contractility, LES tone, and motility (does not affect colon transit time)	**Diabetic** and **postoperative gastroparesis**	Sleepiness, fatigue, headache, insomnia, dizziness, nausea, akathisia, **dystonia,** and tardive dyskinesia	Interacts with **digoxin** and **diabetic agents; contraindicated in small bowel obstruction**

LES, lower esophageal sphincter.

6 The Renal System

DEVELOPMENT

I. Intermediate mesoderm

A. This forms the urogenital ridges on each side of the aorta.
B. The **nephrogenic cord** arises from the urogenital ridge and gives rise, wholly or in part, to the pronephros, the mesonephros, and the metanephros.

II. Pronephros

A. Forms in the fourth week
B. Quickly regresses by the fifth week
C. Nonfunctional

III. Mesonephros

A. Forms late in the fourth week and is functional until the permanent kidney is able to develop
B. The **mesonephric duct** forms from the mesonephros.
   1. Forms the ductus deferens, epididymis, ejaculatory duct, and seminal vesicle in the male
   2. Forms the **ureteric bud** from which the **ureter**, **renal pelvis**, **calyces**, and **collecting tubules** in both the male and female are derived
   3. No important genital or reproductive derivatives of the mesonephric duct specific to females are formed.

QUICK HIT

The entire collecting system arises from the **ureteric bud.** The remainder of the renal system arises from the metanephric mesoderm.

IV. Metanephros

A. Develops into the **adult kidney**
B. Formed during the fifth week from the **ureteric bud** and the metanephric mass (which is induced to form by contact with the ureteric bud) and begins to function in the ninth week
C. Metanephric mesoderm forms the nephrons.
D. "Ascends" from sacral levels to low thoracic levels during its development because of longitudinal growth of the fetus
E. Urogenital sinus forms the **bladder**, which is continuous with allantois. Allantois is equivalent to the median umbilical ligament in the adult.
F. Urethra
   1. Formed from endoderm and urogenital sinus
   2. Distal portion formed from ectoderm

V. Congenital anomalies of the renal system *(Table 6-1)*

TABLE 6-1 **Congenital Anomalies**

Anomaly	Characteristics
Bilateral renal agenesis (Potter syndrome)	• Occurs when the ureteric bud does not form • **Oligohydramnios** • Limb deformities • Facial deformities • **Pulmonary hypoplasia** • Bilateral agenesis is not compatible with life
Accessory renal arteries	• Arise from the aorta • Feed a particular section of the kidney • Are end arteries • **Cutting will produce ischemic infarct** in the area they supply
Congenital polycystic kidney disease	• Multiple small and large cysts causing renal insufficiency • Cysts are "closed"—not continuous with collecting system • Enlarged kidneys palpable on newborn examination • Death within days to weeks
Horseshoe kidney	• Inferior poles of the kidneys are fused • Ascent is arrested at the level of the inferior mesenteric artery • Increases probability of Wilms tumor

QUICK HIT

In the adult male, the ureter passes posterior to the ductus deferens; in the adult female, the ureter passes posterior to the uterine artery.

MNEMONIC

To remember the relationship of the arteries to the ureter, think "water under the bridge"; the ureters (which carry water) are posterior to the ovarian/testicular artery and uterine artery.

QUICK HIT

The left gonadal (testicular or ovarian) vein drains into the left renal vein; the right gonadal vein drains directly into the inferior vena cava.

GROSS DESCRIPTION OF THE KIDNEY

I. Paired adult kidneys weigh approximately 150 g each.

II. They are located posterior to the peritoneum and at approximately the level of the first lumbar vertebra.

III. The right kidney is slightly lower than the left owing to downward displacement by the liver.

IV. The left renal vein lies posterior to the superior mesenteric artery and anterior to the abdominal aorta.

V. The kidney is highly vascularized; it filters more than 1,700 L of blood per day to produce about 1 L of urine.

VI. Kidney and urinary tract *(Figure 6-1)*

VII. Distribution of body water *(Figure 6-2)*

FIGURE 6-1 The kidney and urinary tract

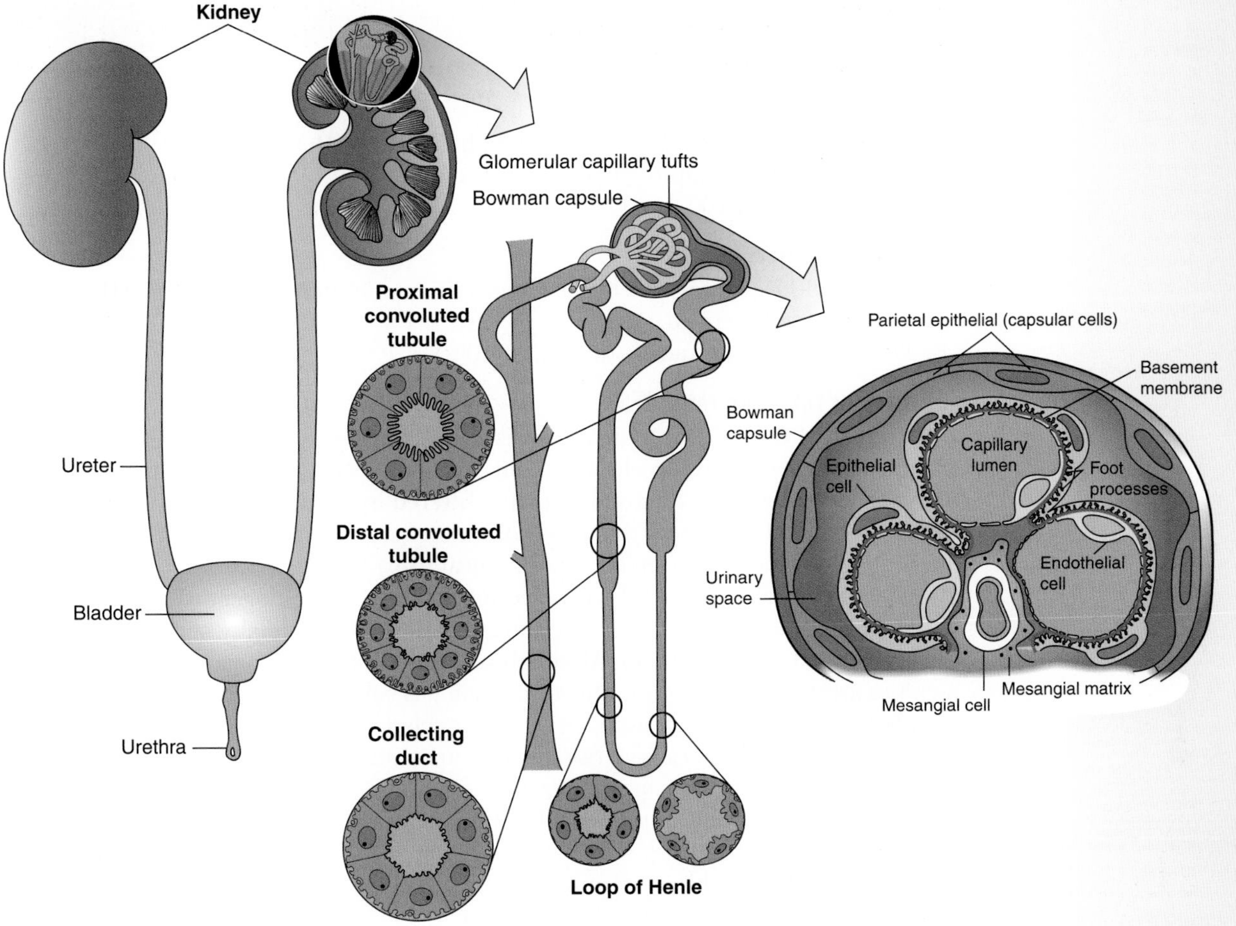
Kidney
Glomerular capillary tufts
Bowman capsule
Proximal convoluted tubule
Parietal epithelial (capsular cells)
Basement membrane
Bowman capsule
Capillary lumen
Epithelial cell
Foot processes
Ureter
Distal convoluted tubule
Endothelial cell
Urinary space
Bladder
Mesangial matrix
Mesangial cell
Urethra
Collecting duct
Loop of Henle

(Adapted with permission from Damjanov I. *A Color Atlas and Textbook of Histopathology.* Baltimore, MD: Lippincott Williams & Wilkins; 1996:258–259.)

FIGURE 6-2 Distribution of body water

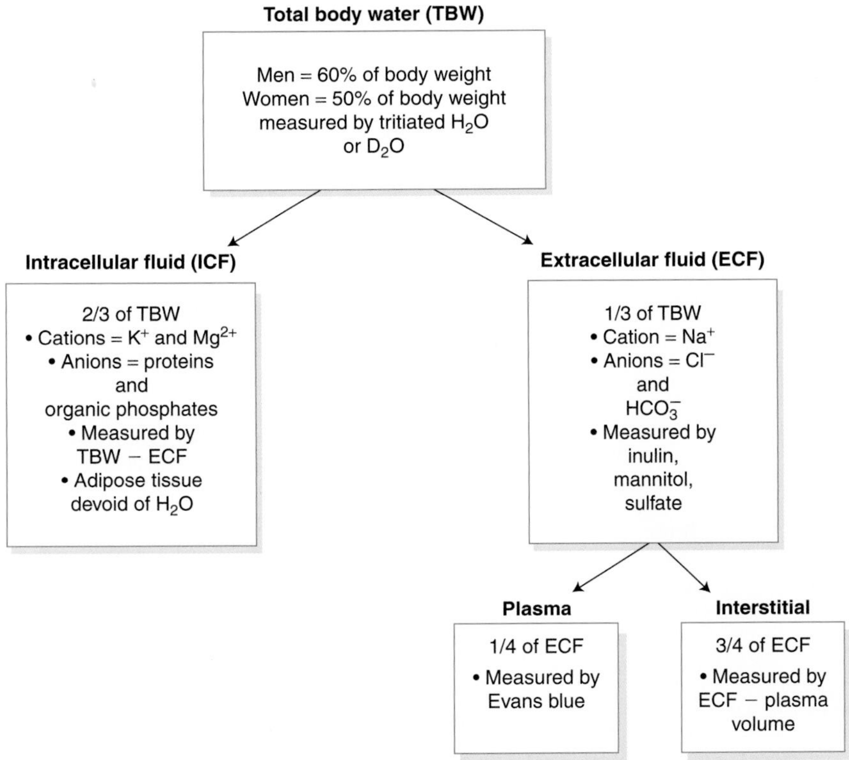
Total body water (TBW)
Men = 60% of body weight
Women = 50% of body weight
measured by tritiated H_2O
or D_2O
Intracellular fluid (ICF)
2/3 of TBW
• Cations = K^+ and Mg^{2+}
• Anions = proteins
and
organic phosphates
• Measured by
TBW − ECF
• Adipose tissue
devoid of H_2O
Extracellular fluid (ECF)
1/3 of TBW
• Cation = Na^+
• Anions = Cl^-
and
HCO_3^-
• Measured by
inulin,
mannitol,
sulfate
Plasma
1/4 of ECF
• Measured by
Evans blue
Interstitial
3/4 of ECF
• Measured by
ECF − plasma
volume

Cl^-, chloride; D_2O, heavy water; HCO_3^-, bicarbonate; H_2O, water; K^+, potassium; Mg^{2+}, magnesium; Na^+, sodium.

NORMAL KIDNEY FUNCTION

I. Renal blood flow (RBF)

A. 25% of cardiac output
B. **RBF = renal plasma flow (RPF)/[1 − hematocrit (Hct)]**
C. Renal vasculature **autoregulates** RBF, keeping it constant even when arterial pressure varies from 100 to 200 mm Hg.

II. Renal plasma flow

A. Effective RPF is measured by clearance of para-aminohippuric acid (**PAH**), which is filtered and secreted.
B. This measurement underestimates by 10%.

III. Glomerular filtration rate (GFR)

A. Normal GFR is 90 to 125 mL/min based on creatinine.
B. It is measured by **inulin** clearance. Inulin is an ideal marker for the measurement of GFR because it is a substance that is **filtered** by the kidney but **not reabsorbed or secreted**. Therefore, urine levels of inulin vary directly with GFR. However, inulin clearance is not practical for clinical use.
C. GFR is clinically measured with **creatinine** clearance. Endogenous creatine is the most common clinical marker because it is **filtered, minimally secreted**, and **not reabsorbed** by the kidneys. Although creatinine excretion is generally 10% to 20% greater than filtration, this discrepancy is cancelled by the overestimation of plasma creatinine. Therefore, creatinine is relatively accurate for GFR calculation.
   1. Decreases in GFR cause a rise in blood urea nitrogen (BUN) and creatinine levels.
   2. GFR decreases with age.
D. GFR is driven by Starling forces (filtration is always favored) (Figure 6-3).
E. Renal clearance
   1. Removal of a substance from the blood by renal excretion
   2. Determined by the following equation:

$$\text{Clearance} = [U \times V]/P \text{ (in mL/min)}$$

where U = concentration of substance in urine in mg/mL
V = urine volume (urine flow rate) in mL/min
P = plasma concentration of substance in mg/mL

FIGURE 6-3 **Starling forces on the glomerular capillary**

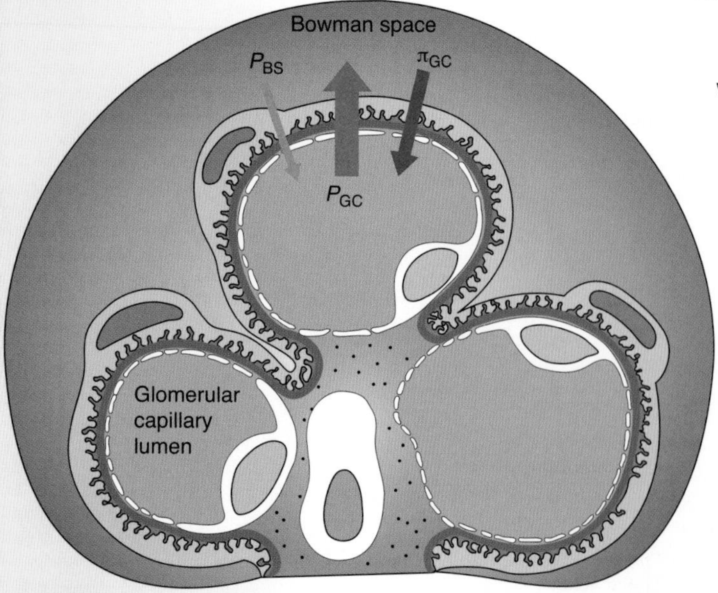

Bowman space
P_{BS}
π_{GC}
P_{GC}
Glomerular capillary lumen

The Starling forces influence the glomerular filtration rate (GFR)

$$GFR = K_F[(P_{GC} - P_{BS}) - (\pi_{GC} - \pi_{BS})]$$

where K_F: The filtration coefficient of the glomerular capillaries

P_{GC}: The hydrostatic pressure exerted by the fluid in the glomerular capillary. A dilated afferent arteriole increases P_{GC}, as does a constricted efferent arteriole.

P_{BS}: The hydrostatic pressure exerted by the fluid in Bowman space. Blockage or constriction of the ureters increases P_{BS}.

π_{GC}: The oncotic pressure of the glomerular capillary. The value of π_{GC} increases along the length of the capillary because the protein concentration in the capillary increases as water is forced into Bowman space.

π_{BS}: The oncotic pressure in Bowman space. This value is usually zero.

Note: One common pitfall to using creatinine is muscle mass. Plasma creatinine varies directly with muscle mass, so individuals with lower **muscle mass** (e.g., emaciated, elderly) may have an artificially higher GFR and individuals with high muscle mass (e.g., bodybuilders) may have an artificially lower GFR. Similarly, with age and loss of muscle mass, GFR may remain stable when in fact there is a decline in glomerular function and a decrease in GFR.

3. Factors that determine clearance
   a. Highly cleared substances (e.g., PAH) are those that are filtered and secreted and not reabsorbed.
   b. Poorly cleared substances are those that are either not filtered (e.g., protein) or are completely reabsorbed (e.g., glucose).
   c. Reabsorption
      - Limited by the number of transporters for certain compounds (e.g., glucose) in various segments of tubule
      - Transport maximum (T_m) is the maximum rate of reabsorption at which the transporters are saturated.
      - At concentrations above T_m, excess is excreted.

> **QUICK HIT**
>
> The T_m for glucose is reached at approximately 350 mg/dL. Greater concentrations result in an osmotic diuresis, such as that seen in diabetics with hyperglycemia.

> **QUICK HIT**
>
> Fanconi syndrome is a **hereditary** or **acquired** dysfunction of the proximal renal tubules. As a result of impaired glucose, amino acid, phosphate, and bicarbonate reabsorption, it manifests clinically as glycosuria, hyperphosphaturia, aminoaciduria, and acidosis.

IV. Filtration fraction (FF)

A. FF = GFR/RPF
B. The normal filtration fraction is 20%.
C. Variables that change FF:
   1. Ureteral obstruction decreases FF.
   2. Increased plasma proteins decrease FF (e.g., multiple myeloma).
   3. Decreased plasma proteins increase FF (e.g., liver failure).
   4. Constriction of efferent arteriole increases FF (e.g., angiotensin II).
   5. Dilation of efferent arteriole decreases FF (e.g., ACE inhibitors).
   6. Constriction of afferent arteriole (e.g., nonsteroidal anti-inflammatory drugs [NSAIDs]) and dilation of afferent arteriole (e.g., prostaglandins) changes GFR and RPF, but the FF remains constant.

> **QUICK HIT**
>
> ACE inhibitors, such as **captopril** and **enalapril,** reduce hypertension by inhibiting the conversion of angiotensin I to angiotensin II, thereby decreasing the release of aldosterone. Angiotensin II receptor blockers, such as losartan and valsartan, prevent angiotensin II from interacting with its receptor. This prevents angiotensin II from causing constriction of efferent arterioles.

V. Innervation and hormones

A. Juxtaglomerular apparatus (JGA) produces renin and is stimulated by the β-sympathetic adrenergics in the kidney and by a fall in pressure of the afferent arteriole.
B. **Renin** cleaves angiotensinogen to **angiotensin I.**
C. Angiotensin I is cleaved to **angiotensin II** by angiotensin-converting enzyme (ACE) in the lung.
   1. Functions of angiotensin II
      a. Stimulates aldosterone release from the zona glomerulosa
      b. Stimulates secretion of antidiuretic hormone (ADH, also known as arginine vasopressin [AVP]) and adrenocorticotropic hormone (ACTH) from the pituitary
      c. Acts as a potent local vasoconstrictor of the renal arterioles at low plasma levels
      d. Acts as a general systemic vasoconstrictor at high plasma levels
      e. Stimulates thirst
      f. Stimulates epinephrine and norepinephrine release from adrenal medulla
   2. Angiotensin II is inactivated to angiotensin III, a potent stimulator of aldosterone secretion but not an effective vasoconstrictor.

VI. Hormones and the nephron *(Figure 6-4)*

VII. Effects of volume change on fluid levels *(Table 6-2)*

A variety of hormones, such as ADH, aldosterone, and atrial natriuretic factor, regulate extracellular and intracellular volumes. Intake and output, as well as hormonal imbalance, can significantly alter the homeostatic fluid balance in the body.

FIGURE 6-4 **Hormones and the nephron**

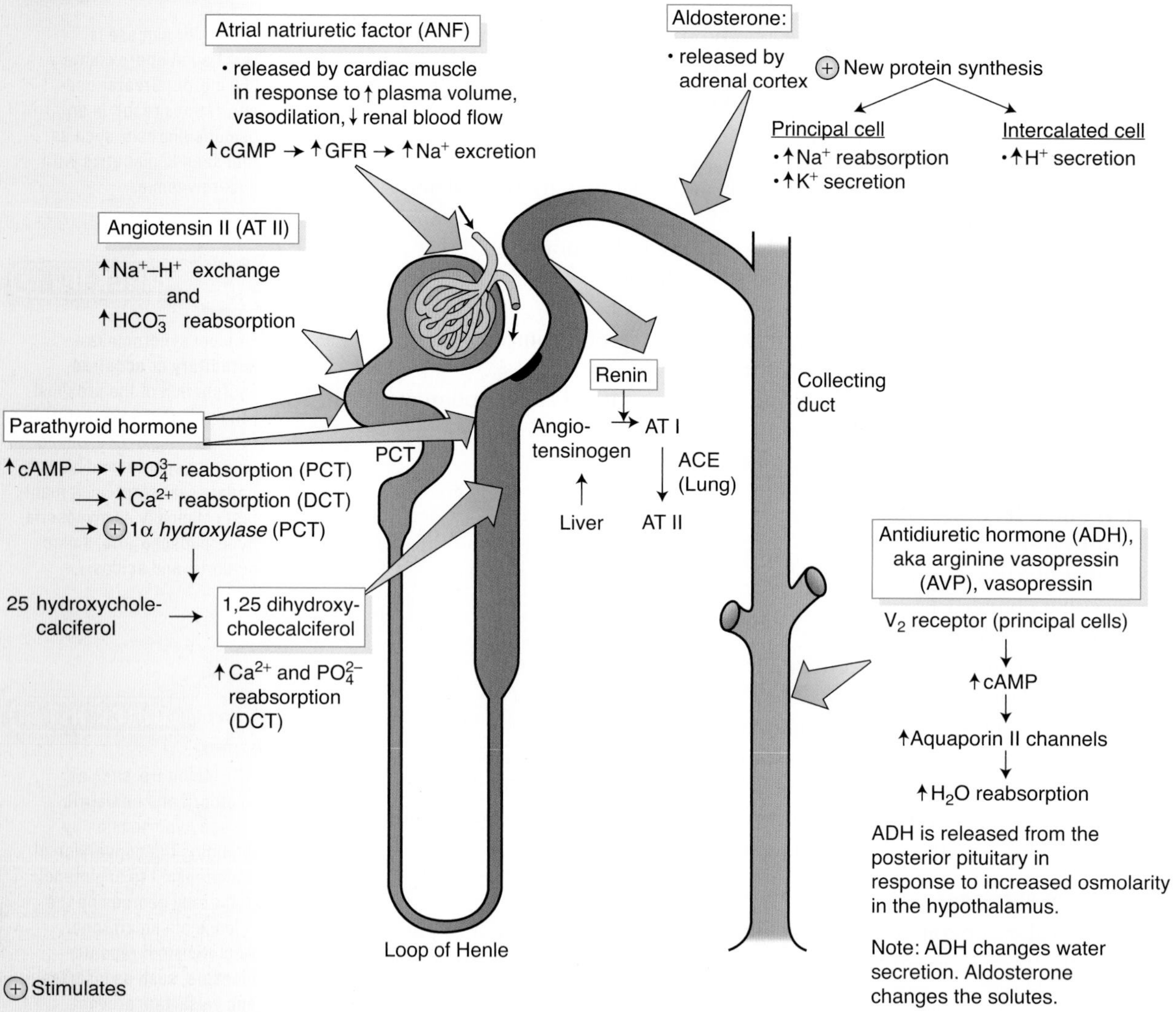

Atrial natriuretic factor (ANF)
• released by cardiac muscle in response to ↑ plasma volume, vasodilation, ↓ renal blood flow
↑cGMP → ↑GFR → ↑Na+ excretion
Aldosterone:
• released by adrenal cortex
+ New protein synthesis
Principal cell
• ↑Na+ reabsorption
• ↑K+ secretion
Intercalated cell
• ↑H+ secretion
Angiotensin II (AT II)
↑Na+–H+ exchange and ↑HCO3− reabsorption
Parathyroid hormone
↑cAMP → ↓PO43− reabsorption (PCT)
→ ↑Ca2+ reabsorption (DCT)
→ + 1α hydroxylase (PCT)
25 hydroxychole-calciferol → 1,25 dihydroxy-cholecalciferol
↑Ca2+ and PO42− reabsorption (DCT)
PCT
Renin
Angio-tensinogen
AT I
ACE (Lung)
Liver
AT II
Collecting duct
Antidiuretic hormone (ADH), aka arginine vasopressin (AVP), vasopressin
V2 receptor (principal cells)
↑cAMP
↑Aquaporin II channels
↑H2O reabsorption
ADH is released from the posterior pituitary in response to increased osmolarity in the hypothalamus.
Note: ADH changes water secretion. Aldosterone changes the solutes.
Loop of Henle
+ Stimulates

ACE, angiotensin-converting enzyme; AT I, angiotensin I; Ca^{2+}, calcium; cAMP, cyclic adenosine monophosphate; cGMP, cyclic guanosine monophosphate; DCT, distal convoluted tubule; GFR, glomerular filtration rate; H^+, hydrogen ion; HCO_3^-, bicarbonate; H_2O, water; K^+, potassium; Na^+, sodium; PCT, proximal convoluted tubule; PO_4^{3-}, phosphate; V2, vasopressin receptor type 2.

TABLE 6-2 **Effects of Volume Change on Fluid Levels**

Type	Key Examples	ECF Volume	ICF Volume	ECF Osmolarity	Hct and Serum [Na^+]
Isosmotic volume expansion	Isotonic fluid infusion (e.g., normal saline or lactated Ringer solution)	↑	No change	No change	↓ Hct – [Na^+]
Isosmotic volume contraction	Diarrhea	↓	No change	No change	↑ Hct – [Na^+]
Hyperosmotic volume expansion	High NaCl intake	↑	↓	↑	↓ Hct ↑ [Na^+]
Hyperosmotic volume contraction	Sweating, fever, diabetes insipidus	↓	↓	↑	– Hct ≠ [Na^+]
Hyposmotic volume expansion	SIADH	↑	↑	↓	– Hct ↓ [Na^+]
Hyposmotic volume contraction	Adrenal insufficiency	↓	↑	↓	↑ Hct ↓ [Na^+]

–, no change; ECF, extracellular fluid; Hct, hematocrit; ICF, intracellular fluid; Na^+, sodium; SIADH, syndrome of inappropriate secretion of antidiuretic hormone.
Reproduced with permission from Costanzo LS. *BRS Physiology.* 2nd ed. Baltimore, MD: Lippincott Williams & Wilkins; 1998:139.

VIII. Electrolyte balance in the nephron *(Figure 6-5)*

Acidosis or alkalosis is determined by evaluating blood pH, arterial partial pressure of carbon dioxide ($Paco_2$,) and bicarbonate (HCO_3^-) concentration. Anion gap (AG) is calculated using the following equation: $AG = Na^+ - (Cl^- + HCO_3^-)$. A normal AG is between 10 and 16 mEq/L. Certain acidotic conditions result in an elevated AG by altering the concentration of anions not considered in the above formula (lactate, β-hydroxybutyrate, formate). Table 6-3 compares acidosis with alkalosis. Table 6-4 outlines the effects of metabolic and respiratory acid–base disturbances.

FIGURE 6-5 Electrolyte balance in the nephron

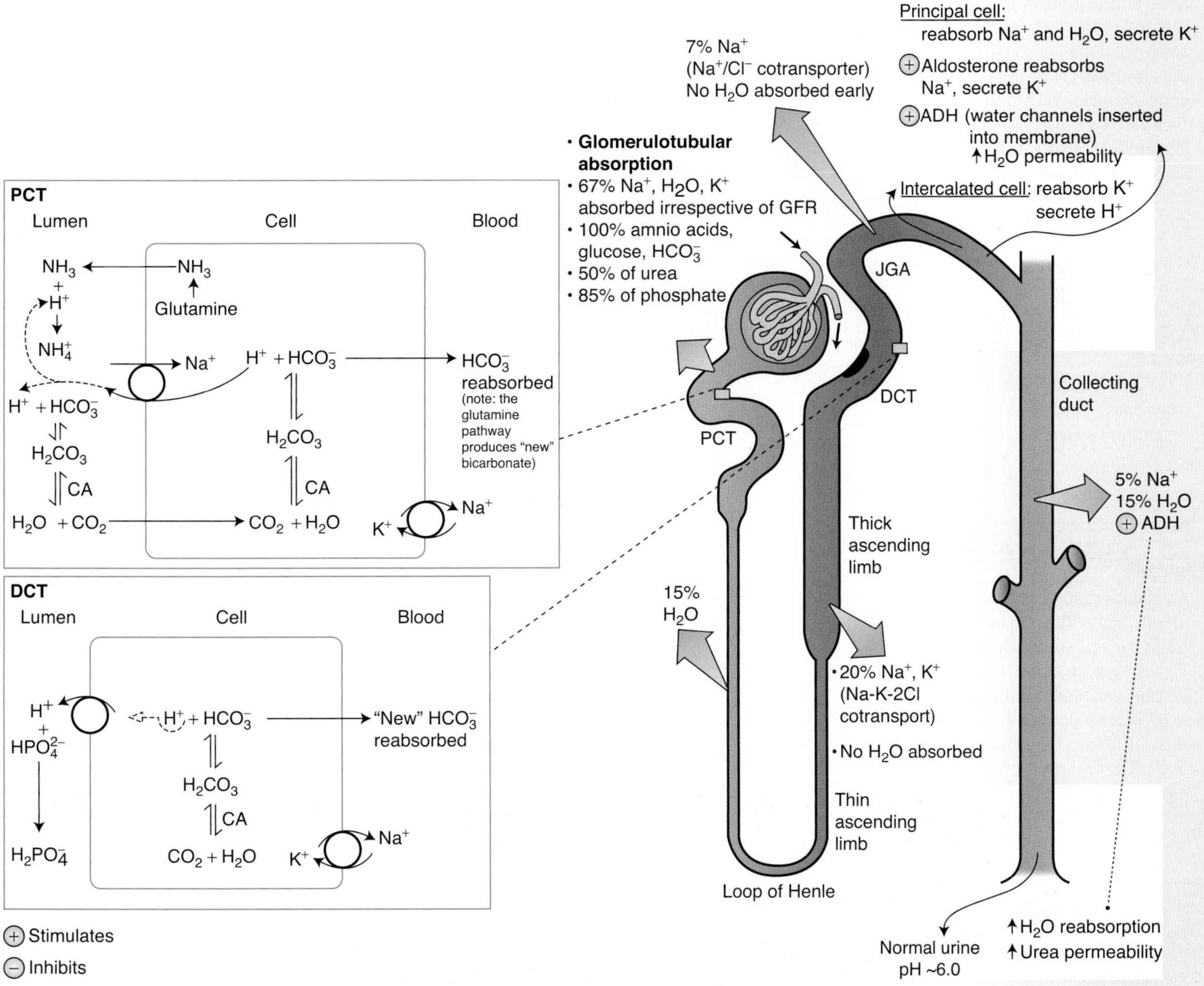
Principal cell:
reabsorb Na+ and H2O, secrete K+
(+) Aldosterone reabsorbs Na+, secrete K+
(+) ADH (water channels inserted into membrane) ↑H2O permeability
Intercalated cell: reabsorb K+ secrete H+
7% Na+ (Na+/Cl− cotransporter) No H2O absorbed early
• Glomerulotubular absorption
• 67% Na+, H2O, K+ absorbed irrespective of GFR
• 100% amnio acids, glucose, HCO3−
• 50% of urea
• 85% of phosphate
JGA
PCT
DCT
Collecting duct
5% Na+
15% H2O
(+) ADH
Thick ascending limb
15% H2O
• 20% Na+, K+ (Na-K-2Cl cotransport)
• No H2O absorbed
Thin ascending limb
Loop of Henle
Normal urine pH ~6.0
↑H2O reabsorption
↑Urea permeability
PCT
Lumen
Cell
Blood
NH3
NH3
Glutamine
H+
NH4+
Na+
H+ + HCO3−
HCO3− reabsorbed
(note: the glutamine pathway produces "new" bicarbonate)
H+ + HCO3−
H2CO3
H2CO3
CA
CA
H2O + CO2
CO2 + H2O
K+
Na+
DCT
Lumen
Cell
Blood
H+
HPO4 2−
H+ + HCO3−
"New" HCO3− reabsorbed
H2CO3
CA
H2PO4−
CO2 + H2O
K+
Na+
(+) Stimulates
(−) Inhibits

ADH, antidiuretic hormone; CA, carbonic anhydrase; Cl^-, chloride; CO_2, carbon dioxide; DCT, distal convoluted tubule; GFR, glomerular filtration rate; H^+, hydrogen ion; HCO_3^-, bicarbonate; H_2CO_3, carbonic acid; H_2O, water; HPO_4^{2-}, $H_2PO_4^-$, two forms of phosphate ions; JGA, juxtaglomerular apparatus; K^+, potassium; Mg^{2+}, magnesium; Na^+, sodium; NH_3, ammonia;
NH_4^+, ammonium; PCT, proximal convoluted tubule.

MNEMONIC

To remember the causes of increased anion gap metabolic acidosis, think **MUDPILES**: **M**ethanol, **U**remia, **D**iabetic ketoacidosis, **P**araldehyde, **I**soniazid or **I**ron tablets, **L**actic acidosis, **E**thylene glycol, **S**alicylates.

QUICK HIT

Renal tubular acidosis (RTA) is characterized by a normal anion gap. Type 1 (distal) RTA is caused by a failure to excrete titratable acid and NH_4^+. Type 2 RTA is caused by renal loss of HCO_3^-. Type 4 RTA is caused by hypoaldosteronism, which leads to poor excretion of NH^{4+} and hyperkalemia.

QUICK HIT

Emphysema and bronchitis often cause chronic respiratory acidosis.

QUICK HIT

A patient's respiratory status affects and is affected by his or her acid–base status. This is because of the reversible conversion of CO_2 to H^+ in the following way: $H_2O + CO_2 \leftrightarrow H_2CO_3 \leftrightarrow HCO_3^- + H^+$. The first reaction is catalyzed by the enzyme carbonic anhydrase.

QUICK HIT

Salicylate (aspirin) overdose causes respiratory alkalosis initially, followed by an increased anion gap metabolic acidosis.

TABLE 6-3 Acidosis and Alkalosis

Metabolic Disturbance	Presentation	Causes
Metabolic acidosis	• Fatigue • Shortness of breath • Abdominal pain • Vomiting • **Kussmaul respirations** • Hypotension • Tachycardia	• Chronic renal failure • Lactic acidosis • Uremia • **Ketoacidosis** • Intoxication (aspirin, methanol, ethylene glycol) • **Diarrhea**[a] • **Renal tubular acidosis**[a] • Acetazolamide[a]
Respiratory acidosis	• **Hypercapnia** • Confusion • Blunted sensation and pain • **Asterixis** • Papilledema	• Respiratory depression by drugs • Cerebral disease • Cardiopulmonary arrest response • Neuromuscular disease (e.g., myasthenia gravis) • Poor ventilation secondary to disease (e.g., asthma, pneumonia, bronchitis, emphysema)
Metabolic alkalosis	• No specific signs or symptoms • Can cause apathy, stupor, and confusion • If coupled with low calcium, can cause tetany	• Diuretics (loop and thiazide) • Vomiting • Milk alkali syndrome • Large intake of alkaline substance • **Cushing syndrome** • Primary aldosteronism
Respiratory alkalosis	• **Hyperventilation** • Numbness • Tingling • Paresthesia • Tetany, if severe	• Asthma • Pneumonia • Pulmonary edema • Heart disease with cyanosis • Pulmonary fibrosis • Aspirin intoxication • **Gram-negative sepsis** • Fever • Anxiety • Pregnancy • Drugs • Conditions that stimulate the medullary respiratory center (e.g., altitude) • Aspirin intoxication (via stimulation of respiratory center)

[a]Normal anion gap acidosis (other acidosis items have an increased anion gap).

TABLE 6-4 **Effects of Metabolic and Respiratory Acid–Base Disturbances**

Primary Disorder	pH	$[H^+]$	$[HCO_3^-]$	PCO_2	Respiratory Compensation	Renal Compensation
Metabolic acidosis	↓	↑	↓[a] (lost by buffering)	↓	Hyperventilation	↑ H^+ excretion (NH_3) ↑ "New" HCO_3^- reabsorption
Metabolic alkalosis	↑	↓	↑[a]	↑	Hypoventilation	↑ HCO_3^- excretion
Acute respiratory acidosis	↓	↑	↑	↑[a]	None	Not yet
Chronic respiratory acidosis	↓ (more normal)	↑	↑↑	↑[a]	None	↑ H^+ excretion (NH_4^+) ↑ "New" HCO_3^- reabsorption
Acute respiratory alkalosis	↑	↓	↓	↓[a]		Not yet
Chronic respiratory alkalosis	↑ (more normal)	↓	↓↓	↓[a]		↓ H^+ excretion ↓ HCO_3^- reabsorption

[a]primary disorder.

↑, increased; ↓, decreased; H^+, hydrogen ion; HCO_3^+, bicarbonate; NH_4^+, ammonium.

Clinical Vignette 6-1

CLINICAL PRESENTATION: A 24-year-old male medical student is brought to the emergency department after being found **unconscious** in his apartment by his roommate. It is unknown whether he suffered any trauma, but the roommate tells you that they just finished exam week at the medical school. There are no signs of injury on examination. The roommate tells you that the patient has no other medical problems. The patient cannot be aroused in the emergency department but does respond to pain. Vital signs: temperature = 100.8° F; **respiration rate (RR) = 35 breaths/min;** blood pressure = 150/90 mm Hg; heart rate = 104 bpm. Pupils are round and reactive to light bilaterally. Laboratory tests reveal the following: WBC = 8.4; Hgb = 14.2; Hct = 30.9; Na = 140; K = 3.8; Cl = 102; **HCO_2 = 13;** BUN = 16; Cr = 0.8; Gluc = 110. Arterial blood gasses are obtained and reveal the following: **pH = 7.19; P_aco_2 = 26; P_ao_2 = 95.**
DIFFERENTIAL: This patient has metabolic acidosis. In approaching a patient with metabolic acidosis, the **first step is the calculation of the AG:** $AG = Na^+ - (Cl^- + HCO_3^-)$. This patient has an increased AG metabolic acidosis (AG >15) for which differentials are diabetic ketoacidosis (DKA), alcoholic ketoacidosis, lactic acidosis, starvation, renal failure, and overdose of salicylate, methanol, or ethylene glycol. Given that the patient is not diabetic and has a glucose of 114 mg/dL, DKA is unlikely. Also, renal function is not impaired. Because the cause is unclear, further testing is necessary.
LABORATORY STUDIES: To determine the cause of the AG metabolic acidosis in this patient, **serum ketone, salicylate, lactate, blood alcohol, methanol,** and **ethylene glycol levels** should be obtained. Next, determine whether this is a primary acid–base disorder or mixed disorder. Using **Winter's formula** [1.5 (measured HCO_3) + 8 ± 2], the expected P_aco_2 level in this patient is 25.5 to 29.5 mm Hg. With a P_aco_2 of 26 mm Hg, this patient has an appropriate respiratory compensation response (RR of 35 breaths/min). If actual P_aco_2 is higher than expected, there is an additional acidotic process occurring. If actual P_aco_2 is lower than expected, then there is an additional alkalotic process occurring.
MANAGEMENT: Management depends on the cause of metabolic acidosis. **Sodium bicarbonate** may be needed in cases of severe acidemia, and **mechanical ventilation** may be required if patient is fatigued from hyperventilation.

The Renal System

MNEMONIC

To remember the hallmark findings of nephrotic syndrome, think **Protein LEAC: Protein**uria, **L**ipid increased, **E**dema, **A**lbumin decreased, **C**holesterol increased.

GLOMERULAR DISEASES

I. Nephrotic syndrome

A. Features
   1. **Proteinuria** of >3.5 g of protein per 24 hours
   2. Hypoalbuminemia
   3. Edema
   4. Hyperlipidemia

B. Etiology
   1. Idiopathic—75%
   2. Systemic disease—25%

C. Common types (Table 6-5)

QUICK HIT

Corticosteroids are often used to help resolve nephritic and nephrotic syndromes.

II. Nephritic syndrome

A. Features
   1. **Hematuria**
   2. Hypertension
   3. Oliguria
   4. Azotemia

B. Common types of nephritic glomerular diseases (Table 6-6)

III. Glomerular deposits in disease *(Figure 6-9)*

TABLE 6-5 Nephrotic Glomerular Diseases

Glomerular Disease	Etiology	Clinical Features	Notes
Minimal change disease (lipoid nephrosis)	Fusion of foot processes on the basement membrane leads to loss of negative charge and changes in the protein selectivity; altered appearance of villi on epithelial cells	Electron microscopy shows **fusion of podocyte foot processes** (Figure 6-6) and lipid-laden renal cortices	**Common in young children** (usually younger than 5 years of age); responds well to steroids; albumin usually selectively secreted
Membranous glomerulonephritis	Idiopathic; secondarily caused by SLE, hepatitis B, syphilis, gold, penicillamine, malignancy	Basement membrane thickening; **"spike and dome"** with **subepithelial IgG and C3 deposits**	Common in young adults
Diabetic nephropathy	Microangiopathy leading to thickening of basement membrane	Basement membrane thickening	Two types: diffuse and nodular glomerulosclerosis; nodular glomerulosclerosis has **Kimmelstiel–Wilson nodules** (Figure 6-7); usually leads to renal failure
Renal amyloidosis	Subendothelial or mesangial amyloid deposits; associated with multiple myeloma	Stains: periodic acid-Schiff (PAS) (−); **Congo Red (+)**	Increasing severity leads to renal failure
Focal and segmental glomerulosclerosis	Has four possible etiologies: idiopathic; superimposed on preexisting pathology; associated with loss of renal mass; secondary to other disorders (e.g., heroin abuse or HIV)	Sclerosis of some glomeruli; only capillary tuft is involved in affected glomeruli	Clinically similar to minimal change disease but affects older population

C3, third component of complement; IgG, immunoglobulin G; SLE, systemic lupus erythematosus.

FIGURE
6-6 Minimal change disease

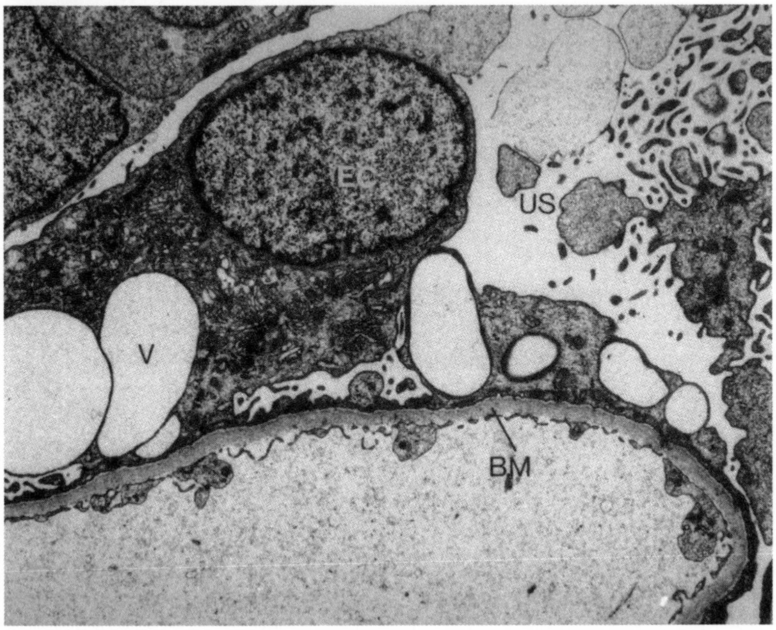
EC
US
V
BM

Electron micrograph showing effacement of the podocyte foot processes. BM, basement membrane; EC, endothelial cell; US, urinary space; V, vacuole. (Reproduced with permission from Rubin E, Farber JL. *Pathology.* 3rd ed. Philadelphia, PA: Lippincott Williams & Wilkins; 1999.)

FIGURE
6-7 Diabetic nodular glomerulosclerosis

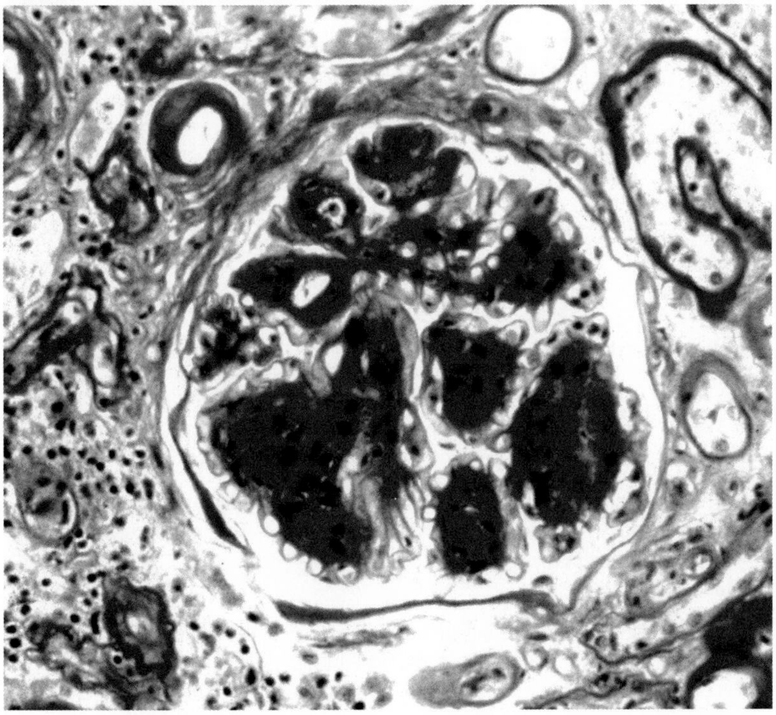

A periodic acid-Schiff stain demonstrates nodular Kimmelstiel-Wilson lesions at the periphery of the glomerulus, which are pathognomonic of diabetic glomerulosclerosis. (Reproduced with permission from Rubin E, Farber JL. *Pathology.* 3rd ed. Philadelphia, PA: Lippincott Williams & Wilkins; 1999.)

TABLE 6-6 **Nephritic Glomerular Diseases**

Disease	Etiology	Special Features	Notes
Poststreptococcal glomerulonephritis	Poststreptococcal pharyngitis or impetigo; hepatitis B; high ASO titer; low C3; type III hypersensitivity	**"Lumpy bumpy"** deposits of antigen- antibody-C3 complexes; subepithelial humps on electron microscopy	Common in children; self-resolving; most common organisms are group A hemolytic streptococci; red cell casts in urine
Rapidly progressive **(crescentic)** glomerulonephritis	**ANCA positive;** poststreptococcal etiology 50%; renal failure within weeks or months	Accumulation of fibrin, macrophages, and PMNs in Bowman capsule; wrinkling of basement membrane on electron microscopy **(crescents)**	If it also involves upper respiratory system, then it is termed **Wegener granulomatosis**
Goodpasture syndrome	**Antiglomerular basement membrane and alveolar basement membrane antibodies** (type II hypersensitivity)	**Linear pattern** of IgG on fluorescence microscopy; may be associated with hemoptysis and pulmonary hemorrhage	Usually **males in their mid-20s**
Alport syndrome	Hereditary structural defect in collagen IV leads to leaky basement membrane	Glomerular basement membrane splitting on electron microscopy	Appears before age 20; associated with deafness and ocular problems
Lupus nephropathy	**Anti-dsDNA**	WHO classifications: • WHO I: normal • WHO II: mesangial proliferation; little clinical relevance • WHO III (focal proliferative): <50% of glomeruli affected • **WHO IV (diffuse proliferative):** worst prognosis; **wire-loop lesions** (Figure 6-8) (subendothelial immune complex deposition of IgM and IgG + C3) • WHO V: membranous glomerulonephritis	Degree of kidney involvement correlates to SLE prognosis; may have nephritic qualities
IgA nephropathy (Berger disease)	IgA deposits in mesangium; hematuria usually follows infection	Mesangial cell proliferation on electron microscopy	Minimal clinical significance; common
Membranoproliferative glomerulonephritis	Type 2 has IgG autoantibody; C3 is reduced in both types	Basement membrane thickens and appears as two layers; **"train-track"** appearance on electron microscopy	Two types: type 1 and type 2 (dense deposit disease); may lead to either nephrotic or nephritic syndromes

ANCA, antineutrophil cytoplasmic antibody; ASO, antistreptolysin-O; C3, third component of complement; dsDNA, double-stranded DNA; Ig, immunoglobulin; PMN, polymorphonuclear leukocyte; SLE, systemic lupus erythematosus; WHO, World Health Organization.

FIGURE 6-8 **Diffuse proliferative lupus nephritis**

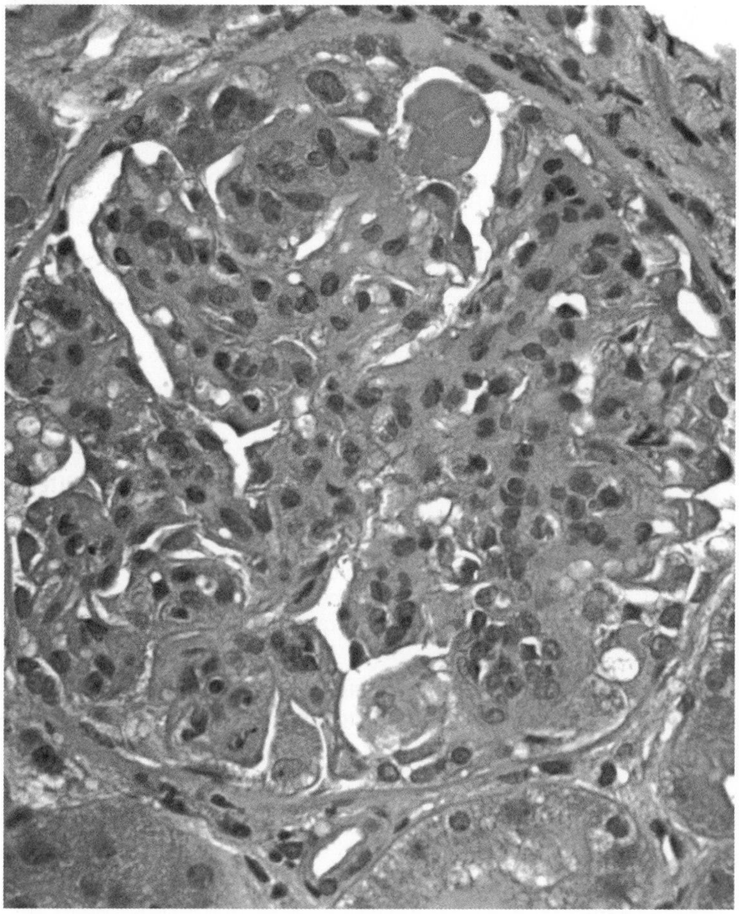

There is a diffuse increase in the cellularity of the glomerulus and thickening of basement membrane. Wire-loop thickening occurs as a result of subendothelial immune complex deposition. (Reproduced with permission from Rubin E, Farber JL. *Pathology*. 3rd ed. Philadelphia, PA: Lippincott Williams & Wilkins; 1999.)

URINARY TRACT INFECTIONS

I. Cystitis

A. Characteristic clinical features
   1. **Dysuria**
   2. **Frequency**
   3. **Urgency**
   4. Suprapubic pain

B. Etiology and pathogenesis
   1. Bacteria gain access to the urinary tract via the urethra.
   2. Cystitis most frequently involves normal colonic flora.
      a. ***Escherichia coli*** is the most common cause (approximately 80%).
      b. *Proteus, Klebsiella,* and *Enterobacter* are also implicated.
      c. *Staphylococcus saprophyticus* causes 10% to 15% of infections in young women.
      d. Nosocomial cystitis is frequently caused by *Pseudomonas* or *Staphylococcus aureus*.
   3. **Women** have a higher incidence of infection because they have shorter urethras.
   4. Other risk factors include sexual activity, pregnancy, urinary obstruction, neurogenic bladder, and vesicoureteral reflux.

FIGURE 6-9 **Glomerular deposits in disease**

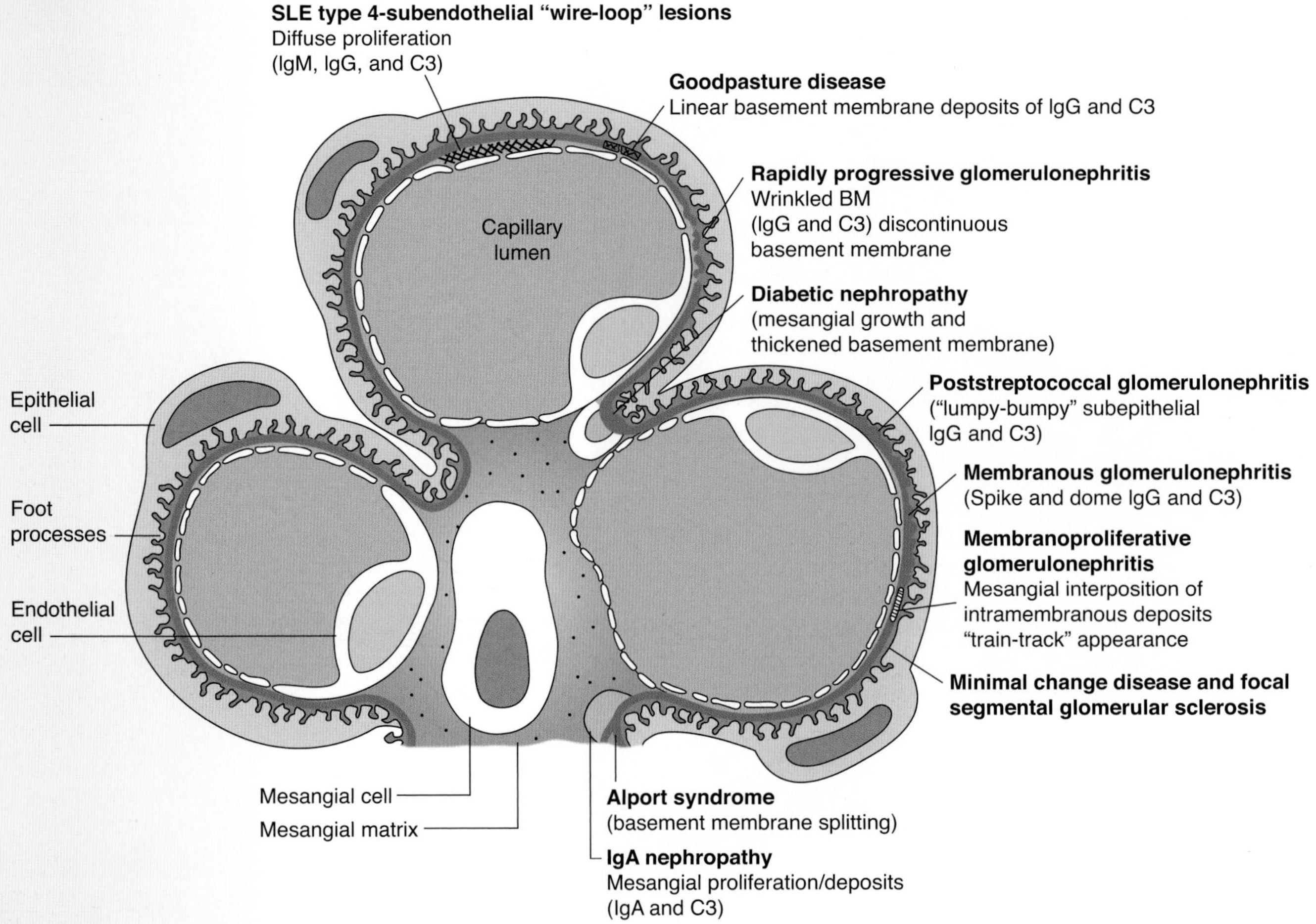
SLE type 4-subendothelial "wire-loop" lesions
Diffuse proliferation
(IgM, IgG, and C3)
Goodpasture disease
Linear basement membrane deposits of IgG and C3
Rapidly progressive glomerulonephritis
Wrinkled BM
(IgG and C3) discontinuous
basement membrane
Capillary
lumen
Diabetic nephropathy
(mesangial growth and
thickened basement membrane)
Poststreptococcal glomerulonephritis
("lumpy-bumpy" subepithelial
IgG and C3)
Epithelial
cell
Membranous glomerulonephritis
(Spike and dome IgG and C3)
Foot
processes
Membranoproliferative
glomerulonephritis
Mesangial interposition of
intramembranous deposits
"train-track" appearance
Endothelial
cell
Minimal change disease and focal
segmental glomerular sclerosis
Mesangial cell
Mesangial matrix
Alport syndrome
(basement membrane splitting)
IgA nephropathy
Mesangial proliferation/deposits
(IgA and C3)

BM, basement membrane; C3, third component of complement; Ig, immunoglobulin; SLE, systemic lupus erythematosus.

The Renal System

Clinical Vignette 6-2

CLINICAL PRESENTATION: A 6-year-old girl presents to her pediatrician with **puffy eyes** of 2 weeks' duration. The mother tells you that the patient has been taking **more naps than usual** and that the pants they had bought recently no longer fit her around the waist. The parents deny any recent upper respiratory infections (URIs). Physical examination shows **periorbital edema, pedal edema, ascites,** and **weight gain.** Cardiothoracic and pulmonary exam is negative, and vital signs are normal.

DIFFERENTIALS: Nephrotic syndrome, glomerulonephritis, congestive heart failure, sinusitis, allergic reaction, hepatic failure. Generalized edema and fatigue are expected in nephrotic syndrome, glomerulonephritis, congestive heart failure (CHF), and hepatic failure. The absence of murmur/gallops/crackles makes CHF less likely. The absence of jaundice makes hepatic failure less likely. A recent URI would suggest glomerulonephritis. Sinusitis is more likely to produce edema localized to periorbital region. Abrupt onset periorbital edema along with conjunctivitis, urticarial rash, wheezing, and rhinorrhea is expected in an allergic reaction. Minimal change disease is the most common cause of nephrotic syndrome in the patient's age group.

LABORATORY STUDIES: **Urinalysis** shows **proteinuria** in both nephrotic and nephritic syndromes but is more severe in nephrotic syndrome. **Hematuria** is seen in nephritic syndrome. **Blood studies** would reveal **hypoalbuminemia** and **hyperlipidemia** in nephrotic syndrome and **azotemia** in nephritic syndrome.

MANAGEMENT: Nephrotic syndrome is best treated by **albumin infusion** followed by **diuretics** and **corticosteroids.** Many children grow out of minimal change disease.

C. Diagnostic findings
1. Characteristic clinical features are present.
2. Pyuria (more than 8 leukocytes/high-power field)
3. Bacterial culture yields **>10^5 organisms/mL**.

D. Treatment
1. Cystitis is treated with antibiotics.
2. Recurrent cystitis may require prophylactic antibiotics.

II. Acute pyelonephritis

A. Characteristic clinical features
1. **Flank pain** or **costovertebral angle tenderness**
2. **Dysuria**
3. **Fever**
4. Chills
5. Nausea and vomiting
6. Diarrhea

B. Etiology and pathogenesis
1. Bacteria **ascend** from an infected urinary bladder to the kidney via the **vesicoureteral reflux**.
2. Infection may also spread **hematogenously** to the kidney (may not necessarily be preceded by acute cystitis).
3. Causative organism is usually *E. coli*.

C. Diagnostic findings
1. Characteristic clinical features are present.
2. Bacteriuria, pyuria, and **white blood cell casts** are seen on urine microscopy.
3. Urine and blood cultures are performed to determine infection.

D. Treatment
1. Treatment is with **antibiotics**, often **intravenously**.
2. Recurrent infection can lead to chronic pyelonephritis. This condition has several complications:
   a. **Scarring and deformity of the renal pelvis and calyces**
   b. Interstitial fibrosis and tubular atrophy
   c. Ischemia of the tubules leading to microscopic "**thyroidization**" of the kidney

MNEMONIC

To remember the most common pathogens of UTIs, think **KEEPS**: ***K**lebsiella, **E**nterobacter, **E.** coil, **P**roteus, **S.** saprophyticus.*

MAJOR CAUSES OF ACUTE RENAL FAILURE *(Figure 6-10)*

I. Prerenal failure is defined as oliguria and an increase in BUN and creatinine with inherently normal renal function.

A. Hypovolemic states
1. Hemorrhage
2. Burns
3. Dehydration
4. Vomiting
5. Diarrhea
6. Diuretics
7. Pancreatitis

B. Low cardiac output states
1. Arrhythmias
2. Pulmonary embolus
3. Myocardial or valvular disease
4. Cardiac tamponade
5. Pulmonary hypertension

C. **Renal vasoconstrictive states** resulting in ischemia may be caused by the following:
1. Cirrhosis with ascites
2. Vasoconstrictive drugs: epinephrine, norepinephrine, cyclosporine, amphotericin B

D. Intrinsic decrease of renal perfusion
1. Cyclooxygenase (COX) inhibitors, NSAIDs
2. Angiotensin-converting enzyme (ACE) inhibitors

QUICK HIT

Cyclooxygenase is inhibited by aspirin and other nonsteroidal anti-inflammatory drugs (NSAIDs) but not by acetaminophen (APAP).

FIGURE 6-10 Etiology of acute renal failure

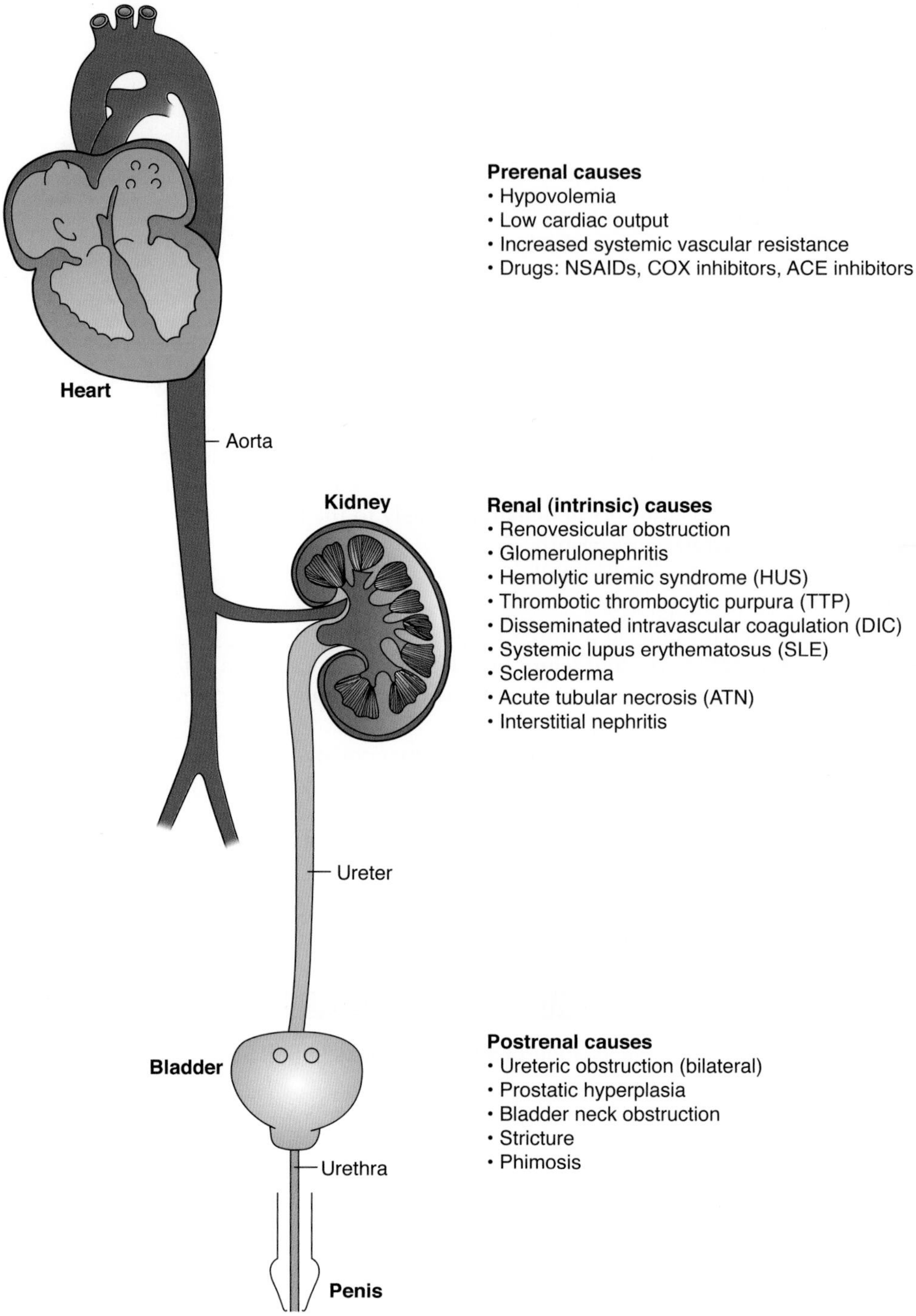
Heart
Aorta
Kidney
Ureter
Bladder
Urethra
Penis
Prerenal causes
• Hypovolemia
• Low cardiac output
• Increased systemic vascular resistance
• Drugs: NSAIDs, COX inhibitors, ACE inhibitors
Renal (intrinsic) causes
• Renovesicular obstruction
• Glomerulonephritis
• Hemolytic uremic syndrome (HUS)
• Thrombotic thrombocytic purpura (TTP)
• Disseminated intravascular coagulation (DIC)
• Systemic lupus erythematosus (SLE)
• Scleroderma
• Acute tubular necrosis (ATN)
• Interstitial nephritis
Postrenal causes
• Ureteric obstruction (bilateral)
• Prostatic hyperplasia
• Bladder neck obstruction
• Stricture
• Phimosis

ACE, angiotensin-converting enzyme; COX, cyclooxygenase; NSAIDs, nonsteroidal anti-inflammatory drugs.

TABLE 6-7 Prerenal versus Intrinsic Renal Failure

	Prerenal Renal Failure	Intrinsic Renal Failure
Fractional excretion of Na^+	<1	>1
Urine sodium concentration	<10 mg/dL	>20 mg/dL
Urine creatinine to plasma creatinine	>40	>20
Urine casts	Hyaline	Muddy brown and granular
Plasma blood urea nitrogen–to–creatinine ratio	>20	<10–15

Na^+, sodium.

QUICK HIT

Fractional excretion of sodium ($FENa^+$ is calculated using the formula:

$$FENa^+ = 100 \times \frac{\frac{\text{urine }[Na^+]}{\text{serum }[Na^+]}}{\frac{\text{urine }[Cr]}{\text{serum }[Cr]}}$$

II. Acute intrinsic renal failure is the inherent malfunction of the renal tissue. It may be glomerular, tubular, or interstitial. Table 6-7 compares prerenal failure with intrinsic renal failure.

A. **Acute tubular necrosis** (ATN)
   1. Drugs that may lead to ATN are exogenous toxins (contrast, cyclosporine, aminoglycosides, ethylene glycol, acetaminophen, heavy metals) or endogenous toxins (myoglobin, uric acid, oxalate).
   2. Ischemia can result in ATN via causes related to prerenal failure.

B. Obstruction of renal vasculature from atherosclerosis, vasculitis, or other factors may also cause acute intrinsic renal failure.

C. Diseases that affect the glomeruli or microvasculature
   1. Disseminated intravascular coagulopathy (DIC)
   2. Glomerulonephritis
   3. Hemolytic uremic syndrome (HUS)
   4. Thrombotic thrombocytopenic purpura (TTP)
   5. Pregnancy
   6. Scleroderma
   7. Systemic lupus erythematosus (SLE)

D. **Interstitial nephritis** can have many causes.
   1. β-Lactams
   2. Sulfonamides
   3. Trimethoprim (TMP)
   4. Rifampin
   5. COX inhibitors
   6. Diuretics
   7. Captopril
   8. Infection
   9. Idiopathic

E. Acute renal transplant rejection is a cause of ATN.

QUICK HIT

Exogenous toxins causing acute tubular necrosis include contrast, cyclosporine, ethylene glycol, and acetaminophen. Endogenous toxins include myoglobin, uric acid, and oxalate.

QUICK HIT

The most **common** cause of acute renal failure (ARF) is therapeutic drugs.

QUICK HIT

HUS and TTP cause a "flea-bitten" kidney.

III. Postrenal failure is bilateral obstruction of the ureters or obstruction of the urethra. It accounts for less than 5% of acute renal failure (ARF) and has a variety of causes.

A. Urolithiasis (see section on stone formation)
B. Prostatic hyperplasia
C. Tumor obstructing the bladder or the ureters bilaterally
D. Neurogenic bladder

QUICK HIT

Renal transplant rejection rates can be decreased by administration of cyclosporine and muromonab-CD3 (OKT3).

CHRONIC RENAL FAILURE AND UREMIA *(Figure 6-11)*

I. Major causes of chronic renal failure (CRF)

A. **Hypertension**
B. **Diabetes mellitus**

FIGURE 6-11 Manifestations of chronic renal failure and uremia

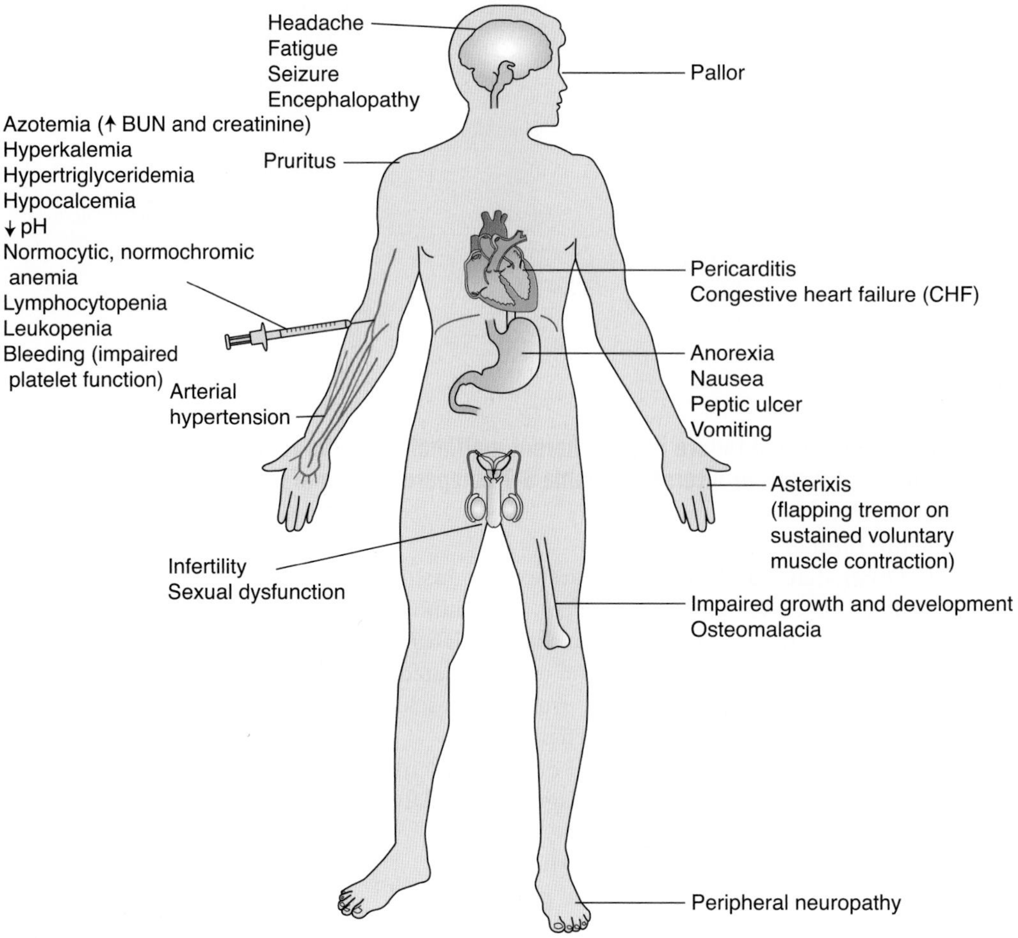
Headache
Fatigue
Seizure
Encephalopathy
Pallor
Azotemia (↑ BUN and creatinine)
Hyperkalemia
Hypertriglyceridemia
Hypocalcemia
↓ pH
Normocytic, normochromic anemia
Lymphocytopenia
Leukopenia
Bleeding (impaired platelet function)
Pruritus
Arterial hypertension
Pericarditis
Congestive heart failure (CHF)
Anorexia
Nausea
Peptic ulcer
Vomiting
Asterixis (flapping tremor on sustained voluntary muscle contraction)
Infertility
Sexual dysfunction
Impaired growth and development
Osteomalacia
Peripheral neuropathy

BUN, blood urea nitrogen.

II. Profound loss of renal function leads to uremia.

A. GFR is reduced to 50% to 65% of normal.

B. Byproducts of amino acid and protein metabolism (especially urea) cause a variety of signs and symptoms.

1. **Endocrine and electrolyte findings**
   a. Hyperkalemia
   b. Hyperphosphatemia
   c. Hypertriglyceridemia
   d. Hyperuricemia
   e. Hypocalcemia and osteomalacia as a result of decreased 1,25-dihydroxycholecalciferol levels
   f. Impaired growth and development
   g. Infertility and sexual dysfunction
   h. Metabolic acidosis
2. **Gastrointestinal findings**
   a. Anorexia
   b. Nausea
   c. Peptic ulcer
   d. Vomiting
3. **Renal findings**: azotemia
4. **Cardiovascular and pulmonary findings**
   a. Arterial hypertension
   b. Congestive heart failure
   c. Pericarditis

QUICK HIT

Uremia causes burr cells. Burr cells are misshapen red blood cells (RBCs) with irregular fingerlike projections from their surface.

5. **Dermatologic findings**
   a. Pallor
   b. Pruritus
   c. "Uremic frost" (crystallized urea on the skin)
6. **Neuromuscular findings**
   a. Asterixis
   b. Headache and fatigue
   c. Peripheral neuropathy
7. **Hematologic findings**
   a. Increased susceptibility to infection
   b. Lymphocytopenia and leukopenia
   c. Normocytic, normochromic anemia

Clinical Vignette 6-3

CLINICAL PRESENTATION: A 55-year-old woman presents to her primary care physician with the chief complaint of **nausea, vomiting,** and **feeling "out of it"** over the past 2 days. She also reports **urinating less frequently** and **weight gain,** although she does not have much of an appetite. Her past medical history is significant for **CHF.** Physical examination reveals generalized edema and a 10-lb weight gain since her last visit 1 month ago.

DIFFERENTIALS: Acute renal failure (ARF), chronic renal failure, acute tubular necrosis. ARF is defined as rapid, progressive decrease in renal function characterized by elevation in blood urea nitrogen/creatinine (BUN/Cr) and possibly oliguria. Renal failure can be prerenal, intrinsic renal, or postrenal. Prerenal failure is caused by insufficient renal perfusion as in CHF, whereas postrenal failure is caused by obstructed renal outflow. Intrinsic renal failure is caused by parenchymal damage to the glomerulus, tubules, interstitium, or vasculature. There are a number of causes for each type of renal failure (Figure 6-10). In this patient, hypovolemia from CHF is the cause of insufficient renal perfusion. Acute tubular necrosis causes 85% of intrinsic renal failure, but we would expect some history of renal ischemia or toxin exposure (see Quick Hit). Chronic renal failure has lab findings in common with ARF, but we would expect clinical manifestations of uremia and multiple instances of abnormal BUN, Cr, and urinalysis.

LABORATORY STUDIES: A urinalysis would be obtained looking for the presence of casts. Presence of muddy brown casts (seen in acute tubular necrosis), red blood cell (RBC) casts (glomerular disease), or white blood cell (WBC) casts (pyelonephritis, acute interstitial nephritis) would not be expected in ARF. **Urine chemistry** consisting of BUN/Cr, fractional excretion of sodium (FENa$^+$), and urine osmolality would also be obtained. In prerenal and postrenal failure, the **BUN:Cr ratio** is typically greater than 20:1 because of increased urea absorption as compared to intrinsic renal failure. In prerenal failure, the FENa$^+$ is less than 1% because the decreased glomerular filtration rate causes massive reabsorption of sodium and water, whereas in intrinsic renal failure, the FENa$^+$ is greater than 2% to 3% because Na is poorly reabsorbed. Similarly, we expect increased **urine osmolality** in prerenal failure because the kidney is able to reabsorb water, whereas we see decreased urine osmolality in intrinsic renal failure because renal water reabsorption is impaired. Also, **renal ultrasound** would be obtained to rule out obstruction. Renal ultrasound showing small, echogenic kidneys are pathognomic of chronic renal failure (CRF).

MANAGEMENT: The most important part of therapy is to follow urinary output: patients with ARF first experience an **oliguric phase** followed by a **diuretic phase.** Approximately 40% of patients go on to a **recovery phase** with normalization of urine output. **Correct fluid imbalance**—some patients with ARF are dehydrated, whereas others are volume overloaded. Correct any **electrolyte abnormalities** and **optimize cardiac output.** Order **dialysis** if symptomatic uremia, acidemia, hyperkalemia, or volume overload develops.

KIDNEY STONE FORMATION *(Figure 6-12)*

FIGURE 6-12 **Comparison of different types of kidney stones**

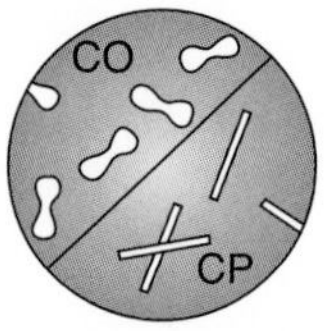
CO
CP

Calcium stones
A. Calcium oxalate (CO) B. Calcium phosphate (CP)

80% of stones
Men
20–30 years of age
Multiple (every 2–3 years)
Familial predisposition
Radiopaque
May be caused by primary hyperthyroidism
CP stones form more readily in alkaline urine pH >6

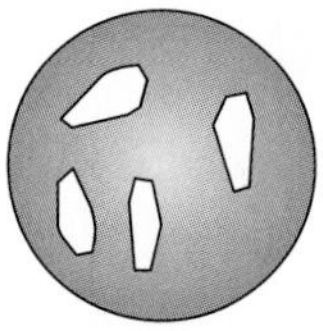

Struvite
12% of stones
Women
Risk factors:
Catheter, UTIs (especially *Proteus*)
May fill renal pelvis and calyces ("staghorn")
Radiopaque

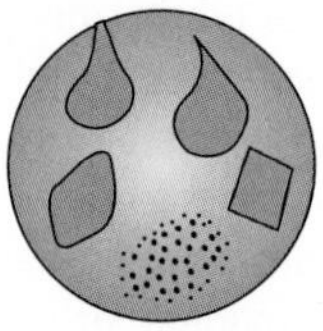

Uric acid
7% of stones
Men
Risk factors:
50% have gout
Strong negative birefringence
Radiolucent
Associated with cell lysis (e.g., chemotherapy, leukemia)
Uric acid increases urine acidity to pH <5.5

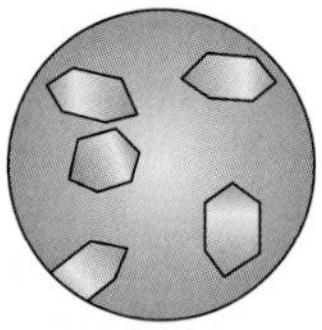

Cystine
1% of stones
Uncommon
Hereditary
Radiopaque (because of sulfur component)
Natural inhibitors of stone formation are (1) citrate, (2) nephrocalcin, (3) Tanim-Hosfall protein (aka uromodulin), and (4) uropontin.

Clinical manifestations of kidney stones include hematuria and flank pain. UTI, urinary tract infection.

AUTOSOMAL DOMINANT POLYCYSTIC KIDNEY DISEASE *(Figure 6-13)*

FIGURE 6-13 **Autosomal dominant polycystic kidney disease (ADPKD) versus normal kidney**

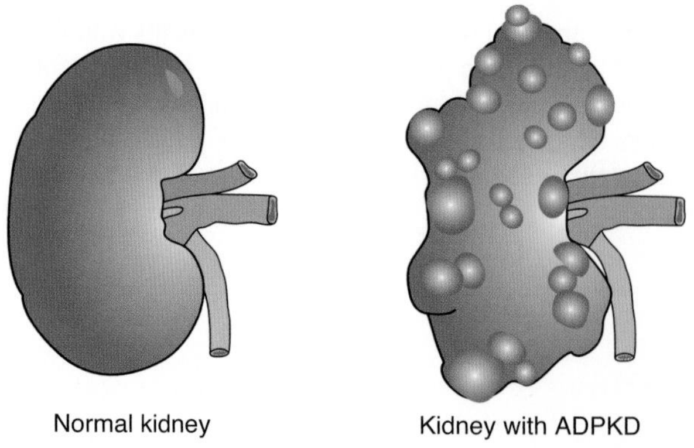
Normal kidney
Kidney with ADPKD

I. Etiology of ADPKD

A. Autosomal dominant
B. Occurs in midlife

II. Clinical features of ADPKD

A. Bilateral
B. Kidney parenchyma is partially replaced with cysts
C. **Hematuria**
D. Hypertension
E. **Large palpable kidneys**
F. Progressively worsening renal function leading to renal failure

III. ADPKD is associated with berry aneurysms of circle of Willis and cystic disease in other organs, especially the liver.

RENAL CANCERS *(Table 6-8)*

I. The classic triad of hematuria, flank pain, and a flank mass is seen only in 10% to 20% of patients with renal cancer. Most are sporadic; however, smoking accounts for 20% to 30% of the cases.

TABLE 6-8 **Renal Cancers**

Maligna	Etiology	Clinical Features	Notes
Renal cell carcinoma	**Smoking;** alteration of chromosome 3 (as seen in **von Hippel–Lindau disease**)	Afflicts men 45-65 years of age; hematuria; mass; pain; fever; **secondary polycythemia;** paraneoplastic syndrome; usually extends from renal poles, with **clear cells**	Most common renal malignancy; may be associated with increased erythropoietin (EPO)
Wilms tumor (nephroblastoma)	Chromosome 11 abnormality; **WAGR**	**Palpable flank mass** in children 2–5 years old; hematuria	Most common renal malignancy of childhood (see following)
Transitional cell carcinoma	Cyclophosphamide treatment; **smoking;** aniline dye exposure; **phenacetin** abuse	Hematuria	Most common tumor of the collecting system

WAGR, Wilms tumor, aniridia, genitourinary abnormalities, and mental retardation.

II. Nephroblastoma (Wilms tumor)

A. **Most common malignant renal tumor in children**
B. Malignant tissue is derived from embryonic nephrogenic tissue.
C. Peak incidence is between 2 and 4 years of age.
D. The **two-hit theory** of oncogenesis, which explains the etiology of Wilms tumor, requires a mutation of both copies of the Wilms tumor-1 (WT-1) tumor-suppressor gene on chromosome 11p.
E. **Characteristic clinical features**
   1. Hematuria
   2. Hypertension
   3. Large abdominal mass
   4. Intestinal obstruction
F. Part of **WAGR syndrome** (**W**ilms tumor, **A**niridia, **G**enital anomalies, mental **R**etardation)

QUICK HIT

In altitude sickness, in order to get enough oxygen, hyperventilation occurs, which causes respiratory alkalosis. Carbonic anhydrase inhibitors speed metabolic compensation by increasing urinary excretion of HCO_3^-, causing metabolic acidosis.

QUICK HIT

Mannitol and other osmotic diuretics also "pull" fluid into the bloodstream, thus decreasing pressure in glaucoma, in cases of **increased intracranial pressure**, and in surgery.

QUICK HIT

Loop diuretics, which have direct **pulmonary vasodilatory** properties, are particularly useful in the treatment of pulmonary edema.

QUICK HIT

Thiazide diuretics are sulfa derivatives and should be used with caution in patients with sulfa drug allergies.

DIURETICS AND FLUID BALANCE

I. Diuretics

A. The diuretics in Figure 6-14 can be grouped into five main categories, each with a different mechanism of action (Table 6-9). The side effects of each type of diuretic are also different, which means that certain diuretics are better suited for certain patients.

FIGURE 6-14 **Effects of diuretics on the nephron**

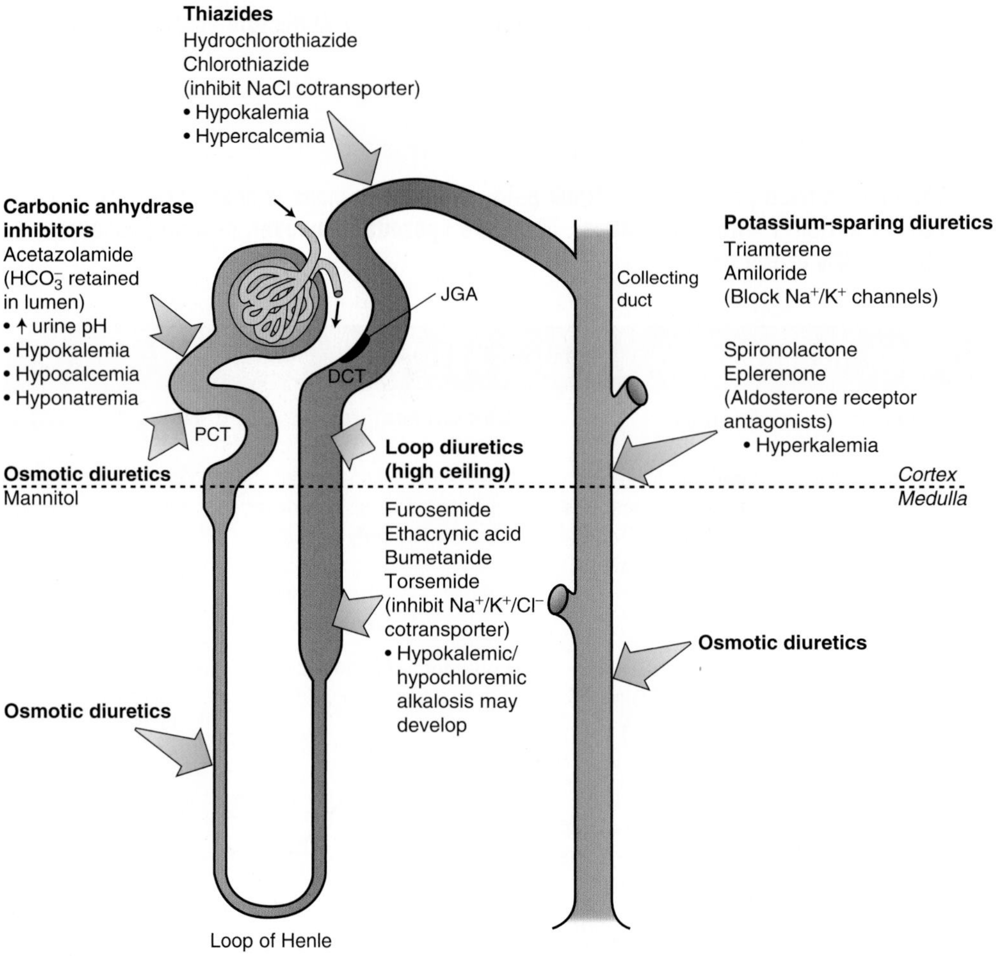
Thiazides
Hydrochlorothiazide
Chlorothiazide
(inhibit NaCl cotransporter)
• Hypokalemia
• Hypercalcemia
Carbonic anhydrase inhibitors
Acetazolamide
(HCO_3^- retained in lumen)
• ↑ urine pH
• Hypokalemia
• Hypocalcemia
• Hyponatremia
JGA
DCT
PCT
Collecting duct
Potassium-sparing diuretics
Triamterene
Amiloride
(Block Na^+/K^+ channels)
Spironolactone
Eplerenone
(Aldosterone receptor antagonists)
• Hyperkalemia
Osmotic diuretics
Mannitol
Loop diuretics (high ceiling)
Cortex
Medulla
Furosemide
Ethacrynic acid
Bumetanide
Torsemide
(inhibit $Na^+/K^+/Cl^-$ cotransporter)
• Hypokalemic/ hypochloremic alkalosis may develop
Osmotic diuretics
Osmotic diuretics
Loop of Henle

Cl^-, chloride; DCT, distal convoluted tubule; HCO_3^-, bicarbonate; JGA, juxtaglomerular apparatus; K^+, potassium; Na^+, sodium; PCT, proximal convoluted tubule.

The Renal System

TABLE **6-9** **Diuretics**

Therapeutic Agent	Mechanism of Action	Electrolytes Lost in Urine	Indications	Side Effects	Notes
Acetazolamide	Carbonic anhydrase inhibitors—Inhibit carbonic anhydrase in **PCT,** which prevents HCO_3^- reabsorption	Na^+ HCO_3^-, K^+	Glaucoma, urinary alkalinization, metabolic alkalosis, altitude sickness	**Hyperchloremic metabolic acidosis, sulfa drug allergy,** neuropathy, ammonium toxicity	Causes decreased secretion of HCO_3^- in aqueous humor
Loop diuretics					
Furosemide, torsemide, bumetanide, ethacrynic acid	Prevents cotransport of Na^+, K^+, and Cl^- in **thick ascending limb** of loop of Henle	Na^+, Cl^-, Ca^{2+}, K^+	**Congestive heart failure,** cirrhosis, nephrotic syndrome, pulmonary edema, hypertension, hypercalcemia	**Ototoxicity, hypokalemic metabolic alkalosis, dehydration, sulfa drug allergy** (not ethacrynic acid), nephritis, gout	Has rapid onset and short duration of action, which is ideal for relieving acute edema
Mannitol	Osmotic diuretic—prevents isosmotic reabsorption of filtrate in **PCT, loop of Henle,** and **collecting tubule**	Na^+ and all other filtered solutes	Shock, drug overdose, decrease intracranial or intraocular pressure; maintenance of urine flow in rhabdomyolysis	Pulmonary edema, dehydration; contraindicated in anuria and congestive heart failure	Results in increased urine volume; readily filtered and not reabsorbed
Potassium-sparing diuretics					
Spironolactone, eplerenone	Binds to intracellular aldosterone steroid receptors in **collecting tubules**	Na^+, Cl^-	Hyperaldosteronism, potassium depletion, congestive heart failure, post-MI	**Hyperkalemic metabolic acidosis, gynecomastia** and antiandrogen effects (spironolactone only)	Results in decreased secretion of K^+ and H^+, which can lead to **hyperkalemic metabolic acidosis**
Triamterene, amiloride	Blocks Na^+ channels in **collecting tubules**	Na^+, Cl^-	Hypertension, potassium depletion	**Hyperkalemic metabolic acidosis,**	Often given in combination with a thiazide
Thiazides					
Hydrochlorothiazide (HCTZ), chlorthalidone,	Inhibit transport of Na^+ and Cl^- into cells of the **DCT**	Na^+, Cl^-, K^+	Hypertension, idiopathic hypercalciuria, nephrogenic diabetes insipidus	**Hypokalemic metabolic alkalosis,** hyponatremia, **hyperglycemia, hyperlipidemia,** hyperuricemia, hypercalcemia, **sulfa drug allergy**	Causes decreased Ca^{2+} excretion, can lead to K^+ wasting with chronic therapy

Ca^{2+}, calcium; Cl^-, chloride; DCT, distal convoluted tubule; HCO_3^-, bicarbonate; K^+, potassium; MI, myocardial infarction; Na^+, sodium; PCT, proximal convoluted tubule.

II. Antidiuretic Hormone (ADH)

A. ADH causes an increase in the expression of **water channels** in the collecting tubule, which results in an increase in the reabsorption of water. Urine output drops, and concentration increases.

B. In the syndrome of inappropriate secretion of antidiuretic hormone (SIADH), **lithium** or **demeclocycline**, which blocks the effects of ADH, can be administered to prevent excessive water retention.

C. In central diabetes insipidus, either **desmopressin** (an ADH analog) or ADH can be given to prevent the excessive loss of dilute urine. These drugs are not useful in the nephrogenic (also known as the peripheral) form of diabetes insipidus, in which the kidneys do not respond to ADH.

The Endocrine System

7

DEVELOPMENT

I. Hypothalamus

A. A division of the **diencephalon**

B. Forms from the embryologic forebrain (see Chapter 2)

II. Pituitary gland consists of two lobes.

A. Anterior lobe: forms from **Rathke pouch**, an ectodermal diverticulum of the primitive mouth that invaginates upward

B. Posterior lobe: forms from an evagination of the **hypothalamus**

III. Thyroid gland

A. It forms from the endoderm of the floor of the pharynx.

B. It begins as a diverticulum that migrates caudally.

C. Thyroid follicular cells are derived from endoderm.

IV. Parathyroid glands

A. **Inferior parathyroid glands** develop from the **third pharyngeal pouch**.

B. **Superior parathyroid glands** develop from the **fourth pharyngeal pouch**.

C. The parathyroid glands migrate caudally and come to lie on the dorsal surface of the thyroid gland.

QUICK HIT

DiGeorge syndrome is a malformation of the third and fourth pharyngeal pouches caused by a mutation of 22q11, leading to a spectrum of disorders including thymic hypoplasia, T-cell deficiency, absent parathyroids, and hypocalcaemia.

V. Adrenal glands

A. **Gross description**

1. Paired adult adrenal glands weigh 4 g each.
2. They are located immediately anterosuperior to the superior renal poles.
3. They are enclosed in renal fascia.

B. **Adrenal cortex**

1. Forms from the mesoderm
2. Includes three major parts
   a. Zona glomerulosa and zona fasciculata are present at birth.
   b. **Zona reticularis** is not completely formed until 3 years of age.

C. Medulla of adrenal gland

1. **Chromaffin cells** form from neural crest cells that invade the adrenal glands during development.
2. These cells are in essence postganglionic neurons of the sympathetic nervous system.

MNEMONIC

Thyroglossal duct cysts are **mid-line** cysts of the neck. B**r**anchi**al** cleft cysts lie **lat**er**al**ly anywhere along the **a**nterior border of the sternocleidomastoid muscle.

VI. Pancreas

A. It forms from a ventral and dorsal bud of endoderm from the foregut.

1. The ventral bud forms the uncinate process and part of the pancreatic head.
2. The dorsal bud forms part of the head, body, and tail.

B. Exocrine pancreas: Acinar cells and ducts form from endoderm surrounded by mesoderm.
C. Endocrine pancreas: Mesodermal cells aggregate to form **pancreatic islet cells**.

VII. Gonads *(see Chapter 8)*

CONGENITAL MALFORMATIONS *(Table 7-1)*

There is a wide spectrum of developmental abnormalities involving the endocrine system. Some of these malformations are anatomic, whereas others are biochemical.

TABLE 7-1 Congenital Malformations

Malformation	Description
Craniopharyngioma	Cystic tumor of the pituitary that forms from the remnants of the **Rathke pouch;** may cause diabetes insipidus
Thyroglossal duct cysts	A remnant of the descending migratory path of the thyroid that persists into adult life Most are asymptomatic, but an infection may cause swelling and produce a progressively enlarging moveable mass
Absence of parathyroid glands	Occurs in **DiGeorge syndrome** (thymic aplasia) (see Chapter 10) Inability to produce parathyroid hormone leads to hypoparathyroidism and hypocalcemia
Congenital adrenal hyperplasia	Figure 7-9
Annular pancreas	Ventral and dorsal pancreatic buds form a ring around the duodenum; may cause **duodenal obstruction**
Accessory pancreatic tissue	Normal pancreatic tissue found within the wall of the stomach; most common type of choristoma (normal tissue found misplaced within another organ)

HORMONES *(Table 7-2)*

Hormones are biologically active chemicals formed in an organ and carried through the blood to act on adjacent cells of the same organ or on a different body part. Hormone function can be localized or systemic. Hormones can alter the activity or structure of the target organ(s) depending on the specificity of the hormone's effects. Hormones play an essential role in homeostasis, reproductive function, and metabolism, and they are vital in nearly every other body system as well.

TABLE 7-2 **Hormones**

Hormone	Secreted by	End-Organ Effects of Hormones	Stimulated by	Inhibited by
GnRH	Hypothalamus	LH/FSH secretion	Puberty	Progesterone, testosterone
FSH	Anterior pituitary gland	Growth of follicles and estrogen secretion (acts on granulosa cells); maturation of sperm (acts on Sertoli cells)	Pulsatile release of GnRH	Constant GnRH release; inhibin
LH	Anterior pituitary gland (basophils)	Ovulation; formation of corpus luteum; estrogen/progesterone synthesis (acts on theca lutein cells); synthesis/secretion of testosterone (acts on Leydig cells)	Pulsatile release of GnRH	Constant GnRH release; progesterone, testosterone
Estrogen	Ovary (granulosa cells)	Proliferative phase of menstrual cycle; development of female reproductive organs	FSH	Estrogen
Progesterone	Ovary (granulosa lutein cells)	Breast development; secretory activity during luteal phase	LH	Progesterone
Testosterone	Testes (Leydig cells)	Spermatogenesis; conversion of testosterone to dihydrotestosterone via 5α-reductase stimulates development of secondary male sex characteristics	LH	Testosterone
hCG	Placenta (syncytiotrophoblast)	Increased estrogen/progesterone synthesis; maintains corpus luteum secretion of estrogen and progesterone	Trophoblast differentiation after implantation of fertilized egg	
ACTH	Anterior pituitary	Synthesis and secretion of adrenal cortical hormones	CRH, stress	Cortisol
Cortisol (glucocorticoids)	Adrenal cortex (zona fasciculata)	Anti-inflammatory effects (via inhibition of phospholipase A2); immunosuppressive effects; stimulation of gluconeogenesis; increased blood sugar	ACTH	Cortisol
Aldosterone	Adrenal cortex (zona glomerulosa)	Increased renal sodium reabsorption and potassium secretion; increase in blood volume	Decrease in blood volume; angiotensin II; hyperkalemia; hyponatremia	Hypernatremia, hypokalemia, fluid overload
TSH	Anterior pituitary	Synthesis and secretion of thyroid hormone (T_4, T_3)	TRH	T_4, T_3

(continued)

QUICK HIT

Luteinizing hormone (LH), follicle-stimulating hormone (FSH), human chorionic gonadotropin (hCG), and thyrotropin-releasing hormone (TRH) are hormones consisting of two subunits: α and β. The α subunits in these hormones are identical, whereas the β subunit is unique for each.

QUICK HIT

Finasteride, a 5α-reductase inhibitor, is used in the treatment of benign prostatic hyperplasia. Flutamide, a competitive androgen receptor blocker, is used to treat prostatic carcinoma.

QUICK HIT

Antibodies specific for βhCG are used in pregnancy tests. Increased βhCG can be detected 1 to 2 weeks after conception.

QUICK HIT

The hormone hCG is increased in normal pregnancy, hydatidiform moles, choriocarcinomas, gestational tumors, ectopic pregnancy, and pseudocyesis.

QUICK HIT

The anti-inflammatory effect of cortisol is mediated by its induction of **lipocortin**, which inhibits phospholipase A2 and prostaglandin synthesis. Cortisol also inhibits the production of interleukin-2 (IL-2).

TABLE 7-2 **Hormones** *(Continued)*

Hormone	Secreted by	End-Organ Effects of Hormones	Stimulated by	Inhibited by
T_4, T_3	Thyroid	Growth; maturation of CNS; increased basal metabolic rate, cardiac output, and nutrient use	TSH, estrogen	Somatostatin, dopamine
Somatostatin (somatotropin-inhibiting hormone)	Hypothalamus	Inhibited secretion of growth hormone	Growth hormone, somatomedins (IGF)	
GH (somatotropin)	Anterior pituitary (acidophils)	Decreased glucose uptake; increased protein synthesis, growth, organ size, and lean body mass	GHRH, exercise, sleep, puberty, hypoglycemia, estrogen, stress, endogenous opiates	Somatomedins (IGF), somatostatin, obesity, pregnancy, hyperglycemia
Prolactin	Anterior pituitary (acidophils)	Stimulation of milk production and secretion; breast development; inhibition of ovulation	Prolactin-stimulating factor, TRH	Prolactin-inhibiting factor (dopamine)
Oxytocin	Hypothalamus via posterior pituitary	Milk ejection from breast (milk letdown); uterine contraction	Suckling, sex, dilation of the cervix	Alcohol, stress
PTH	Parathyroid gland (chief cells)	Increased serum calcium; increased renal calcium absorption; inhibition of phosphate reabsorption; activates vitamin D to increase intestinal calcium absorption	Decreased serum calcium, mild decreased serum magnesium	Severe decrease in serum magnesium
Vitamin D (1,25 dihydroxy-cholecalciferol)	Kidney (active form produced by activity of 1α-hydroxylase), sun-exposed skin	Increased intestinal calcium and phosphorus absorption; increased bone calcium resorption; increased kidney phosphate and calcium reabsorption	Decreased serum calcium, increased PTH, decreased serum phosphate	
ADH (vasopressin)	Hypothalamus via posterior pituitary	Increased water permeability in distal tubules and collecting duct to regulate osmolarity (V2 receptor); constriction of vascular smooth muscle (V1 receptor)	Volume contraction, nicotine, opiates, increased serum osmolarity	Ethanol, ANF, decreased serum osmolarity
ANF	Atrial myocytes	Vasodilation to decrease systemic BP, increase urinary Na^+ and H_2O excretion	Atrial stretch due to blood volume increase	ANF
Glucagon	Pancreatic islet cells (α cells)	Increased blood glucose; increased glycogenolysis and gluconeogenesis in the liver; increased lipolysis and ketone production	Decreased blood glucose; increased amino acids, ACh	Increased blood glucose; insulin; somatostatin
Insulin	Pancreatic islet cells (β cells)	Decreased blood glucose caused by increased uptake into muscle and fat; decreased glycogenolysis and gluconeogenesis; increased protein synthesis; increased fat deposition; inhibition of lipolysis	Increased blood glucose, amino acids; glucagon; ACh	Decreased blood glucose; somatostatin
Leptin	Fat cells	Reduced food intake (satiety); inhibits the arcuate nucleus and lateral nucleus of the hypothalamus, stimulates the ventromedial nucleus of the hypothalamus	Obesity, overeating, pregnancy	Fasting

ACh, acetylcholine; ACTH, adrenocorticotropic hormone; ADH, antidiuretic hormone; ANP, atrial natriuretic peptide; BP, blood pressure; CNS, central nervous system; CRH, corticotropin-releasing hormone; FSH, follicle-stimulating hormone; GH, growth hormone; GHRH, growth hormone–releasing hormone; GnRH, gonadotropin-releasing hormone; hCG, human chorionic gonadotropin; IGF, insulin-like growth factor; LH, luteinizing hormone; PTH, parathyroid hormone; T_3, triiodothyronine; T_4, thyroxine; TRH, thyrotropin-releasing hormone; TSH, thyroid-stimulating hormone.

I. Hormones of the hypothalamic–pituitary axis *(Figure 7-1)*

II. Hormones of the adrenal gland *(Figure 7-2)*

III. Hormone second-messenger system

The second-messenger system is the process by which extracellular signals are translated into cellular responses. Biologically active chemicals, such as hormones, bind to receptor sites on the cell membrane, resulting in phosphorylation of intracellular proteins or changes in ion channel conductivity and subsequent cellular modulation (Table 7-3 and Figure 7-3).

FIGURE 7-1 Hormones of the hypothalamic–pituitary axis

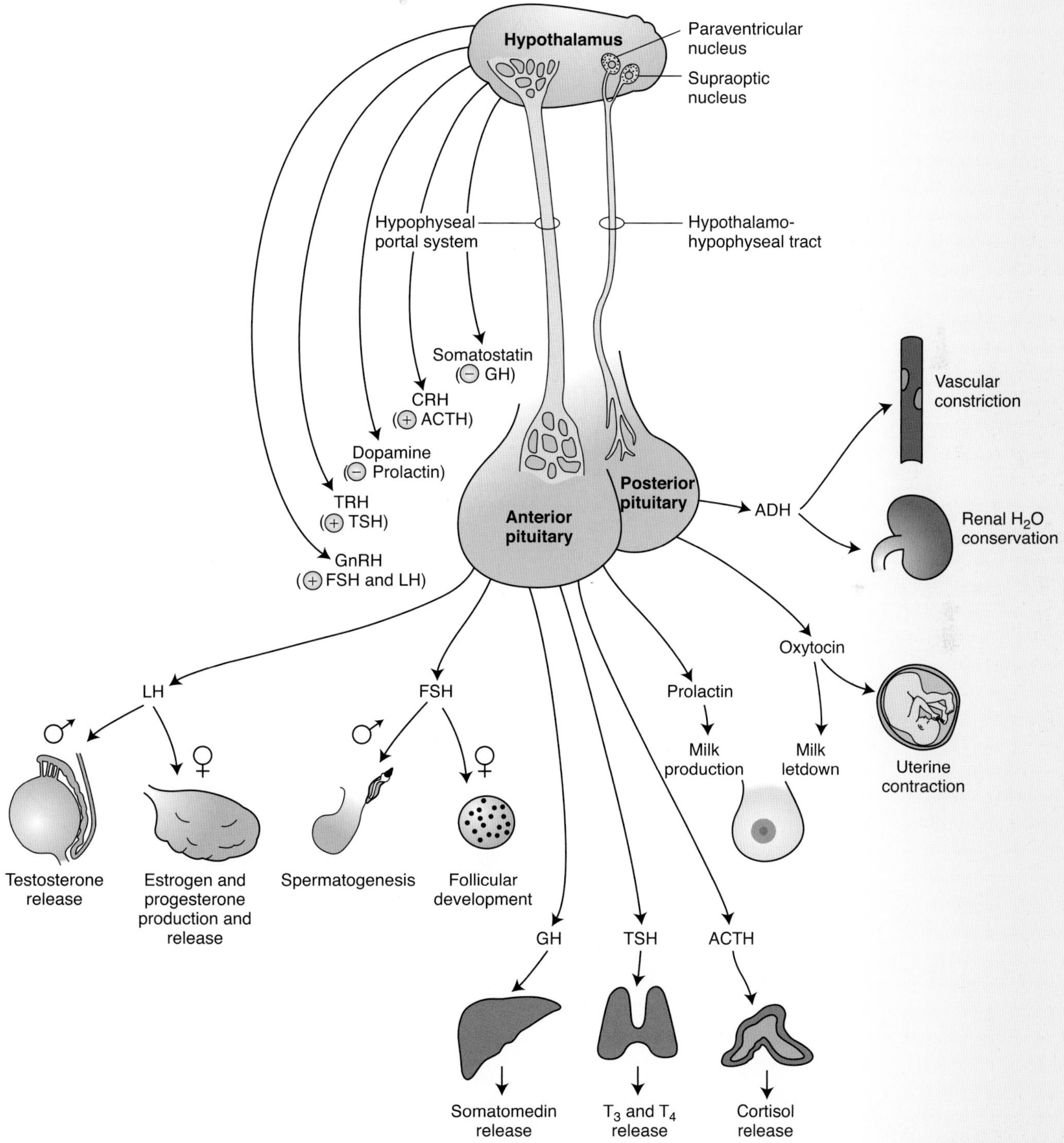

Hypothalamus
Paraventricular nucleus
Supraoptic nucleus
Hypophyseal portal system
Hypothalamo-hypophyseal tract
Somatostatin (⊖ GH)
CRH (⊕ ACTH)
Dopamine (⊖ Prolactin)
TRH (⊕ TSH)
GnRH (⊕ FSH and LH)
Anterior pituitary
Posterior pituitary
ADH
Vascular constriction
Renal H_2O conservation
Oxytocin
Uterine contraction
Milk letdown
Prolactin
Milk production
LH
FSH
♂
♀
Testosterone release
Estrogen and progesterone production and release
Spermatogenesis
Follicular development
GH
TSH
ACTH
Somatomedin release
T_3 and T_4 release
Cortisol release

ACTH, adrenocorticotropic hormone; ADH, antidiuretic hormone; CRH, corticotropin-releasing hormone; FSH, follicle-stimulating hormone; GH, growth hormone; GnRH, gonadotropin-releasing hormone; LH, luteinizing hormone; T_3, triiodothyronine; T_4, thyroxine; TRH, thyrotropin-releasing hormone; TSH, thyroid-stimulating hormone.

MNEMONIC

To remember the anatomic layers of the adrenal cortex, think **GFR: G**lomerulosa, **F**asciculata, and **R**eticularis. To remember the hormones produced by each layer, think **"the deeper you go, the sweeter it gets":** aldosterone (**salt** hormone), glucocorticoid (**sugar** hormone), and androgens (**sex** hormone).

FIGURE 7-2 **Hormones of the adrenal gland**

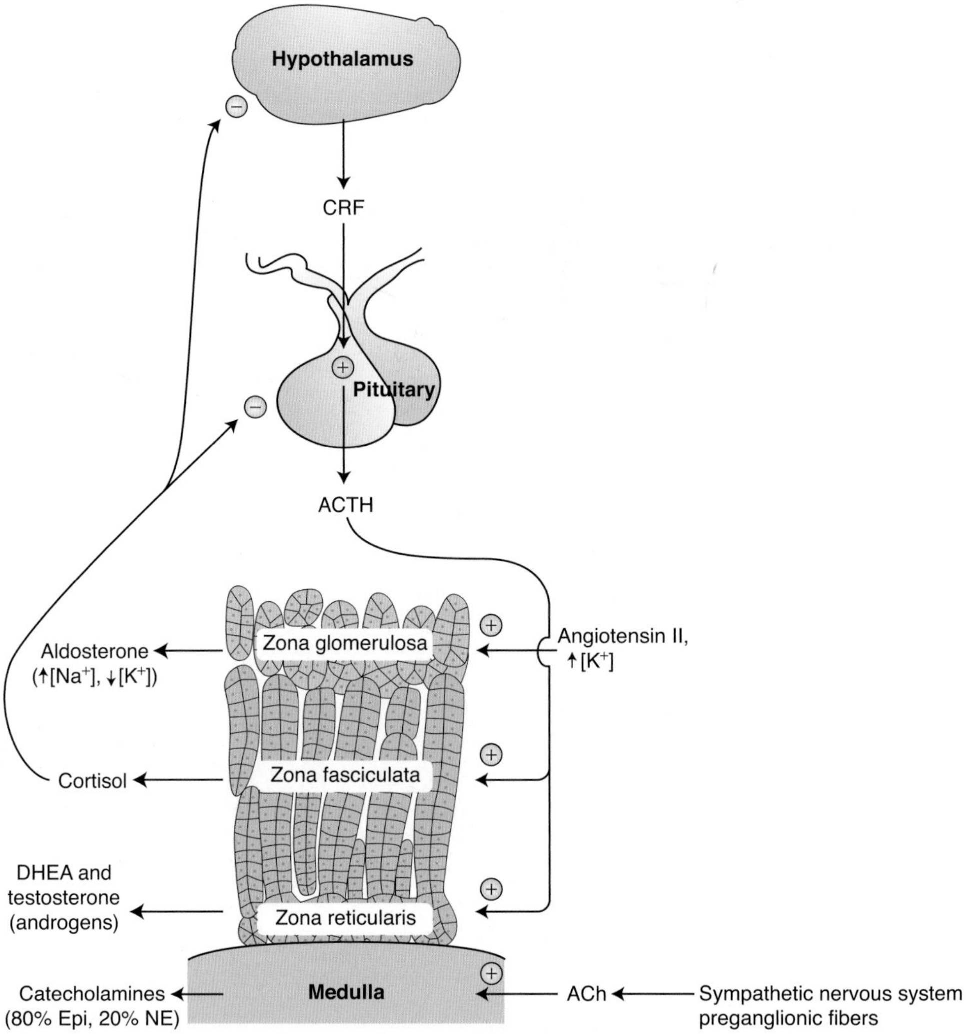
Hypothalamus
CRF
Pituitary
ACTH
Zona glomerulosa
Aldosterone
(↑[Na+], ↓[K+])
Angiotensin II,
↑[K+]
Zona fasciculata
Cortisol
Zona reticularis
DHEA and
testosterone
(androgens)
Medulla
Catecholamines
(80% Epi, 20% NE)
ACh
Sympathetic nervous system
preganglionic fibers

ACh, acetylcholine; ACTH, adrenocorticotropic hormone; CRF, corticotropin-releasing factor; DHEA, dehydroepiandrosterone; Epi, epinephrine; NE, norepinephrine.

TABLE 7-3 **Hormone Second-messenger Systems**

cAMP	cGMP	IP3	Steroid	Tyrosine Kinase
β_1-agonists	ANF	α_1-agonists	Aldosterone	Insulin
β_2-agonists	EDRF	GnRH	Estrogen	IGF-1
LH		TRH	Glucocorticoids	Prolactin
FSH		GHRH	Testosterone	GH
TSH		Angiotensin II	Progesterone	
ADH (V_2)		ADH (V_1)	Thyroid	
hCG		Oxytocin	Vitamin D	
CRH				
PTH				
Calcitonin				
Glucagon				

ADH, antidiuretic hormone; ANF, atrial natriuretic factor (also known as ANP, atrial natriuretic peptide); cAMP, cyclic adenosine monophosphate; cGMP, cyclic guanine monophosphate; CRH, corticotropin-releasing hormone; EDRF, endothelium-derived relaxing factor; FSH, follicle-stimulating hormone; GH, growth hormone; GHRH, growth hormone–releasing factor; GnRH, gonadotropin-releasing hormone; hCG, human chorionic gonadotropin; IGF, insulin-like growth factor; IP3, inositol-1,4,5-triphosphate; LH, luteinizing hormone; PTH, parathyroid hormone; TRH, thyrotropin-releasing hormone; TSH, thyroid-stimulating hormone.

FIGURE 7-3 **Hormone second-messenger systems**

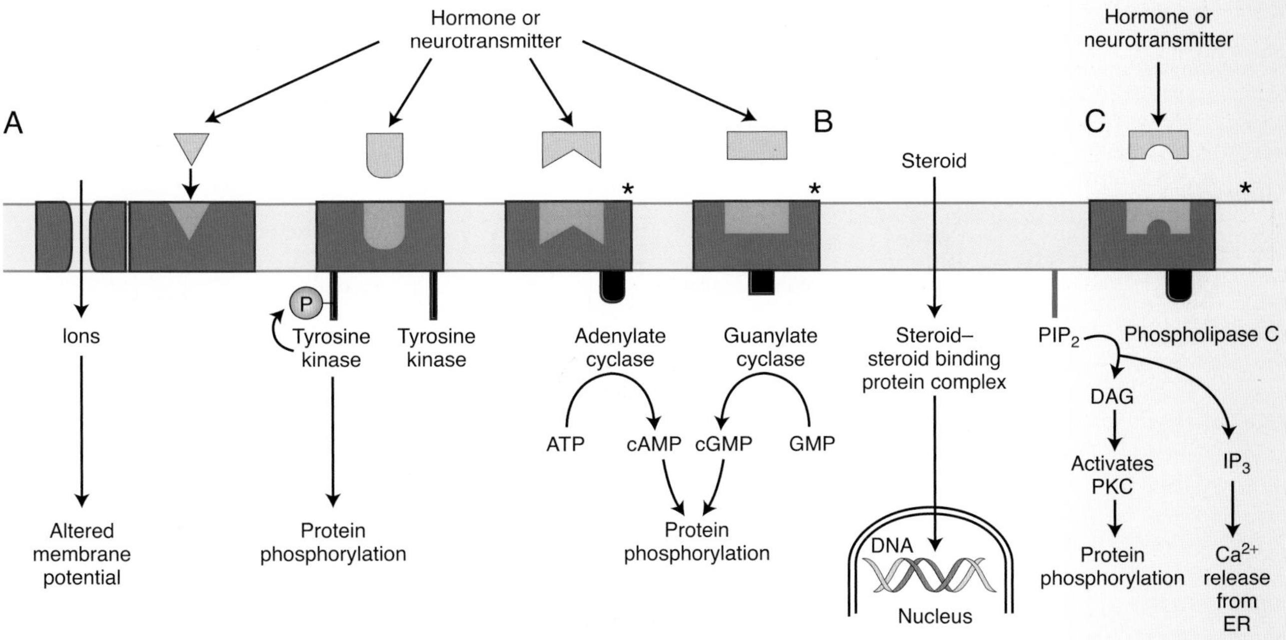

Hormone or
neurotransmitter
A
B
C
Hormone or
neurotransmitter
Steroid
*
*
*
P
Ions
Tyrosine
kinase
Tyrosine
kinase
Adenylate
cyclase
Guanylate
cyclase
Steroid–
steroid binding
protein complex
PIP2
Phospholipase C
DAG
ATP
cAMP
cGMP
GMP
Activates
PKC
IP3
Altered
membrane
potential
Protein
phosphorylation
Protein
phosphorylation
DNA
Nucleus
Protein
phosphorylation
Ca2+
release
from
ER

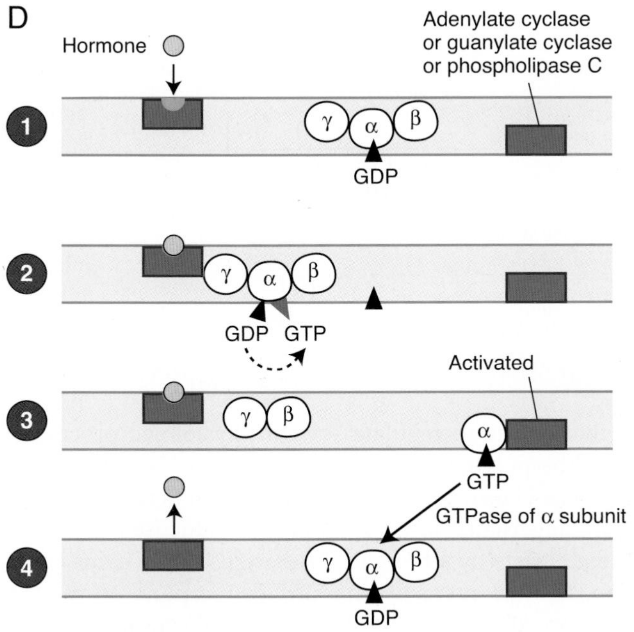

D
Hormone
Adenylate cyclase
or guanylate cyclase
or phospholipase C
1
γ
α
β
GDP
2
GDP
GTP
3
Activated
α
GTP
GTPase of α subunit
4
GDP

A. Peptide mechanism. Peptide binds to hormone receptor site and influences various second-messenger systems. These hormones are typically short acting and do not involve gene regulation, in contrast to steroid hormones, which have a slower onset of action.

B. Steroid mechanism. Lipid-soluble steroid penetrates cell membrane and binds to steroid-binding protein. This complex enters the nucleus and influences DNA synthesis.

C. Phospholipase C mechanism

D. G-protein mechanism.

1. Messenger system before hormone binding
2. After hormone binding, GTP replaces GDP on G-protein.
3. GTP, attached to α subunit, dissociates from the β–γ complex and converts ATP to cAMP.
4. Hormone is released from binding site and complex returns to inactive state when GTPase cleaves GTP to GDP.

*Mechanism utilizing a G-protein, as shown in D.

ATP, adenosine triphosphate; cAMP, cyclic adenosine monophosphate; cGMP, cyclic guanosine monophosphate; DAG, diacylglycerol; ER, endoplasmic reticulum; GDP, guanosine 5′-diphosphate; GTP, guanosine triphosphate; GMP, guanosine monophosphate; IP_3, inositol triphosphate; PKC, protein kinase C.

G-Protein Class	Action	Examples
G_q	Activates phospholipase C → cleaves phosopholipids to form PIP_2, which is subsequently cleaved into DAG and IP3. DAG activates protein kinase C. IP3 increases intracellular calcium, which also has downstream effects (including activating protein kinase C).	H_1, α_1, V_1, M_1, M_3
G_s	Stimulates adenylyl cyclase → converts ATP to cAMP, which activates protein kinase A	β_1, β_2, D_1, H_2, V_2
G_i	Inhibits adenylyl cyclase → decreased cAMP production → decreased activity of protein kinase A	M_2, α_2, D_2

ATP, adenosine triphosphate; cAMP, cyclic adenosine monophosphate; DAG, diacylglycerol; IP_3, inositol triphosphate; PIP_2, phosphatidylinositol 4,5-bisphosphate;

CALCIUM HOMEOSTASIS *(Figure 7-4)*

FIGURE 7-4 Calcium homeostasis

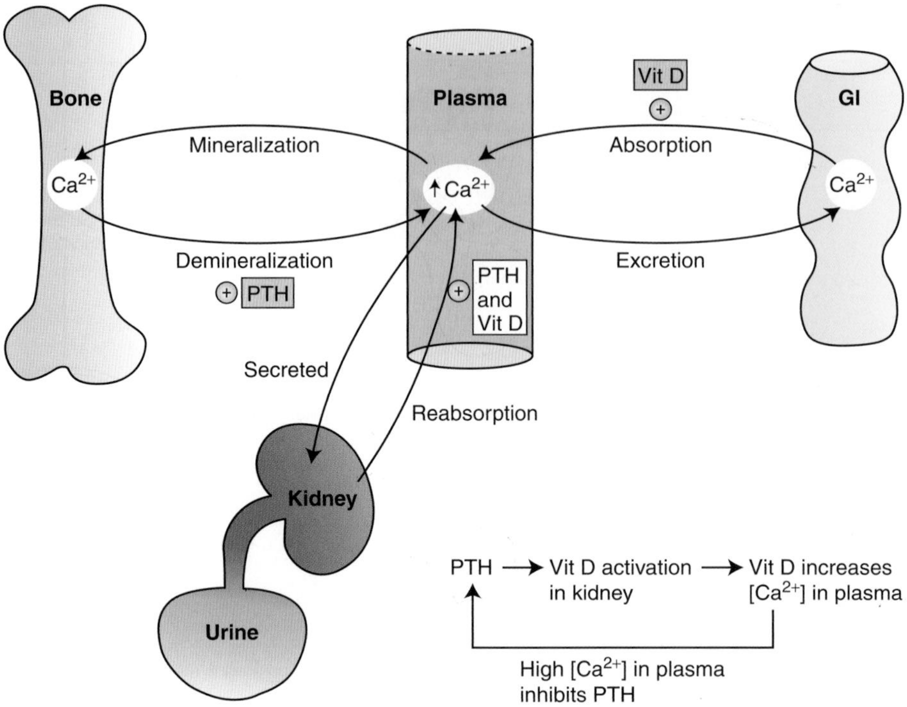

Bone
Ca2+
Mineralization
Demineralization
+ PTH
Plasma
↑Ca2+
PTH and Vit D
Vit D
Absorption
Excretion
GI
Ca2+
Secreted
Reabsorption
Kidney
Urine
PTH → Vit D activation in kidney → Vit D increases [Ca2+] in plasma
High [Ca2+] in plasma inhibits PTH

Ca^{2+}, calcium; GI, gastrointestinal tract; PTH, parathyroid hormone; Vit D, vitamin D.

QUICK HIT

Somatostatin is also secreted in the brain, gastrointestinal (GI) tract, and δ cells of the pancreas. It functions to decrease systemic secretion of insulin, glucagon, and gastrin.

QUICK HIT

Glucose enters cells through facilitated transporters designated glucose transporter (GLUT)-1 through GLUT-5. These transporters have the following locations:
GLUT 1: erythrocytes, blood–brain barrier
GLUT 2: liver, kidney, pancreatic β cell, intestinal mucosa
GLUT 3: neurons
GLUT 4*: adipose tissue, skeletal and cardiac muscle
GLUT 5: intestinal epithelium

*insulin-responsive transport to membrane

INSULIN AND GLUCAGON

Insulin is a polypeptide hormone that serves to regulate several physiologic processes. Its primary role, in conjunction with the polypeptide hormone glucagon, is to **maintain blood glucose levels**. When blood glucose levels rise after a meal, insulin is released from the β cells of the pancreatic islets of Langerhans in proportion to the glucose concentration of blood. Innervation of pancreatic islets by a branch of the vagus nerve helps coordinate insulin release with digestion. Insulin interacts with surface receptors on muscle and adipose tissue and stimulates glucose absorption and triacylglycerol synthesis. In the liver, insulin inhibits gluconeogenesis and glycogen breakdown.

Insulin is formed by two polypeptides linked by disulfide bridges (Figure 7-5). The insulin receptor is **tyrosine kinase** linked; binding of insulin to the α subunit causes phosphorylation of the tyrosine kinase connected to the β subunit. This stimulates recruitment of glucose transporters (GLUTs) to the cell membrane (GLUT-4 in skeletal muscle) and increases the uptake of glucose (Figure 7-6). Glucagon counteracts the actions of insulin. It is a single polypeptide secreted by the β cells of the islets of Langerhans. Glucagon is secreted in response to low blood glucose, increased amino acids in the blood, and epinephrine. Glucagon secretion leads to a rise in blood glucose concentration via **gluconeogenesis** and **glycogenolysis**. Release of glucagon is inhibited by insulin. Glucagon is also responsible for the formation of ketone bodies, and increased uptake of amino acids by the liver muscle is not responsive to glucagon.

- **Blood Levels of Glucose, Insulin, and Glucagon after a High-Carbohydrate Meal** (Figure 7-7)

FIGURE 7-5 **Formation of insulin**

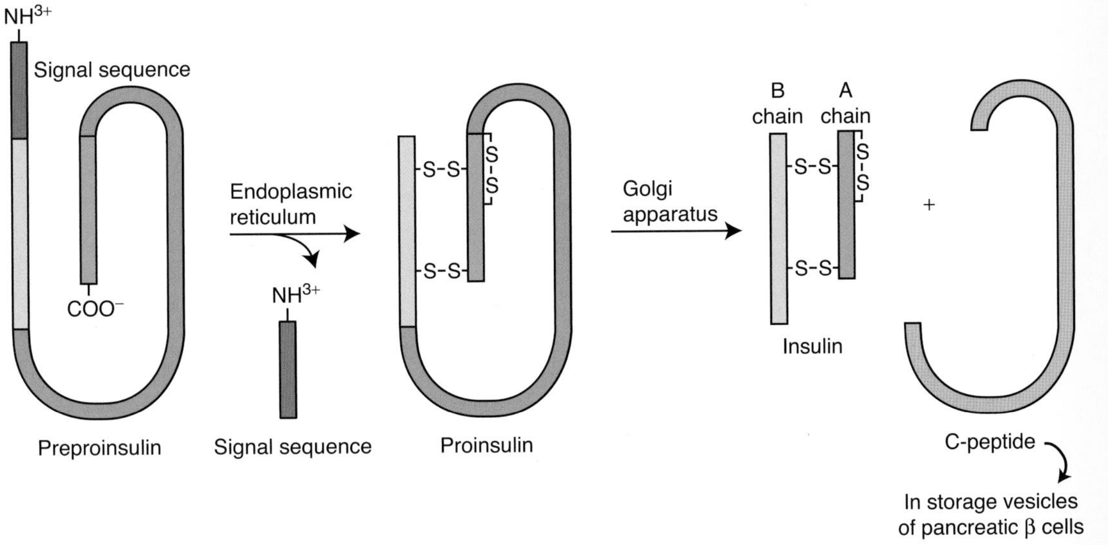
NH3+
Signal sequence
COO−
Endoplasmic reticulum
NH3+
-S-S-
S-S
-S-S-
Golgi apparatus
B chain
A chain
-S-S-
S-S
-S-S-
+
Insulin
Preproinsulin
Signal sequence
Proinsulin
C-peptide
In storage vesicles of pancreatic β cells

FIGURE 7-6 **Insulin recruitment of glucose transporters**

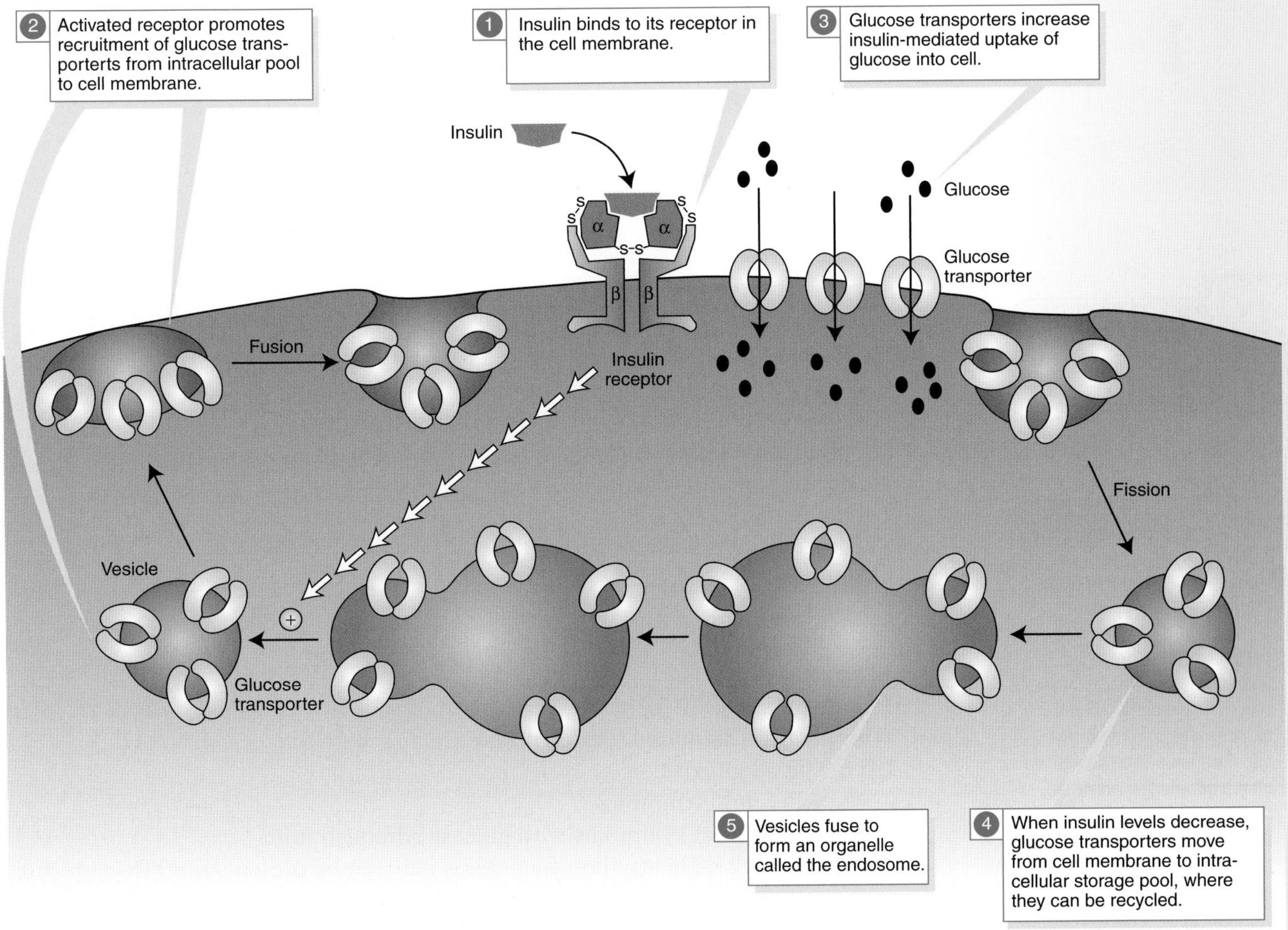
2 Activated receptor promotes recruitment of glucose transporterts from intracellular pool to cell membrane.
1 Insulin binds to its receptor in the cell membrane.
3 Glucose transporters increase insulin-mediated uptake of glucose into cell.
Insulin
Glucose
Glucose transporter
α
α
β
β
Insulin receptor
Fusion
Fission
Vesicle
Glucose transporter
5 Vesicles fuse to form an organelle called the endosome.
4 When insulin levels decrease, glucose transporters move from cell membrane to intracellular storage pool, where they can be recycled.

(Adapted with permission from Champe PC, Harvey RA. *Lippincott's Illustrated Reviews: Biochemistry.* 2nd ed. Philadelphia, PA: Lippincott-Raven; 1994:274.)

FIGURE 7-7 Blood levels of glucose, insulin, and glucagon after a high-carbohydrate meal

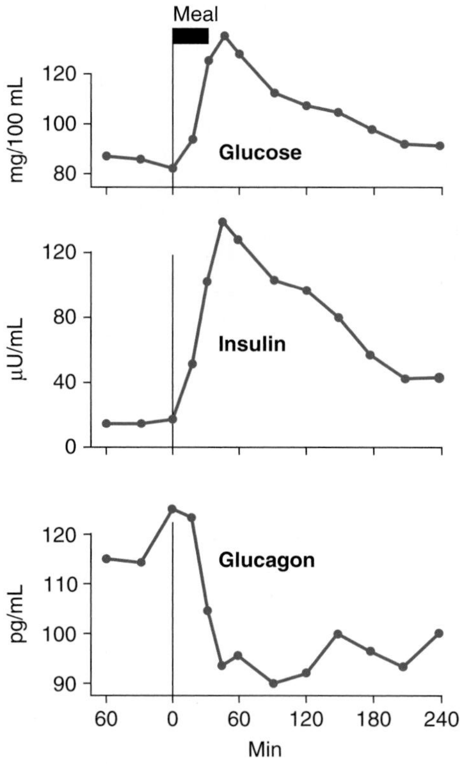
Meal
120
100
80
mg/100 mL
Glucose
120
80
40
0
μU/mL
Insulin
120
110
100
90
pg/mL
Glucagon
60
0
60
120
180
240
Min

(Adapted with permission from Champe PC, Harvey RA. *Lippincott's Illustrated Reviews: Biochemistry.* 2nd ed. Philadelphia, PA: Lippincott-Raven; 1994:272.)

QUICK HIT

In factitious hyperinsulinism, C-peptide levels will be low.

QUICK HIT

Hypoglycemia triggers the release of anti-insulin hormones such as glucagon, cortisol, growth hormone, epinephrine, and norepinephrine to help maintain blood glucose levels. Epinephrine and norepinephrine also turn on the adrenergic response, resulting in symptoms of sweating, anxiety, palpitations, and tremor. Decreased availability of glucose to the central nervous system (CNS) eventually results in neuroglycopenic symptoms of lethargy, confusion, slurred speech, coma, and death.

BLOOD GLUCOSE LEVELS

I. Hypoglycemia

A. Causes
  1. Excess insulin administration (in a diabetic patient)
  2. Sulfonylurea administration
  3. Alcohol ingestion
  4. Insulinoma
  5. Factitious hyperinsulinism

B. **Symptoms**
  1. Sweating
  2. Palpitations
  3. Anxiety
  4. Tremor

C. **Whipple triad** (required for diagnosis)
  1. Low blood glucose
  2. Hypoglycemic symptoms
  3. Improvement of symptoms with glucose administration

D. In patients with diabetes, these symptoms may not be present, and blood glucose may be allowed to drop to dangerous levels; coma or death may result.

E. Therapy
  1. Glucose or intravenous (IV) dextrose should be given after measuring blood glucose levels.
  2. Glucagon should be administered.
  3. Epinephrine is sometimes appropriate therapy.

Clinical Vignette 7-1

CLINICAL PRESENTATION: A 4-year-old boy presents to the emergency department having woken up this morning feeling **lethargic** and **confused**. The child's past medical history is significant for two prior episodes of hypoglycemia. The patient's parents also report **resting tremor**. Mother denies **seizure activity, loss of consciousness**, and recent trauma. Mother did urine dipstick, which showed glucose level of 42 mg/dL (low). Parents administered glucose orally and brought the patient to the emergency department. Physical examination revealed an **anxious, diaphoretic** child with **slurred speech**. No hepatomegaly. Vital signs: Temperature = 97.5° F; heart rate = 119 bpm; respiration rate = 30 breaths/min; blood pressure = 109/55 mm Hg; oxygen saturation = 99% on room air.

DIFFERENTIALS: Hyperinsulinism, fatty acid oxidation defect, glycogen storage disease, glycogen synthesis defect, gluconeogenesis defect, glucagon deficiency, cortisol deficiency, and growth hormone deficiency. Figure 7-8 groups the various causes of hypoglycemia in the child by pathophysiology.

LABORATORY STUDIES: **Urine ketones** should be assessed via urinalysis. If urine ketones are low, it indicates the presence of a hyperinsulinemic state or a defect in fatty acid oxidation (resulting in an inability to produce ketones). These are best differentiated by obtaining an **insulin level**. If urine ketones are high, further workup is necessary to differentiate liver metabolism from endocrine defects. Consequently, **serum lactate, pyruvate, liver function tests,** and **uric acid** levels should be obtained to help rule out possibilities such as maple syrup urine disease, glycogenolysis defect, glycogen storage disease, and gluconeogenesis defect. Also, **serum cortisol** levels should be obtained to rule out cortisol deficiency. Eventually, the patient should be screened for **growth hormone** and **pituitary hormones**.

MANAGEMENT: Key point is to **treat first** and evaluate lab studies later. After blood samples are drawn, a quick bedside glucose reading should be done. If hypoglycemia is mild and the patient is able to tolerate oral dosing, treat with **oral glucose**. If severe hypoglycemia occurs and/or if the patient is unable to tolerate oral dosing, provide dextrose bolus followed by appropriate **maintenance infusion**.

FIGURE 7-8 **Causes of hypoglycemia**

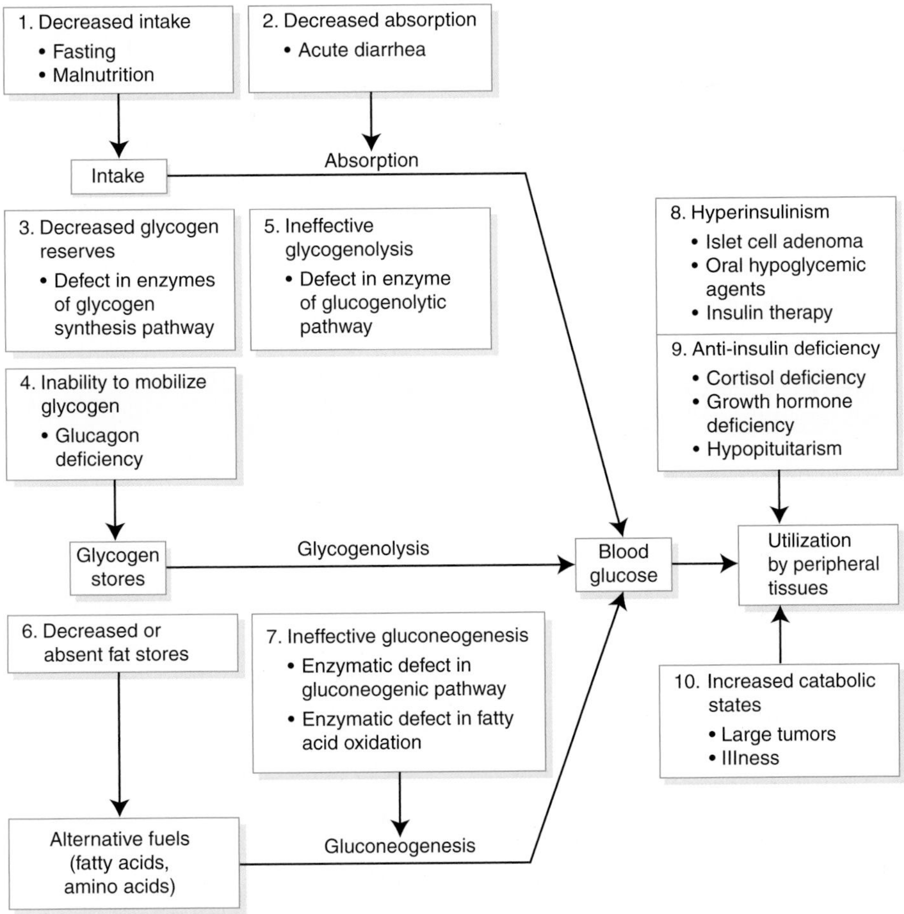
1. Decreased intake
• Fasting
• Malnutrition
2. Decreased absorption
• Acute diarrhea
Intake
Absorption
3. Decreased glycogen reserves
• Defect in enzymes of glycogen synthesis pathway
5. Ineffective glycogenolysis
• Defect in enzyme of glucogenolytic pathway
8. Hyperinsulinism
• Islet cell adenoma
• Oral hypoglycemic agents
• Insulin therapy
9. Anti-insulin deficiency
• Cortisol deficiency
• Growth hormone deficiency
• Hypopituitarism
4. Inability to mobilize glycogen
• Glucagon deficiency
Glycogen stores
Glycogenolysis
Blood glucose
Utilization by peripheral tissues
6. Decreased or absent fat stores
7. Ineffective gluconeogenesis
• Enzymatic defect in gluconeogenic pathway
• Enzymatic defect in fatty acid oxidation
10. Increased catabolic states
• Large tumors
• Illness
Alternative fuels (fatty acids, amino acids)
Gluconeogenesis

II. Hyperglycemia

A. Causes
   1. Diabetes mellitus
   2. Chronic pancreatitis
   3. Acromegaly
   4. Cushing syndrome
   5. Adverse drug reactions
      a. Furosemide
      b. Glucocorticoids
      c. Growth hormone
      d. Oral contraceptives
      e. Thiazides

B. Acute symptoms
   1. Ketoacidosis or hyperosmolar hyperglycemic nonketotic syndrome (see Table 7-6)
   2. Polyuria
   3. Polydipsia
   4. Polyphagia
   5. Weight loss
   6. Encephalopathy
      a. Tremulousness
      b. Convulsions
      c. Coma

The chronic symptoms of hyperglycemia mimic the chronic complications of diabetes (Table 7-7).

DIABETES MELLITUS

Diabetes mellitus (or, simply, diabetes) refers to a group of disorders that are characterized by hyperglycemia and affect 1% to 2% of the U.S. population. Although the pathogenesis of these disorders is varied, individuals with diabetes lack the ability to produce sufficient insulin or respond to secreted insulin in order to meet their metabolic needs. Furthermore, all patients with diabetes are vulnerable to complications such as nephropathy, neuropathy, and retinopathy. Monitoring and control of blood sugar, insulin replacement, proper diet, and exercise can significantly reduce the morbidity and mortality of this disease.

I. Diagnosis of diabetes mellitus *(Table 7-4)*

TABLE 7-4 **Diagnosis of Diabetes Mellitus**

	Normal	IFG	IGT	DM
Random blood glucose (mg/dL)	<200			≥200 (with symptoms)
Fasting blood glucose (mg/dL)	<100	100–125		≥126 (on 2 occasions)
Blood glucose after oral glucose tolerance test (mg/dL)	<140		140–199	≥200
Hemoglobin A_{1c} (%)	<5.7	5.7–6.4	5.7–6.4	≥6.5

DM, diabetes mellitus; IFG, impaired fasting glucose; IGT, impaired glucose tolerance.

II. Type 1 versus type 2 diabetes mellitus *(Table 7-5)*

TABLE 7-5 Type 1 versus Type 2 Diabetes Mellitus

	Type 1 Diabetes (15%)	Type 2 Diabetes (85%)
Cause	Possible **autoimmunity** to β cells triggered by viral cause	Increased **insulin resistance**, decreased receptors, or decreased conversion of proinsulin to insulin
Chromosomal association	6 (HLA-DRQ, HLA-DR3/DR4)	Unknown
Family history	Weak predictor	Strong predictor
Age of onset	Younger than 25 years of age	Older than 40 years of age
Body habitus	Normal to thin	Obese
Plasma insulin	Low	Normal to high
Plasma glucagon	High but suppressible	High and resistant to suppression
Pancreas morphology	Atrophy and fibrosis; β-cell depletion	Atrophy and amyloid deposits; variable β-cell population
Acute complication (Table 7-6)	Ketoacidosis	Hyperosmolar hyperglycemic nonketotic state
Common symptoms	**Polydipsia**, **polyuria**, **polyphagia** (**symptoms of hyperglycemia**)	Variable: from asymptomatic to polydipsia, polyuria, and polyphagia
Response to insulin therapy	Responsive	Variable
Response to oral therapy	Unresponsive	Responsive

HLA-DQ, human leukocyte antigen-DQ.

QUICK HIT

Rubella, mumps, and coxsackie are viral agents that can trigger the autoimmune response of the body to pancreatic β cells and cause type 1 diabetes (also called juvenile-onset diabetes).

QUICK HIT

Individuals with insulin resistance often have elevated fibrinogen and plasminogen activator inhibitors, making them susceptible to thrombosis.

QUICK HIT

Type 1 diabetes can be distinguished from type 2 by low C-peptide levels, which also indicates the need for treatment with insulin.

III. Diabetic ketoacidosis and hyperosmolar hyperglycemic nonketotic syndrome *(Table 7-6)*

TABLE 7-6 Diabetic Ketoacidosis and Hyperosmolar Hyperglycemic Nonketotic Syndrome

	DKA	HHNS
Pathology	Increased serum **ketones**; anion gap metabolic acidosis (pH <7.2); **hyperglycemia** (glucose 300–800 mg/dL because of increased production and decreased uptake)	**Hyperglycemia** (>600 mg/dL); **hyperosmolarity** (>320 mg/dL); pH >7.3
Patient	Type 1 diabetes	Type 2 diabetes
Precipitating event	**Infection**, **insufficient insulin** (new-onset diabetes, medication reduction/omission), severe medical illness (MI, stroke, trauma), dehydration, alcohol or drug abuse, corticosteroids	**Infection**, **dehydration**, medication noncompliance, severe illness (MI, stroke, trauma), alcohol or drug abuse, corticosteroids
Clinical presentation	Nausea and vomiting, **Kussmaul respiration**, abdominal pain, fruity breath odor, osmotic diuresis, shock, coma	Confusion, possibly seizures or coma, nausea and vomiting, osmotic diuresis
Mortality	10%	17%
Treatment	Insulin, saline, K^+ replacement	Saline (essential), insulin

DKA, diabetic ketoacidosis; HHNS, hyperosmolar hyperglycemic nonketotic state; MI, myocardial infarction.

QUICK HIT

The ketone bodies (**acetoacetate**, **β-hydroxybutyrate**) are produced by the liver from acetyl coenzyme A (CoA) in the fasting state. The body (including the brain after 4 to 5 days) uses the ketone bodies for energy instead of glucose and amino acids. Red blood cells (RBCs), however, can only use glucose.

QUICK HIT

In DKA, there is insufficient insulin to inhibit lipolysis at the adipocytes, which liberate stored fatty acids that are subsequently taken up by the liver and converted to ketones to meet the body's energy demands. In HHNS, however, there tends to be minimal ketosis because there is sufficient insulin to inhibit lipolysis and production of ketones.

QUICK HIT

Kussmaul respirations are deep and labored but may be either rapid or slow.

IV. Chronic symptoms of diabetes *(Table 7-7)*

TABLE 7-7 Chronic Symptoms of Diabetes Mellitus

Anatomic Location	Clinical Features
Red blood cells	**Glycation (HbA_{1c})**; measure of long-term control of diabetes (reflects past 3 months)
Blood vessels/ cardiovascular system	**Atherosclerosis**, dyslipidemia, coronary artery disease, gangrene, peripheral vascular disease
Eyes	**Retinopathy**, hemorrhage, hard exudates, cotton-wool spots, cataracts, glaucoma
GI tract	Constipation, **gastroparesis**
Kidneys	Nephropathy, **nodular sclerosis**, **Kimmelstiel–Wilson nodules**, chronic renal failure, azotemia
Penis	**Erectile dysfunction** as a result of autonomic neuropathy
Extremities	**Stocking-glove peripheral neuropathy**, nonhealing ulcers

GI, gastrointestinal.

V. Treatment of diabetes mellitus *(Table 7-8 and 7-9)*

The goal of treatment of both type 1 and type 2 diabetes mellitus is steady control of blood glucose levels. However, because the pathogenesis underlying these two disease processes is different, the therapy is also different.

Type 1 diabetes mellitus, which can be viewed simply as a total deficiency of insulin, may be treated with careful administration of exogenous insulin. This agent has been the only treatment option for type 1 diabetes mellitus for many years and remains so today. However, advances have been made in both the type of insulin and the method of delivery. To maintain steady glucose levels, different preparations of human insulin have been designed, each with a characteristic rate of onset and duration of action (Table 7-8). Insulin, a peptide hormone, cannot be given orally. It is typically administered subcutaneously and, in emergencies, intravenously.

Some combination of these types of insulin usually can be found that provides adequate glucose control during both the fed and fasting states. Treatment of type 1 diabetes mellitus is essentially a balancing act—too much insulin causes hypoglycemia, and too little leads to hyperglycemia, which, over time, leads to the long-term complications of diabetes mellitus.

TABLE 7-8 Commonly Used Insulin Preparations

Insulin Preparation	Onset of Activity	Time of Peak Activity	Duration of Action
Insulin lispro	5–15 minutes	1–2 hours	3–4 hours
Insulin aspart	5–15 minutes	1–2 hours	3–4 hours
Insulin glulisine	5–15 minutes	1–2 hours	3–4 hours
Regular insulin	30 minutes	2–4 hours	6–8 hours
NPH (neutral protamine Hagedorn) insulin	1–2 hours	4–12 hours	18–24 hours
Insulin detemir	3–4 hours	3–9 hours	6–24 hours
Insulin glargine	3–4 hours	No peak	24 hours or longer

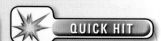

TABLE 7-9 Therapeutic Agents for Diabetes

Therapeutic Agent (common name, if relevant) [trade name, where appropriate]	Class—Pharmacology and Pharmacokinetics	Indications	Side Effects or Adverse Effects	Contraindications or Precautions to Consider; Notes
Insulin				
Lispro [Humalog], **aspart** [Novolog], **glulisine** [Apidra]	**Rapid-acting insulin**—see *mechanism for regular insulin*	**Diabetes mellitus** (typically **Type 1**), **hyperkalemia, stress-induced hyperglycemia**	**Hypoglycemia** (diaphoresis, vertigo, tachycardia), insulin allergy, insulin antibodies, lipodystrophy	
Regular insulin [Humulin R, Novolin R]	**Short-acting insulin—liver:** Promotes glucose storage as glycogen, increases triglyceride synthesis **Muscle:** facilitates protein and glycogen synthesis **Adipose tissue:** improves triglyceride storage by activating plasma lipoprotein lipase; reduces circulating free fatty acids	**Diabetes mellitus** (typically **Type 1**), **hyperkalemia, stress-induced hyperglycemia**	**Hypoglycemia** (diaphoresis, vertigo, tachycardia), insulin allergy, insulin antibodies, lipodystrophy	
NPH [Humulin N, Novolin N]	**Intermediate-acting insulin**—*see mechanism for insulin*	**Diabetes mellitus** (typically **Type 1**)	**Hypoglycemia** (diaphoresis, vertigo, tachycardia), insulin allergy, insulin antibodies, lipodystrophy	
Glargine [Lantus], detemir [Levemir]	**Long-acting insulin**—*see mechanism for regular insulin*	**Diabetes mellitus** (typically **Type 1**)	**Hypoglycemia** (diaphoresis, vertigo, tachycardia), insulin allergy, insulin antibodies, lipodystrophy	
Sulfonylureas				
Tolbutamide, chlorpropamide	**First-generation sulfonylureas**—closes potassium channel in β-cell membrane → reduces K^+ efflux, increases Ca^{2+} influx → increases secretion of insulin	Oral treatment for **type 2 diabetes**	**Hypoglycemia,** GI disturbances, muscle weakness, mental confusion	Rarely used due to toxicity
Glyburide [DiaBeta, Micronase], **glimepiride** [Amaryl], **glipizide** [Glucotrol]	**Second generation sulfonylureas**—closes potassium channel in pancreatic β-islet cell membrane → reduces K^+ efflux, increases Ca^{2+} influx → increases secretion of insulin	Oral treatment for **type 2 diabetes**	**Hypoglycemia,** GI disturbances, muscle weakness, mental confusion, weight gain	Not useful in Type 1 diabetes mellitus because it requires some β cell function.
Biguanides				
Metformin [Glucophage]	**Biguanide—decreases hepatic gluconeogenesis,** increases glycolysis → decreases serum glucose levels	**First-line** oral treatment for **type 2 diabetes**	**Lactic acidosis,** GI upset (diarrhea, nausea, abdominal pain), metallic taste; decreased vitamin B_{12} absorption	Stop drug in patients undergoing studies or procedures involving contrast; **contraindicated in patients with renal dysfunction**
Thiazolidinediones				
Pioglitazone [Actos], **rosiglitazone** [Avandia]	**Glitazones—bind PPARγ receptors; improve target cell sensitivity to insulin**	Oral treatment for **type 2 diabetes**	**Weight gain, edema,** rare hepatotoxicity, increases LDL and triglycerides; rosiglitazone may increase the risk of MI	Contraindicated in CHF

(continued)

TABLE 7-9 **Therapeutic Agents for Diabetes** *(Continued)*

Therapeutic Agent (common name, if relevant) [trade name, where appropriate]	Class—Pharmacology and Pharmacokinetics	Indications	Side Effects or Adverse Effects	Contraindications or Precautions to Consider; Notes
Other				
Sitagliptin [Januvia], **saxagliptin** [Onglyza], **linagliptin** [Tradjenta]	**DPP-IV inhibitors**—prevents degradation of incretin hormones → decreased glucagon, increased insulin, delays gastric emptying	Oral treatment for **type 2 diabetes**	Diarrhea, constipation, edema	
Exenatide [Byetta]	**Incretin mimetic**—agonizes GLP-1 receptors → decreases glucagon, increases insulin, delays gastric emptying	Injectable treatment for **type 2 diabetes**	Mild weight loss, nausea, hypoglycemia, constipation, slight risk of pancreatitis	Derived from exendin, a hormone found in Gila monster saliva
Liraglutide [Victoza]	**Incretin mimetic**—synthetic GLP-1 analog → decreases glucagon, increases insulin, delays gastric emptying	Injectable treatment for **type 2 diabetes**	Mild weight loss, nausea, vomiting, diarrhea, slight risk of pancreatitis	Increased incidence of medullary thyroid cancer in animal models
Pramlintide [Symlin]	**Analog of amylin**, a pancreatic hormone secreted with insulin that decreases glucagon and delays gastric empyting	Injectable treatment for **type 2 diabetes**	Nausea, vomiting, hypoglycemia	
α-Glucosidase inhibitors				
Acarbose [Precose] **miglitol**	**α-Glucosidase inhibitor**—inhibit intestinal brush border enzyme α-glucosidase → delays sugar hydrolysis and glucose absorption from gut → decreases **postprandial hyperglycemia**	Oral treatment for **type 2 diabetes** postprandially	**GI effects** (flatulence, cramps, diarrhea); may reduce absorption of iron	

CHF, congestive heart failure; DPP-IV, dipeptidyl peptidase-IV; GI, gastrointestinal; GLP-1, glucagon-like peptide-1; LDL, low-density lipoprotein; NPH, neutral protamine Hagedorn; PPARγ, peroxisome proliferator-activated receptor gamma.

Type 2 diabetes mellitus, which is more complex than type 1 disease, is characterized primarily by insulin resistance. In some cases, a strict regimen of diet and exercise completely reverses the course of the disease. In many cases, however, drugs are required to control blood sugar levels. The most commonly used drugs in type 2 diabetes mellitus are metformin and the insulin sensitizers. **Metformin**, in the biguanide class of agents, is considered by many to be the first-line drug of choice in type 2 diabetes mellitus and acts primarily by decreasing hepatic glucose production. Advantages include the very low risk of hypoglycemia as well as the weight loss and improvement in lipid profiles in many patients. The one feared adverse reaction is lactic acidosis, a rare but serious complication. Also, nausea and diarrhea are side effects of this medication.

Pioglitazone and **rosiglitazone**, of the thiazolidinedione class, are the two most common insulin sensitizers. Like metformin, these agents can be used alone or as part of a multidrug regimen for diabetic blood sugar control. Both drugs have a low risk of hypoglycemia. However, they have been known to exacerbate congestive heart failure, and frequent monitoring of liver function is required. Rosiglitazone may increase the risk of myocardial infarction (MI) and cardiovascular events.

Sulfonylureas were once the mainstay of treatment for type 2 diabetes, but they are used less frequently today. These drugs, which include agents such as glipizide and glyburide, act by increasing the release of insulin from the pancreas. To a lesser extent, these agents also decrease glucagon levels and increase insulin binding at target sites in the periphery. The primary side effect of these drugs is hypoglycemia.

Clinical Vignette 7-2

CLINICAL PRESENTATION: An 8-year-old female child presents to the emergency department with complaints of several days of **vomiting** and **thirst**. The mother also reports that the patient has **not been acting like herself** lately and has been **urinating** more than usual. The patient recently recovered from an **upper respiratory infection** with high fevers. On examination, the patient is breathing rapidly and deeply (**Kussmaul respirations**), and a **sweet smell** is noticed on her breath. Her **skin and oral mucosa are dry**.

DIFFERENTIALS: Diabetic ketoacidosis (DKA), hyperosmolar hyperglycemic nonketotic state (HHNS), gastroenteritis, hypoglycemic coma, metabolic acidosis (from causes other than DKA).

LABORATORY STUDIES: A **urinalysis** should be obtained with interest in glucose and ketone levels—high glucose and ketone levels suggest DKA. **In HHNS, the glucose levels are elevated but there is no ketosis.** HHNS is more often seen more in type 2 diabetics, and DKA is more often seen in type 1 diabetics. A **blood chemistry** would also be key in differentiating causes; in DKA, it would show high glucose, high ketones, and an acidotic profile with low pH, low bicarbonate, and elevated anion gap from the ketones (organic acids). Also in DKA, serum potassium is high because the acidosis causes a shift of serum hydrogen ions into cells in exchange for intracellular potassium ions. Serum sodium appears decreased because hyperglycemia increases serum osmolality shifting water out of cells. Blood glucose and serum osmolality are significantly higher in HHNS than in DKA, and ketones are not found because there are sufficient levels of insulin to prevent lipolysis, thereby preventing ketogenesis. HHNS usually presents with a nonacidotic profile. Metabolic acidosis can also cause vomiting, Kussmaul respirations, a low blood pH, and bicarbonate. Causes of metabolic acidosis with a normal anion gap include diarrhea, renal tubular acidosis, or acetazolamide overdose. Causes of metabolic acidosis with an elevated anion gap include chronic renal failure, lactic acidosis, DKA, uremia, salicylate overdose, methanol ingestion, and ethylene glycol ingestion. To determine the cause of the metabolic acidosis in this patient, **salicylate, lactate, blood alcohol, methanol**, and **ethylene glycol levels** should be obtained. Finally, in gastroenteritis, a metabolic alkalosis from the vomiting is expected. In hypoglycemic coma, the glucose levels are low.

MANAGEMENT: Three-tiered approach: (1) **Rehydration**—a fluid bolus is indicated because the patient is severely dehydrated. Monitor rehydration status by noting resolution of mental status changes. The most common complication of this treatment is **cerebral edema** from too rapid a change in serum osmolality. (2) **Insulin**—to facilitate peripheral uptake of glucose, decrease ketone body formation. (3) **Potassium replacement**—although blood studies show high serum potassium levels, that is misleading because the acidosis caused the potassium to shift out of cells and the body is actually potassium starved.

OBESITY

Obesity is a multifactorial disease with a variable genetic component and is associated with diet, lifestyle, drugs, and endocrine disorders. Multiple therapeutic strategies including diet, exercise, bariatric surgery, and drugs can be attempted. Table 7-10 summarizes pharmacological agents available in treating obesity.

TABLE **7-10** **Therapeutic Agents for Obesity**

Therapeutic Agent (common name, if relevant) [trade name, where appropriate)	Class—Pharmacology and Pharmacokinetics	Indications	Side Effects or Adverse Effects	Contraindications or Precautions to Consider; Notes
Orlistat	**Inhibits pancreatic lipases** → alters fat metabolism	**Obesity** (long term)	**Steatorrhea**, GI irritation, reduced absorption of fat-soluble vitamins, and headache	**Used in conjunction with modified diet**
Phentermine	**Sympathomimetic**—stimulates the release of norepinephrine	Obesity (short term)	Hypertension, tachycardia, euphoria, tremulor	Contraindicated in patients with cardiovascular disease or with history of drug abuse.

GI, gastrointestinal.

PITUITARY DISORDERS *(Table 7-11)*

The pituitary gland sits in the sella turcica. The anterior portion is regulated by the hypothalamus. The posterior portion contains extensions of hypothalamic neurons. Excess prolactin can result from estrogen therapy or drugs, such as antipsychotics, that interfere with dopamine (prolactin-inhibiting hormone).

QUICK HIT

Sheehan syndrome is panhypopituitarism caused by postpartum pituitary necrosis resulting from blood loss and ischemia during childbirth.

TABLE 7-11 **Pituitary Disorders**

Disorder	Etiology	Clinical Features	Laboratory Diagnosis	Treatment
Prolactinoma	Lactotrophic (chromophobic) anterior pituitary tumor; **most common** pituitary tumor	Decreased libido, vision changes, amenorrhea, gynecomastia, galactorrhea, virilization	Minimal or no increase in serum prolactin after TRH given	Bromocriptine or surgery
Acromegaly (adults)/ gigantism (children)	Somatotrophic (acidophilic) anterior pituitary adenoma	Prominent forehead, jaw; **large hands, feet; enlargement of viscera;** hyperglycemia; renal failure; hypertension; mental disturbances	Excess growth hormones and somatomedins (IGF-1)	Transsphenoidal surgery, bromocriptine, radiation, or octreotide
Cushing disease	Hypersecretion of ACTH from basophilic adenoma of pituitary	(Table 7-13)	Suppression of ACTH secretion during high-dose dexamethasone test	Surgery or pituitary irradiation
Panhypopituitarism (Simmonds disease, Sheehan syndrome)	Pituitary tumors, ischemia, trauma; DIC; sickle cell anemia	Marked wasting, **panhypopituitarism,** headache, vomiting	Decreased levels of FSH, LH, ACTH, TSH	Hormone replacement
SIADH	Pituitary hypersecretion; ectopic production of ADH **(small cell lung cancer)**	Decreased urinary output, fatigue, mental disturbances	Hyponatremia, high urine osmolality	Fluid restriction
Diabetes insipidus	**Central** (neurogenic): ADH insufficiency **Nephrogenic**: lack of end-organ (kidney) response	Dehydration, thirst, polyuria, recent trauma to the head or anoxia	(Table 7-12); hypernatremia	Central: desmopressin (DDAVP) replaces ADH. Nephrogenic: fluid restriction and thiazide response diuretics (works by a paradoxical effect)

ACTH, adrenocorticotropic hormone; ADH, antidiuretic hormone (vasopressin); DDAVP, 1-deamino-8-D-arginine vasopressin; DIC, disseminated intravascular coagulation; FSH, follicle-stimulating hormone; IGF-1, insulin-like growth factor-1; LH, luteinizing hormone; SIADH, syndrome of inappropriate secretion of antidiuretic hormone; TRH, thyrotropin-releasing hormone; TSH, thyroid-stimulating hormone.

DIABETES INSIPIDUS *(Table 7-12)*

Diabetes insipidus is a disease characterized by excessive low-osmolality urine output. There are two forms: central and nephrogenic.

TABLE 7-12 Diabetes Insipidus

	Urine Osmolality Greater than 280 mOsm/kg with Dehydration	Response to Antidiuretic Hormone after Dehydration
Normal	+	–
Central diabetes insipidus	–	+
Partial diabetes insipidus	+	+
Nephrogenic diabetes insipidus	–	–
Primary polydipsia	+	+

THE ADRENAL GLANDS

I. Congenital adrenal hyperplasia *(Figure 7-9)*

The adrenal glands are anatomically divided into a medulla and a cortex. The cortex itself is divided into three anatomic layers. The four anatomic layers of the adrenal glands are responsible for various metabolic functions in the body.

II. Adrenal cortex pathology *(Table 7-13)*

TABLE 7-13 Adrenal Cortex Pathology

Disease	Etiology	Clinical Features
Cushing syndrome	Excess cortisol as a result of **iatrogenic corticosteroid therapy (most common cause),** adrenal adenoma (more common than carcinoma); ectopic ACTH from neoplasm (especially **small cell lung carcinoma**)	Peripheral muscle wasting and weakness; **central obesity** with rounds facies and increased fat deposition at upper back, easy bruising with abdominal striae; bone demineralization, osteoporosis, psychosis, acne; hirsutism; hyperglycemia; hypertension
Cushing disease	Excess cortisol as a result of **pituitary hypersecretion of ACTH;** bilateral hyperplasia of adrenal cortex; **second most common** cause of Cushing syndrome	Identical to Cushing syndrome
Conn syndrome (primary hyperaldosteronism)	Adrenal cortex **adenoma** (more common than hyperplasia, which is more common than carcinoma), sodium retention, **low plasma renin**	**Hypertension,** hypokalemic alkalosis
Secondary hyperaldosteronism	Renal tumors, renal ischemia, edematous conditions (cirrhosis, nephrotic syndromes, congestive heart failure), **increased plasma renin**	**Hypertension,** hypokalemic alkalosis

(continued)

MNEMONIC

Both nephrogenic and central diabetes insipidus present with dilute urine after dehydration. In diagnosing these subtypes of diabetes insipidus, think after administering antidiuretic hormone: **C**oncentrated urine = **Central**; **N**o effect = **N**ephrogenic.

QUICK HIT

Surprisingly, diabetes insipidus can be treated with hydrochlorothiazide (a diuretic).

QUICK HIT

Primary polydipsia, a psychological condition of drinking excess water, causes a decrease in plasma osmolality, and thus can be differentiated from diabetes insipidus, which causes an increase in plasma osmolality. Patients who present with primary polydipsia are generally young or middle-aged women with a history of neurosis.

QUICK HIT

Diabetes insipidus may be transiently induced during pregnancy due to greater metabolism of vasopressin (ADH).

QUICK HIT

21-Hydroxylase deficiency is the **most common** adrenal enzyme deficiency.

QUICK HIT

Small cell lung carcinoma is a potential source for ectopic ACTH production resulting in paraneoplastic syndrome.

QUICK HIT

Hyperpigmentation in Addison disease is caused by increased production of proopiomelanocortin (POMC) by the pituitary. POMC is enzymatically split to yield adrenocorticotropin hormone (ACTH) and melanocyte-stimulating hormone **(MSH).**

TABLE 7-13 **Adrenal Cortex Pathology** *(Continued)*

Disease	Etiology	Clinical Features
Addison disease	Most commonly **idiopathic** cortisol deficiency; possibly autoimmune; may be caused by tumor, infections (i.e., tuberculosis)	**Hypotension,** low serum sodium, **hyperpigmentation,** increased serum potassium
Waterhouse–Friderichsen syndrome	***Neisseria meningitidis*** infection leads to disseminated intravascular coagulation (**DIC**); hemorrhagic adrenal **necrosis** and circulation collapse	Acute hypotension and salt wasting; **shock;** more common in children; death within hours if not treated

ACTH, adrenocorticotropic hormone.

FIGURE 7-9 **Congenital adrenal hyperplasia**

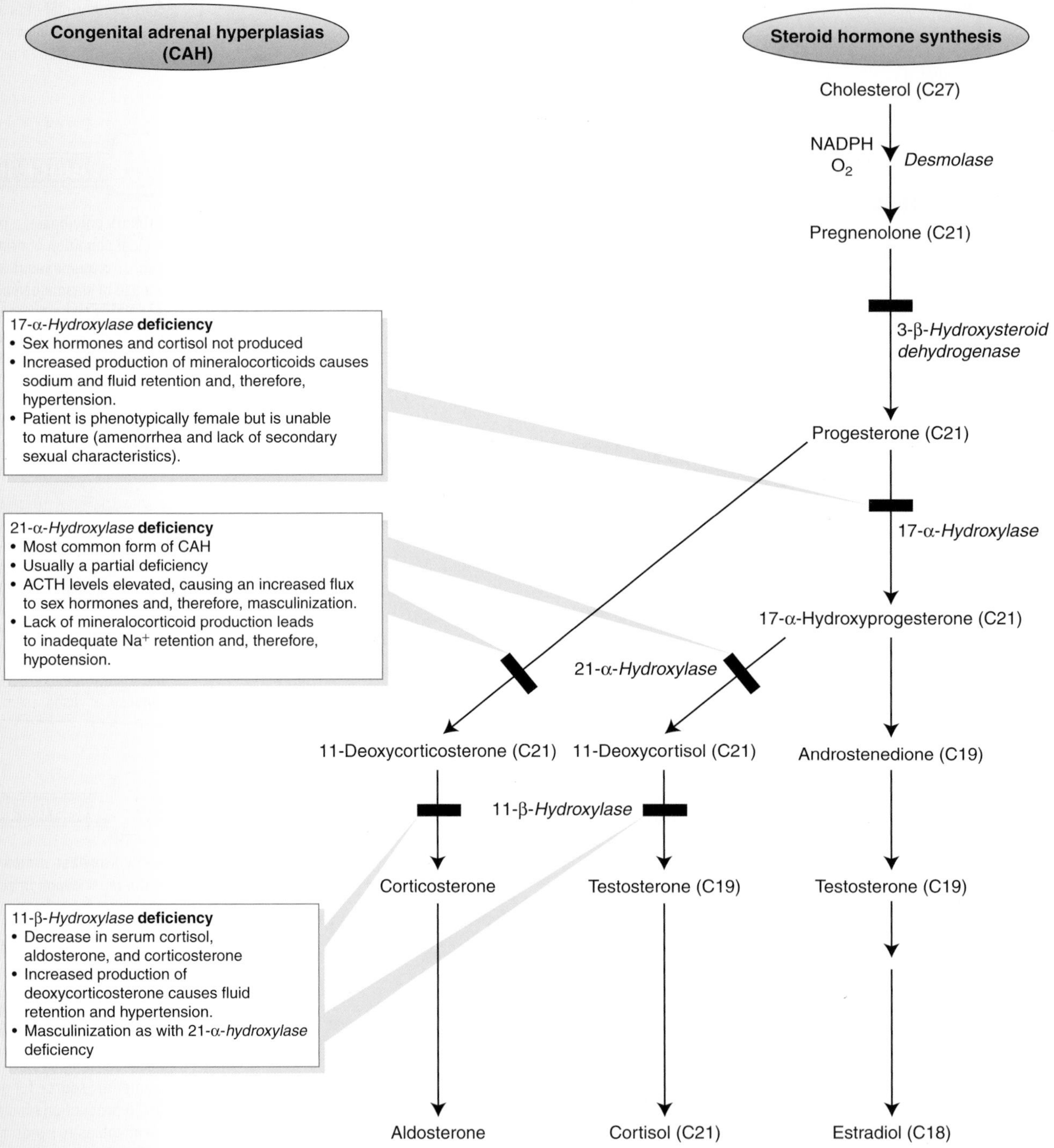

Congenital adrenal hyperplasias (CAH)
Steroid hormone synthesis
Cholesterol (C27)
NADPH
O2
Desmolase
Pregnenolone (C21)
3-β-Hydroxysteroid dehydrogenase
Progesterone (C21)
17-α-Hydroxylase
17-α-Hydroxyprogesterone (C21)
21-α-Hydroxylase
11-Deoxycorticosterone (C21)
11-Deoxycortisol (C21)
Androstenedione (C19)
11-β-Hydroxylase
Corticosterone
Testosterone (C19)
Testosterone (C19)
Aldosterone
Cortisol (C21)
Estradiol (C18)
17-α-Hydroxylase deficiency
• Sex hormones and cortisol not produced
• Increased production of mineralocorticoids causes sodium and fluid retention and, therefore, hypertension.
• Patient is phenotypically female but is unable to mature (amenorrhea and lack of secondary sexual characteristics).
21-α-Hydroxylase deficiency
• Most common form of CAH
• Usually a partial deficiency
• ACTH levels elevated, causing an increased flux to sex hormones and, therefore, masculinization.
• Lack of mineralocorticoid production leads to inadequate Na+ retention and, therefore, hypotension.
11-β-Hydroxylase deficiency
• Decrease in serum cortisol, aldosterone, and corticosterone
• Increased production of deoxycorticosterone causes fluid retention and hypertension.
• Masculinization as with 21-α-hydroxylase deficiency

ACTH, adrenocorticotropic hormone; NADPH, reduced nicotinamide adenine dinucleotide phosphate.

III. Adrenal medulla pathology *(Table 7-14)*

TABLE 7-14 Adrenal Medulla Tumors

Tumor	Pathology	Clinical Manifestation
Neuroblastoma	**Malignant**; excess catecholamine secretion; N-*myc* (oncogene) amplification	**Children**; degree of N-*myc* amplification related to prognosis; abdominal pain, constipation, possibly some hypertension
Pheochromocytoma	**Benign** (10% malignant); tumor of chromaffin cells; seen in MEN 2a and 2b	**Adults**; hypertension (usually paroxysmal); palpitations, sweating, and headache; increased urinary vanillylmandelic acid **(VMA)**

MEN 2a and 2b, multiple endocrine neoplasia types 2a and 2b.

QUICK HIT

The pheochromocytoma rule of 10s: 10% are malignant, 10% multiple, 10% bilateral, 10% familial, 10% extra-adrenal, and 10% children.

Clinical Vignette 7-3

CLINICAL PRESENTATION: A 37-year-old woman presents to her primary care physician with a chief complaint of **weight gain, fatigue, acne,** and **hirsutism.** After further questions, the patient reports that she has not had her period for 3 months. Her past medical history is significant for a bone marrow transplantation, for which the patient is currently on medication. Patient denies a family history of diabetes or hypertension. Physical examination reveals **central obesity, abdominal striae, bruising** on thighs and buttocks, and **muscle weakness.** Vital signs: Temperature = 97.5° F; heart rate = 80 bpm; respiration rate = 20 breaths/min; **blood pressure =140/90 mm Hg.**

DIFFERENTIAL: Iatrogenic Cushing syndrome, adrenocorticotropic hormone (ACTH)–producing pituitary adenoma (Cushing **disease**), adrenal adenoma, ectopic ACTH production, and obesity. This patient is exhibiting signs and symptoms of high cortisol termed *Cushing syndrome.* Some findings (i.e., **obesity, hypertension, osteoporosis, diabetes mellitus**) are nonspecific and less helpful in diagnosis of Cushing syndrome. **Easy bruising, striae, virilization,** and **myopathy** are more helpful in the diagnosis. Also, patients with **Cushing disease** can have **hyperpigmentation** as a result of elevated ACTH levels, whereas patients with **Cushing syndrome** due to other causes will not have hyperpigmentation. The most common cause of Cushing syndrome is an unfavorable response to prescribed steroids; patient's recent transplantation history suggests the possibility that she received immunosuppressive steroids.

LABORATORY STUDIES: Figure 7-10 outlines the approach. The first step is to determine whether cortisol levels are elevated in this patient, which can be done via a **urine 24-hour free cortisol level** or an **overnight dexamethasone suppression test.** In this latter test, dexamethasone is given at night, and serum cortisol levels are measured in the morning. In normal individuals, dexamethasone should suppress the pituitary–adrenal axis, resulting in decreased cortisol in the morning. In Cushing syndrome, the serum cortisol remains elevated. The next step is to determine the cause of the cortisol elevation, which could be from (a) **increased ACTH production** at the level of the pituitary or ectopically, (b) **increased cortisol production** at the level of the adrenal gland, or (c) **exogenous cortisol** in the form of prednisone. To determine the cause, measure **ACTH levels,** which would be low in the case of exogenous cortisol and adrenal adenoma, because cortisol feedback inhibits the pituitary from secreting ACTH. Knowing which medications the patient is using helps in differentiating these causes. ACTH levels are high in patients with obesity, patients with ectopic ACTH production, or pituitary ACTH adenoma. The key differentiating factor is that **low-dose dexamethasone** will suppress ACTH production in obese individuals, **high-dose dexamethasone** will suppress ACTH production in pituitary adenoma cases, and nothing will suppress ACTH levels in the patients with ectopic ACTH production.

MANAGEMENT: This patient most likely has iatrogenic Cushing syndrome, which is remedied by **tapering of the glucocorticoid.** Pituitary or adrenal adenoma requires **surgical removal of the neoplasm.**

MNEMONIC

To remember the side effects of glucocorticoids, think CUSHINGOID:
Cataract
Ulcers
Skin: striae, thinning, bruising
Hypertension/**H**irsutism/**H**yperglycemia
Infections
Necrosis (avascular necrosis of the femoral head)
Glycosuria
Osteoporosis/Obesity
Immunosuppression
Diabetes

FIGURE 7-10 Approach to Cushing syndrome

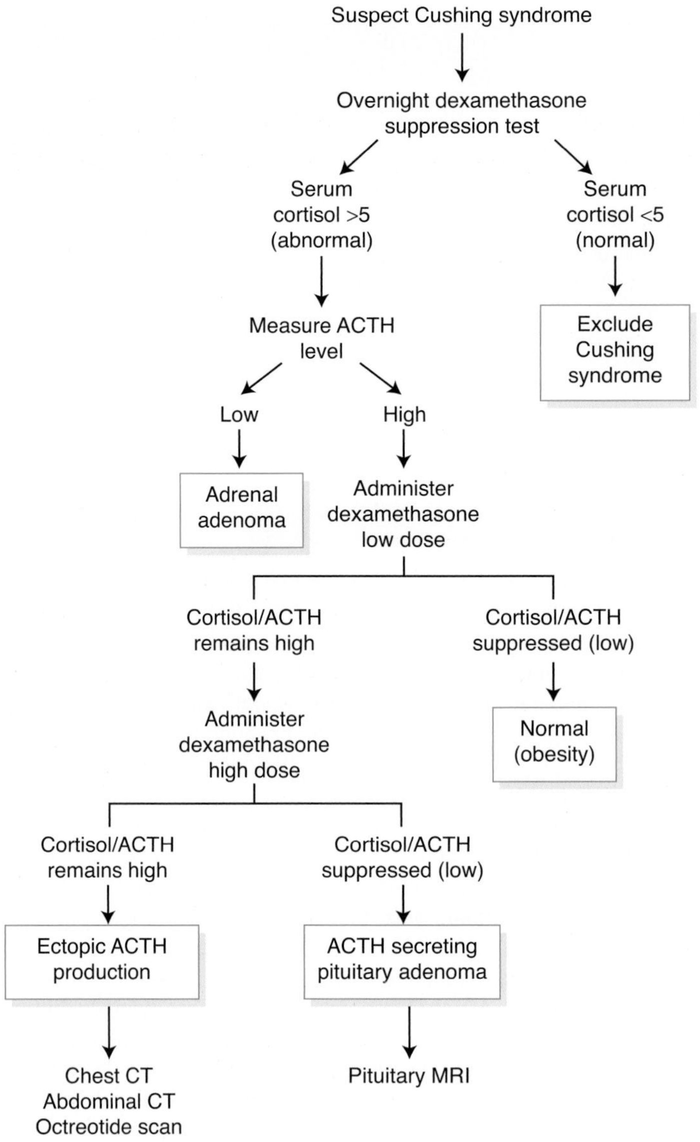
Suspect Cushing syndrome
Overnight dexamethasone suppression test
Serum cortisol >5 (abnormal)
Serum cortisol <5 (normal)
Exclude Cushing syndrome
Measure ACTH level
Low
High
Adrenal adenoma
Administer dexamethasone low dose
Cortisol/ACTH remains high
Cortisol/ACTH suppressed (low)
Normal (obesity)
Administer dexamethasone high dose
Cortisol/ACTH remains high
Cortisol/ACTH suppressed (low)
Ectopic ACTH production
ACTH secreting pituitary adenoma
Chest CT
Abdominal CT
Octreotide scan
Pituitary MRI

ACTH, adrenocorticotropic hormone; CT, computed tomography; MRI, magnetic resonance imaging.

THERAPEUTIC AGENTS FOR THE HYPOTHALAMUS, PITUITARY, AND ADRENAL GLANDS *(Table 7-15)*

TABLE 7-15 **Therapeutic Agents for Hypothalamic, Pituitary, and Adrenal Conditions**

Therapeutic Agent (common name, if relevant) [trade name, where appropriate]	Class—Pharmacology and Pharmacokinetics	Indications	Side Effects or Adverse Effects	Contraindications or Precautions to Consider; Notes
Growth hormone (somatropin, somatrem)	**Synthetic analog of growth hormone—causes liver to produce insulin-like growth factors (somatomedins)**	Replacement therapy in children with **growth hormone deficiency, Turner syndrome; burn victims**		Should not be used in patients with closed epiphyses
Growth hormone–releasing hormone (GHRH)	**Synthetic analog of GHRH—stimulates release of GH**	**Dwarfism**	**Pain at injection**	
Octreotide [Sandostatin]	**Synthetic analog of somatostatin**—decreases release of GH, gastrin, secretin, VIP, CCK, glucagon, insulin	**Acromegaly, glucagonoma, insulinoma, carcinoid syndrome**	Nausea, cramps, gallstones	
Oxytocin [Pitocin, Syntocinon]	**Synthetic analog of oxytocin—stimulates uterine contraction and contraction of breast myoepithelial cells; milk letdown reflex**	**Induces labor; control uterine hemorrhage**		
Desmopressin (DDAVP)	**Synthetic analog of ADH**—recruits water channels to luminal membrane in collecting duct	Central diabetes insipidus, nocturnal enuresis, von Willebrand disease	Overhydration; allergic reaction; larger doses result in pallor, diarrhea, hypertension; coronary constriction; chronic rhinopharyngitis	**Synthetic analog to vasopressin; intranasal administration**
Prednisone, hydrocortisone, triamcinolone, dexamethasone, beclomethasone	**Glucocorticoid**—inhibits protein synthesis; reduces lymph node and spleen size; inhibits cell cycle activity of lymphoid cells; lyses T cells; suppresses antibody, prostaglandin, and leukotriene synthesis; blocks monocyte production of IL-1	Addison disease, rheumatic arthritis, autoimmune disorders, allergic reaction, asthma, organ transplantation (especially during rejection crisis)	**Osteoporosis, Cushingoid reaction, acne, psychosis, glucose intolerance, infection, hypertension, cataracts, peptic ulcers**	

ADH, antidiuretic hormone; CCK, cholecystokinin; GH, growth hormone; IL-1, interleukin 1; VIP, vasoactive intestinal peptide.

THYROID

I. Formation of thyroid hormone *(Figure 7-11)*

QUICK HIT

Thyroxine (T_4) is converted to triiodothyronine (T_3) in the periphery, with T_3 being 35 times more potent than T_4. T_4 has a half-life of 5 to 7 days, whereas T_3 has a half-life of 1 day.

FIGURE 7-11 Formation of thyroid hormone

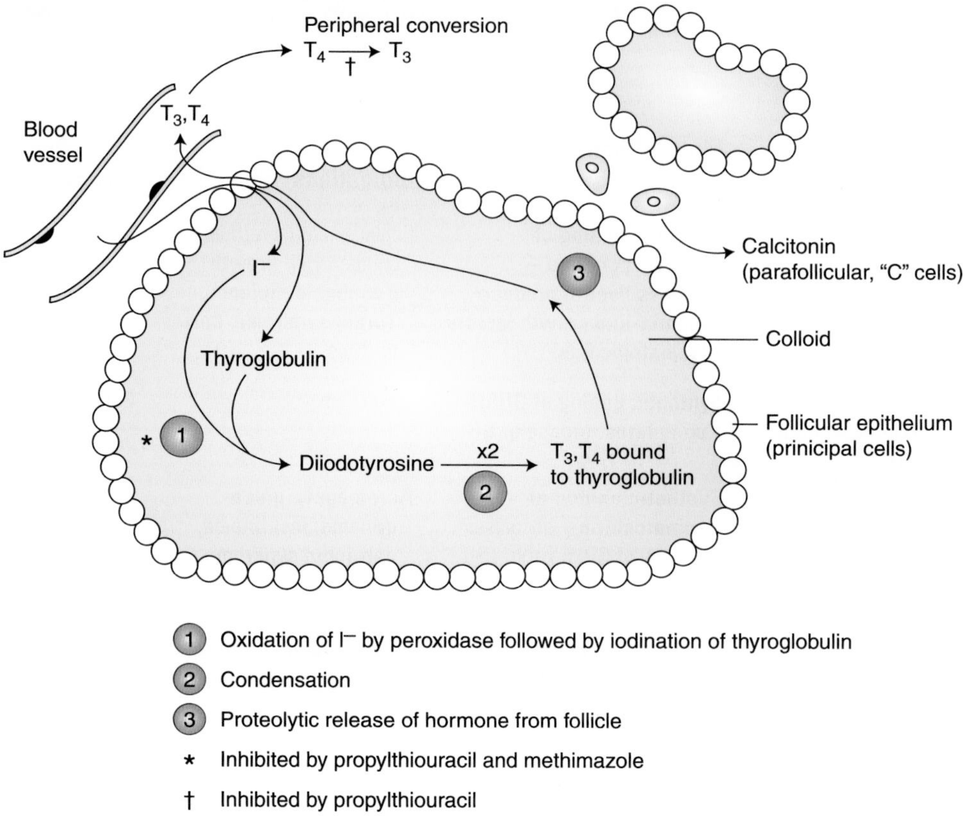

Peripheral conversion
T4 → T3
†
T3,T4
Blood vessel
I−
Thyroglobulin
*
1
Diiodotyrosine
x2
2
T3,T4 bound to thyroglobulin
3
Calcitonin (parafollicular, "C" cells)
Colloid
Follicular epithelium (prinicipal cells)
1 Oxidation of I− by peroxidase followed by iodination of thyroglobulin
2 Condensation
3 Proteolytic release of hormone from follicle
* Inhibited by propylthiouracil and methimazole
† Inhibited by propylthiouracil

T_3, triiodothyronine; T_4, thyroxine.

II. Myxedema

A. Can be described as hypothyroidism of the adult
B. Causes
   1. Hashimoto thyroiditis (see the following)
   2. Idiopathic causes
   3. Iodine deficiency
      a. A problem in geographic areas with poor nutrition
      b. Deficiency in pregnant women can lead to cretinism in the child (see the following).
   4. Paradoxically, high doses of iodine lead to a decrease in thyroid hormone production.
   5. **Overirradiation** of the thyroid using iodine-131 for treatment of hyperthyroidism.
C. Clinical features of the hypothyroid state
   1. Cold intolerance
   2. Weight gain
   3. Constipation
   4. Lowering of voice
   5. Menorrhagia
   6. Slowed mental and physical function
   7. Dry skin with coarse and brittle hair
   8. Reflexes showing slow return phase ("hung reflex")
D. Treatment is usually with levothyroxine (T_4)

QUICK HIT

Because of its long half-life, T_4 is ideal as a hormone replacement in patients with hypothyroidism. Even with once-a-day dosing, steady serum levels of T_4 and T_3 can be achieved.

III. Cretinism

A. Can be describe as **hypothyroidism** of the **fetus or child**

B. Causes

1. **Iodine-deficient diet** in the mother or during the early life of the child
2. Thyroid-related enzyme deficiency
3. Thyroid developmental defect
4. Failure of thyroid descent during development
5. Transfer of antithyroid antibodies from the mother with an autoimmune disease to the fetus

C. Clinical features

1. Impaired physical growth
2. Mental retardation
3. Enlarged tongue
4. Enlarged, distended abdomen

> **QUICK HIT**
>
> Because of the devastating effects that hypothyroidism can have on children (**cretinism**), thyroid hormone levels (along with galactosemia and phenylketonuria) are routinely evaluated at birth in the United States.

IV. Hashimoto thyroiditis

A. An **autoimmune** disorder causing **hypothyroidism** and a **painless goiter**

1. Dense infiltrate of lymphocytes into the thyroid gland
2. Antithyroglobulin and antithyroid peroxidase (formerly antimicrosomal) antibodies
3. **5:1 female predominance**
4. Incidence increases with age.
5. Associated with human leukocyte antigen-DR5 (**HLA-DR5**) and **HLA-B5**

B. Is the **most common form of hypothyroidism in those with adequate iodine** intake

C. Clinical features

1. Slowly progressing course with stages of euthyroid state, hyperthyroid state, and hypothyroid state
2. May lead to a scarred and shrunken gland in hypothyroid state
3. Microscopically, thyroid resembles lymph node

D. Associated with other autoimmune disorders

1. Diabetes mellitus
2. Pernicious anemia
3. Sjögren syndrome

V. Subacute (de Quervain) thyroiditis

A. Transient hyperthyroidism with painful goiter

1. Focal destruction of thyroid
2. Granulomatous inflammation
3. 3:1 female predominance
4. Associated with HLA-B35

B. Causes—possibly as a result of recent viral infection with coxsackie virus, echovirus, adenovirus, measles, or mumps

C. Clinical features

1. Acute febrile state
2. Rapid, painful enlargement of the thyroid
3. Transient hyperthyroidism owing to gland destruction

D. Self-limited disease

VI. Graves disease

A. **Autoimmune** disorder causing **hyperthyroidism** and **goiter**

1. Thyroid-stimulating immunoglobulin (**TSI**) is an immunoglobulin G (IgG) antibody to the thyroid-stimulating hormone (TSH) receptor.
2. Binding of TSI to the TSH receptor stimulates thyroid hormone production and hyperplasia of the thyroid gland.
3. It is associated with **HLA-DR3** and **HLA-B8**.
4. It has a **4:1 female** predominance.

B. Clinical features of Graves disease
   1. Hyperthyroidism and goiter caused by autoimmune immunoglobulins
      a. Increased total thyroxine (T_4)
      b. Increased triiodothyronine (T_3)
      c. Decreased TSH level
      d. Increased resin radioactive T_3 uptake
      e. Increased radioactive iodine
   2. Exophthalmos, proptosis
   3. Warm, moist, and flushed skin
   4. Thin, fine hair
   5. Cardiovascular system
      a. Increased heart rate and cardiac output
      b. **Palpitations and fibrillations**
   6. Muscle atrophy.
      a. Weakening of skeletal muscles occurs.
      b. Vital capacity of lungs decreases owing to weakened respiratory muscles.
   7. **Weight loss** occurs despite an increased appetite.
   8. Diarrhea is common.
   9. Menstrual flow may decrease or stop.

C. Treatment (Table 7-16)
   1. Antithyroid drugs (e.g., propylthiouracil or methimazole)
   2. A **β-blocker** to reduce the cardiac effects
   3. Radioactive iodine (iodine-131)
   4. Surgery

QUICK HIT

Care must be taken when performing thyroid or parathyroid surgery because the **recurrent laryngeal nerves** run directly posterior to these glands. Cutting the recurrent nerve leads to paralysis of the muscles used for speech (**except the cricothyroid**) and hoarseness on the affected side.

QUICK HIT

If a patient presents with hypocalcemic symptoms status post thyroidectomy, think of accidental removal of the parathyroid glands.

TABLE **7-16** **Therapeutic Agents for Thyroid Disorders**

Therapeutic Agent (common name, if relevant) [trade name, where appropriate]	Class—Pharmacology and Pharmacokinetics	Indications	Side Effects or Adverse Effects	Contraindications or Precautions to Consider; Notes
Propylthiouracil (PTU)	Antithyroid agent—inhibits peroxidase enzyme in thyroid → decreases synthesis of thyroid hormone; also blocks peripheral conversion of T_4 to T_3	**Hyperthyroidism**	**Agranulocytosis**	**Crosses the placenta and can cause fetal goiter and hypothyroidism;** preferred to methimazole in treating pregnant females with moderate to severe hyperthyroidism
Methimazole [Tapazole]	Antithyroid agent—inhibits peroxidase enzyme in thyroid → decreases synthesis of thyroid hormone	**Hyperthyroidism**	**Agranulocytosis**	**Crosses the placenta;** can cause fetal goiter, hypothyroidism, and aplasia cutis (fetal scalp defect).
Levothyroxine (T_4) [Synthroid, Levothroid]	Synthetic analog of thyroxine (T_4)	**Hypothyroidism**	Tachycardia, heat intolerance, tremors, arrhythmia	
Triiodothyronine (T_3) [Triostat]	Synthetic analog of thyroid hormone T_3	**Hypothyroidism**	Tachycardia, heat intolerance, tremors, arrhythmia	

Clinical Vignette 7-4

CLINICAL PRESENTATION: A 40-year-old woman presents to your office with a 20-lb **weight loss** over the past 2 months despite **eating more.** She also reports **irregular menses, diarrhea,** and **difficulty sleeping and concentrating.** She denies chest pain and palpitations. Physical examination reveals **warm, moist skin** and **resting hand tremor.** Neck examination shows a **diffusely enlarged, nontender thyroid gland.** Vital signs: Temperature = 99.0° F; respiration rate = 20 breaths/min; **heart rate = 99 bpm; blood pressure = 140/90 mm Hg.**

DIFFERENTIALS: Hyperthyroidism (Graves disease, factitious hyperthyroidism, subacute thyroiditis, multinodular goiter, thyroid adenoma), Hashimoto thyroiditis, menopause, panic disorder, and pheochromocytoma. The patient's symptoms are indicative of thyrotoxicosis. Of all the causes of thyrotoxicosis listed previously, **exophthalmos** and **thyroid bruit** occur only in Graves disease. Also, although Hashimoto thyroiditis eventually results in hypothyroidism, early findings in the disease are consistent with hyperthyroidism.

LABORATORY STUDIES: Figure 7-12 outlines the approach to determining a cause of hyperthyroidism in a patient. **Serum thyroid-stimulating hormone (TSH) and triiodothyronine (T_3)/thyroxine (T_4)** should be obtained. These tests would show elevated T_3/T_4 and suppressed TSH in hyperthyroidism and would be normal in menopause, panic disorder, and pheochromocytoma. A **thyroid scan with radioactive iodide uptake** is useful for distinguishing between the various causes of hyperthyroidism listed previously. A negative scan would be expected for subacute thyroiditis and factitious hyperthyroidism. These can be further differentiated by a thorough history and physical examination. The patient with subacute thyroiditis has a tender thyroid, systemic flulike symptoms, and possible history of recent viral infection. Factitious hyperthyroidism is more often seen in healthcare workers with access to T_3/T_4 who are abusing it for weight loss purposes. A positive scan of different types would be observed in Graves disease, multinodular goiter, and thyroid adenoma. In Graves disease, a diffuse hot scan would be seen, whereas in multinodular goiter, several nodules—both hot and cold—would be visualized. In thyroid adenoma, only one such hot nodule would be seen. Graves disease can be further supported by presence of **thyroid-stimulating immunoglobulin G,** which binds to thyrotropin receptors on the thyroid gland. These lab studies would be normal in menopause and panic disorder. Normal **urine metanephrines** and **vanillylmandelic acid** would rule out pheochromocytoma.

FIGURE 7-12 **Approach to thyrotoxicosis**

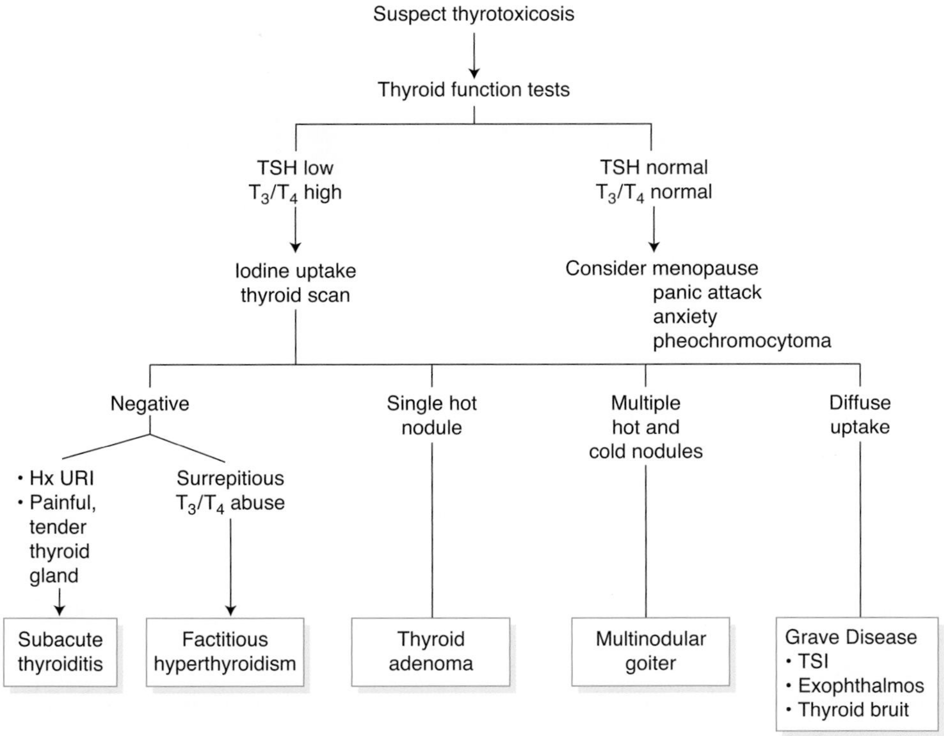
Suspect thyrotoxicosis
Thyroid function tests
TSH low
T3/T4 high
TSH normal
T3/T4 normal
Iodine uptake
thyroid scan
Consider menopause
panic attack
anxiety
pheochromocytoma
Negative
Single hot nodule
Multiple hot and cold nodules
Diffuse uptake
• Hx URI
• Painful, tender thyroid gland
Surrepitious T3/T4 abuse
Subacute thyroiditis
Factitious hyperthyroidism
Thyroid adenoma
Multinodular goiter
Grave Disease
• TSI
• Exophthalmos
• Thyroid bruit

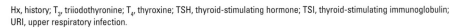

Hx, history; T_3, triiodothyronine; T_4, thyroxine; TSH, thyroid-stimulating hormone; TSI, thyroid-stimulating immunoglobulin; URI, upper respiratory infection.

QUICK HIT

Thyrotoxicosis factitia is a factitious disorder in which the patient intentionally self-administers excess thyroid hormone (levothyroxine) to simulate the symptoms of hyperthyroidism.

VII. Thyroid neoplasms *(Table 7-17)*

TABLE 7-17 Thyroid Carcinomas

Tumor	Description
Papillary carcinoma	• **Most common** thyroid cancer • **Best prognosis** of the thyroid cancers • **3:1 female predominance** • Usually occurs in third to fifth decade of life • **Associated with radiation exposure** in childhood, associated with *RET* oncogene mutation • "Ground glass" nuclei of neoplastic cells, also called "Orphan Annie eyes" due to the way the chromatin disperses • **Psammoma bodies** may be present • Forms papillary projections covered with cuboidal epithelium within glandular spaces
Follicular carcinoma	• Good prognosis, although worse than papillary • **3:1 female predominance** • More common in iodine-deficient areas • **Associated with *RAS* oncogene mutation** in 40% of cases • Uniform cuboidal cells lining follicles • Lacks the distinctive nuclear features of papillary carcinoma
Medullary carcinoma	• Parafollicular (C) cell neoplasm • **Secretes calcitonin,** no hypercalcemia or hypocalcemia • Associated with MEN 2a and MEN 2b • **Associated with *RET* oncogene mutation**
Anaplastic thyroid carcinoma	• Anaplastic, undifferentiated neoplasm • More common in older patients • Rapidly fatal

MEN 2a and 2b, multiple endocrine neoplasia types 2a and 2b.

MNEMONIC

To remember the symptoms of hypercalcemia, think:
Bones: pain in bones
Stones: renal stones
Groans: abdominal pain
Psychic moans/overtones: confused state

PARATHYROID PATHOLOGY *(Table 7-18)*

TABLE 7-18 Parathyroid Disorders

Condition	Etiology	Clinical Features
Primary hyperparathyroidism	**Adenoma** (most common); hyperplasia more common than carcinoma; seen in **MEN 1** and **MEN 2a;** excess parathyroid hormone (PTH); **hypercalcemia**	**Osteitis fibrosa cystica** (cystic "brown tumors" of bone); **renal calculi** and nephrocalcinosis; duodenal ulcers
Secondary hyperparathyroidism	**Hypocalcemia** caused by **chronic renal failure** (loss of vitamin D activation); parathyroid hyperplasia; excess PTH; high alkaline phosphatase; ectopic PTH (squamous cell lung carcinoma)	Cystic bone lesions; metastatic **calcification** of organs
Hypoparathyroidism	Most commonly secondary to **thyroidectomy;** seen in DiGeorge syndrome; **hypocalcemia**	Tetany; positive **Chvostek** and **Trousseau** signs
Pseudohypoparathyroidism	Autosomal recessive; deficient organ response to PTH	**Short stature;** underdeveloped fourth and fifth digits

MEN 1 and 2a, multiple endoplasmic neoplasia types 1 and 2a.

MULTIPLE ENDOCRINE NEOPLASIA (MEN) SYNDROMES *(Table 7-19)*

TABLE 7-19 Multiple Endocrine Neoplasia Syndromes

Type 1 (Wermer)	Type 2a (Sipple)	Type 2b
Parathyroid hyperplasia, pituitary adenomas, pancreatic tumors, angiofibromas	**Medullary thyroid carcinoma, parathyroid hyperplasia, pheochromocytoma**	**Mucosal neuromas** (particularly of the GI tract), **medullary thyroid carcinoma, pheochromocytoma**, marfanoid body habitus

GI, gastrointestinal.

QUICK HIT

The multiple endocrine neoplasia (MEN) syndromes are autosomal dominant conditions in which more than one endocrine organ is affected by either hyperplasia or neoplasia.

MNEMONIC

MEN 1 is a disease of **3 Ps**: **P**ituitary, **P**arathyroid, and **P**ancreas.

MNEMONIC

MEN 2a is a disease of **1 M and 2 Ps**: **M**edullary thyroid carcinoma, **P**arathyroid, and **P**heochromocytoma.

MNEMONIC

MEN 2b is a disease of **2 Ms and 1 P**: **M**ucosal neuromas, **M**edullary thyroid carcinoma, and **P**heochromocytoma.

8 The Reproductive System

DETERMINATION OF SEX

Before the seventh week of gestation, the fetal gonads are not differentiated into either the male or female genotype. Primordial germ cells migrate into the genital ridge mesoderm to form testes and ovaries. The presence or absence of the Y chromosome and the sex-determining region of the Y chromosome (SRY) determine gonadal differentiation. Therefore, the "default" gender is female if there is no SRY region on an active Y chromosome. Gender determination, which occurs after the seventh week, depends on the type of gonads present.

FEMALE REPRODUCTIVE SYSTEM DEVELOPMENT

I. Ovaries and other female reproductive structures

A. Primordial follicles contain primary **oocytes (XX genotype)** and follicular (granulosa) cells, which form the ovaries.
B. As the upper abdomen grows, the ovaries "descend" toward the perineum.
C. The gubernaculum assists in this descent and then becomes the ovarian ligament and the round ligament of the uterus.
D. The **paramesonephric ducts** develop into the fallopian tubes and eventually into the uterus.

II. Vagina and uterus *(Figure 8-1)*

III. Breasts

A. Only the main lactiferous ducts develop during the fetal life.
B. Glands enlarge during puberty owing to the increased levels of estrogens, progestins, prolactin, and growth hormone.

FIGURE 8-1 **Development of the female genital tract**

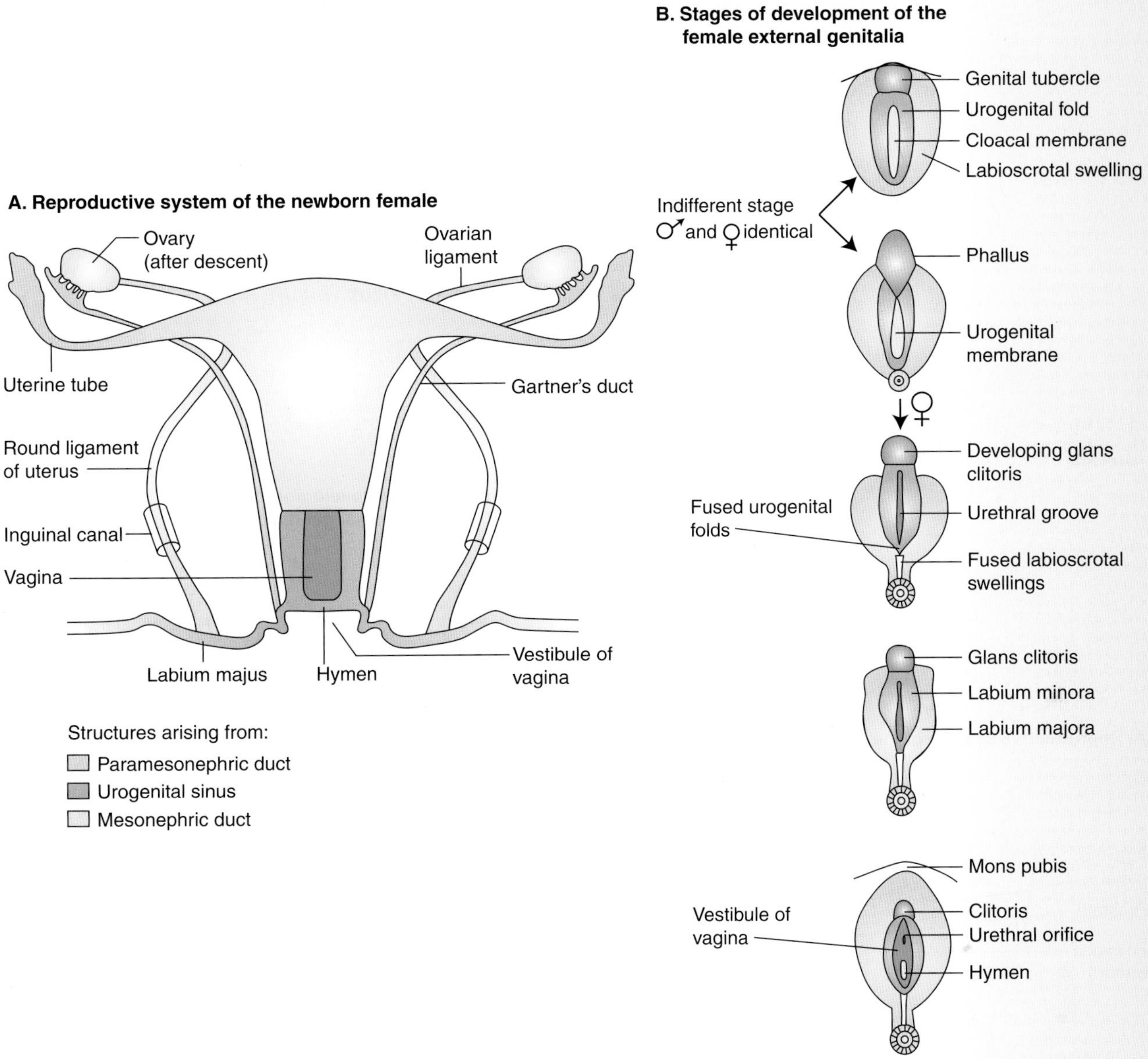
A. Reproductive system of the newborn female
Ovary
(after descent)
Ovarian
ligament
Uterine tube
Gartner's duct
Round ligament
of uterus
Inguinal canal
Vagina
Labium majus
Hymen
Vestibule of
vagina
Structures arising from:
Paramesonephric duct
Urogenital sinus
Mesonephric duct
B. Stages of development of the
female external genitalia
Genital tubercle
Urogenital fold
Cloacal membrane
Labioscrotal swelling
Indifferent stage
♂ and ♀ identical
Phallus
Urogenital
membrane
♀
Developing glans
clitoris
Fused urogenital
folds
Urethral groove
Fused labioscrotal
swellings
Glans clitoris
Labium minora
Labium majora
Mons pubis
Vestibule of
vagina
Clitoris
Urethral orifice
Hymen

(Adapted with permission from Moore KL, Persaud TVN. *The Developing Human: Clinically Oriented Embryology.* 6th ed. Philadelphia, PA: WB Saunders; 1998.)

MALE REPRODUCTIVE SYSTEM DEVELOPMENT

I. Testes and other male reproductive organs

A. Primary sex cords contain primordial germ cells of **XY genotype**. The Y chromosome codes for the testes-determining factor that allows for male gonadal differentiation (i.e., formation of medullary cords and seminiferous tubules).

B. Müllerian-inhibiting factor (**MIF**) is secreted by **Sertoli cells**. MIF causes regression of the Müllerian (paramesonephric) ducts and their associated female genital structures (uterine tubes and uterus).

C. The mesonephric ducts, under the influence of testosterone, become the ductus deferens, the seminal vesicles, and the ejaculatory ducts in the adult male.

II. The prostate gland forms from the urogenital sinus *(Figure 8-2)*

FIGURE 8-2 Development of the male genital tract

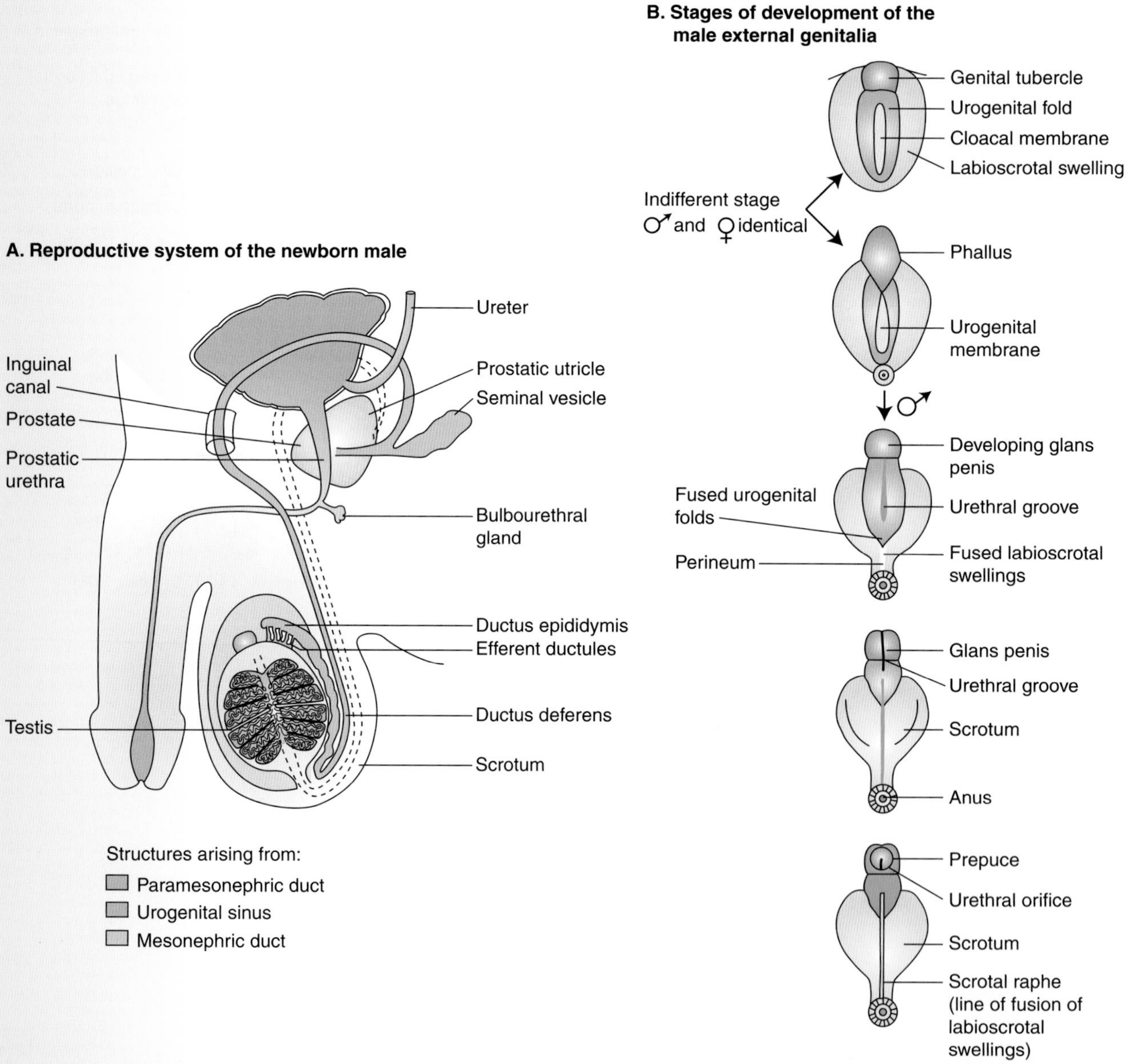
A. Reproductive system of the newborn male
Ureter
Inguinal canal
Prostatic utricle
Seminal vesicle
Prostate
Prostatic urethra
Bulbourethral gland
Ductus epididymis
Efferent ductules
Ductus deferens
Testis
Scrotum
Structures arising from:
Paramesonephric duct
Urogenital sinus
Mesonephric duct
B. Stages of development of the male external genitalia
Genital tubercle
Urogenital fold
Cloacal membrane
Labioscrotal swelling
Indifferent stage
♂ and ♀ identical
Phallus
Urogenital membrane
♂
Developing glans penis
Fused urogenital folds
Urethral groove
Perineum
Fused labioscrotal swellings
Glans penis
Urethral groove
Scrotum
Anus
Prepuce
Urethral orifice
Scrotum
Scrotal raphe (line of fusion of labioscrotal swellings)

(Adapted with permission from Moore KL, Persaud TVN. *The Developing Human: Clinically Oriented Embryology.* 6th ed. Philadelphia, PA: WB Saunders; 1998.)

III. External genitalia

A. Dihydrotestosterone (DHT) is responsible for the masculinization of genitalia.
B. The genital tubercle enlarges to become the glans penis.
C. The urogenital fold becomes the shaft of the penis.
D. The labioscrotal swellings fuse in the midline and become the scrotum.

- **Spermatogenesis versus Oogenesis** (Figure 8-3)
- **Important Anatomic Features of the Perineum** (Figure 8-4)

FIGURE 8-3 **Spermatogenesis versus oogenesis**

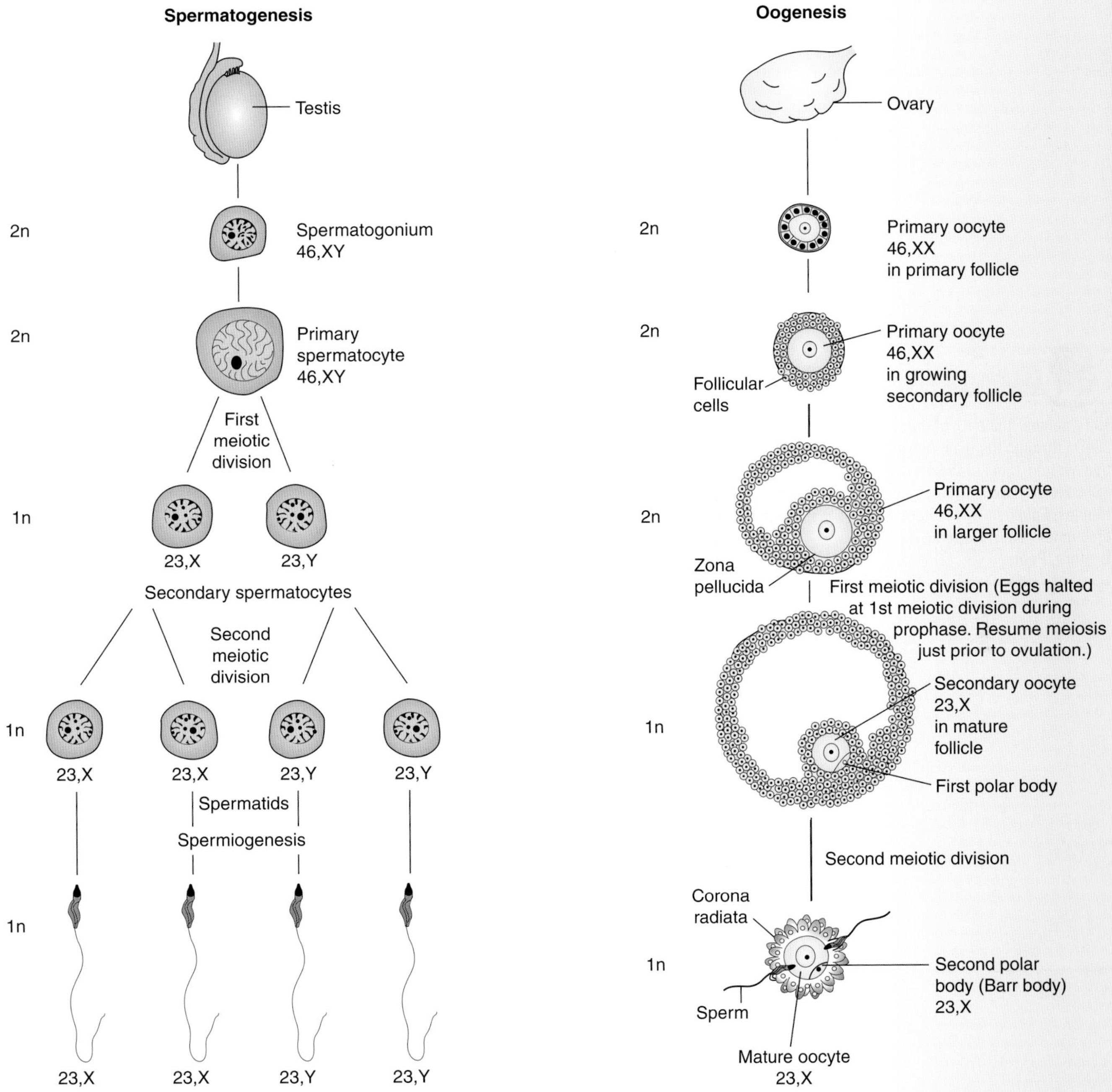

Spermatogenesis
Testis
2n
Spermatogonium 46,XY
2n
Primary spermatocyte 46,XY
First meiotic division
1n
23,X
23,Y
Secondary spermatocytes
Second meiotic division
1n
23,X
23,X
23,Y
23,Y
Spermatids
Spermiogenesis
1n
23,X
23,X
23,Y
23,Y
Oogenesis
Ovary
2n
Primary oocyte 46,XX in primary follicle
2n
Primary oocyte 46,XX in growing secondary follicle
Follicular cells
2n
Primary oocyte 46,XX in larger follicle
Zona pellucida
First meiotic division (Eggs halted at 1st meiotic division during prophase. Resume meiosis just prior to ovulation.)
1n
Secondary oocyte 23,X in mature follicle
First polar body
Second meiotic division
Corona radiata
1n
Second polar body (Barr body) 23,X
Sperm
Mature oocyte 23,X

(Adapted with permission from Moore KL, Persaud TVN. *The Developing Human: Clinically Oriented Embryology.* 6th ed. Philadelphia, PA: WB Saunders; 1998.)

QUICK HIT

Puberty in males, usually occurring at age 15, is marked by an increased testosterone, leading to a greater hair distribution, growth of genitalia, nocturnal emissions, deepening of the voice, and increased muscle mass. Precocious puberty in males has a similar pathology to that in females, with the exception that it has a later age of onset.

MNEMONIC

To remember the path of the sperm through the male reproductive system, think of the phrase "SEVEN UP": **S**eminiferous tubules, **E**pididymis, **V**as deferens, **E**jaculatory duct, **N**othing, **U**rethra, **P**enis.

FIGURE 8-4 Important anatomic features of the perineum

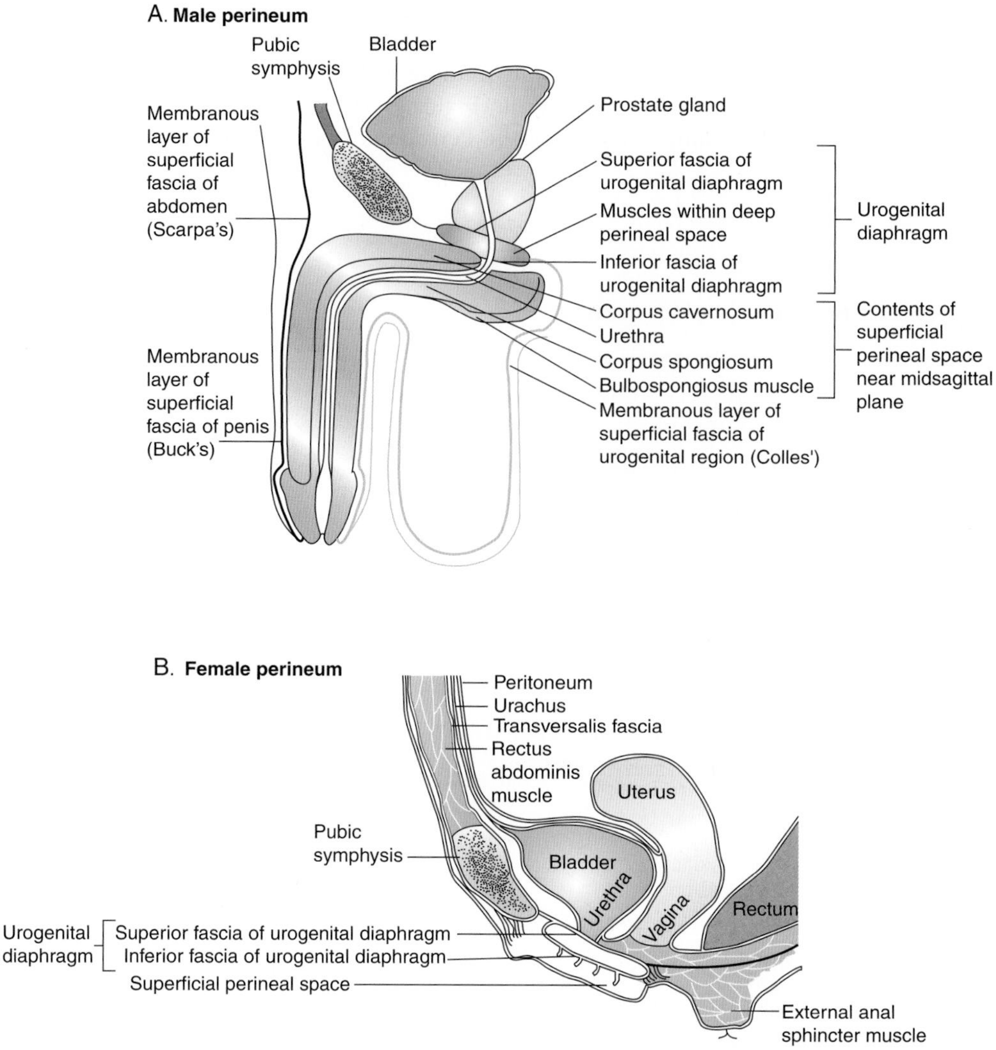
A. Male perineum
Pubic symphysis
Bladder
Membranous layer of superficial fascia of abdomen (Scarpa's)
Prostate gland
Superior fascia of urogenital diaphragm
Muscles within deep perineal space
Inferior fascia of urogenital diaphragm
Urogenital diaphragm
Corpus cavernosum
Urethra
Corpus spongiosum
Bulbospongiosus muscle
Contents of superficial perineal space near midsagittal plane
Membranous layer of superficial fascia of penis (Buck's)
Membranous layer of superficial fascia of urogenital region (Colles')
B. Female perineum
Peritoneum
Urachus
Transversalis fascia
Rectus abdominis muscle
Uterus
Pubic symphysis
Bladder
Urethra
Vagina
Rectum
Urogenital diaphragm
Superior fascia of urogenital diaphragm
Inferior fascia of urogenital diaphragm
Superficial perineal space
External anal sphincter muscle

CONGENITAL MALFORMATIONS

Congenital malformations are most often caused by exposure to teratogens during the third to eighth weeks of pregnancy, which is the period of organogenesis (Table 8-1).

TABLE **8-1** **Congenital Malformations**

Malformation	Clinical Features
Hypospadias	• Urethra opens on the **ventral** side of the penis • Spongy urethra does not form properly or the **urogenital folds** do not fuse • Paucity of hormone receptors or too little hormone produced from the testes may play a role • More common than epispadias
Epispadias	• Urethra opens on the **dorsum** of the penis
Undescended testis (cryptorchidism)	• Most are of unknown cause • May be unilateral or bilateral • Most testes descend before 1 year of life • If testes remain undescended, **sterility or testicular cancer** can result
Congenital inguinal hernia (indirect hernia)	• A communication is formed between the **tunica vaginalis** (adjacent to the testis) and the peritoneal cavity • A loop of intestine may herniate into the opening and become entrapped, resulting in obstruction
True hermaphroditism	• **Both testicular** and **ovarian tissue** are present • External genitalia are ambiguous • Usually 46,XX
Female pseudohermaphroditism	• XX genotype with **virilization** of the external genitalia is present • The cause is **excess androgen exposure** • This malformation is most often caused by congenital adrenal hyperplasia, a **21-hydroxylase deficiency** (autosomal recessive disease with low cortisol and high ACTH)
Male pseudohermaphroditism	• XY genotype with varying ambiguities of the external genitalia • The cause is a **lack of MIF and testosterone**
Androgen insensitivity syndrome (testicular feminization)	• **XY** genotype with female phenotype • Caused by a **defective androgen receptor** • Vagina ends blindly (no uterus) • Normal female pubertal development occurs but pubic hair is scant and there are no menses
Double uterus completely	• The cause is failure of the **paramesonephric ducts** to fuse • The condition may appear in two forms: uterus divided internally by a thin septum or a division of only the superior part of the uterus (bicornuate uterus)
Kallmann syndrome	• A deficiency of GnRH results in decreased FSH and LH • No secondary sexual characteristics are present • Associated with hypoplasia of the olfactory bulbs **(anosmia)**

ACTH, adrenocorticotropic hormone; FSH, follicle-stimulating hormone; GnRH, gonadotropin-releasing hormone; LH, luteinizing hormone; MIF, müllerian-inhibiting factor.

QUICK HIT

Epispadias is associated with exstrophy of the bladder.

QUICK HIT

Congenital inguinal hernia is associated with cryptorchidism.

QUICK HIT

In androgen insensitivity syndrome (AIS), affected individuals have normal testes with normal production of testosterone and normal conversion to DHT, which differentiates this condition from 5α-reductase deficiency. Because the testes produce normal amounts of MIF, affected individuals do not have fallopian tubes, a uterus, or a proximal (upper) vagina. In AIS, the external female genitalia and breasts develop by default because of the **lack of responsiveness of androgen receptors to DHT** during development. In 5α-reductase deficiency, **lack of DHT** results in a female genotype. At puberty in these individuals, a testosterone surge results in adequate levels of DHT, resulting in growth of male genitalia and "penis at 12" syndrome.

GENETIC ABNORMALITIES

The incidence of genetic abnormalities as a result of aberrant chromosomes significantly increases when the mother is older than 35 years of age. In these patients, additional consideration should be given to genetic testing.

- **Genetic Abnormalities Caused by Abnormal Somatic Chromosomes** (Table 8-2)
- **Genetic Abnormalities Caused by Abnormal Sex Chromosomes** (Table 8-3)

QUICK HIT

There is an increased incidence of trisomy 21 in women older than 35 years of age. The incidence of the Robertsonian translocation type of Down syndrome is familial and does not increase with the age of the mother.

QUICK HIT

Down syndrome is the most common genetic cause of mental retardation in males; fragile X is the second most common.

TABLE 8-2 Genetic Abnormalities Caused by Abnormal Somatic Chromosomes

Syndrome	Genotype	Description
Down syndrome	Trisomy 21 (95%) or Robertsonian translocation of 14 and 21	• **Mental retardation** • Epicanthal folds • Large tongue • Brushfield spots on iris • Simian crease in hands • Increased incidence of congenital heart disease, acute leukemia, and dementia of the Alzheimer type later in life
Edward syndrome	Trisomy 18	• Duodenal atresia • Mental retardation • Micrognathia • **Rocker bottom feet** • Second digit overlaps third and fourth • Increased incidence of congenital heart disease
Patau syndrome	Trisomy 13	• Mental retardation • Microphthalmia • Polydactyly • Cleft lip and palate
Cri du chat syndrome	Deletion of 5p (5p−)	• Catlike cry • Mental retardation • Microcephaly • Hypertelorism

MNEMONIC

To remember that fragile X is due to trinucleotide repeat **CGG**, think: "**S**ee **G**iant **G**onads."

TABLE 8-3 Genetic Abnormalities Caused by Abnormal Sex Chromosomes

Syndrome	Genotype	Description
Turner syndrome	45,XO	• **Monosomy** of the X chromosome • Absence of Barr body • Short stature • Webbed neck • Widely spaced nipples • Wide, "shield-like" chest • Wide carrying angle of arms • Lack of sexual maturity • Amenorrhea • Coarctation of the aorta
Klinefelter syndrome	47,XXY	• Tall with long limbs • Often presents with gynecomastia • Hyalinization of seminiferous tubules • Hypogonadism, lack of spermatogenesis leading to sterility • One Barr body

(continued)

TABLE 8-3 Genetic Abnormalities Caused by Abnormal Sex Chromosomes (Continued)

Syndrome	Genotype	Description
XYY syndrome	47,XYY	• Normal-appearing male, often tall • Often associated with **aggressive behavior** • May be overrepresented in the population of incarcerated males
XXX syndrome	47,XXX	• Usually asymptomatic • Rarely associated with **menstrual irregularities** and mild mental retardation • Two Barr bodies
Fragile X syndrome	46,XY	• The end of the X chromosome appears delicate • **Macroorchidism** • Common cause of **mental retardation** • Long face • Low-set, large ears
Prader–Willi syndrome	−15q12 (no paternal contribution, imprinting disorder)	• Obesity • **Hyperphagia** • **Hypogonadism** • Short stature • Mental retardation
Angelman syndrome	−15q12 (no maternal contribution, imprinting disorder)	• Ataxia • Mental retardation • **Inappropriate laughter** • Patient appears to act like a **"happy puppet"**

MENARCHE, MENSTRUATION, AND MENOPAUSE

I. Menarche

A. First menstruation; usually occurs between **11 and 14 years of age**

B. Follows thelarche (development of breast buds) by 2 years

C. Precocious puberty

1. Pubertal changes before 9 years of age in boys and 8 years of age in girls.
2. True precocious puberty
    a. Early but normal pubertal development
    b. Precocious puberty is **usually familial and not pathologic.**
    c. May cause emotional and social adjustment problems
3. Incomplete precocious puberty
    a. Premature development of a single pubertal characteristic
    b. Types
        - Premature thelarche: breast budding before 8 years of age
        - Premature adrenarche: growth of axillary hair
        - Premature pubarche: growth of pubic hair
    c. Generally self-limited
4. Etiology
    a. Central—increased follicle-stimulating hormone (FSH) and luteinizing hormone (LH) (from the pituitary) lead to sex steroid production by the gonads.
    b. Peripheral—caused by increased sex steroids not driven by pituitary gonadotropins (gonadal tumors, adrenal pathology, exogenous estrogens, etc.)

QUICK HIT

Breast surgery should not be performed in girls with precocious puberty because the excision of a "lump" in premature thelarche leads to the loss of an entire breast.

MNEMONIC

Associate **4** with the female reproductive system: **4** is the normal pH of the vagina; **40** weeks is the normal gestation period; **400** oocytes are released between menarche and menopause; **400,000** oocytes are present at puberty.

QUICK HIT

In understanding Müllerian duct agenesis and androgen insensitivity syndrome, it is important to remember that the ovaries and the lower vagina are not derived from the Müllerian system. The ovaries are derived from germ cells that migrate from the primitive yolk sac into the mesenchyme of the peritoneal cavity and subsequently develop into ova and supporting cells. The lower one-third of the vagina arises from the sinovaginal bulb, which fuses with the Müllerian-derived upper two-thirds to form the complete vagina.

QUICK HIT

There are four causes of primary amenorrhea in the female: Turner syndrome (XO), Müllerian duct agenesis (XX), outflow obstruction (imperforate hymen, transverse vaginal septum) (XX), and androgen insensitivity syndrome (XY).

MNEMONIC

Remember the function of luteinizing hormone (**LH**) and follicle-stimulating hormone (**FSH**) in the male; **LH** stimulates **L**eydig cells to produce testosterone and **FSH** stimulates **S**permatogenesis.

II. Menstruation and fertilization

FIGURE 8-5 Hormone function within the menstrual cycle

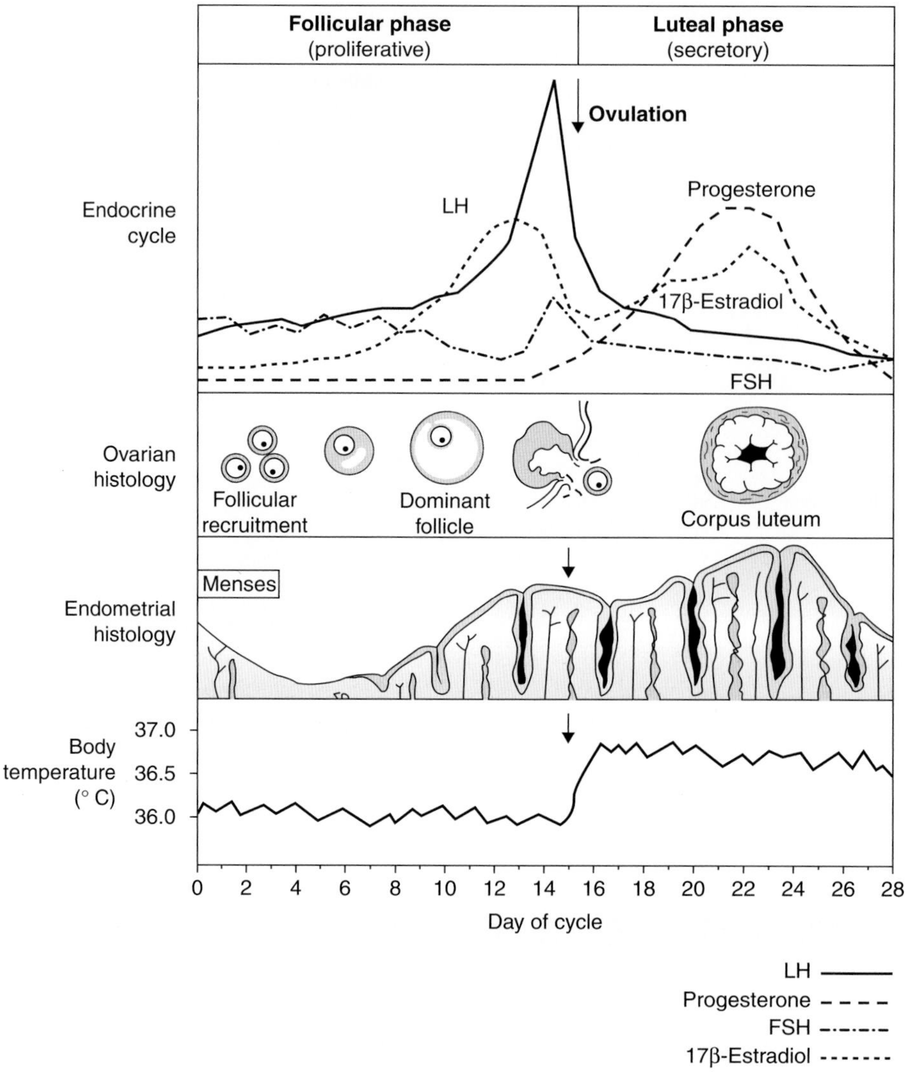

Follicular phase
(proliferative)
Luteal phase
(secretory)
Ovulation
Endocrine cycle
LH
Progesterone
17β-Estradiol
FSH
Ovarian histology
Follicular recruitment
Dominant follicle
Corpus luteum
Menses
Endometrial histology
Body temperature (° C)
37.0
36.5
36.0
0 2 4 6 8 10 12 14 16 18 20 22 24 26 28
Day of cycle
LH
Progesterone
FSH
17β-Estradiol

FSH, follicle-stimulating hormone; LH, luteinizing hormone.

A. Hormone formation and function (Figure 8-5)
   1. Ovarian **steroids** are synthesized from **cholesterol**.
   2. LH from the pituitary regulates the conversion of cholesterol to pregnenolone (the first step in estrogen synthesis) in the theca cells.
   3. FSH from the pituitary regulates the final step in estrogen synthesis in the granulosa cells.
   4. Estrogen
      a. Secreted by the follicular cells of the **ovary**
      b. Induces development of the secondary sex characteristics
         - Binds to the estrogen receptor
         - Activated estrogen-receptor complex interacts with nuclear chromatin.
         - Initiates hormone-specific RNA synthesis
         - Results in protein synthesis
      c. Stimulates uterine growth and development
      d. Induces proliferation of endometrium
      e. Causes thickening of the vaginal mucosa

f. Induces development of the breast ductal system
g. Causes bone growth (increased osteoblastic activity and decreased osteoclastic activity)

5. Progesterone
   a. Secreted by the **corpus luteum** produced in response to LH
   b. Converts proliferative endometrium to secretory endometrium
   c. Inhibits uterine contractions
   d. Increases the viscosity of cervical mucus
   e. Increases the basal body temperature
   f. Induces the development of breast glandular system

B. Menstrual cycle (Figure 8-6)
   1. One cycle is defined as the time from the onset of one menses to the next, with an average of **28 days**.
   2. Characteristic changes in the ovary lead to ovulation and hormone production (Figure 8-7).

FIGURE **8-6** **The menstrual cycle**

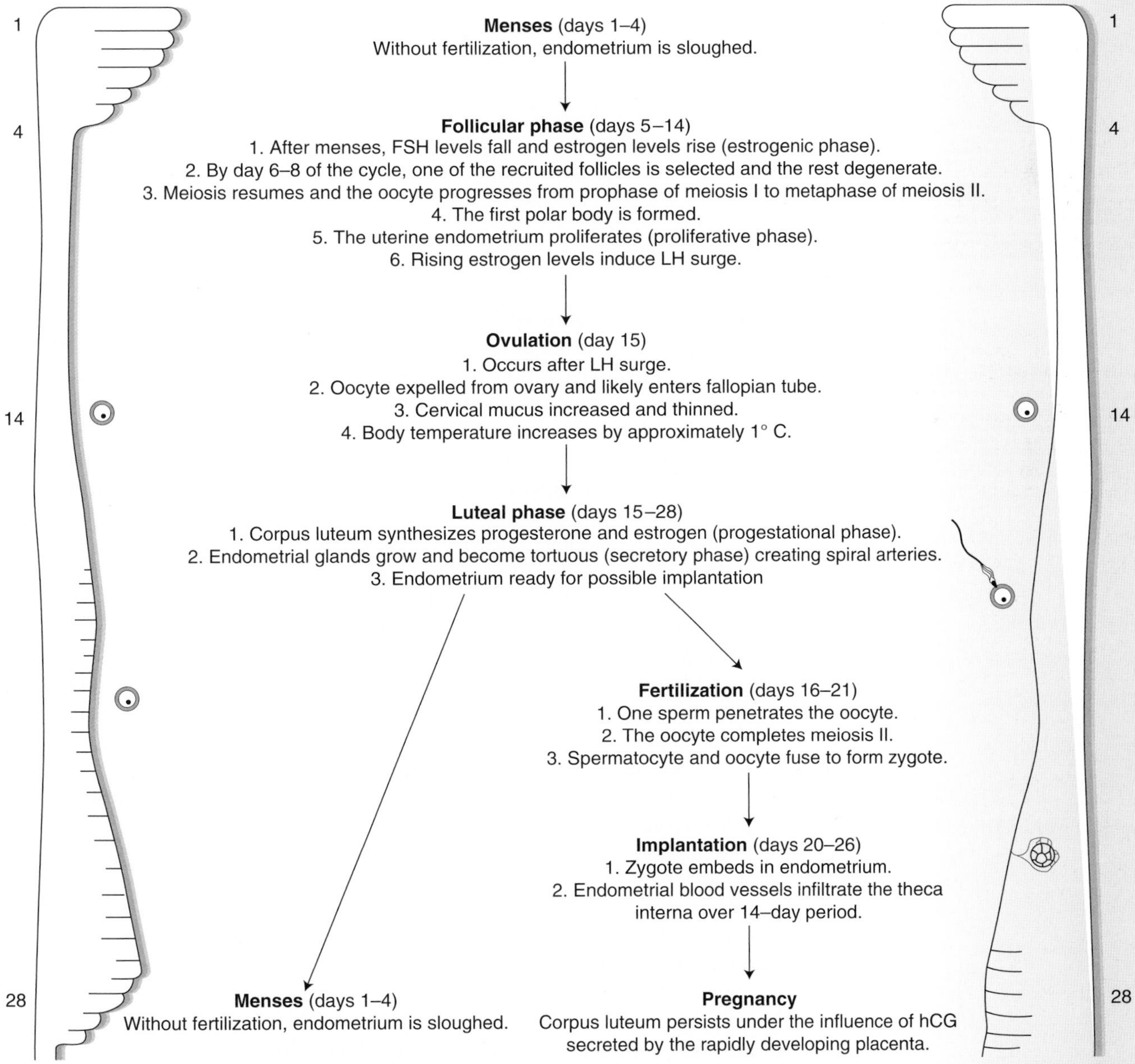
1
4
14
28
Menses (days 1–4)
Without fertilization, endometrium is sloughed.
Follicular phase (days 5–14)
1. After menses, FSH levels fall and estrogen levels rise (estrogenic phase).
2. By day 6–8 of the cycle, one of the recruited follicles is selected and the rest degenerate.
3. Meiosis resumes and the oocyte progresses from prophase of meiosis I to metaphase of meiosis II.
4. The first polar body is formed.
5. The uterine endometrium proliferates (proliferative phase).
6. Rising estrogen levels induce LH surge.
Ovulation (day 15)
1. Occurs after LH surge.
2. Oocyte expelled from ovary and likely enters fallopian tube.
3. Cervical mucus increased and thinned.
4. Body temperature increases by approximately 1° C.
Luteal phase (days 15–28)
1. Corpus luteum synthesizes progesterone and estrogen (progestational phase).
2. Endometrial glands grow and become tortuous (secretory phase) creating spiral arteries.
3. Endometrium ready for possible implantation
Fertilization (days 16–21)
1. One sperm penetrates the oocyte.
2. The oocyte completes meiosis II.
3. Spermatocyte and oocyte fuse to form zygote.
Implantation (days 20–26)
1. Zygote embeds in endometrium.
2. Endometrial blood vessels infiltrate the theca interna over 14–day period.
Menses (days 1–4)
Without fertilization, endometrium is sloughed.
Pregnancy
Corpus luteum persists under the influence of hCG secreted by the rapidly developing placenta.

FSH, follicle-stimulating hormone; hCG, human chorionic gonadotropin; LH, luteinizing hormone.

FIGURE 8-7 Developmental changes in the ovary

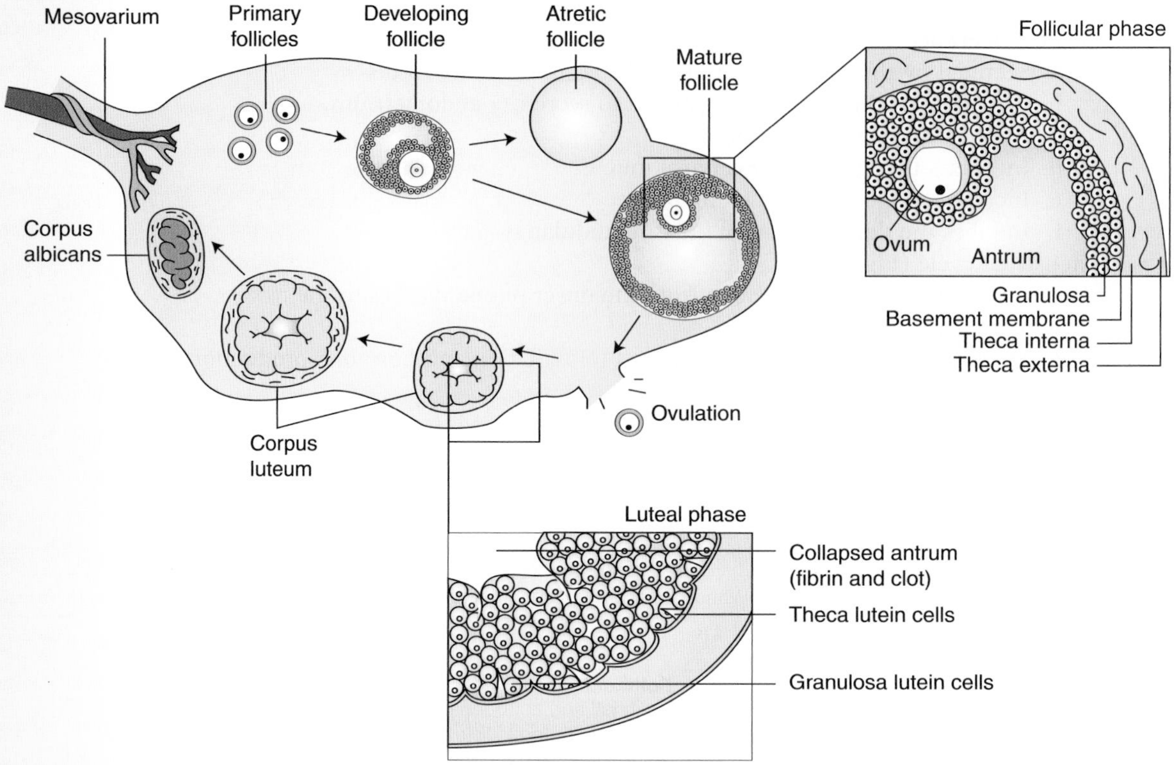
Mesovarium
Primary follicles
Developing follicle
Atretic follicle
Mature follicle
Follicular phase
Ovum
Antrum
Granulosa
Basement membrane
Theca interna
Theca externa
Corpus albicans
Corpus luteum
Ovulation
Luteal phase
Collapsed antrum (fibrin and clot)
Theca lutein cells
Granulosa lutein cells

C. **Disorders**
1. **Abnormal uterine bleeding**
   a. Functional menstrual disorders, characterized as excessive bleeding either during ("menorrhagia") or between ("metrorrhagia") menstrual periods
   b. Most common gynecologic problem during reproductive years
   c. Causes
      - Organic lesions (polyps, fibroids)
      - Hormonal dysregulation (anovulatory cycles, polycystic ovary syndrome, functional ovarian cysts)
      - Neoplasia (endometrial hyperplasia, cancer)
      - Abnormal pregnancy (ectopic pregnancy, abortion)
2. **Polycystic ovary syndrome** (Stein–Leventhal syndrome)
   a. Triad of:
      - **Androgen excess** (hirsutism, acne)
      - **Ovulatory dysfunction** or anovulation (causing secondary amenorrhea)
      - Characteristic **appearance of the ovaries on ultrasound** (stromal fibrosis and small follicular cysts)
   b. Also associated with obesity and insulin resistance
   c. Increased LH and testosterone, increased estrogen (from aromatization of testosterone in adipose tissue), decreased FSH
   d. Endometrial hyperplasia is common; increased risk of endometrial adenocarcinoma
   e. Treat with weight loss; clomiphene or metformin for infertility/anovulation; oral contraceptives or progesterone; spironolactone for androgen excess
3. **Endometriosis**
   a. Nonneoplastic endometrial tissue located outside the uterus
   b. Responds to hormonal variations of menstrual cycle
   c. Most commonly occurs on the ovaries (bilateral)
   d. Presents as pain before and during menstruation

e. Multiple, small, hemosiderin-filled endometrial implants; "powder burns"; scarring; adhesions; endometriomas (large, blood-filled sacs called "**chocolate cysts**")
f. May result in infertility
g. Treat with oral contraceptive pills (OCPs), leuprolide, and/or surgical excision. Danazol, a mild androgen, is rarely used anymore because of side effects.

4. **Amenorrhea** (Figures 8-8 and 8-9)
   a. **Primary amenorrhea**: absence of menarche in a woman by age 16 years
   - Genetic (Turner syndrome, androgen insensitivity syndrome)
   - Structural (imperforate hymen, Müllerian duct agenesis)
   - Delayed puberty

   b. **Secondary amenorrhea**: cessation of menstruation for >3 months in a woman of reproductive age with cyclic periods or >6 months in a woman with irregular periods
   - Pregnancy
   - Ovarian failure
   - Polycystic ovary syndrome
   - Thyroid disorders
   - Athleticism
   - Anorexia
   - Stress

FIGURE 8-8 Causes of amenorrhea

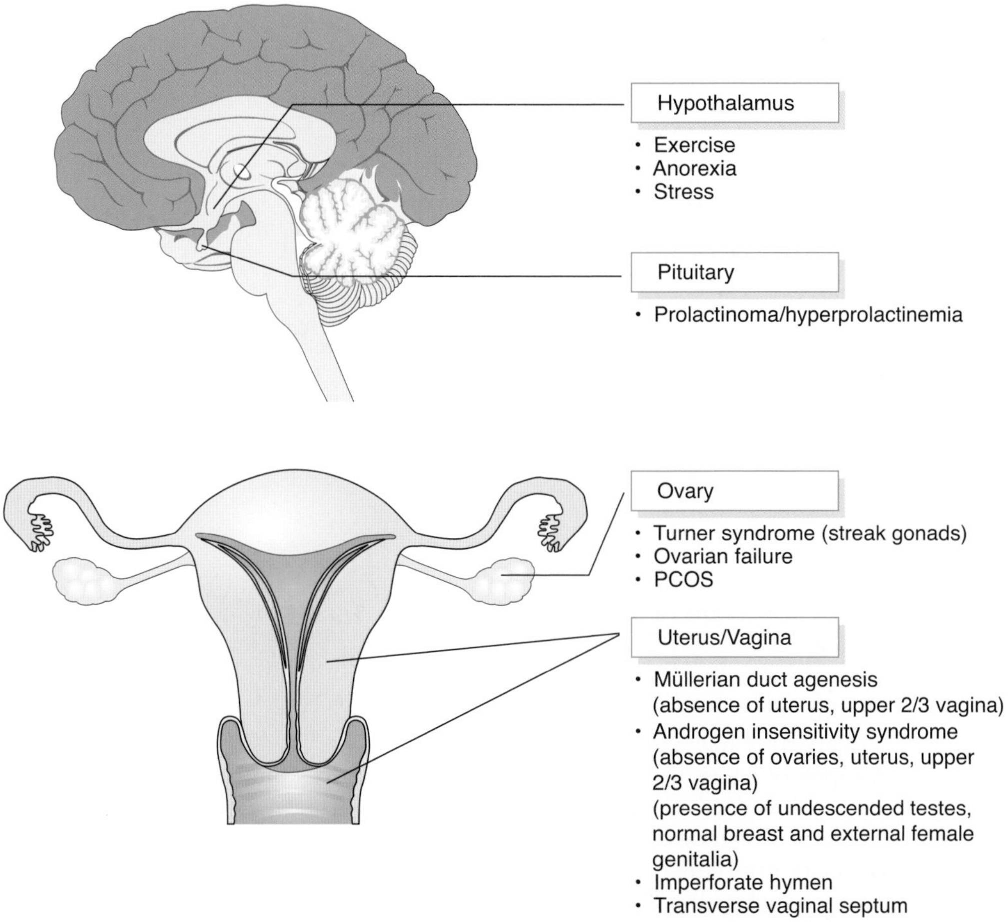
Hypothalamus
• Exercise
• Anorexia
• Stress
Pituitary
• Prolactinoma/hyperprolactinemia
Ovary
• Turner syndrome (streak gonads)
• Ovarian failure
• PCOS
Uterus/Vagina
• Müllerian duct agenesis (absence of uterus, upper 2/3 vagina)
• Androgen insensitivity syndrome (absence of ovaries, uterus, upper 2/3 vagina) (presence of undescended testes, normal breast and external female genitalia)
• Imperforate hymen
• Transverse vaginal septum

In approaching the various causes of amenorrhea, it is easiest to conceptualize them within the hypothalamic-pituitary-ovarian-uterine framework. It is postulated that stress, exercise, and anorexia act at the level of the hypothalamus to stop the menstrual cycle. Prolactin tumors at the pituitary level disrupt the neuroendocrine regulation of gonadotropin-releasing hormone, resulting in an abnormal menstrual function. At the ovarian level, ovarian failure, polycystic ovary syndrome (PCOS) , and streak gonads of Turner syndrome result in menstrual dysfunction. Müllerian duct agenesis, imperforate hymen, and androgen insensitivity syndrome are abnormalities at the uterine and vaginal level.

FIGURE 8-9 **Approach to amenorrhea**

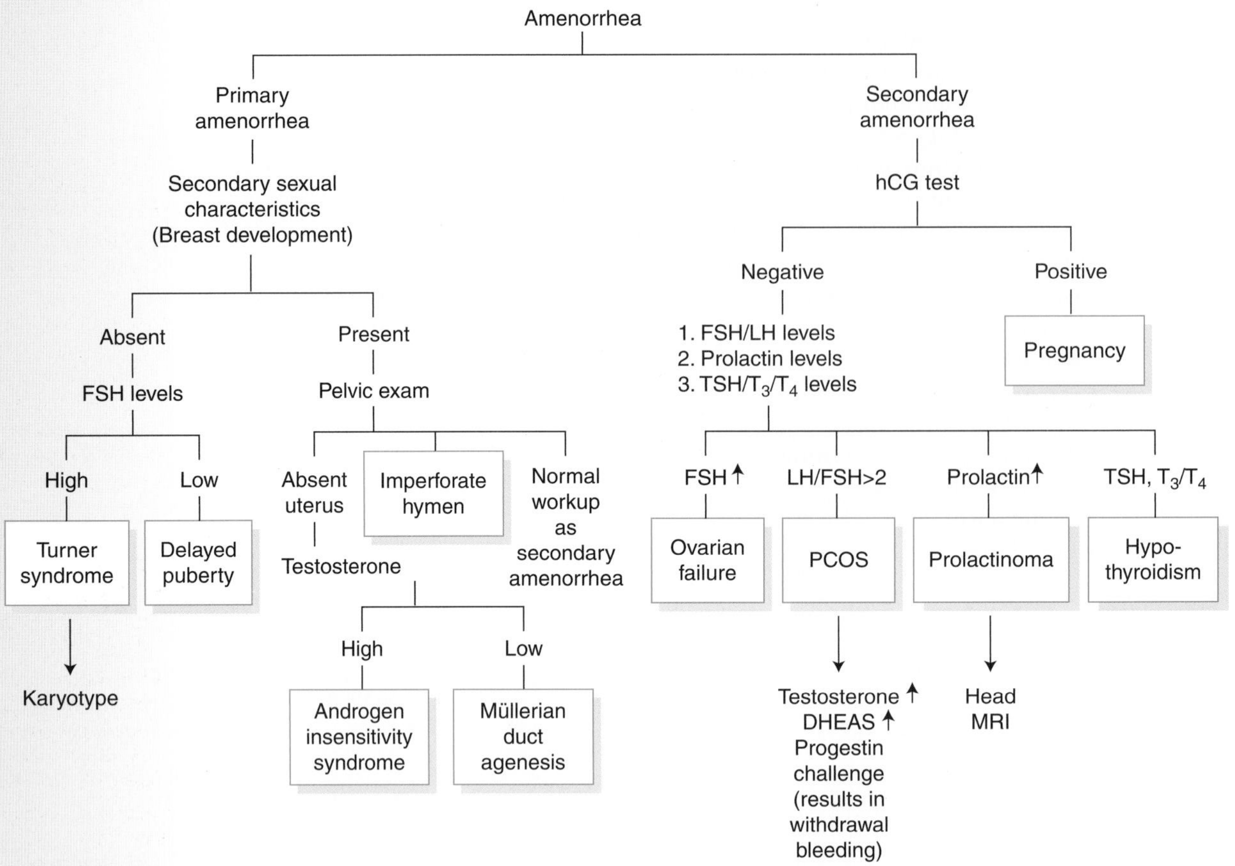

Amenorrhea
Primary amenorrhea
Secondary amenorrhea
Secondary sexual characteristics (Breast development)
hCG test
Negative
Positive
Absent
Present
1. FSH/LH levels
2. Prolactin levels
3. TSH/T3/T4 levels
Pregnancy
FSH levels
Pelvic exam
High
Low
Absent uterus
Imperforate hymen
Normal workup as secondary amenorrhea
FSH ↑
LH/FSH>2
Prolactin ↑
TSH, T3/T4
Turner syndrome
Delayed puberty
Testosterone
Ovarian failure
PCOS
Prolactinoma
Hypo-thyroidism
Karyotype
High
Low
Androgen insensitivity syndrome
Müllerian duct agenesis
Testosterone ↑
DHEAS ↑
Progestin challenge (results in withdrawal bleeding)
Head MRI

DHEAS, dehydroepiandrosterone sulfate; FSH, follicle-stimulating hormone; hCG, human chorionic gonadotropin; LH, luteinizing hormone; MRI, magnetic resonance imaging; PCOS, polycystic ovary syndrome; T_3, triiodothyronine; T_4, thyroxine; TSH, thyroid-stimulating hormone.

III. Menopause

A. Last physiologic menstrual cycle usually occurs in the **early 50s** (mean age is 51½ years).

B. Estrogen levels fall (because of the reduced ovarian function) and FSH levels increase.

C. Early signs
   1. Anxiety
   2. Mood swings
   3. Irritability
   4. Depression
   5. **Hot flashes**: bouts of flushing and sweating

D. Late signs
   1. Vaginal dryness
   2. Painful intercourse
   3. Urinary tract infections
   4. Atrophy of breast tissue because of lack of estrogen stimulation
   5. **Osteoporosis**
   6. **Decreased high-density lipoprotein** (HDL), leading to an increased risk of **coronary artery disease**

E. Management of patients who are menopausal or postmenopausal may involve estrogen replacement therapy.
   1. Effects
      a. Decreases sleep disturbances
      b. Increases HDL and decreases low-density lipoprotein (LDL)
      c. Decreases postmenopausal vaginal atrophy

d. Decreases bone resorption and osteoporosis
e. Decreases frequency of "hot flashes" by reestablishing hypothalamic control of norepinephrine secretion

2. Risks and contraindications
a. History of estrogen-dependent cancer
b. Increased risk of breast and endometrial cancer
c. In women with an intact uterus, estrogen increases the risk of developing endometrial carcinoma. Therefore, estrogen is combined with progestin to decrease the effects of unopposed estrogen.
d. Women's Health Initiative showed that estrogen increased the absolute risk of stroke by 0.13% when compared to placebo.

IV. Oral contraceptives

A. Agents that interfere with ovulation to prevent pregnancy
B. Combination pills contain progestin and estrogen.
1. The estrogen component suppresses ovulation.
2. The progestin component thickens the cervical mucus, reducing the passage of sperm.

C. Other agents
1. Progestin-only
a. Available as pills, intramuscular (IM) injection, or progestin implants
b. Progestin-only pills have higher failure rates; injections and implant devices have lower failure rates than combination oral contraceptives.
c. Increased rate of menstrual irregularities

2. Mifepristone (RU 486), a progestin antagonist
a. Results in fetal abortion when given early in pregnancy (within first 6 weeks)
b. Interferes with progesterone and decreases human chorionic gonadotropin (hCG)

D. Side effects
1. Cardiovascular disease
a. Women older than 35 years of age who smoke are at greatest risk from thromboembolism.
b. Progestin-predominant preparations can lead to an increase in the LDL:HDL ratio.

2. Benign liver hepatomas and hemangiomas
3. Gallbladder disease
4. Emotional changes

PREGNANCY AND ITS ASSOCIATED COMPLICATIONS

I. Normal pregnancy

A. For clinical purposes, assume that a **woman of childbearing age is pregnant** unless proven otherwise.
B. Normal gestation is **40 weeks**.
C. Clinical signs include missed periods, swollen breasts, fatigue, nausea, and **elevated** β-human chorionic gonadotropin (**β-hCG**) (serum).
D. Hormonal regulation
1. During fertilization, **β-hCG** produced by the placenta **prevents corpus luteum regression**.
2. During the first trimester, the corpus luteum produces estrogen and progesterone.
3. Second and third trimester
a. Progesterone is produced by the placenta.
b. Estrogen production is regulated by the interplay among the fetal adrenal gland, fetal liver, and placenta.

4. The initiating event in parturition is unknown, but delivery can be induced by oxytocin.

QUICK HIT

Clomiphene interferes with the negative feedback provided by estrogen to the brain and causes an increase in gonadotropin-releasing hormone (GnRH). This leads to stimulation of ovulation and can be used to treat infertility associated with anovulatory cycles.

QUICK HIT

Taking oral contraceptives provides other benefits, such as decreased risk of dysmenorrhea, iron deficiency anemia, ectopic pregnancy, benign breast disease, endometrial cancer, ovarian cysts, ovarian cancer, and postmenopausal hip fracture.

QUICK HIT

A pudendal nerve block can be performed to alleviate the pain of childbirth. One hand is inserted into the vagina to locate the ischial spine, which is used as a landmark, while the other hand inserts a needle, which contains anesthetic for the pudendal nerve, which crosses the ischial spine at this level, thus anesthetizing the skin lateral to the vaginal opening.

QUICK HIT

The narrowest diameter that the fetus must transverse during birth is the pelvic outlet, from ischial spine to ischial spine (interspinous distance).

Clinical Vignette 8-1

CLINICAL PRESENTATION: A 17-year-old girl presents to her primary care physician with the chief complaint that she has not **had her period for several months.** She previously had fairly regular menses, with menarche at age 13. She is the daughter of a **middle class family,** an **excellent student,** and **active in track** outside of class. Physical examination shows a well-developed female with **normal external female genitalia.** Pelvic examination is deferred.

DIFFERENTIALS: Pregnancy, anorexia nervosa, exercise, pituitary prolactinoma, polycystic ovary syndrome, ovarian failure, Turner syndrome, and hypothyroidism. **Any female who reports missing her period should be evaluated for pregnancy.** The first step in approaching amenorrhea is to determine whether the patient has had periods in the past (secondary amenorrhea) or has never experienced menstruation (primary amenorrhea). There are four diagnoses unique to primary amenorrhea: Turner syndrome, Müllerian duct agenesis, imperforate hymen, and androgen insensitivity syndrome. These disorders can be ruled out in this case because the patient has a history of periods. (*Note:* Mosaic Turner syndrome can have some menstrual bleeding prior to the cessation of periods.) Figure 8-8 shows the various causes of amenorrhea. On the USMLE, look for certain symptoms that suggest some disorders over others: hirsutism (polycystic ovary syndrome [PCOS]), obesity (PCOS), galactorrhea (prolactinoma), webbed neck (Turner), widely spaced nipples (Turner), presence of abdominal masses (testes in androgen insensitivity syndrome), and renal anomalies (Müllerian duct agenesis). Pelvic examination would be helpful in assessing imperforate hymen, androgen insensitivity syndrome (blind-ending short vaginal canal and absence of uterus and ovaries), and Müllerian duct agenesis (blind-ending short vaginal canal and absence of uterus).

LABORATORY STUDIES: In approaching secondary amenorrhea (Figure 8-9), first obtain a **pregnancy test.** If negative, a battery of tests would be performed, including **follicle-stimulating hormone (FSH), luteinizing hormone (LH), thyroid-stimulating hormone (TSH)/triiodothyronine (T_3)/levothyroxine (T_4), and prolactin levels** to rule out hypothyroidism and prolactinoma, respectively. FSH and LH levels are expected to be high in cases of ovarian defects (Turner syndrome, ovarian failure, and PCOS) and low to normal in defects at the hypothalamic/pituitary level (pituitary tumors, anorexia, and athleticism). To further differentiate among these, if LH/FSH >2, it suggests PCOS, and **testosterone** and dehydroepiandrosterone sulfate **(DHEAS) levels** should be measured (will likely be elevated). Also, progestin challenge should induce withdrawal from menstrual bleeding. Turner syndrome with ovarian failure can be distinguished by karyotype. In cases of suspected anatomical abnormalities, a pelvic ultrasound should be performed.

MANAGEMENT: Most treatments of secondary amenorrhea are directed to correct the underlying disease process via surgery or restore ovulatory cycle via estrogen–progestin therapy. PCOS is treated based on the reproductive desire of the female—**spironolactone** with **clomiphene citrate** is used if the patient is interested in conceiving; otherwise, **oral contraception** may be used.

5. Lactation
    a. Estrogen and progesterone block the effect of prolactin on the breast.
    b. Prolactin levels rise throughout pregnancy and suppress ovulation.
    c. Estrogen/progesterone levels fall after delivery.

E. Prenatal diagnostic procedures
1. **Amniocentesis** is an aspiration of fluid from the amniotic sac at $\geq$15 weeks' gestation.
    a. α-Fetoprotein (**AFP**) assay for neural tube defects
    b. **Spectrophotometry** to determine hemolytic disease of the newborn (see Chapter 10)
    c. Sex chromatin studies for X-linked disease
    d. **Cell culture** studies for chromosomal abnormalities
    e. Enzyme and DNA analysis
    f. Infection testing (cytomegalovirus [CMV] or *Toxoplasma* DNA)
2. Maternal serum AFP
    a. Elevated in neural tube defects
    b. Reduced in Down syndrome

MNEMONIC

Remember the causes of **I**ncreased **M**aternal **S**erum **A**lpha **F**eto**P**rotein: **I**ntestinal obstruction, **M**ultiple gestation/**M**yeloschisis, **S**pina bifida cystica, **A**nencephaly/**A**bdominal wall defects, **F**etal deaths, and **P**lacental abruption.

3. Chorionic villus sampling
    a. It can be performed at 10 weeks of pregnancy.
    b. Cells are aspirated from the chorionic villus.
    c. Cells are evaluated for genetic abnormalities.
4. **Ultrasound**
    a. Measures fetal size, determines sex, and diagnoses fetal malformations

F. Apgar score
1. It is used for physical assessment of child 1 minute and 5 minutes after birth.
2. Five categories are scored 0, 1, or 2, with 2 being indicative of better performance.
    a. Color (blue = 0, trunk pink = 1, all pink = 2)
    b. Heart rate (0 = 0, <100 = 1, 100+ = 2)
    c. Reflexes (none = 0, grimace = 1, grimace and irritable = 2)
    d. Muscle tone (none = 0, some = 1, active = 2)
    e. Respiration (none = 0, irregular = 1, regular = 2)

MNEMONIC

To remember the 5 parts of the Apgar score, think **APGAR**: Appearance, Pulse, Grimace, Activity, Respiration.

II. Abnormal placental attachment

A. **Abruptio placentae**
1. Placenta separates from the uterine wall before parturition.
2. It is associated with painful bleeding in the third trimester.
3. It usually leads to fetal **death**.
4. It may result in hemorrhage and disseminated intravascular coagulation (DIC) in mother.

B. **Placenta accreta**
1. Direct connection of the myometrium to placenta after loss of decidua basalis
2. Caused by prior surgery or trauma during pregnancy
3. Improper separation results in massive **hemorrhage**

C. **Placenta previa**
1. Placenta attaches to the lower uterus and blocks the cervical os.
2. It is associated with **painless bleeding** in the third trimester.

III. Ectopic pregnancy

A. Risk factors
1. **Pelvic inflammatory disease (PID)** (e.g., chronic salpingitis)
2. Previous surgery
3. Endometriosis
4. Previous ectopic pregnancy

B. Clinical features
1. Amenorrhea
2. Pelvic pain and cervical tenderness
3. Tissue mass (usually in the fallopian tubes)
4. Elevated β-hCG levels without intrauterine pregnancy

QUICK HIT

Eclampsia may be treated with magnesium sulfate. However, the treatment of choice for a complete cure is the delivery of the fetus, if feasible.

IV. Preeclampsia

A. Diagnosis requires only **hypertension** and any **proteinuria** during pregnancy. It is often associated with **edema**.
B. Most common in the last trimester of first pregnancy
C. May result in eclampsia if untreated
1. Eclampsia has manifestations similar to preeclampsia, but it also includes seizures and possibly DIC.
2. **HELLP syndrome** is a severe, atypical variant of eclampsia, characterized by Hypertension, Elevated Liver enzymes, and Low Platelets.

QUICK HIT

Hydatidiform moles are the most common precursors of gestational choriocarcinoma (a malignant neoplasm of trophoblastic cells).

V. Hydatidiform mole

A. A benign placental tumor resembling a **"cluster of grapes,"** with a marked increase in β-hCG
B. Manifests as vaginal bleeding and an increase in uterine size
C. "Snowstorm" pattern seen on ultrasound

D. Two types
  1. **Complete mole**
     a. Diploid XX karyotype
     b. No embryo present
     c. Completely paternal in origin
  2. **Partial mole**
     a. Triploid karyotype (XXX, XXY, or XYY)
     b. Embryonic parts may be present

VI. Gestational diabetes

A. Insulin resistance occurs in normal pregnancy.
B. The diagnosis is made using a 3-hour 100-g oral glucose tolerance test, if the patient's serum glucose exceeds two of the four following criteria (exact cutoffs may vary by institution):
  1. Fasting >105 mg/dL
  2. 1 hour >190 mg/dL
  3. 2 hours >165 mg/dL
  4. 3 hours >145 mg/dL
C. High blood glucose leads to hyperglycemia in the fetus, macrosomia (enlarged body), increased risk of birth trauma, and increased likelihood of cesarean section because of the large size of fetus.
D. Neonatal hypoglycemia can occur because the infant's increased insulin production is too great.

VII. Infections causing birth defects (TORCHES)

A. The **TORCHES** are **T**oxoplasmosis, **O**ther infections, **R**ubella, **C**ytomegalovirus infection, **HE**rpes simplex, and **S**yphilis.
B. This group of infectious organisms can cause birth defects if the mother is infected during pregnancy, especially in the first trimester.
  1. Infection with herpes simplex more commonly occurs during the passage through the birth canal.
C. Important agents in the "other" category are HIV, hepatitis B, and parvovirus B19.

GYNECOLOGIC DIAGNOSTIC TESTS

I. Wet mount

A. Vaginal epithelial scrapings placed on a glass slide with a drop of saline
B. Microbes detected
  1. *Trichomonas* appears as a pear-shaped, flagellated organism with sporadic movement.
  2. Bacterial vaginosis appears as vaginal epithelium with spotting and stippling (**clue cells**).

II. Potassium hydroxide (KOH) preparation

A. KOH is added to a microscope slide prepared with vaginal epithelial scrapings.
B. Epithelium is dissolved with KOH.
C. Microbes detected
  1. *Candida,* which is resistant to KOH, remains on the slide and is identified by its **budding cells with short hyphae**.
  2. KOH reacts with bacterial amines, producing a "fishy odor" characteristic of bacterial vaginosis (whiff test).

III. Papanicolaou (Pap) smear

A. Cells from the cervix are scraped and fixed onto a glass slide.
B. Human papilloma virus (HPV) is characterized by **koilocytes** (large epithelial cells with perinuclear clearing).
C. Precancerous lesions detected: cervical intraepithelial neoplasia (**CIN**) 1, 2, and 3

D. Cancers detected
1. Invasive **squamous cell carcinoma** (most common)
2. Cervical adenocarcinoma

SEXUALLY TRANSMITTED DISEASES

Between 20% and 50% of those patients with one sexually transmitted disease (STD) will have a coexisting infection with another. The sexual partners of those diagnosed with an STD should be treated. Physicians should encourage their patients to make partners aware of potential STD risk and urge them to seek diagnosis and treatment (Table 8-4).

TABLE 8-4 **Sexually Transmitted Diseases**

Microbe	Disease
Klebsiella granulomatis	Granuloma inguinale; biopsy shows **Donovan bodies**
Chlamydia trachomatis	Urethritis; **acute pelvic inflammatory disease;** cervicitis; serotypes L1, L2, and L3 cause lymphogranuloma venereum, with ulcerative lesions of the genitalia
Gardnerella vaginalis	Vulvovaginitis, bacterial vaginosis
Haemophilus ducreyi	Chancroid; **painful** ulcerative lesions of the genitalia
Herpes simplex virus-2	Genital herpes; urethritis; **painful** ulcerative lesions of the genitalia
HIV types 1 and 2	**AIDS**
Human papilloma virus (especially serotypes 6 and 11)	**Genital or anal warts** (condyloma acuminatum) of vulva
Human papilloma virus (especially serotypes 16, 18, 31, and 45)	**Squamous cell carcinoma** of cervix, vagina, anus, or penis; CIN
Neisseria gonorrhoeae	Urethritis; **acute pelvic inflammatory disease;** cervicitis; pharyngitis; monoarticular **arthritis**
Treponema pallidum	Syphilis: Primary syphilis—chancres (**painless** ulcerative lesions of the genitalia) Secondary syphilis—gray, wartlike lesions on the genitalia (condyloma lata); rash on palms and soles Tertiary syphilis—neurologic manifestations such as tabes dorsalis and ascending aortic aneurysm
Trichomonas vaginalis	Vulvovaginitis; male urethritis

CIN, cervical intraepithelial neoplasia.

FEMALE GYNECOLOGIC NEOPLASMS

Tumors of the gynecologic organs may manifest themselves as abnormal uterine bleeding and, as such, a heightened level of suspicion must be maintained with this presentation. Many of these neoplasms can be detected, and even prevented (as is the case with cervical cancer), by routine gynecologic examinations.

I. **Ovarian neoplasms of epithelial cell origin** *(Table 8-5)*

II. **Ovarian neoplasms of germ cell origin** *(Table 8-6)*

III. **Tumors of the uterus (cervix and body)** *(Table 8-7)*

IV. **Tumors of the vulva and vagina** *(Table 8-8)*

QUICK HIT

Chlamydia is the most common bacterial sexually transmitted disease (STD) in the world in part because of the fact that it goes undetected so frequently. If a person is diagnosed with gonorrhea, treatment for gonorrhea should be supplemented with chlamydia therapy for both the patient and his or her partner.

MNEMONIC

To remember the painful ulcers of the genitalia, think in *Haemophilus ducreyi* "you do cry," and HSV**2** is painful, **too.** Syphi**lis** is pain**less**.

QUICK HIT

Some nonsexually transmitted infections of the genitourinary tract include *Candida albicans,* which causes vulvovaginitis; *Staphylococcus aureus,* which can result in toxic shock syndrome; and *Escherichia coli* and *Staphylococcus saprophyticus,* both of which can cause urinary tract infections (UTIs).

QUICK HIT

Salpingitis, often associated with PID, can lead to infertility if left untreated.

QUICK HIT

PID can be diagnosed via bimanual pelvic examination eliciting **"the chandelier sign"** (exquisite cervical motion tenderness).

MNEMONIC

Remember the features of *Trichomonas* with the four Fs: **F**lagella, **F**rothy discharge, **F**ishy odor, and **F**lagyl (treatment).

QUICK HIT

Toxic shock syndrome can result from bacterial (*Staphylococcus aureus*) overgrowth on tampons. The enterotoxin involved acts as a supertoxin, causing excess activation of T-helper cells, resulting in an increased cytokine production and septic shock.

QUICK HIT

Of ovarian neoplasms, 75% are epithelial in origin. These tumors are usually seen in middle-aged to elderly women.

QUICK HIT

CA-125 (cancer antigen 125) is elevated in more than 80% of ovarian carcinomas.

QUICK HIT

Germ cell tumors account for only 25% of ovarian neoplasms, but they are the most common ovarian tumors found in women younger than 20 years of age.

TABLE 8-5 Ovarian Neoplasms of Epithelial Cell Origin

Neoplasm	Morphology	Clinical Presentation
Serous cystadenoma	Cystic	Benign; frequently bilateral
Serous cystadenocarcinoma	Cystic	Malignant; frequently bilateral; most common (50% of ovarian neoplasms)
Mucinous cystadenoma	Mucin-filled cysts	Benign
Mucinous cystadenocarcinoma	Mucin-filled cysts	Malignant; **pseudomyxoma peritonei** (diffuse peritoneal metastasis secreting mucin)
Endometrioid adenocarcinoma	Resembles endometrium	Malignant
Brenner tumor	Resembles **transitional epithelium**	Benign; rare tumor
Clear cell cancer	Abundant **clear cytoplasm**	Usually unilateral; rare

TABLE 8-6 Ovarian Neoplasms of Germ Cell Origin

Neoplasm	Morphology	Clinical Features
Dysgerminoma	Large cells with clear cytoplasm	Malignant; **equivalent of seminoma;** occurs in children
Endodermal sinus (yolk sac)	Resembles yolk sac	Malignant; produces **AFP**
Immature teratoma	Elements from multiple embryonic layers; poorly differentiated; resembles fetal or embryonic tissue	Malignant
Mature teratoma (dermoid cyst)	Elements from multiple embryonic layers, including hair, bone, tooth, and nervous tissue; duplication of maternal genetics; resembles adult tissue	**Most common germ cell neoplasm** (90%); **benign** (versus malignant in males)
Monodermal teratoma	Elements from multiple embryonic layers; one tissue type develops, most commonly thyroid tissue **(struma ovarii)**	Benign; hyperthyroidism
Choriocarcinoma	Usually seen in combination with other germ cell tumors	Malignant; produces **(β-hCG)**
Granulosa-theca tumor	Lipid-laden cells; fibroblast proliferation; cuboidal cells in cords; eosinophilic follicles **(Call–Exner bodies)**	Benign; may secrete estrogen, leading to precocious puberty or endometrial hyperplasia or carcinoma
Thecoma fibroma	Fibroblast proliferation	Benign; rare; in combination with ascites and hydrothorax, referred to as **Meigs syndrome**
Sertoli–Leydig cell tumor	Tubules containing Sertoli and Leydig cells	Produces testosterone; virilization
Metastasis	Most commonly from gastrointestinal tract, breast, or ovary; **Krukenberg tumor,** primary from stomach with signet-ring cells bilaterally	Only 5% of ovarian neoplasms

AFP, α-fetoprotein; hCG, human chorionic gonadotropin.

TABLE 8-7 **Tumors of the Uterus (Cervix and Body)**

Neoplasm	Clinical Features
Cervical intraepithelial neoplasia (CIN)	• May be classified as CIN I, CIN II, or CIN III • Neoplastic changes in the endometrium beginning at the **squamocolumnar junction** • CIN I: mild dysplasia extending less than one-third the thickness of the epithelium • CIN II: cells appear more malignant with increased mitotic figures and variation in nuclear size; approximately two-thirds of the epithelium involved • CIN III: also called carcinoma in situ; involves the full thickness of the cervical epithelium • Associated with HPV 16, 18, 31, 33, and 45 infection
Squamous cell carcinoma of the cervix	• Evolves from a progression of CIN • Increased incidence is associated with **early sexual activity** and **multiple sex partners**, smoking, and immunosuppression
Leiomyoma	• Benign tumor of the uterine body • The **most common tumor of women** (the most common malignancy in women is breast cancer) • Often multiple • Size increases with pregnancy and decreases with menopause
Leiomyosarcoma	• Uncommon • Does not arise from a preexisting dysplastic or neoplastic condition (fibroids)
Endometrial carcinoma	• The **most common malignancy** of the female genital tract • Associated with nulliparity • More often found in older women • Exogenous **estrogen** administration or estrogen-producing tumors may be the predisposing factors • Other risk factors are diabetes, tamoxifen, hypertension, and obesity • Usually presents as vaginal bleeding

HPV, human papilloma virus.

TABLE 8-8 **Tumors of the Vulva and Vagina**

Tumor	Description
Papillary hidradenoma	• **Most common** benign tumor of the vulva • Often presents as an ulcerated and bleeding nodule • Originates from apocrine sweat glands • Can easily be surgically removed
Squamous cell carcinoma of the vulva	• Similar to squamous cell carcinoma of the cervix • Highest occurrence in **older women** • Vulvar dystrophy precedes carcinoma • Associated with the infections of HPV 16, 18, 31, 33, and 45
Paget disease of the vulva	• Noninvasive intraepithelial adenocarcinoma, similar to Paget disease of the breast • Not always associated with underlying adenocarcinoma (unlike Paget disease of the breast)
Malignant melanoma	• Similar to malignant melanoma of the skin • 10% of malignant tumors of the vulva
Squamous cell carcinoma of the vagina	• The vagina is rarely a primary site of cancer formation • Usually an extension of squamous cell carcinoma of the cervix
Clear cell adenocarcinoma	• A rare malignant tumor • Occurs in the daughters of women given **diethylstilbestrol (DES)** during pregnancy
Sarcoma botryoides	• A type of rhabdomyosarcoma • Usually occurs in **girls younger than 5** years of age • **"Bunch of grapes"** that protrude from the vagina

HPV, human papilloma virus.

QUICK HIT

Estrogens can be synthesized by adipose tissue. This may be partially responsible for predisposing obese women to endometrial carcinoma.

QUICK HIT

Male breast cancer represents 1% of all breast cancers.

BREAST PATHOLOGY

Risk factors for breast cancer include being older than 45 years of age, nulliparity, early menarche, late menopause, high-fat diet, *HER-2*/neu oncogene activation, first-degree relative with positive history, and a history of breast cancer in the contralateral breast (Table 8-9).

TABLE 8-9 **Breast Pathology**

Condition	Pathology	Clinical Features
Acute mastitis	Entry of ***Staphylococcus aureus*** through nipple; focal cellulitis versus abscess	Most often occurs during **nursing;** may be caused by eczema
Fibrocystic changes	Breast mass; tender during menstruation; usually **bilateral; "blue-domed"** cysts	**Most common breast disorder;** nonneoplastic hypertrophy of breast tissue that is hormonally mediated; predisposition to cancer only if there is evidence of cellular atypia
Fibroadenoma	Painless; rubbery mass	Benign; **most common tumor in patients younger than 25 years of age;** not a precursor to malignancy
Intraductal papilloma	Tumor of the lactiferous ducts	May present as **serous discharge** or bloody discharge; benign, small risk of cancer
Phyllodes tumor	Large, bulky mass; cysts; leaflike projections; ulceration of the skin	Malignant potential, though most are benign; may recur
Ductal carcinoma in situ (DCIS)	Tumor cells fill the ducts but do not penetrate basement membrane; **comedocarcinoma** associated with caseous necrosis and cheesy discharge	Malignant; may progress to invasive
Lobular carcinoma in situ (LCIS)	Tumor cells do not penetrate basement membrane; estrogen-receptor (ER) and progesterone-receptor (PR) positive	Malignant; no palpable lesion—**usually found incidentally** on breast biopsy; associated with infiltrating ductal cancers arising from other lesions
Infiltrating ductal carcinoma	Firm mass; cells may form glands; fibrous stroma	Malignant; **most common** carcinoma of the breast; may be progression of ductal carcinoma in situ
Infiltrating lobular carcinoma	Cells line up **"single file"; inactivation of E-cadherin**	Malignant; often multiple and bilateral**; bloody discharge**
Paget disease	Superficial lesion of nipple or areola; **Paget cells** in epidermis (large cell with marginal clearing seen)	Malignant; indicative of **underlying ductal carcinoma**
Medullary carcinoma	Soft, fleshy tumor; characterized by lymphocytic infiltrate	Malignant
Inflammatory breast cancer	Inflammatory changes superimposed on any histologic type of breast cancer	Findings may include peau d'orange, dimpling of the breast, nipple retraction

QUICK HIT

Breast cancer is the **most common cancer** of women but the second leading cause of cancer death after lung cancer. The most common location is the upper outer quadrant.

QUICK HIT

The presence of estrogen or progesterone receptors on breast cancer reflects a good prognosis because of the ability to use hormonal (antiestrogen) therapy.

QUICK HIT

Gynecomastia (enlargement of the breast tissue in males) can be caused by marijuana, alcoholism, cimetidine, ketoconazole, spironolactone, and digitalis.

QUICK HIT

Tamoxifen, a selective estrogen receptor modulator, can be used to treat advanced breast cancer in postmenopausal women. It can lead to the regression of estrogen-stimulated tumors in some cases.

PROSTATE PATHOLOGY *(Figure 8-10)*

FIGURE 8-10 The prostate

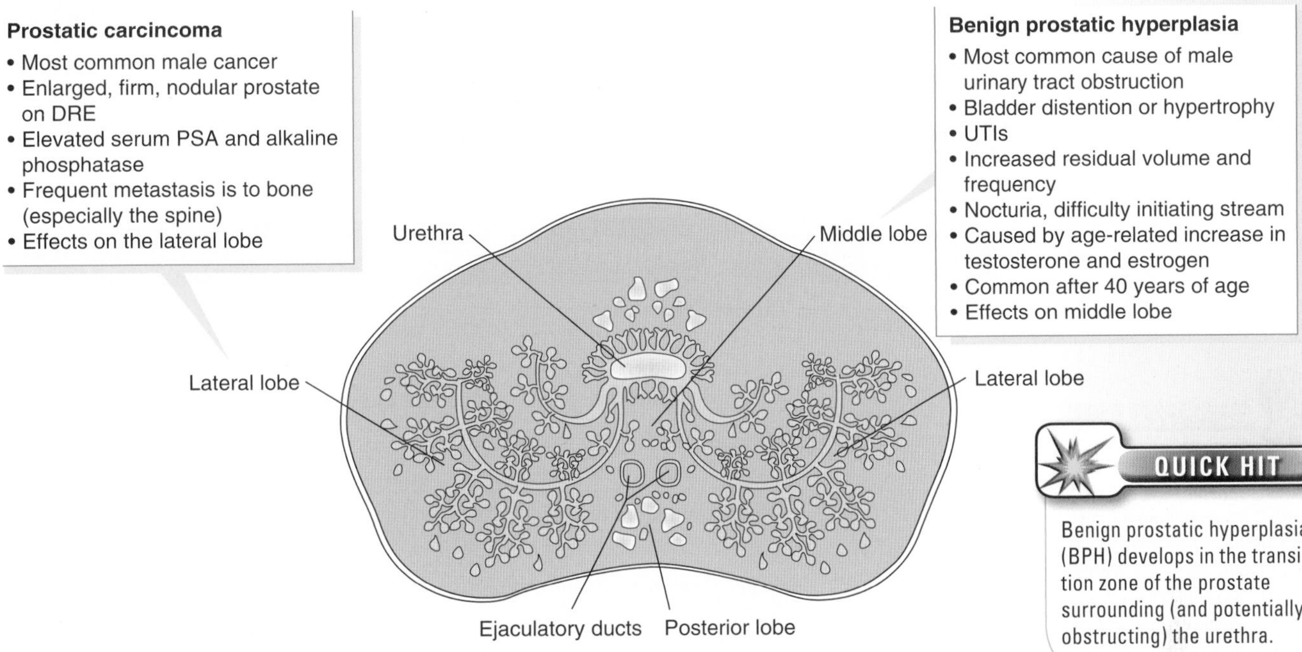
Prostatic carcincoma
• Most common male cancer
• Enlarged, firm, nodular prostate on DRE
• Elevated serum PSA and alkaline phosphatase
• Frequent metastasis is to bone (especially the spine)
• Effects on the lateral lobe
Benign prostatic hyperplasia
• Most common cause of male urinary tract obstruction
• Bladder distention or hypertrophy
• UTIs
• Increased residual volume and frequency
• Nocturia, difficulty initiating stream
• Caused by age-related increase in testosterone and estrogen
• Common after 40 years of age
• Effects on middle lobe
Urethra
Middle lobe
Lateral lobe
Lateral lobe
Ejaculatory ducts
Posterior lobe

DRE, digital rectal examination; PSA, prostate-specific antigen; UTI, urinary tract infection.

QUICK HIT

Benign prostatic hyperplasia (BPH) develops in the transition zone of the prostate surrounding (and potentially obstructing) the urethra.

QUICK HIT

BPH is not a precancerous disorder, and it cannot be accurately diagnosed by measuring prostate-specific antigen (PSA).

QUICK HIT

Prostate cancer is the second most common cause of cancer death in males. The leading cause is lung cancer.

QUICK HIT

The digital rectal examination is essential because many of the male pelvic organs can be assessed. When the examining finger is introduced into the rectum, anal tone (S_2S_4 innervation) can be evaluated. Anteriorly, from inferior to superior, lies the lower border of the prostate, the posterior aspect of the prostate, and the bladder, if distended.

Clinical Vignette 8-2

CLINICAL PRESENTATION: A 55-year-old man presents to his primary care physician with the chief complaint of **frequent urination** that has increased over the past few months. Although he feels an **urgent need to urinate immediately,** the patient finds that he has a **weak urinary stream** with **intermittent flow** and that he is **straining to urinate,** with resulting feeling of **incomplete emptying.** Also, the patient reports **waking to urinate** at night and has noted **some blood in his urine** lately. Rectal examination deferred reveals an enlarged prostate with no nodules palpable. Otherwise, the physical examination is benign and the vital signs are stable.

DIFFERENTIAL: Benign prostatic hyperplasia (BPH), urethral strictures, urinary tract infection, bladder cancer, bladder stone, and bladder trauma. Lower urinary tract symptoms can be best remembered by the mnemonic **WISE FUN. WISE** refers to the obstructive symptoms: **W**eak urinary stream, **I**ntermittent flow, **S**training to urinate, and incomplete **E**mptying. **FUN** refers to the irritative symptoms: **F**requency, **U**rgency, and **N**octuria. BPH can present with any of these lower urinary tract symptoms and also hematuria. Urethral strictures can also result in obstructive symptoms, urinary tract infection (UTI) in irritative symptoms, and bladder cancer/stones/trauma in hematuria.

LABORATORY STUDIES: **Urinalysis** and **urine culture** should be obtained to rule out urinary tract infection. Also, **ultrasound** is useful for determining the bladder and prostate size but is not commonly used in initial evaluation of uncomplicated cases. More precise measurements of prostate can be made via **transrectal ultrasound,** which is indicated in select patients.

MANAGEMENT: An **α-blocker** relaxes the prostatic smooth muscle and is the first-line treatment for BPH. The most common side effect is dizziness. A **5α-reductase** inhibitor (finasteride) reduces symptoms by reducing the volume of the prostate. If pharmacologic therapy is unsuccessful, **transurethral resection of the prostate** is the gold standard surgical procedure for the treatment of BPH. Open radical prostatectomy is a cancer operation and is ***not*** indicated for benign prostatic obstruction.

TESTICULAR PATHOLOGY

Anatomic disorders of the testis occur more often in young children, whereas the infectious and neoplastic diseases are more likely to occur in the young adult, sexually active population. Routine testicular examinations can often prevent and detect serious complications. When detected early, testicular neoplasms are one of the most curable cancers.

I. Testicular disorders *(Table 8-10)*

II. Testicular neoplasms *(Table 8-11)*

MNEMONIC

To remember the layers of the scrotum, consider the phrase "Some Darn Englishman Called It The Testis"; from superficial to deep: **S**kin, **D**artos, **E**xternal spermatic fascia, **C**remaster, **I**nternal spermatic fascia, **T**unica vaginalis, and **T**estis.

TABLE **8-10** Testicular Disorders

Disorder	Clinical Features
Hydrocele	• **Serous fluid** collects in the tunica vaginalis • Caused by **patency** between the peritoneal cavity and the tunica vaginalis
Hematocele	• **Blood** collects in the tunica vaginalis • Usually caused by **trauma**
Varicocele	• **Engorgement of the veins** of the spermatic cord • Most noticeable when patient is standing
Spermatocele	• Epididymal cyst containing **sperm**
Cryptorchidism	• **Failure** of one or both of the testes to **descend** • Increased incidence of **germ cell testicular cancer** such as seminoma and embryonal carcinoma (see testicular neoplasms [Table 8-11]) • Failure of descent leads to testicular **atrophy, sterility,** and increased risk of **germ cell neoplasia**
Testicular torsion	• **Twisting** of the spermatic cord • If untreated, will result in **testicular** necrosis
Orchitis	• Testicular infection and inflammation • May be viral or bacterial in origin • Can lead to **sterility if bilateral**
Epididymitis	• **Inflammation and infection** of the epididymis • Most often caused by ***Neisseria gonorrhoeae, Chlamydia trachomatis,*** *Escherichia coli, and Mycobacterium tuberculosis*

TABLE **8-11** Testicular Neoplasms

Neoplasm	Site of Origin; Morphology	Clinical Features
Seminoma	Germ cell; arranged in lobules or nests	Malignant; incidence highest in 35–40-year-olds; painless enlargement of testis; **most common germ cell tumor;** similar to dysgerminoma of the ovary; radiosensitive and curable
Embryonal carcinoma	Germ cell; variable morphology with papillary convolutions	Malignant; highest incidence in men in their 20s; more aggressive than seminomas; very common in mixed tumors
Yolk sac tumor (endodermal sinus tumor)	Germ cell; anastomosing cords; malignant; presents with pain or metastasis; similar to ovarian tumor; peak incidence in childhood (infants to 3 years of age); increased **AFP**	

(continued)

TABLE 8-11 **Testicular Neoplasms** *(Continued)*

Neoplasm	Site of Origin; Morphology	Clinical Features
Teratoma	Two or more embryonic layers; **multiple tissue types** such as cartilage, epithelium, liver, and muscle	Malignant; occurs at any age but more common in children; mature: heterogeneous tissue in organoid fashion; immature: incompletely differentiated
Mixed germ cell tumor	Variable	Malignant; aggressive; more than one neoplastic pattern; **most common**
Leydig cell tumor (interstitial)	Testicular stroma; intracytoplasmic **Reinke crystals**	Benign; produces androgens, estrogens, or corticosteroids; often seen with **precocious puberty** or gynecomastia; similar to ovarian Sertoli–Leydig cell tumor
Sertoli cell tumor	Testicular stroma; forms cordlike structures	Benign; minor endocrine abnormalities; similar to ovarian Sertoli–Leydig cell tumor
Choriocarcinoma	Trophoblastic cells; villous structures resembling placenta	Malignant; hemorrhagic; **β-hCG** elevated; peaks in early adulthood

AFP, α-fetoprotein; hCG, human chorionic gonadotropin.

HIV

I. Etiology *(Figure 8-11)*

A. HIV-1 (more common) or HIV-2 **retrovirus**
B. Transmitted by:
  1. Sexual contact
  2. **Intravenous (IV) drug abusers** sharing needles
  3. Contact with bodily fluids (blood, semen, breast milk, etc.)
  4. Mother to fetus (transplacentally)
C. Not transmitted through:
  1. Casual contact
  2. Toilet seats
  3. Kissing
  4. Mosquitoes
D. Occupational risk to healthcare workers is low. A needle stick with an HIV-positive patient's blood carries a **0.3% chance of transmission**.

II. Pathology

A. Primary infection
  1. Transmitted virus infects **T-helper lymphocytes** (cluster of differentiation 4 [CD4]) via the interaction of viral proteins **gp120** and **gp41** with each other and the CD4 marker (Figure 8-11 and Table 8-12).
  2. The virus also infects macrophages and monocytes (proposed portal of entry into the central nervous system).
  3. Viremia is accompanied by the "**acute retroviral syndrome**" (a flulike illness).
  4. The first month is the **window period** as p24 antigen is not yet detectable in the blood (patient is contagious).
B. Chronic infection
  1. Immune response lowers viral blood counts, but active replication persists.
  2. No clinical symptoms for up to 10 years (latent period).
  3. CD4 count steadily declines.
  4. Near end of the latent period, constitutional symptoms develop
    a. Weight loss
    b. Fever
    c. Night sweats
    d. Adenopathy

QUICK HIT

The gene encoding the gp120 envelope protein mutates rapidly, protecting the HIV from elimination by providing **genetic variation**.

FIGURE 8-11 **Replication of HIV and its effect**

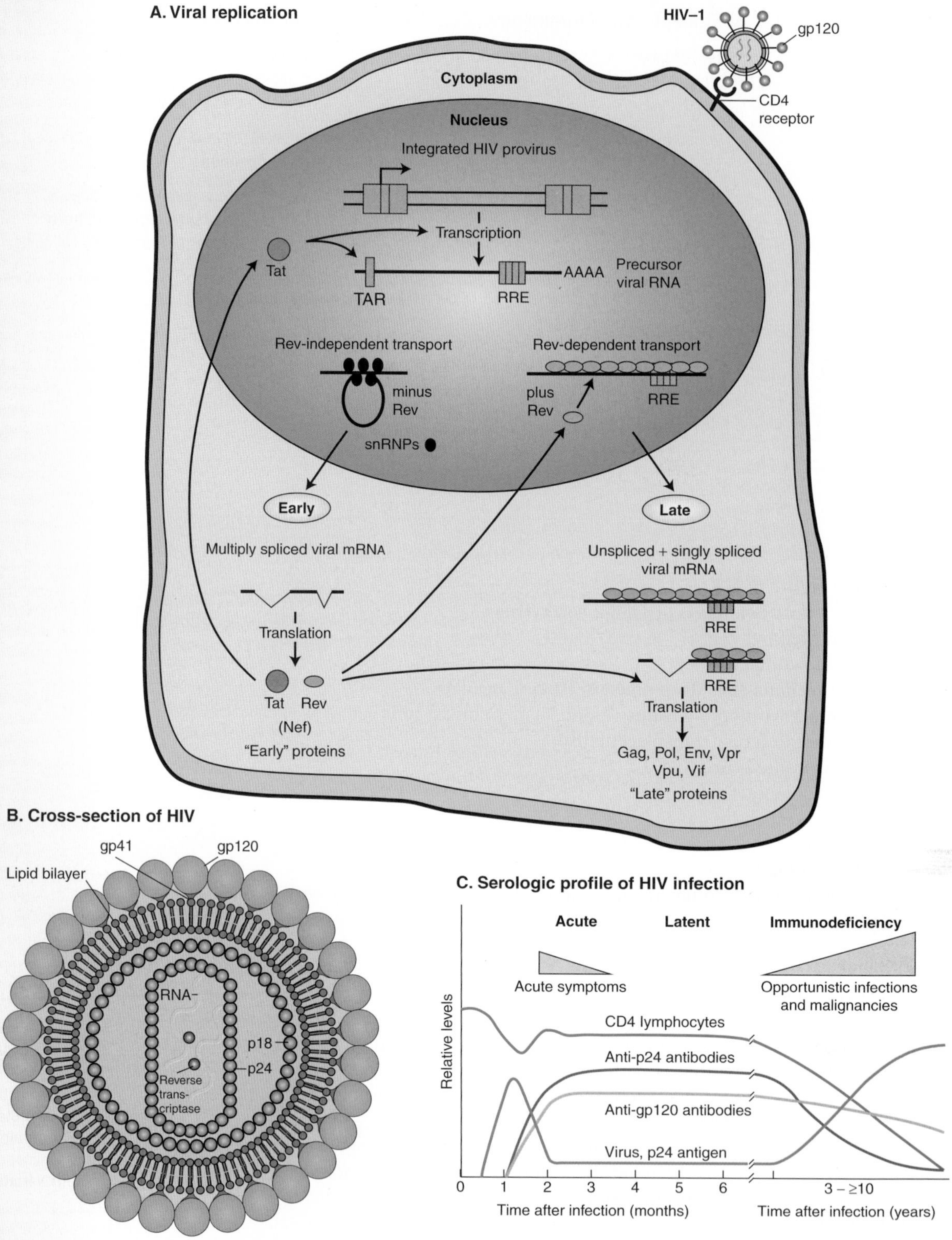
A. Viral replication
HIV–1
gp120
CD4 receptor
Cytoplasm
Nucleus
Integrated HIV provirus
Transcription
Tat
TAR
RRE
AAAA
Precursor viral RNA
Rev-independent transport
minus Rev
snRNPs
Rev-dependent transport
plus Rev
RRE
Early
Multiply spliced viral mRNA
Translation
Tat Rev
(Nef)
"Early" proteins
Late
Unspliced + singly spliced viral mRNA
RRE
RRE
Translation
Gag, Pol, Env, Vpr
Vpu, Vif
"Late" proteins
B. Cross-section of HIV
gp41
gp120
Lipid bilayer
RNA
p18
p24
Reverse trans-criptase
C. Serologic profile of HIV infection
Acute
Latent
Immunodeficiency
Acute symptoms
Opportunistic infections and malignancies
CD4 lymphocytes
Anti-p24 antibodies
Anti-gp120 antibodies
Virus, p24 antigen
Relative levels
0 1 2 3 4 5 6
3 – ≥10
Time after infection (months)
Time after infection (years)

Env, envelope protein; Gag, group-specific core antigen; gp, glycoprotein; mRNA, messenger RNA; nef, negative factor; Pol, polymerase; Rev, regulator of viral protein expression; RRE, Rev response element; snRNP, small nuclear ribonucleoprotein particle; TAR, trans-activation response; TAT, transcriptional transactivator; Vif, viral infectivity; Vpr, viral protein R; Vpu, viral protein U.

TABLE 8-12 **HIV Proteins and Function**

Gene	Product and Function
gag	Viral core proteins p17 and p24
pol	Protease, integrase, reverse transcriptase, and RNase H
env	gp120 and gp41
tat	Transcriptional transactivator (increases gene expression); essential for replication
rev	Transition from early to late gene expression; protein transport from nucleus to cytoplasm; essential for replication
nef	Transcriptional silencer; may produce latent infection
vif	Viral infectivity gene; cell-to-cell transmission
vpu	Viral protein U; viral particle export
vpr	Viral protein R; activates viral and cellular promoters

C. AIDS
1. Defined as a **CD4 count of ≤200 cells/mL** or the presence of certain **opportunistic** infections
2. Infections typically seen with AIDS
   a. ***Pneumocystis jirovecii* pneumonia** (80%)
   b. **Kaposi sarcoma** (human herpes virus [HHV]-8)
   c. B-cell lymphoma (brain and bone marrow)
   d. *Toxoplasma gondii* (brain tissue infection)
   e. CMV (leads to retinitis)
   f. *Cryptococcus neoformans* (meningeal infection)
   g. *Mycobacterium avium-intracellulare* (MAI)
   h. Tuberculosis (TB)
   i. *Candida albicans* (thrush, esophagitis)
   j. *Cryptosporidium* (chronic diarrhea)

D. Epidemiology
1. In the United States, during the 1980s, the infection first spread among **male homosexuals**.
2. **IV drug abusers** and **hemophiliacs** (before tests were developed to screen blood) were the next populations affected.
3. **Heterosexual** transmission is rising in the United States and is now the leading cause of infection in Africa.

E. Laboratory diagnosis
1. The **enzyme-linked immunosorbent assay (ELISA) test** for antibodies lends a presumptive diagnosis (screening test).
2. This must be confirmed by the **Western blot** test, which demonstrates antibodies to gp41 or p24 (Figure 8-11).

III. Treatment *(Table 8-13)*

A. Agents used in the treatment of HIV include **protease inhibitors**, **nucleoside reverse transcriptase inhibitors**, **non-nucleoside reverse transcriptase inhibitors**, **integrase strand transfer inhibitors**, **C-C chemokine receptor type 5 (CCR5) antagonists**, and **fusion inhibitors**.

B. Combination therapy has drastically improved HIV treatment by forestalling the development of resistance to medication and is referred to as **highly active antiretroviral therapy (HAART)**.
1. Two reverse transcriptase inhibitors are combined with a third agent—often a protease inhibitor or non-nucleoside reverse transcriptase inhibitor.
2. Therapy should be initiated before compromise of the immune system occurs.
3. Ideally, therapy should be based on the genotype or phenotype results from the particular virus isolated from the patient.

TABLE 8-13 Therapeutic Agents in HIV

Therapeutic Agent (common name, if relevant)	Class—Pharmacology and Pharmacokinetics	Indications	Side Effects or Adverse Effects	Contraindications or Precautions to Consider; Notes
Saquinavir (SQV), ritonavir (RTV), indinavir (IDV), nelfinavir, amprenavir, lopinavir, atazanavir, tipranavir, darunavir	**Protease inhibitor**—protease responsible for final step of viral proliferation; inhibits protease in progeny virions → assembly of nonfunctional viruses	**HAART**	**GI irritation (nausea and diarrhea), hyperglycemia, hyperlipidemia, lipodystrophy, thrombocytopenia (indinavir)**	**All protease inhibitors ending in -navir; metabolism occurs by CYP450**
Zidovudine (ZDV; formerly azidothymidine [AZT]	**NRTI—guanosine analog →** inhibits viral reverse transcriptase → prevents integration of DNA copy of viral genome into host DNA	**HAART; HIV pregnant women** to reduce fetal transmission	**Neutropenia, anemia** (megaloblastic anemia), **peripheral neuropathy, pancreatitis, and lactic acidosis**	**Effects of bone marrow suppression such as neutropenia and anemia can be reduced by the addition of GM-CSF**
Abacavir (ABC)	**NRTI—guanosine analog** (similar to Zidovudine)	**HAART**	**Neutropenia, anemia, peripheral neuropathy, pancreatitis, lactic acidosis, hypersensitivity reaction (can be fatal)**	Check HLA-B*5701 test prior to starting ABC to avoid giving to patients at risk for hypersensitivity reactions
Didanosine (ddI)	**NRTI—guanosine analog;** (similar to Zidovudine)	**HAART**	**Neutropenia, anemia, peripheral neuropathy, pancreatitis, and lactic acidosis**	
Lamivudine (3TC)	**NRTI—cytidine analog →** inhibits viral reverse transcriptase → prevents integration of DNA copy of the viral genome into the host DNA	**HAART**	**Neutropenia, anemia, peripheral neuropathy, pancreatitis, and lactic acidosis**	
Emtricitabine (FTC)	**NRTI—cytidine analog** (similar to Lamivudine)	**HAART**	**Neutropenia, anemia, peripheral neuropathy, pancreatitis, and lactic acidosis**	
Tenofovir disoproxil fumarate (TDF)	**Nucleotide reverse transcriptase inhibitor—adenosine analog →** inhibits viral reverse transcriptase	**HAART**	**Nausea, vomiting, headache, renal dysfunction**	
Nevirapine, efavirenz, delavirdine, etravirine	**NNRTI**—binds viral reverse transcriptase and inhibits the movement of protein domains → terminates viral DNA synthesis → prevents integration of viral genome into the host DNA	**HAART;** noncompetitive inhibitors of reverse transcriptase	**Neutropenia, anemia, peripheral neuropathy, and rash** Efavirenz: depression, dizziness, vivid dreams, **teratogenic**	
Raltegravir	**Integrase inhibitor**—inhibits the final step in integration of viral DNA into host DNA	**HAART**	**Neutropenia, pancreatitis, hepatotoxicity, hyperglycemia**	
Enfuvirtide	**Fusion inhibitor**—binds viral gp41 subunit → inhibits conformation change (required for fusion with CD4 cell) → blocks viral entry and replication	**Patients on antiretroviral therapy with persistent viral replication**	**Hypersensitivity reactions; reaction at injection site; bacterial pneumonia**	**Used in combination with other antiretroviral drugs**
Maraviroc	**CCR5 antagonist**—inhibits viral CCR5 coreceptor → blocks viral entry to host cell	**Patients on antiretroviral therapy with persistent viral replication**	**Fever, cough, upper respiratory infections, peripheral neuropathy, dizziness**	

CCR5, C-C chemokine receptor type 5; CD4, cluster of differentiation 4; CYP450, cytochrome P450; GI, gastrointestinal; GM-CSF, granulocyte macrophage colony-stimulating factor; HAART, highly active antiretroviral therapy; NNRTI, non-nucleoside reverse transcriptase inhibitor; NRTI, nucleoside reverse transcriptase inhibitor.

PSYCHOSOCIAL DEVELOPMENT *(Figure 8-12)*

FIGURE 8-12 Stages of development

	Infancy (0–1 y)	Toddler (1–3 y)	School age (3–11 y)	Adolescence (11–20 y)	Early adulthood (20–40 y)	Middle adulthood (40–60 y)	Late adulthood (60–80 y)
Freud	Oral	Anal	Phallic-oedipal (3–6 y); latency (6–11 y)	Genital			
Erikson	Trust versus mistrust	Autonomy versus shame and doubt	Initiative versus guilt (3–6 y); industry versus inferiority	Identity versus role confusion	Intimacy versus isolation	Generativity versus stagnation	Ego integrity versus despair
Piaget	Sensorimotor (0–2 y)	Preoperational (2–7 y)	Concrete operations (7–11 y)	Formal operations			
Characteristics	Reflexes: • Palmar grasp (0–2 m) • Rooting (0–3 m) • Babinski (0–12 m) Milestones: • Turn over (5 m) • Sit (6 m) • Walk (12 m)	Terrible two's ("no"); band-aid (2–4 y); parallel play (2–4 y); balance on one foot (2 y); climb stairs (3 y)	Cooperative play (4–7 y); conservation of mass (7–11 y); button clothes (4 y); throw a ball (4 y);	First menstruation (11 y); first ejaculation (13 y); peer pressure	New family; children; role in society solidified; period of reassessment	Height of career; midlife crises; menopause (45–55 y)	Depression (ECT); women outlive men by 6–8 y; Kübler-Ross (stages of grief and dying) • Denial • Anger • Bargaining • Depression • Acceptance

ECT, electroconvulsive therapy.

THE FAMILY UNIT AND RELATED CONCEPTS

I. Postpartum depression

A. Up to 50% of all women develop a short-lived depression after giving birth (postpartum blues).

B. Etiology
  1. Change in hormone levels
  2. Increased responsibility
  3. Fatigue

C. Major depression is seen in 5% to 10% of all women after childbirth.

II. Attachment of the child to the mother

A. **Anaclitic depression**: sustained absence of mother when child is between 6 and 12 months of age leads to a withdrawn and unresponsive infant.

B. **Harlow** showed that monkeys raised in **isolation** do not develop normally.
  1. Males are more affected than females.
  2. Recovery is not possible if isolation lasts longer than 6 months.

C. **Bowlby** showed that **physical contact** between the mother and the child is crucial to development.

D. **Spitz** observed that children **without proper mothering** are slow to develop and have a greater number of medical problems.

E. **Mahler** documented the development as a process in which the infant **separates** from the mother.
  1. Normal autistic phase (0 to 1 month): infant has little interaction
  2. Symbiotic phase (15 months): infant is close to mother
  3. Separation–individuation phase (5 to 16 months): child realizes individuality and begins to explore the environment.

III. Child abuse

A. It includes physical abuse, sexual abuse, and emotional neglect.
B. Risk factors
  1. Substance abuse by parents
  2. Poverty
  3. Marital problems or single-parent home
C. Physical abuse is marked by numerous fractures, bruises, subdural hematomas, or burns (at various stages of healing).
D. Sexual abuse of children is marked by trauma to the genitalia, sexually transmitted diseases, or urinary tract infections.
E. Abuse predisposes the child to posttraumatic stress disorder (PTSD), dissociative disorders, depression, anorexia, phobias, and personality disorders.
F. Physician intervention is necessary and obligatory.

IV. Family therapy

A. Involves all members of a family even though only one person might have a problem
B. Identifies dysfunctional behavior and encourages communication and problem solving
C. Based on the concept that the family system is composed of subsystems in which boundaries are established and mutual accommodation occurs

SEXUALITY

I. Gender

A. **Gender identity** is an individual's sense of being male or female, whereas **gender role** is the expression of one's gender.
B. Sexual orientation is a physical preference for one or both genders (heterosexual, homosexual, and bisexual).
C. Psychological factors play a role in gender identity and sexual orientation.
  1. **Transsexual**: a person who has the sense of being in the wrong-sex body and has a strong desire to correct it
  2. **Homosexual**: a person who has a sexual preference for same-sex individuals
  3. **Transvestite**: a man who dresses in women's clothing for pleasure, usually heterosexual

II. Sexual dysfunction

A. Premature ejaculation (early climax without reaching plateau phase) is the **most common** male sexual disorder.
B. The most common sexual dysfunction in women is **sexual arousal disorder**, in which lubrication cannot be maintained throughout the sexual act.
C. Impotence (in men)
  1. Failure to achieve erection or ejaculation
  2. Usually has an organic component but may be psychogenic (e.g., caused by stress or anxiety)
    a. It is often related to alcohol abuse.
    b. It may also result from medical problems such as diabetes or illicit drug use.
    c. Psychogenic cause can be confirmed by observing erections during rapid eye movement (REM) sleep.
D. Vaginismus (in women)
  1. Spasm in the outer third of the vagina
  2. Difficulty during intercourse or pelvic examination
  3. Often results from rape, incest, or abuse
E. Paraphilias (Table 8-14)

MNEMONIC

To remember the four phases of normal sexual response, think **EXPLORE: EX**citation, **PL**ateau, **O**rgasm, and **RE**solution.

QUICK HIT

Penile erection is achieved via two crucial steps: (a) parasympathetic-mediated relaxation of arterioles to the penis and (b) mechanical compression of the venous outflow channels.

TABLE 8-14 **Paraphilias**

Category	Description (How Sexual Pleasure is Derived)
Exhibitionism	Exposing one's genitalia
Fetishism	Inanimate objects (e.g., women's high-heeled shoes or undergarments)
Frotteurism	Furtively rubbing genitalia against a woman (e.g., pushing up against a woman in a crowded subway)
Necrophilia	Corpses
Pedophilia	Children
Masochism	Receiving physical or psychological pain and humiliation
Sadism	Inducing physical or psychological pain and humiliation in others
Transvestic fetishism	Wearing women's clothing (such men are still attracted to women)
Voyeurism	Furtively watching individuals engaged in intercourse or seductive activities
Zoophilia	Animals

QUICK HIT

Pedophilia is the **most common** paraphilia and needs to be reported to the authorities on discovery by the physician if the patient acts on this desire.

Clinical Vignette 8-3

CLINICAL PRESENTATION: A 45-year-old man presents to his primary care physician for his yearly physical examination. His past medical history is significant for **diabetes, hypertension,** and **hypercholesterolemia**. He has been keeping physically fit with **lengthy bike rides**. He has not cut back on his tobacco usage and smokes 0.5 pack per day for 5 years. As you review the systems, he tells you that he has had **increasing difficulty achieving a firm erection**. He denies any **recent penile or perineal trauma, surgery, or radiation**. Vital signs: temperature = 97.4° F; respiration rate = 20 breaths/min; blood pressure = 150/90 mm Hg; and heart rate = 85 bpm.

DIFFERENTIALS: Erectile dysfunction (ED) from vascular, neurologic, iatrogenic, traumatic, or psychogenic origin. It is important to note that the bolded items in this patient's history are the risk factors for ED.

LABORATORY STUDIES: Direct injection of prostaglandin E_1 into the corpora should result in a normal erection within minutes if the penile vasculature is normal. **Nocturnal penile tumescence testing** is useful in distinguishing psychogenic from organic impotence. Inadequate nocturnal erections suggest organic dysfunction, whereas normal erection during rapid eye movement (REM) sleep suggests psychogenic etiology. Given his diabetic history, formal **neurologic testing** may be needed.

MANAGEMENT: All patients with ED should be given an empiric trial of **sildenafil** as long as they do not have any contraindications. Contraindications include use of nitrates, active cardiac disease, or hypertension. **Phosphodiesterase inhibitors** such as sildenafil increase cyclic guanosine monophosphate (cGMP), which relaxes the smooth muscle surrounding the penile arterioles with resulting dilation of vasculature and erection. Patients with ED refractory to therapy with oral phosphodiesterase inhibitors should be referred to urology for other therapies such as **vacuum constriction device, prostaglandin E_1 injections,** and surgical placement of a **penile prosthesis.**

QUICK HIT

The core set of symptoms in PTSD is reexperiencing the traumatic event, avoidance, numbing, and arousal or hypervigilance.

RAPE

I. An act of sexual aggression in which the penis penetrates the outer vulva.

II. Rapists tend to be male and tend to rape women of their own race.

A. Roughly, half of the assailants are Black and half are White.
B. Use of weapons and alcohol is common.
C. Rapists are usually young (younger than 25 years of age).
D. Rapes are underreported (usually only 39% of total).
   1. Victims are generally 15 to 30 years of age.
   2. Rape usually occurs inside the woman's home by an individual whom she knows.
E. Rape usually results in rape trauma syndrome, which involves emotional lability for more than 1 year.
   1. Group therapy and support are important treatment modalities.
   2. PTSD may occur even after treatment.
      a. PTSD occurs in a subgroup of individuals exposed to trauma.
      b. Usually develops in adolescents or young adults.

QUICK HIT

The death of a child or the suicide of a spouse is the most severe psychological stressor.

QUICK HIT

Divorced White males older than 65 years of age who have a plan and are taking three or more medications have the highest risk of suicide.

SUICIDE

I. Third-leading cause of death in persons 15 to 24 years of age and eighth leading cause of death in the United States.

II. Women attempt suicide three times more often than men, but men are four times more successful owing to the lethality of the method used.

III. Gay and lesbian youths have a threefold increased risk of suicide because of increased societal pressures and stigmata.

IV. Marriage reduces the risk of suicide.

V. Professional women may be at an increased risk for suicide.

VI. Suicide risk should be assessed during the mental status examination.

A. Patients with a suicide plan are at higher risk.
B. Indications for hospitalization include impulsiveness, lack of social support, and a plan.

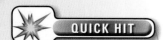

THERAPEUTIC AGENTS FOR THE REPRODUCTIVE SYSTEM *(Table 8-15)*

TABLE 8-15 Therapeutic Agents for the Reproductive System

Therapeutic Agent (common name, if relevant) [trade name, where appropriate]	Class—Pharmacology and Pharmacokinetics	Indications	Side Effects or Adverse Effects	Contraindications or Precautions to Consider; Notes
Hormone antagonists				
Finasteride [Proscar]	**Antiandrogen—5α-reductase inhibitor** → decreases the conversion of testosterone to dihydrotestosterone	**Benign prostatic hyperplasia;** male-pattern baldness	Decreased libido, decreased ejaculate volume	
Flutamide [Eulexin]	**Antiandrogen**—nonsteroidal, competitive androgen receptor blocker	**Metastatic prostate cancer**		

(continued)

TABLE 8-15 **Therapeutic Agents for the Reproductive System** *(Continued)*

Therapeutic Agent (common name, if relevant) [trade name, where appropriate]	Class—Pharmacology and Pharmacokinetics	Indications	Side Effects or Adverse Effects	Contraindications or Precautions to Consider; Notes
Ketoconazole [Nizoral]	**Antiandrogen**—inhibits ergosterol (steroid) synthesis → inhibits adrenal and gonadal steroid synthesis; also prevents cell membrane formation	**Prostate carcinoma, fungal infections**	Nausea, vomiting, diarrhea, rash, headache, anorexia, thrombocytopenia, gynecomastia, hepatotoxic	**Inhibits cytochrome P450**
Spironolactone [Aldactone]	**Antiandrogen**—inhibits steroid binding	**Hirsutism in women, acne in women;** hyperaldosteronism, hypokalemia, hypertension, edema, and CHF	Gynecomastia, breast pain, hyperkalemia, impotence, menstrual irregularities	
Mifepristone (RU-486)	**Antiprogesterone**—synthetic steroid, progesterone receptor blocker → blocks the effects of progesterone → myometrium contraction	**Termination of intrauterine pregnancy**	**Heavy bleeding, uterine cramping,** GI effects (nausea, vomiting, and anorexia)	Controversial "morning after" drug
Anastrozole [Arimidex]	Aromatase inhibitor	**Breast cancer** in postmenopausal women; endometriosis	Hot flashes, nausea, vomiting	Can be used in ER-positive or hormone receptor–unknown breast cancer
Hormone agonists				
Methyltestosterone [Android, Virilon]	**Androgen**—androgen receptor agonist	**In males: hypogonadism, delayed puberty** (promotes secondary sex characteristics), impotence; **In females: estrogen receptor positive breast cancer**	**Masculinization (hirsutism), testicular atrophy,** prostate hyperplasia, prostate cancer, impotence, **stunted growth** (premature epiphyseal plate closure), hyperlipidemia	Decreased testicular testosterone leading to Leydig cell inhibition and gonadal atrophy
Ethinyl estradiol, diethylstilbestrol (DES), mestranol	**Estrogen**—bind estrogen receptor	**In women: hypogonadism, ovarian failure,** menstrual abnormalities; **contraception** **In men: androgen-dependent prostate cancer**	**Endometrial cancer, bleeding, thrombosis**	Used in combination with progestin in patients with intact uterus; increased risk of endometrial cancer with unopposed estrogen therapy; females exposed to DES in utero have an increased risk of **vaginal clear cell adenocarcinoma**
Progesterone, norethindrone, levonorgestrel [Plan B], **norgestimate, desogestrel, gestodene**	**Progesterone**—bind progesterone receptors	**Endometrial cancer;** amenorrhea; abnormal uterine bleeding; **prevention of pregnancy**		Also used to prevent endometrial hyperplasia in postmenopausal women taking estrogen

(continued)

The Reproductive System

TABLE 8-15 **Therapeutic Agents for the Reproductive System** *(Continued)*

Therapeutic Agent (common name, if relevant) [trade name, where appropriate]	Class—Pharmacology and Pharmacokinetics	Indications	Side Effects or Adverse Effects	Contraindications or Precautions to Consider; Notes
Partial agonists and antagonists				
Clomiphene [Clomid]	**Selective estrogen receptor modulator**—binds estrogen receptors in pituitary → prevents normal feedback inhibition, increases LH and FSH release from the pituitary → stimulates ovulation	**Infertility—stimulates ovulation; PCOS**	**Hot flashes, ovarian enlargement, multiple gestation pregnancy, visual disturbances**	
Tamoxifen	**Selective estrogen receptor modular—competitively binds estrogen receptors; breast (estrogen antagonist):** prevents proliferation of estrogen receptor positive tumor cells; **endometrium (partial agonist); bone (agonist):** decreases bone turnover, increases bone density	**Treats estrogen-dependent breast cancer in postmenopausal women;** reduces contralateral breast cancer	**May increase the risk of endometrial cancer; hot flashes;** flushing; increased risk of blood clots	
Raloxifene [Evista]	**Selective estrogen receptor modulator—breast (estrogen antagonist); endometrium (estrogen antagonist):** prevents the proliferation of endometrium; **bone (estrogen agonist):** decreases bone turnover, increases bone density; **cardiovascular (estrogen agonist):** decreases LDL	**Osteoporosis, breast cancer**	**Hot flashes,** sinusitis, weight gain, muscle pain, leg cramps, **increased risk of blood clots**	Unlike estrogen, raloxifene **does not decrease HDL**
Other				
Leuprolide [Lupron]	**GnRH analog**—agonist (when given pulsatile), antagonist (when given continuously)	**Infertility** (given pulsatile), **prostate cancer** (given continuous), **uterine fibroids,** endometriosis, precocious puberty	Nausea, vomiting, antiandrogen effects (testicular atrophy), menopausal symptoms	
Sildenafil [Viagra], **vardenafil** [Levitra], **tadalafil** [Cialis]	**Phosphodiesterase type 5 inhibitor (cGMP-specific)**—increased cGMP → smooth muscle relaxation → increased blood flow in the corpus cavernosum → penile erection	**Erectile dysfunction**	**Abnormal vision** (impaired blue-green color vision), UTIs, **cardiovascular events, priapism, dyspepsia,** headache, flushing	Risk of hypotension (fatal) in a patient taking nitrates
Misoprostol [Cytotec]	**Prostaglandin—PGE_1 analog** → cervical dilation, uterine contractions	**Induction of labor,** termination of pregnancy		
Dinoprostone	Prostaglandin—PGE_2 analog → cervical dilation, uterine contraction	Induction of labor, termination of pregnancy		
Ritodrine, terbutaline	β agonist → uterine relaxation	Inhibits preterm labor; used to treat uterine hyperstimulation in labor		

(continued)

TABLE 8-15 **Therapeutic Agents for the Reproductive System** *(Continued)*

Therapeutic Agent (common name, if relevant) [trade name, where appropriate]	Class—Pharmacology and Pharmacokinetics	Indications	Side Effects or Adverse Effects	Contraindications or Precautions to Consider; Notes
Combination oral contraceptives	**Combination of estrogen and progesterone—estrogen →** inhibits midcycle surge of gonadotropin secretion → prevents ovulation; **progesterone →** alters endometrium cervical mucus, tube motility, and peristalsis → less suitable for sperm penetration and implantation	**Contraception, acne, hirsutism, PCOS**		Contraindicated in patients with stroke or prior thromboembolic event, estrogen-dependent tumor, pregnancy, hypertriglyceridemia, **heavy smokers;** avoid use in women with migraines with aura and poorly controlled hypertension
Hormone replacement therapy	**Combination of estrogen and progesterone**	**Menopause** (relief of symptoms), osteoporosis, vulvar/vaginal atrophy, hypoestrogenism (hypogonadism)	Possible increased risk of **stroke**	Combination of progesterone and estrogen is used because **unopposed estrogen increases the risk of endometrial cancer**

cGMP, cyclic guanosine monophosphate; CHF, congestive heart failure; ER, estrogen receptor; FSH, follicle-stimulating hormone; GI, gastrointestinal; GnRH, gonadotropin-releasing hormone; HDL, high-density lipoprotein; LDL, low-density lipoprotein; LH, luteinizing hormone; PCOS, polycystic ovary syndrome; PGE, prostaglandin E; UTI, urinary tract infection.

9 The Musculoskeletal System

DEVELOPMENT

I. Bone formation

A. **Endochondral bone**
   1. Forms over a cartilage frame
   2. Becomes the **long bones** of the skeleton (e.g., **femur**)

B. **Membranous bone**
   1. Forms without a cartilage frame
   2. Becomes the **flat bones** of the skeleton (e.g., bones of the cranium)

II. Skeletal muscle

A. It derives from **somites**.
B. Each somite produces its own **myotome**.
C. Each somite produces its own **dermatome**.

III. Pharyngeal arches

Begin to develop in the **fourth week** and originate from **neural crest cells**.

A. **Arch 1**
   1. Innervated by the mandibular branch of the trigeminal nerve (**cranial nerve** [CN] V)
   2. Gives rise to the following muscles:
      a. Muscles of mastication (temporalis, masseter, lateral pterygoid, medial pterygoid)
      b. Two tensor muscles (tensor veli palatini, tensor tympani)
      c. Two other muscles (mylohyoid, anterior belly of the digastric)
   3. Gives rise to the following skeletal structures:
      a. Malleus
      b. Incus
   4. Gives rise to the following ligamentous structures:
      a. Anterior ligament of malleus
      b. Sphenomandibular ligament

B. **Arch 2**
   1. Innervated by the facial nerve (**CN VII**)
   2. Gives rise to the following muscles:
      a. Muscles of facial expression (orbicularis oculi, orbicularis oris, buccinator)
      b. Three other muscles (stylohyoid, stapedius, and the posterior belly of the digastric)
   3. Gives rise to the following skeletal structures:
      a. Greater cornu of hyoid bone
      b. Inferior portion of the body of hyoid bone

C. **Arch 3**
   1. Innervated by the glossopharyngeal nerve (**CN IX**)
   2. Gives rise to the stylopharyngeus muscle
   3. Gives rise to the following skeletal structures:
      a. Greater cornu of the hyoid bone
      b. Lower portion of the body of hyoid bone

D. **Arch 4**
   1. Innervated by the vagus nerve (pharyngeal and superior laryngeal branches of CN X)
   2. Gives rise to the following muscles:
      a. Cricothyroid muscle
      b. All the muscles of the soft palate and pharynx except the stylopharyngeus muscle (arch 3) and tensor veli palatini (arch 1)

E. **Arch 6**
   1. Innervated by the vagus nerve (recurrent laryngeal branch of CN X)
   2. Gives rise to the intrinsic muscles of the larynx except the cricothyroid

F. **Arch 4 and Arch 6** fuse to give rise to the thyroid, cricoids, arytenoids, corniculate, and cuneiform cartilages.

BONE FUNCTION AND METABOLISM *(Figure 9-1)*

I. Osteoblasts

A. They synthesize type I collagen and bone matrix proteins to form an unmineralized osteoid (Figure 9-2).

FIGURE 9-1 **Bone histology**

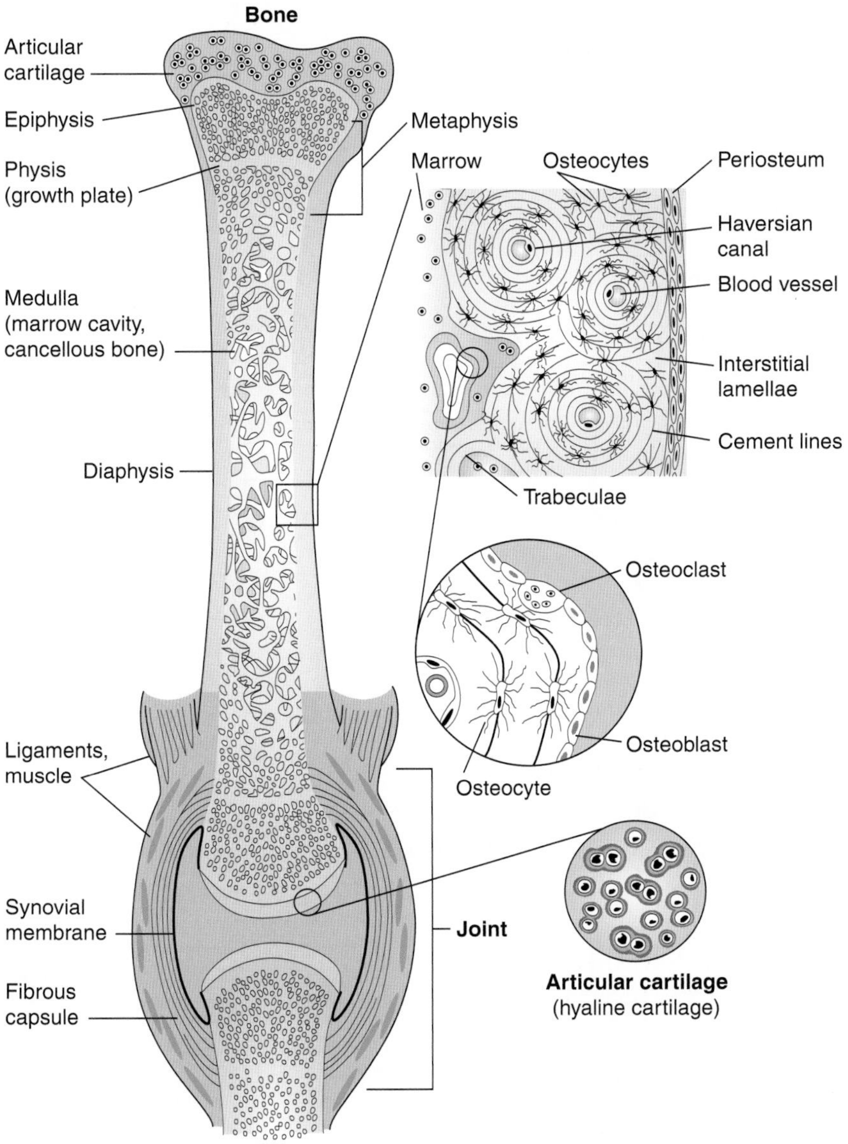
Bone
Articular cartilage
Epiphysis
Physis (growth plate)
Medulla (marrow cavity, cancellous bone)
Diaphysis
Ligaments, muscle
Synovial membrane
Fibrous capsule
Metaphysis
Marrow
Osteocytes
Periosteum
Haversian canal
Blood vessel
Interstitial lamellae
Cement lines
Trabeculae
Osteoclast
Osteoblast
Osteocyte
Joint
Articular cartilage
(hyaline cartilage)

(Adapted with permission from Damjanov IM. *Histology: A Color Atlas and Textbook.* Baltimore, MD: Lippincott Williams & Wilkins; 1996:422.)

QUICK HIT

All the intrinsic muscles of the pharynx, except the cricothyroid, are innervated by the recurrent laryngeal branches of the vagus nerve. Consequently, bilateral injury to the recurrent laryngeal nerves leaves the cricothyroid unopposed, and the vocal cords become tense and adducted.

QUICK HIT

Of all the intrinsic muscles of the larynx (posterior cricoarytenoid, lateral cricoarytenoid, arytenoid, thyroarytenoid, cricothyroid, transverse arytenoid, oblique arytenoid, and vocal muscle), the posterior cricoarytenoid muscle is the only muscle that **abducts** the vocal cords.

QUICK HIT

Exogenous estrogen administration (hormone replacement therapy) slows the rate of bone loss that occurs after menopause by stimulating osteoblasts via estrogen receptors.

FIGURE 9-2 **Collagen synthesis**

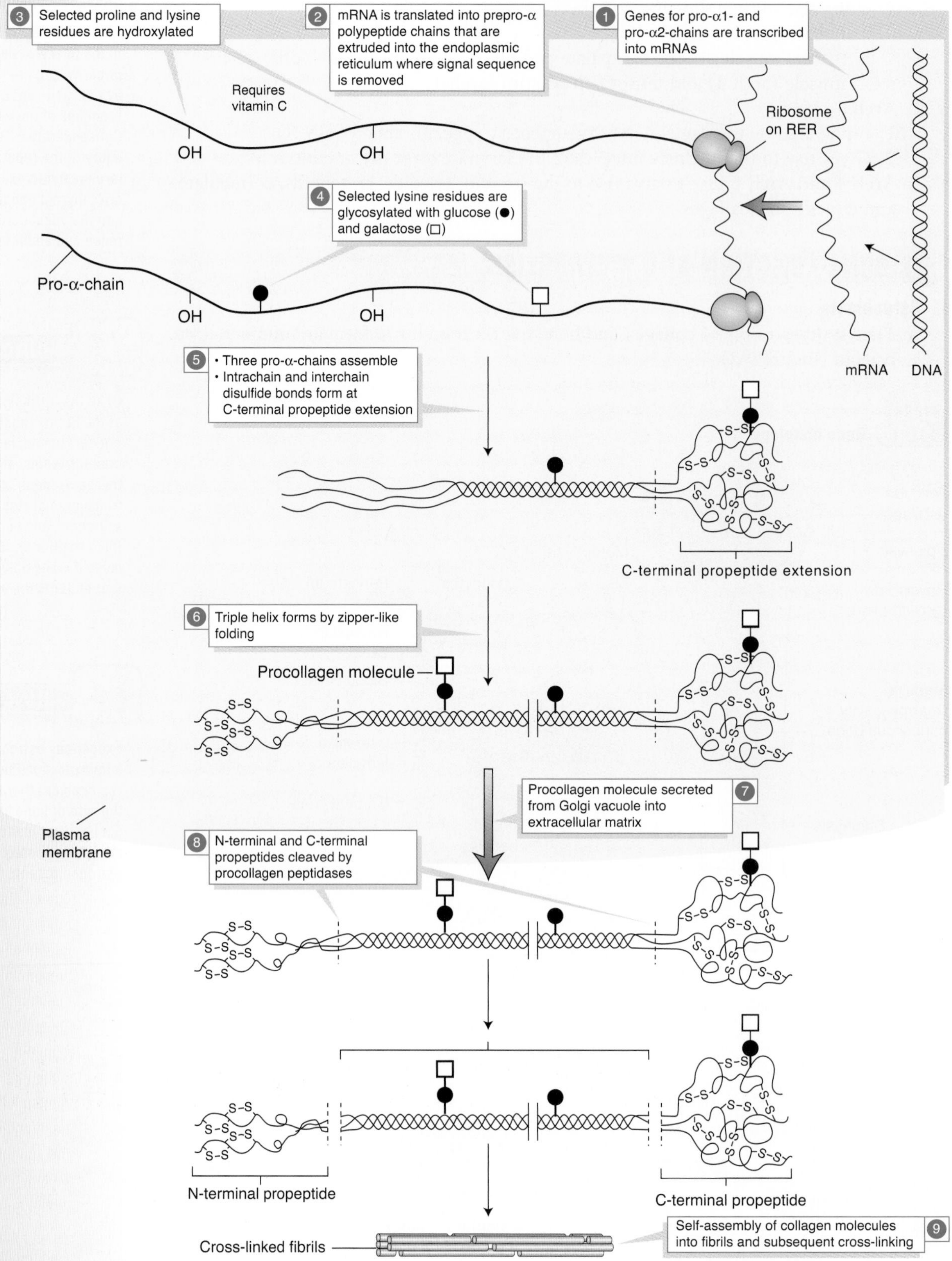

1 Genes for pro-α1- and pro-α2-chains are transcribed into mRNAs
2 mRNA is translated into prepro-α polypeptide chains that are extruded into the endoplasmic reticulum where signal sequence is removed
3 Selected proline and lysine residues are hydroxylated
Requires vitamin C
OH
OH
Ribosome on RER
4 Selected lysine residues are glycosylated with glucose (●) and galactose (□)
Pro-α-chain
mRNA
DNA
5 • Three pro-α-chains assemble • Intrachain and interchain disulfide bonds form at C-terminal propeptide extension
S-S
C-terminal propeptide extension
6 Triple helix forms by zipper-like folding
Procollagen molecule
7 Procollagen molecule secreted from Golgi vacuole into extracellular matrix
Plasma membrane
8 N-terminal and C-terminal propeptides cleaved by procollagen peptidases
N-terminal propeptide
C-terminal propeptide
Cross-linked fibrils
9 Self-assembly of collagen molecules into fibrils and subsequent cross-linking

mRNA, messenger RNA; RER, rough endoplasmic reticulum. (Adapted from Champe PC, Harvey RA. *Lippincott's Illustrated Reviews: Biochemistry.* 2nd ed. Philadelphia, PA: Lippincott-Raven; 1994:41. Used by permission of Lippincott Williams & Wilkins.)

B. Calcium (Ca^{2+}) and phosphate are deposited on the cartilaginous matrix to form mineralized bone.
C. Blood supply goes to osteoblasts via vessels within the **haversian canals**.
D. When osteoblasts become surrounded by bone matrix, they become **osteocytes**.

II. Osteocytes

A. Occupy a space called lacuna
B. Communicate with other osteocytes via cytoplasmic extensions called canaliculi
C. Are influenced by parathyroid hormone (**PTH**) to stimulate osteoclastic bone resorption
D. Resorption allows Ca^{2+} to be transferred rapidly into the blood.
E. Are not directly involved in bone resorption

III. Osteoclasts

A. Multinucleated cells formed from monocytes, which are responsible for bone resorption
B. Contain acid phosphatase
C. Resorb bone under influence of PTH

QUICK HIT

Tartrate-resistant acid phosphatase (TRAP) is used as an indicator of osteoclast activity and also as a marker for hairy cell leukemia.

IV. Hormonal control (also see Chapter 7)

A. **Parathyroid hormone**
1. Release is stimulated by hypocalcemia and hypophosphatemia
2. Stimulates osteoclastic activity causing osteolysis and release of Ca^{2+} from bone
3. Promotes the reabsorption of Ca^{2+} in the distal tubule of the kidney
4. Inhibits phosphate (PO_4^{3-}) reabsorption in the proximal tubule of the kidney
5. Converts vitamin D to its active form, 1,25-dihydroxycholecalciferol
6. Raises blood calcium and lowers blood phosphate

B. **Calcitonin**
1. Inhibits osteoclasts, which inhibits bone resorption
2. Lowers blood calcium

C. **Vitamin D**
1. Assists PTH in the resorption of bone
2. Increases Ca^{2+} absorption from the intestine
3. Increases Ca^{2+} reabsorption from the kidney
4. Increases PO_4^{3-} reabsorption from the kidney
5. Raises blood calcium and phosphate
6. Has net effect on bone growth

BONE, CARTILAGE, AND JOINT DISEASE

In the healthy adult, bone mass peaks between 20 and 25 years of age. Peak bone mass is typically higher in males and blacks. Bone diseases can adversely affect the mass and strength of the skeleton, predisposing the patient to fractures.

- **Diseases That Affect Bone Formation** (Table 9-1)

TABLE **9-1** **Diseases that Affect Bone Formation**

Disease	Etiology	Clinical Features
Osteitis fibrosa cystica (von Recklinghausen disease of bone)	Caused by increased levels of **PTH;** primary or secondary hyperparathyroidism	Cystic spaces in the bone that are lined with osteoclasts; often colored brown owing to hemorrhage, hence the name **"brown tumor of bone"**
Achondroplasia (dwarfism)	Caused by failure of long bones to elongate because of narrow epiphyseal plates and sealing of these plates with the metaphysis; **autosomal dominant** disease; **most common cause of dwarfism;** linked to activating mutation in gene for fibroblast growth factor-3 receptor	Short limbs; normal-size head and trunk

(continued)

TABLE 9-1 **Diseases that Affect Bone Formation**

Disease	Etiology	Clinical Features
Osteogenesis imperfecta ("brittle bone disease")	Group of gene mutations that cause **defective type I collagen synthesis;** most common type of mutation is **autosomal dominant**	Multiple fractures occur with only minor trauma; **blue sclera;** deformities of teeth and skin; deafness
Osteopetrosis ("marble bone disease")	**Defective osteoclasts** cause a decrease in reabsorption leading to **increased bone density;** the most severe form is autosomal recessive	Multiple **fractures** despite increased density; narrowing of marrow spaces causes anemia; narrowing of other cavities causes blindness, deafness, and cranial nerve compression
Paget disease of bone	Increased osteoblastic and osteoclastic activity by an unknown cause; occurs most commonly in the elderly; may involve one or more bones	**Skeletal deformities;** complications include bone pain owing to fracture, multiple arteriovenous (AV) shunts in bone causing high output cardiac failure, hearing loss as a result of thickening of bony structures in ear; may lead to osteosarcoma; increased levels of serum alkaline phosphatase; three phases of disease: • Osteolytic phase—resorption owing to osteoclasts • Mixed phase—osteoclastic and osteoblastic activity leads to a **mosaic pattern** in the bone • Late phase—increase in bone density as a result of osteoblastic activity

PTH, parathyroid hormone.

Clinical Vignette 9-1

CLINICAL PRESENTATION: A 4-year-old child with the chief complaint of "belly pain" is brought to the emergency department by his mother. As you begin his physical examination, you note that the child is short for his age and that there are multiple ecchymoses on his lower extremities. The mother reports that her son bruises easily. A head, ear, eye, nose, and throat examination shows multiple dental caries and blue sclera. Physical examination shows that the abdomen is soft, nontender, and nondistended. There are normoactive bowel sounds. The patient is without organomegaly or masses. Temperature = 98.6° F; heart rate = 80 bpm; respiration rate = 18 breaths/min; blood pressure = 100/80 mm Hg.

DIFFERENTIALS: Osteogenesis imperfecta (OI), child abuse, child neglect. Short stature, multiple ecchymoses, and dental caries can be seen in each of the listed differentials. However, blue sclera is a characteristic finding of OI. Also, child abuse can be differentiated from OI based on nonskeletal manifestations such as retinal hemorrhage, intracranial bleeding, and splenic trauma.

DIAGNOSTIC WORKUP: **Radiographs** should be obtained of the skull, chest, long bones, and pelvis, looking for **type of fracture** as well as **osteopenia** (seen in OI). Diaphyseal fractures (break in the midshaft of long bone) and metaphyseal fractures (appear as corner chip of bone edge) suggest child abuse. In addition to multiple fractures, osteopenia would be seen on radiograph in OI. In child abuse, serial plain films should show healing and remineralization. In OI, fractures continue to occur in protective custody. In difficult cases, **collagen synthesis analysis** would show abnormal findings in OI.

MANAGEMENT: Medical therapy of OI is supportive, and in some cases, surgical interventions are done to improve weight bearing.

METABOLIC AND INFECTIOUS BONE DISEASE *(Table 9-2)*

TABLE 9-2 Metabolic and Infectious Bone Disease

Disease	Etiology	Clinical Features
Osteoporosis	**Primary:** ***Type I:*** postmenopausal, with excess loss of trabecular bone ***Type II:*** men and women >70 years of age, with loss of trabecular and cortical bone **Secondary:** Physical inactivity, increased parathyroid levels, hypercortisolism, hyperthyroidism, vitamin D deficiency, hypocalcemia	**Bone mineral density** is 2.5 or more standard deviations **below** normal; **decrease in bone mass** leads to fractures (especially of the weight-bearing bones of the spine); radiolucent bone seen on radiograph; DEXA scan positive
Scurvy	Lack of vitamin C intake; defective **proline and lysine hydroxylation** in collagen synthesis (Figure 9-2)	Impaired bone formation and lesions result; painful subperiosteal hemorrhage; osteoporosis; bleeding gums; poor wound healing
Rickets (children); osteomalacia (adults)	Impaired calcification of bone because of deficiency of vitamin D; if caused by renal disease, termed "renal osteodystrophy"	**Children:** Skeletal malformations Craniotabes (thinned and softened bones of the skull) Late fontanelle closure Decreased height Rachitic rosary (costochondral junction thickening resembling string of beads) Pigeon breast owing to a protruding sternum **Adults:** Fractures Radiolucency on radiography
Avascular necrosis	Death of osteocytes and fat necrosis via the following mechanisms: vascular compression, vascular interruption (fracture), thrombosis (sickle cell disease, caisson disease), vessel injury	Joint pain; osteoarthritis; sites include head of the femur, shoulder, knee
Pyogenic osteomyelitis	Infection of bone most often caused by ***Staphylococcus aureus;*** routes of infection include hematogenous extension from adjacent infection, open fracture, or surgery	Acute febrile illness; pain; tenderness; usually affects metaphysis of distal femur, proximal tibia, and proximal humerus; forms sequestrum and involucrum
Tuberculous osteomyelitis	Tuberculous infection spreads to bone from elsewhere in body	Seen in hips, long bones, hands, feet, and vertebrae **(Pott disease)**

DEXA, dual energy X-ray absorptiometry.

I. Bisphosphonates

The bisphosphonates, which include alendronate, risedronate, ibandronate, pamidronate, and etidronate, inhibit osteoclast-mediated bone resorption by binding to hydroxyapatite. The bisphosphonates are most commonly used to prevent or treat postmenopausal osteoporosis but can also be used for Paget disease and steroid-induced osteoporosis.

QUICK HIT

Osteoporosis versus osteopenia: Osteoporosis is a loss of bone that predisposes to fractures; osteopenia is detectable loss of bone via resorption.

QUICK HIT

Dual-energy X-ray absorptiometry (DEXA) scan is the gold standard for diagnosis of osteoporosis.

QUICK HIT

Osteochondrosis is avascular necrosis of epiphysis sites in children. **Legg–Calvé–Perthes disease** is avascular necrosis of the femoral head in children and often presents with limp. **Osgood–Schlatter disease** is an inflammation at the insertion site of the patellar tendon on the tibial apophysis.

QUICK HIT

The most common cause of avascular necrosis is steroid-induced vascular compression, most commonly occurring in the femoral head.

QUICK HIT

Patients with sickle disease contract osteomyelitis as a result of *Salmonella,* whereas intravenous drug users may be infected with *Pseudomonas.* However, *Staphylococcus aureus* continues to be the most common cause of osteomyelitis in both these groups of patients.

II. Tumors of bone and cartilage *(Table 9-3)*

Tumors of the bone and cartilage, although rare, occur most commonly in the lower extremities of young males. Metastases are more common than primary tumors of the bone. Tumors of the prostate, breast, and lung account for 80% of bone metastases.

TABLE 9-3 Tumors of Bone and Cartilage

Tumor	Morphology	Clinical Features
Osteochondroma	Benign bone tumor; **most common benign tumor;** originates in metaphysis of long bones; growth of mature bone (exostosis) with a cartilaginous cap	Most common in men younger than 25 years of age; usually occurs on the lower end of the femur or upper end of the tibia
Giant cell tumor	Benign bone tumor; spindle-shaped cells with multinuclear giant cells; most commonly occur in the epiphysis of the distal femur or proximal tibia	Most common in women 20–55 years of age; has **"soap bubble"** appearance on radiograph; usually occurs on the lower end of the femur or upper end of the tibia
Osteoma	Benign bone tumor; mature bone (dense tissue)	Most common in men; affects skull or facial bones; protrudes from surface; associated with Gardner syndrome
Osteoid osteoma	Benign bone tumor; **nidus** rimmed by osteoblasts and surrounded by vascular, spindled stroma; $<$2 cm in diameter	Most common in men 20–30 years of age; occurs near the ends of the tibia and femur; painful due to excess prostaglandin E_2 production; radiolucent **nidus** is seen on radiograph
Osteosarcoma	Malignant mesenchymal bone tumor; malignant cells produce bone matrix; origin usually in metaphyseal long bones; destructive masses with hemorrhage and necrosis; retinoblastoma, Paget disease, radiation exposure are risk factors	Bimodal distribution, most common in boys in their teenage years and in elderly; usually occurs in tibia or femur near the knee; local pain; tenderness; swelling; metastasizes to lung first; growth under bone results in the **Codman triangle and a "sunburst" appearance** on radiograph
Chondrosarcoma	Malignant cartilage tumor; lobulated translucent tumors; necrosis; calcification	Most common in men usually 40 years of age or older; central skeleton is affected such as the pelvis, ribs, shoulders, spine; radiograph shows localized area of bone destruction
Ewing sarcoma	Malignant small round cell tumors of bone and soft tissue; **t(11;22);** sheets of small round cells producing **Homer-Wright pseudorosettes;** histologically similar to lymphoma, small cell carcinoma, rhabdomyosarcoma	Most common in boys 10–15 years of age; occurs in long bones, ribs, pelvis, scapula; early metastasis; responds to chemotherapy; painful, warm, swollen mass; "onion skin" appearance on radiograph
Fibrous dysplasia	Benign; bone replaced haphazardly by fibrous tissue	**"Chinese figures"** configuration on radiograph. Three types: Single bone involvement; Several bones involved; Several bones involved, along with precocious puberty and café au lait spots
Metastasis	Malignant; usually lytic lesions unless arising from prostate or breast	Originate from prostate, breast, kidney, lung; ectopic hormone production **(parathyroid hormone-related protein [PTHrP])**

QUICK HIT

Osteochondromas generally do not undergo malignant transformation to chondrosarcoma, except in the familial variety, which is characterized by multiple lesions.

QUICK HIT

Gardner syndrome is an autosomal dominant disorder characterized by multiple colonic polyps associated with other tumors such as osteomas of the skull, fibromas, thyroid cancer, epidermoid cysts, and sebaceous cysts.

QUICK HIT

In osteosarcoma, a "sunburst" appearance on radiography is due to calcified streaks that radiate from a tumor. Codman triangle is due to periosteum lifting away from the bone due to an underlying tumor.

QUICK HIT

The most common bone sarcoma in children is an osteosarcoma, followed by Ewing sarcoma.

QUICK HIT

Predisposing factors for osteosarcoma include Paget disease of the bone, mutations of the p53 gene on chromosome 17 (Li–Fraumeni syndrome), familial retinoblastoma, radiation, and bone infarcts.

QUICK HIT

The most common malignancy of the skeleton is metastatic tumors.

III. Arthritic joint disease *(Table 9-4)*

The etiology of arthritic joint diseases is not well understood. For this reason, treatment is often palliative rather than curative.

Two factors to consider in the differential diagnosis of an acutely painful joint include infection and urate deposition. These two entities may be distinguished from each other, in part, by aspiration of the joint fluid with evaluation for white blood cells (WBCs), bacteria on Gram stain, or crystals.

QUICK HIT

Seventy-five percent of the population demonstrates radiographic evidence of osteoarthritis by age 65.

QUICK HIT

Osteoarthritis may affect only one joint and can affect the distal interphalangeal (DIP) joints of the hands. Rheumatoid arthritis is bilaterally symmetric and does not affect the DIP joints. Also, rheumatoid arthritis is characterized by joint stiffness in the morning that is relieved as the day goes on, whereas osteoarthritis pain gets worse as the day goes on.

QUICK HIT

Disease-modifying antirheumatic drugs (DMARDs) such as chemotherapy agents (**methotrexate**), antimalarials (**hydroxychloroquine**), and tumor necrosis factor (TNF) inhibitors (**Etanercept, Infliximab**) are standard of care for rheumatoid arthritis.

QUICK HIT

Radiographic evidence of osteoarthritis include **joint space narrowing, osteophytes,** and **subchondral cysts.**

MNEMONIC

To remember **Reiter syndrome:** "Can't see" (uveitis), "can't pee" (urethritis), "can't climb a tree" (arthritis).

TABLE 9-4 **Arthritic Joint Disease**

Disease	Etiology	Clinical Features
Osteoarthritis (degenerative joint disease)	Degeneration of joint articular cartilage followed by growth of surrounding bone; the **most common type of arthritis;** primary type has no specific risk factor; secondary type related to trauma, metabolic disorder, or inflammatory arthropathy; knee is the most common site	Pain in joint after use, improves with rest, stiffness in the morning or after a period of immobility; **"Joint mice"** form from pieces of torn and frayed joint cartilage and broken pieces of osteophytes; erosion of cartilage results in **eburnation** (polishing) of the underlying bone; cysts visible in bone on radiograph; Heberden nodes are osteophytes at the DIP joint; Bouchard nodes are osteophytes of the PIP joints
Rheumatoid arthritis	Symmetrical, chronic inflammation of the synovium with edema and cellular infiltrate, leading to the destruction of articular cartilage of joints, most likely because of autoimmune reaction; synovial hypertrophy and hyperplasia; granulation tissue **(pannus)** over articular cartilage; **rheumatoid factor**—IgM autoantibody against the Fc receptor located on IgG; more common in women; associated with **HLA-DR4**	Ulnar deviation of MCP joints, **swan-neck,** and **boutonnière** deformity develop owing to inflammation, muscle atrophy, and contracture; **DIP joints are spared;** morning stiffness that improves throughout the day; subcutaneous rheumatoid nodules; systemic symptoms such as fever, weight loss, fatigue
Ankylosing spondylitis	Unknown cause; high association with **HLA-B27;** negative rheumatoid factor; males are more commonly affected	Bilateral sacroiliitis (inflammation of the sacroiliac joint) noted; chronic low back pain and stiffness; improves with movement; calcification of spinal ligaments and fusion of the facet joints produces a **"bamboo spine";** may produce extraskeletal manifestations of **apical lung fibrosis, aortic insufficiency,** or **cauda equina syndrome**
Psoriatic arthritis	Unknown cause; may present similar to rheumatoid arthritis; HLA-B27 association; **no rheumatoid factor;** no male or female preponderance	**Asymmetric** involvement of **DIP joints,** PIP joints, feet, ankles, and knees; **"pencil-in-a-cup"** deformity of the proximal phalanges
Reiter syndrome	Caused by reaction to systemic illness that originated either enteropathically or urogenitally; HLA-B27 association; most common in males, usually 20–40 years of age	Classic triad of genitourinary inflammation **(urethritis),** ocular inflammation **(conjunctivitis),** and acute asymmetric **arthritis**

(continued)

QUICK HIT

Lesch–Nyhan syndrome is an **X-linked deficiency** of **hypoxanthine-guanine phosphoribosyl transferase** (HGPRT) that results in elevated levels of uric acid and manifests as mental retardation, gout, and self-mutilation. It can be treated with allopurinol, which blocks xanthine oxidase, an important enzyme in the formation of uric acid.

QUICK HIT

Pseudogout, caused by **calcium pyrophosphate** crystals, resembles gout in its presentation. However, calcium pyrophosphate crystals have weak **positive birefringence** under polarized light.

TABLE 9-4 **Arthritic Joint Disease** *(Continued)*

Disease	Etiology	Clinical Features
Gout	Inflammatory reaction in joints caused by monosodium **urate crystal** deposition; IgG opsonization of the crystals followed by phagocytosis stimulates inflammation; pathogenesis includes increased uric acid production such as Lesch–Nyhan syndrome (hypoxanthine-guanine phosphoribosyltransferase deficiency), increased activity of phosphoribosyl pyrophosphate (PRPP) synthetase, and decreased uric acid secretion such as diuretics; acidosis; often precipitated by a large, high-protein meal or by drinking excessive amounts of alcohol	First MTP joint involvement is called **podagra; tophi** (nodules of fibrous tissue and crystals) occur near the joints, on the ear, and on the Achilles tendon; renal damage may occur when crystals deposit in collecting tubules; urate crystals have **strong negative birefringence** under polarized light and are **needle shaped**. For treatment, see Table 9-5.

DIP, distal interphalangeal; HLA, human leukocyte antigen; Ig, immunoglobulin; MCP, metacarpophalangeal; MTP, metatarsophalangeal; PIP, proximal interphalangeal.

IV. Gout is a condition in which uric acid crystals in joints trigger intermittent inflammatory reactions. The etiologic process can be blocked at different stages (Table 9-5).

A. Inhibition of the production of uric acid from the breakdown of DNA **purines**

B. Increased excretion of uric acid in the urine

C. Blunting the body's **inflammatory response** to the gout crystals (the body's reaction to gout crystals actually causes the pain and damage associated with gout)

TABLE 9-5 **Drugs Used to Treat Gout**

Therapeutic Agent	Mechanism of Action	Indications	Side Effects	Notes
Allopurinol	Inhibition of uric acid production—**competitive inhibitor of xanthine oxidase**, decreases conversion of **xanthine to uric acid**	Chronic gout therapy; lymphoma, leukemia (prevents tumor lysis associated urate nephropathy), uric acid stones	Rash, fever, diarrhea, occasional peripheral neuritis; enhances effect of azathioprine	Should not be used to treat acute gout
Probenecid	Increased secretion of uric acid (uricosuric)—small dose inhibits uric acid secretion; large dose inhibits uric acid reabsorption (i.e., promotes excretion)	Chronic gout therapy	**Caution: should not be used in patients with sulfa allergies**	Should not be used to treat acute gout or patients with uric acid stones
Colchicine	Anti-inflammatory—interrupts **microtubule formation**, thereby interfering with normal mitosis and inhibiting WBC migration and phagocytosis	Acute gout therapy	Diarrhea (common)	

(continued)

TABLE 9-5 **Drugs Used to Treat Gout** *(Continued)*

Therapeutic Agent	Mechanism of Action	Indications	Side Effects	Notes
NSAIDs (e.g., indomethacin)	Decrease **prostaglandin** production, thereby interrupting the inflammatory process	Acute therapy	Bone marrow suppression and renal damage (indomethacin); GI distress and ulceration	
Celecoxib	Selectively inhibits cyclooxygenase-2 (COX-2)	Acute therapy	Sulfa allergy; renal damage	Less toxic to GI mucosa than NSAIDs
Glucocorticoids (prednisone)	Suppresses prostaglandin and leukotriene synthesis	Acute therapy	Osteoporosis, Cushingoid reaction, psychosis, glucose intolerance, infection, hypertension, cataracts	

GI, gastrointestinal; NSAID, nonsteroidal anti-inflammatory drug; WBC, white blood cell.

Clinical Vignette 9-2

CLINICAL PRESENTATION: A 45-year-old man presents to the emergency department with severe pain in his left **great toe** that began suddenly yesterday evening. He reports **exquisite tenderness,** saying "even the bed sheet touching my toe was intolerable." The patient also reports that yesterday afternoon, he had "gone out with the boys" and estimates drinking five to six **beers.** Patient denies both pain in other joints and having felt pain like this before. Physical examination shows swelling, erythema, rubor, and tenderness of the left great toe. His past medical history is significant for osteoarthritis of the left knee for which he takes ibuprofen. Temperature = 98.5° F; blood pressure = 135/70 mm Hg; heart rate = 85 bpm; respiration rate = 21 breaths/min.

DIFFERENTIALS: Septic arthritis, cellulitis, gout, pseudogout. Osteoarthritis and rheumatoid arthritis are ruled out in this case because they typically present as pain in multiple joints. Polyarticular pain should be thought of as inflammatory (showing signs of rubor, swelling, and erythema as in rheumatoid arthritis) and noninflammatory (as in osteoarthritis). Septic arthritis is unlikely in this case because of the location of the pain and the lack of fever. Based on the location of the pain, occurrence after a diet rich in purines, and the examination, this patient most likely is experiencing an acute gouty attack.

LABORATORY STUDIES: Appropriate workup of monoarticular pain includes **synovial fluid aspiration and analysis.** If the fluid is **inflammatory** (white blood cells >5,000), the fluid should be further evaluated by **crystal analysis** (positive in gout and pseudogout), **Gram stain,** and **culture** (showing bacteria in infectious arthritis). **Complete blood count (CBC), erythrocyte sedimentation rate (ESR),** and **blood cultures** should also be obtained to rule out septic arthritis.

MANAGEMENT: Acute gout is treated by **nonsteroidal anti-inflammatory** drugs (NSAIDs; indomethacin is traditionally used, aspirin aggravates the problem), **colchicines** (if the patient did not respond to NSAIDs), and **corticosteroids** (if patient cannot tolerate NSAIDs or colchicine). Prophylactic therapy would not be initiated in this patient because this is his first acute gouty attack. Prophylactic therapy is indicated after two gouty attacks and consists of **uricosuric drugs** or **allopurinol,** depending on the amount of uric acid excreted in urine over 24 hours. Never give allopurinol for acute gout; it makes it worse.

The Musculoskeletal System

V. Infectious joint disease *(Table 9-6)*

TABLE 9-6 **Infectious Joint Disease**

Disease	Etiology	Clinical Features
Nongonococcal septic arthritis	Inflammation of joints; most commonly ***Staphylococcus aureus*** and *Streptococcus species*	Monoarticular arthritis, usually affecting the knee; chills and fever; **positive Gram stain** and cultures of synovial fluid
Gonococcal septic arthritis	Inflammation of joints and other systemic effects secondary to dissemination of sexually acquired gonococcal infection; **most common form of arthritis in sexually active adults**	Monoarticular arthritis, usually affects the knee; chills and fever; rash (including papules and pustules); Gram stain and synovial fluid cultures often negative
Lyme disease	Infection with *Borrelia burgdorferi*, which is transmitted by the tick *Ixodes dammini*; arthritis occurs late in the disease	**Erythema chronicum migrans**, a characteristic expanding bull's-eye rash; knees are most common site of arthritis; may cause myocardial, pericardial, and neurologic manifestations

> **QUICK HIT**
> **SLE** has a female-to-male ratio of 2:1 and is more common in African-American women.

> **QUICK HIT**
> Presence of antibodies against double-stranded DNA antibodies and Smith (Sm) antigen is practically diagnostic of SLE.

> **QUICK HIT**
> In vitro, the hypocoagulable state is caused by antibodies that react with the cardiolipin test substrate. However, this reaction does not occur in vivo because the patient with SLE is prone to excessive clotting, not excessive bleeding.

> **QUICK HIT**
> **Antihistone antibodies** are associated with drug-induced lupus. Common drugs that cause drug-induced lupus: hydralazine, procainamide, isoniazid, chlorpromazine, methyldopa, and quinidine.

SYSTEMIC LUPUS ERYTHEMATOSUS

I. Prototypical connective tissue disorder that more frequently affects women

II. Clinical features

A. Fever, lymphadenopathy, weight loss, and general malaise
B. **Immune complex deposition** in the vessels of almost all organs
C. Pulmonary fibrosis characterized by interstitial fibrosis or diffuse alveolitis
D. **Libman–Sacks endocarditis**
   1. **Mitral valve** affected
   2. Sterile verrucous lesions seen on both sides of the leaflets
E. Pericarditis and pleuritis
F. Glomerular disease
   1. May range from mild to diffuse proliferative change
   2. Subendothelial and mesangial immune complex deposits
   3. Endothelial proliferation (wire loops) and thickened basement membranes (membranous glomerulonephritis)
G. Arthralgia and arthritis
H. Vasospasm of small vessels, especially of the fingers (**Raynaud phenomenon**)
I. **Cotton-wool spot lesions in fundus of eye**
J. Skin rash
   1. Characteristic **butterfly rash** over the malar eminences of the face
   2. Rashes can also be prevalent elsewhere on the body
   3. Rashes associated with exposure to sunlight (photosensitivity)

III. Laboratory findings

A. Antinuclear antibodies (ANAs) are seen in almost all cases.
   1. ANA is a sensitive marker, but it is not specific for systemic lupus erythematosus (SLE).
   2. Presence of antibodies to **double-stranded DNA** is highly specific for SLE.
   3. Antibodies to **Smith (Sm) antigen** are also specific for SLE.

B. Decreased level of complement (C3 and C4) in the serum
C. Skin biopsies show immune complex deposition.
D. **False-positive test for syphilis**
E. **Hypercoagulable** state in vivo owing to antiphospholipid antibodies

QUICK HIT

In vitro, the hypocoagulable state is caused by antibodies that react with the cardiolipin test substrate. However, this reaction does not occur in vivo because the SLE patient is prone to excessive clotting, not excessive bleeding.

OTHER CONNECTIVE TISSUE DISORDERS *(Table 9-7)*

Inherited disorders of the bone, skin, cartilage, and blood vessels are some of the most common genetic conditions in humans. These diseases are characterized by widespread manifestations.

TABLE 9-7 Other Connective Tissue Disorders

Disease	Etiology	Clinical Features
Marfan syndrome	Abnormality of **fibrillin** (a glycoprotein in microfibrils) due to mutations in the FBN1 gene on chromosome 15; results in skeletal, visual, and cardiovascular defects; **autosomal dominant** inheritance	Abnormally long fingers **(arachnodactyly)**, arms, and legs; hyperextensible joints; tall and thin body habitus; high palate; ocular lens dislocation **(ectopia lentis)**; cardiovascular defects including mitral valve prolapse, proximal aorta aneurysm, aortic valve insufficiency, and **aortic dissection**
Ehlers–Danlos syndrome	Genetic defect in type I and type III **collagen and elastin** formation	Frequent hemorrhage, **hyperextensibility of joints** and skin, fragility of tissue, poor wound healing
Progressive systemic sclerosis (scleroderma)	Diffuse fibrosis and degeneration of almost every organ owing to autoimmune reaction; **anti- scl70** (ANA); anticentromere antibody present in **CREST** (**c**alcinosis cutis, **R**aynaud phenomenon, **e**sophageal dysfunction, **s**clerodactyly, and **t**elangiectasia); occurs more frequently in women	Hypertrophy of subcutaneous collagen leads to thickened skin, fixed facial expression, clawlike hand (sclerodactyly); Raynaud phenomenon; fibrosis of esophagus, GI tract, lungs, heart, and kidney
Sjögren syndrome	Autoimmune reaction; **anti-SSA (anti-Ro)** and **anti-SSB (anti-La)** antibodies; anti-SSB antibody is highly specific; occurs more often in women Enlarged parotid glands as a consequence of lymphocytic infiltration; hypergammaglobulinemia	Classic triad: • Dry eyes (xerophthalmia) • Dry mouth **(xerostomia)** • Presence of **other connective tissue or autoimmune disease** (often rheumatoid arthritis)
Polymyositis	Autoimmune inflammatory disorder; occurs more frequently in women; often **associated with malignancy**	Weakness in the proximal muscles of the extremities; high level of creatine kinase in serum; termed **dermatomyositis** when skin is involved
Mixed connective tissue disease	Autoimmune disorder; occurs more frequently in women; renal involvement is rare (as opposed to other connective tissue diseases); antinuclear ribonucleic protein **(anti-nRNP)** is a highly specific ANA	Raynaud phenomenon, arthralgia, muscle inflammation, esophageal dysmotility

ANA, antinuclear antibodies; *FBN1*, fibrillin-1; GI, gastrointestinal.

QUICK HIT

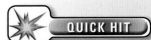

Most common cause of sudden death in Ehlers-Danlos syndrome is aortic dissection.

QUICK HIT

Hypertrophic osteoarthropathy, which manifests as clubbing of the digits and periostitis, is one of the sequelae of systemic disorders such as chronic lung disease, cirrhosis, inflammatory bowel disease, and congenital cyanotic heart disease.

QUICK HIT

Xerostomia and xerophthalmia alone are characteristic of **sicca syndrome**, which is also autoimmune in nature.

Clinical Vignette 9-3

CLINICAL PRESENTATION: A 35-year-old woman presents to her primary care physician complaining of **joint pain** in her wrist, ankle, and knee for the past several months. She also reports a **painful intermittent rash** of the same duration on her **face** that **worsens in the sun**. The patient also tells you that she has noted that her **fingers oddly become very pale, turn blue,** and then **bright red** while in the **cold outdoors.** Review of systems is positive for **fatigue and weight loss.** A head, ear, eye, nose, and throat (HEENT) examination shows an **erythematous rash over the cheeks and nasal bridge, sparing the nasolabial folds, hair thinning along the crown, and ulceration of the oral mucosa.** Examination of the forearm shows a **raised erythematous patch** with some **scaling**. Temperature = 100.2° F; blood pressure = 145/90 mm Hg; heart rate = 75 bpm; respiration rate = 20 breaths/min.
DIFFERENTIALS: SLE, drug-induced lupus, discoid lupus, mixed connective tissue disease (MCTD), scleroderma. The arthralgia, malar rash, discoid lesions on sun-exposed arms, alopecia, weight loss, oral ulcers, and mild fever all suggest SLE. **Drug-induced lupus** could be ruled out from a detailed medication history (see Quick Hit for list of drugs). Although Raynaud phenomenon is observed in SLE, it also occurs in **scleroderma. MCTD** is a disorder in which features of SLE, systemic sclerosis, dermatomyositis, polymyositis, and Sjögren syndrome can coexist and overlap. Serologic studies should be performed to differentiate these further.
LABORATORY STUDIES: When given serologic studies on the USMLE, look for the following results: A **positive antinuclear antibody (ANA)** screening test occurs in SLE, rheumatoid arthritis, scleroderma, Sjögren syndrome, MCTD, polymyositis, dermatomyositis, and drug-induced lupus. **A negative ANA** screening test suggests that the diagnosis is likely not SLE. Presence of either **anti–double-stranded DNA (dsDNA)** or **anti-Sm antibody** is diagnostic of SLE. **Antihistone antibodies** are present in 100% of cases of drug-induced lupus. If negative, drug-induced lupus can be excluded. Ribonucleoprotein (RNP) antibodies are a specific marker of MCTD. **Positive anti-scl70** indicates scleroderma, and positive **anticentromere antibody** specifically indicates CREST (calcinosis cutis, Raynaud phenomenon, esophageal motility disorder, sclerodactyly, and telangiectasia) syndrome. **Complete blood count** studies show anemia, leukopenia, lymphopenia, or thrombocytopenia in SLE. Also, **serum electrolytes** with **blood urea nitrogen (BUN)** and **creatinine** should be ordered to detect renal disease. In SLE, a **urinalysis** should also be performed, looking for **proteinuria** (evaluate further for nephrotic syndrome), **cellular casts,** and **hematuria** (evaluate further for glomerulonephritis).
MANAGEMENT: Depends on severity and type of symptoms: **mild symptoms**—NSAIDS; **acute exacerbations**—local/systemic corticosteroids; **constitutional, cutaneous, articular symptoms**—antimalarial agents (hydroxychloroquine); **active glomerulonephritis**—cytotoxic agents cyclophosphamide). Monitor for renal disease and hypertension.

BRACHIAL PLEXUS *(Figure 9-3)*

- **Lesions of the brachial plexus and its branches** (Table 9-8)
- **Nerve damage and regeneration** (Figure 9-4)

FIGURE 9-3 **Brachial plexus**

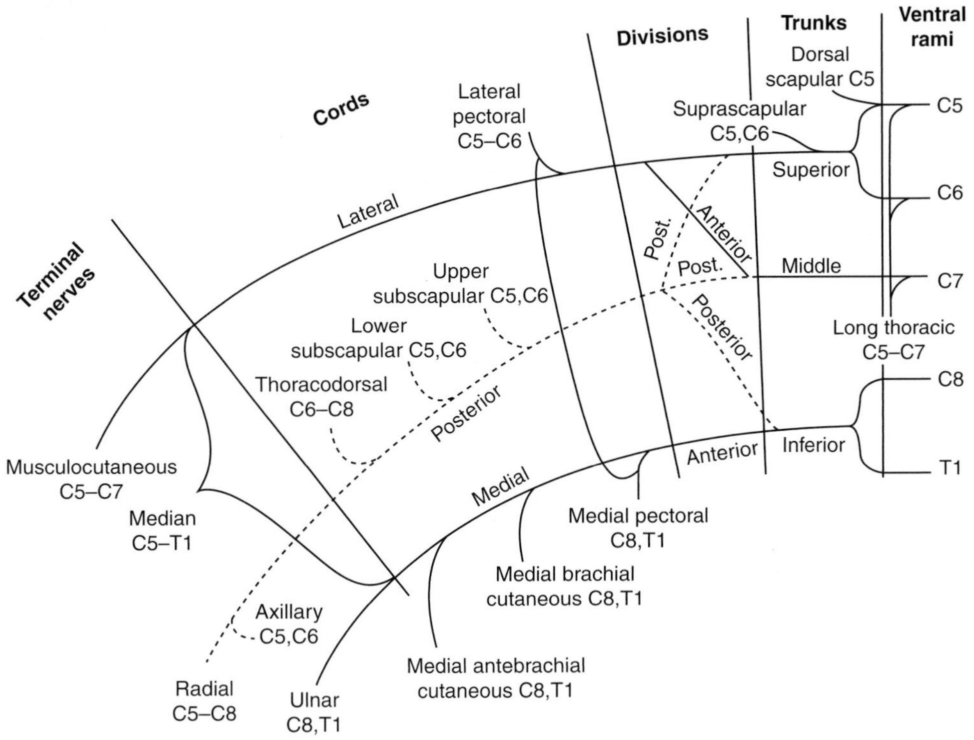
Ventral rami
Trunks
Divisions
Cords
Terminal nerves
Dorsal scapular C5
Suprascapular C5,C6
Lateral pectoral C5–C6
C5
C6
C7
C8
T1
Superior
Middle
Inferior
Anterior
Post.
Posterior
Lateral
Medial
Upper subscapular C5,C6
Lower subscapular C5,C6
Thoracodorsal C6–C8
Long thoracic C5–C7
Musculocutaneous C5–C7
Median C5–T1
Axillary C5,C6
Radial C5–C8
Ulnar C8,T1
Medial antebrachial cutaneous C8,T1
Medial brachial cutaneous C8,T1
Medial pectoral C8,T1

C, cervical vertebra; Post, posterior; T, thoracic vertebra.

MNEMONIC

To remember the parts of the brachial plexus: "Real Texans Drink Cold Beer" (Roots, Trunks, Divisions, Cords, Branches).

TABLE 9-8 **Lesions of the Brachial Plexus and its Branches**

Disorder	Lesion	Cause	Clinical Features
Erb–Duchenne palsy	Upper brachial plexus (C5 and C6)	**Hyperabduction** of the arm (such as trauma, shoulder dystocia during delivery)	**"Waiter's tip"** position (arm extended and adducted, forearm pronated)
Klumpke palsy	Lower brachial plexus (C8–T1)	**Hyperabduction** of the arm (shoulder dystocia during delivery)	Claw hand from ulnar nerve involvement; wrist and hand dysfunction; associated with **Horner syndrome**
Claw hand	Ulnar nerve	Occurs in children with **epiphyseal separation** of the medial epicondyle of the humerus	Weak finger adduction; medial hand numbness; dysfunction of fourth and fifth digit flexion
Radial nerve palsy	Radial nerve	**Fracture of midhumerus**	**Wrist drop;** inability to extend wrist or fingers; loss of sensation from dorsum of hand
Carpal tunnel syndrome	Median nerve	**Repetitive wrist motion** (swelling within the flexor retinaculum compresses the median nerve)	Wrist flexion elicits pain; wrist extension relieves pain; symptoms worse at night

(continued)

QUICK HIT

Wrist drop also occurs in lead poisoning.

QUICK HIT

Contents of the carpal tunnel include tendons of flexor digitorum profundus, flexor digitorum superficialis, flexor pollicis longus, and the median nerve.

QUICK HIT

Lateral winging is caused by accessory nerve lesions leading to trapezius paralysis.

QUICK HIT

Posterior dislocations of the shoulder are common in seizure disorders and injuries caused by electrocution.

QUICK HIT

The median nerve can also be damaged in fractures of the distal third of the humerus and elbow (causing total loss of thumb opposition) or slashing of the wrist.

MNEMONIC

To remember the nerves affected by humerus fracture location, think ARM fracture from superior to inferior: **A**xillary-head of humerus; **R**adial-mid shaft of humerus; **M**edian-supracondylar/distal third of humerus.

TABLE 9-8 **Lesions of the Brachial Plexus and its Branches** *(Continued)*

Disorder	Lesion	Cause	Clinical Features
Medial winging of the scapula	Long thoracic nerve	Surgery (e.g., **mastectomy**)	Limited arm abduction and flexion; **serratus anterior paralysis;** medial scapula protrudes if patient pushes against a wall
Shoulder dislocation	Axillary nerve	**Anterior dislocation** (owing to forced abduction and extension)	Loss of innervation to deltoid; compromised shoulder flexion and extension; palpable depression under acromion
Surgical neck fracture of the humerus	Axillary nerve	A fall landing on the elbow	Loss of innervation to deltoid; compromised shoulder flexion and extension; palpable depression under acromion

FIGURE 9-4 **Nerve damage and regeneration**

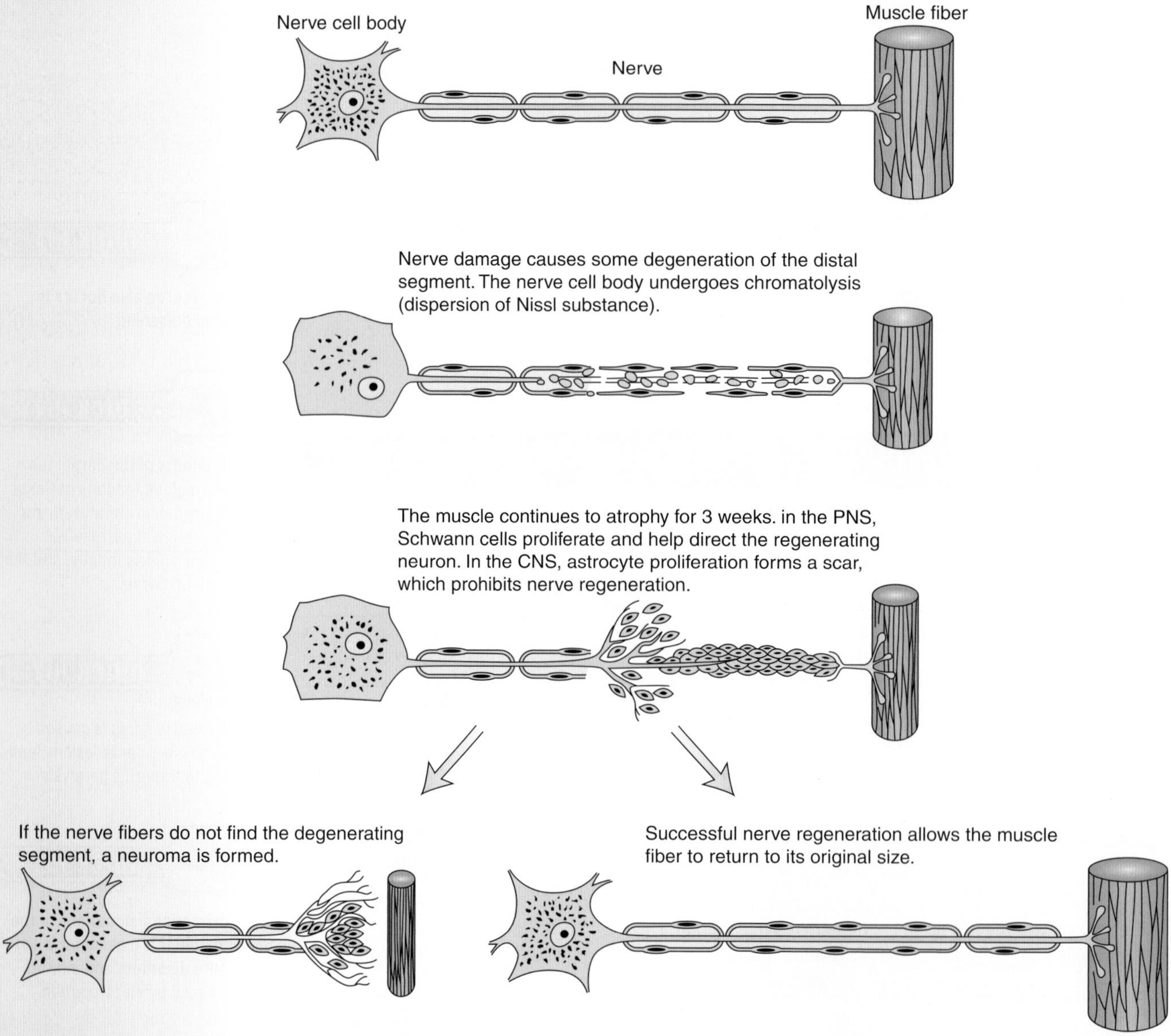
Nerve cell body
Muscle fiber
Nerve
Nerve damage causes some degeneration of the distal segment. The nerve cell body undergoes chromatolysis (dispersion of Nissl substance).
The muscle continues to atrophy for 3 weeks. in the PNS, Schwann cells proliferate and help direct the regenerating neuron. In the CNS, astrocyte proliferation forms a scar, which prohibits nerve regeneration.
If the nerve fibers do not find the degenerating segment, a neuroma is formed.
Successful nerve regeneration allows the muscle fiber to return to its original size.

CNS, central nervous system; PNS, peripheral nervous system.

LUMBOSACRAL PLEXUS *(Figure 9-5)*

I. The lumbosacral plexus, which consists of the ventral rami of L1–S4, supplies the lower extremity.

FIGURE 9-5 **Lumbosacral plexus**

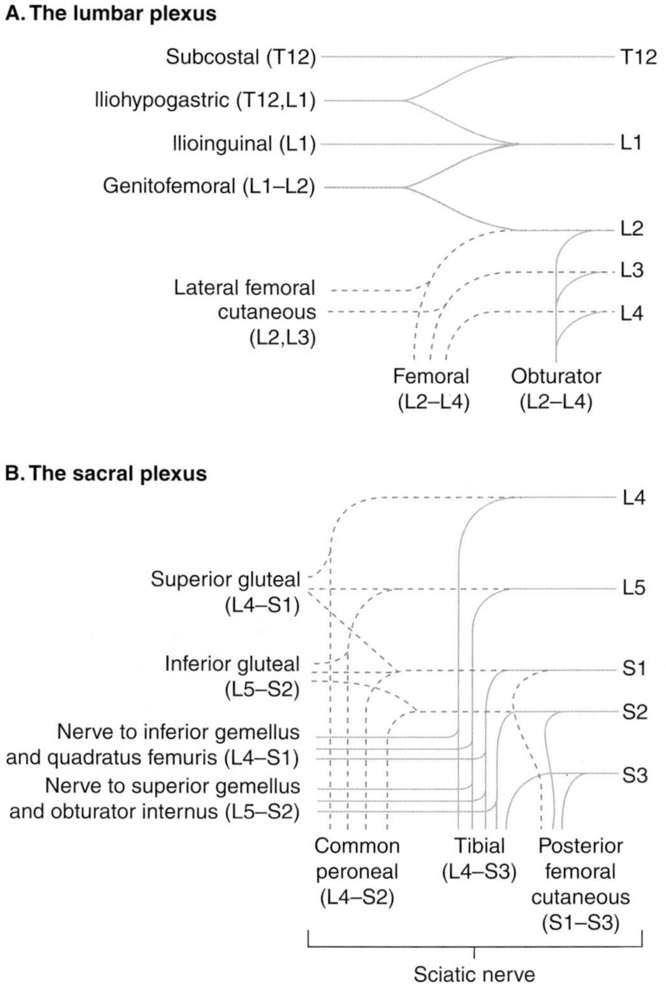
A. The lumbar plexus
Subcostal (T12)
Iliohypogastric (T12,L1)
Ilioinguinal (L1)
Genitofemoral (L1–L2)
Lateral femoral cutaneous (L2,L3)
T12
L1
L2
L3
L4
Femoral (L2–L4)
Obturator (L2–L4)
B. The sacral plexus
L4
L5
S1
S2
S3
Superior gluteal (L4–S1)
Inferior gluteal (L5–S2)
Nerve to inferior gemellus and quadratus femuris (L4–S1)
Nerve to superior gemellus and obturator internus (L5–S2)
Common peroneal (L4–S2)
Tibial (L4–S3)
Posterior femoral cutaneous (S1–S3)
Sciatic nerve

L, lumbar vertebra; S, sacral vertebra; T, thoracic vertebra.

QUICK HIT

All the nerves of the sacral plexus and the pudendal nerve (S2–S4) emerge from the pelvis through the greater sciatic foramen below the piriformis muscle except the superior gluteal nerve, which passes above the piriformis.

II. Motor and sensory functions of the lumbosacral plexus

Sacral plexus lesions are commonly caused by locally invading or metastasizing carcinoma from pelvic organs (e.g., bladder, prostate, ovaries). Knowledge of the motor and sensory functions of the sacral plexus can assist in determining the deficits resulting from complications of these tumors (Tables 9-9 and 9-10).

TABLE 9-9 Segmental Nerve Functions of the Lumbosacral Plexus

Spinal Nerve	Muscle Innervation	Muscle Test	Sensory Function
L1	Cremaster	Cremasteric reflex	Inguinal region
L2	Iliopsoas	Hip flexion	Upper anteromedial thigh
L3	Medial thigh Quadriceps femoris	Hip adduction Knee extension	Lower anteromedial thigh
L4	Tibialis anterior	Ankle dorsiflexion	Anteromedial leg
L5	Extensor hallucis longus	Great toe extension	Anterolateral leg, medial dorsal foot, plantar region of great toe
S1	Gastrocnemius, soleus Posterior thigh Gluteus maximus	Ankle plantarflexion Hip extension, knee flexion Power hip extension, external rotation	Heel region, plantar foot, lateral dorsal foot
S2	Gastrocnemius, soleus Foot intrinsics	Ankle plantarflexion Abduction and adduction of toes	Posterior upper thigh and leg
S3–S4	External anal sphincter Bulbospongiosus	External anal sphincter tone Bulbospongiosus reflex	Circumanal and perineal region

TABLE 9-10 Peripheral Nerve Functions of the Sacral Plexus

Nerve	Muscle Innervation	Muscle Test	Sensory Function
Genitofemoral	Cremaster	Cremasteric reflex	Skin below middle of inguinal ligament
Lateral femoral cutaneous	None	None	Skin of lateral thigh
Femoral	Anterior thigh (quadriceps)	Knee extension	Skin of anteromedial thigh and leg
Obturator	Medial thigh	Hip adduction	Hip joint and medial skin of knee
Superior gluteal	Gluteus medius, gluteus minimus	Hip abduction and internal rotation	None
Inferior gluteal	Gluteus maximus	Power hip extension and external rotation	None
Posterior femoral cutaneous	None	None	Skin of posterior thigh and upper leg
Superficial peroneal	Lateral leg	Foot eversion	Skin of anterolateral leg and dorsum of foot
Deep peroneal	Anterior leg	Ankle dorsiflexion, foot inversion, metatarso-phalangeal joint extension	Skin of dorsum of web space between great and second toes
Tibial	Posterior thigh, gastrocnemius, soleus, deep posterior leg, planar muscles	Hip extensions, knee flexion, foot inversion, toe flexion	Skin of posterior leg and plantar foot

OTHER TRAUMATIC INJURIES *(Table 9-11)*

Musculoskeletal dysfunction can be caused by dearrangement of bone, nerve, musculature, or any combination of these elements. Insult to the body can result in problems that are acute (e.g., a torn anterior cruciate ligament) or chronic (e.g., tennis elbow).

QUICK HIT

Symptoms of compartment syndrome include the "5 Ps": pain, pallor, paresthesia, paralysis, and pulselessness.

QUICK HIT

Ankle sprain grading system: Grade I: stretching of the ligament(s); Grade II: partial tear of the ligament(s); Grade III: complete tear of the ligament(s).

TABLE 9-11 Other Traumatic Injuries

Injury	Description
Anterior cruciate ligament (ACL) tear	Positive **anterior drawer sign** (lower leg pulled forward with knee flexed); often manifests as **"terrible triad"** (i.e., torn medial collateral ligament, medial meniscus damage, and torn ACL), which occurs due to a force to the knee directed laterally to medially
Clavicle fracture	**Middle third** of clavicle; upward displacement of proximal fragment due to the sternocleidomastoid muscle; downward displacement of distal fragment; severe pain
Compartment syndrome	Fascial sheets separate the limbs into anterior and posterior compartments; hemorrhage into these compartments owing to crush injury or fracture, results in **compression of neurovascular structures** and further complications; emergent fasciotomy is needed
Inversion sprain of ankle	**Most common ankle injury;** results from forced inversion; stretches or tears lateral ligaments (especially the **anterior talofibular**)
Scaphoid fracture	Tenderness in the anatomical snuffbox; may lead to **avascular necrosis** if left untreated; easily missed on radiographs
Scoliosis	Complex lateral deviation and torsion of the spine; may be idiopathic or congenital or may result from a short leg, hip displacement, or polio
Shoulder separation	Downward displacement of the clavicle as a result of laxity of the acromioclavicular and coracoclavicular ligaments
Subacromial bursitis	Inflammation of the subacromial bursa; **most common bursitis** in the body
Tennis elbow (lateral epicondylitis)	Sprain of radial collateral ligament (lateral epicondyle); pain on wrist extension and forearm supination
Golfer's elbow (medial epicondylitis)	Overuse of the pronator teres, palmaris longus, and flexor carpi radialis; causes sprain of their tendinous insertion on the anterior medial epicondyle; pain on wrist flexion

(continued)

QUICK HIT

Scaphoid fractures tend to occur with a fall on an outstretched hand, which causes dorsiflexion and exposes the scaphoid bone.

QUICK HIT

The anatomic snuffbox is bounded dorsally by the extensor pollicis longus and on the palmar side by the extensor pollicis brevis and the abductor pollicis longus, with the scaphoid and the trapezium bones creating the base.

QUICK HIT

The artery supplying the scaphoid first goes distally then curves proximally, making the proximal aspect of the scaphoid susceptible to avascular necrosis.

QUICK HIT

Golf elbow has manifestations similar to those of tennis elbow, except that it involves the medial epicondyle.

QUICK HIT

The Trendelenburg sign results in downward tilting of the pelvis to the side opposite that of injury when standing on the foot of the injured side secondary to weakness or paralysis of the gluteus muscle. It can also be seen in a hip dislocation or a fracture of the neck of the femur.

TABLE 9-11 **Other Traumatic Injuries** *(Continued)*

Injury	Description
Waddling gait	Limp caused by superior gluteal nerve injury affecting gluteus medius and gluteus minimus; inability to abduct thigh; results in **Trendelenburg sign**

PAIN MANAGEMENT *(Figure 9-6) (Table 9-12)*

I. Musculoskeletal conditions, such as fractures and soft-tissue injuries, can result in significant disability, pain, and inflammation. Medical management of this pain and discomfort involves the use of nonnarcotic and narcotic preparations.

II. Acetaminophen

Acetaminophen (Tylenol) is a nonnarcotic analgesic with antipyretic and analgesic properties. It has little anti-inflammatory action. After acetaminophen is absorbed by the gastrointestinal (GI) tract, it is metabolized in the liver. In therapeutic doses, acetaminophen has minimal significant adverse effects. However, in large doses, depletion of liver **glutathione** levels may occur, resulting in hepatic necrosis as a result of the excess *N*-acetyl-*p*-benzoquinoneimine (NAPQI). Treatment for acetaminophen overdose is aerosolized *N*-**acetylcysteine, which regenerates the depleted levels of glutathione**.

QUICK HIT

Drugs such as carbamazepine, rifampin, and isoniazid can increase the action of liver enzymes, thus increasing the metabolism and reducing the effectiveness of acetaminophen.

III. Nonsteroidal anti-inflammatory drugs (NSAIDs)

NSAIDs are similar to acetaminophen in that they have **antipyretic** and **analgesic** properties. In addition, these agents have **anti-inflammatory** effects. NSAIDs act by inhibiting cyclooxygenase (COX) enzymes (Figure 9-6).

QUICK HIT

It is believed that prostaglandin E_2 (PGE_2) sensitizes the nerve endings to the action of bradykinin, histamine, and other chemical mediators.

FIGURE 9-6 **Mechanism of action of nonsteroidal anti-inflammatory drugs**

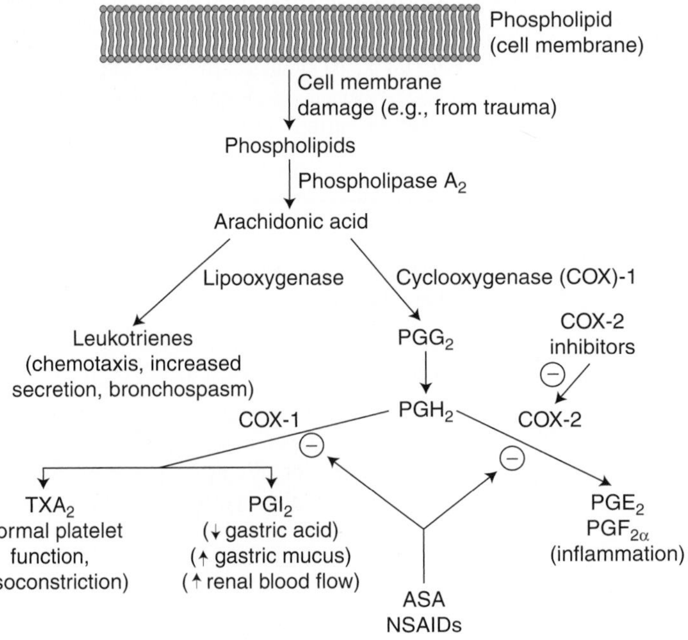

Phospholipid (cell membrane)
Cell membrane damage (e.g., from trauma)
Phospholipids
Phospholipase A2
Arachidonic acid
Lipooxygenase
Cyclooxygenase (COX)-1
Leukotrienes (chemotaxis, increased secretion, bronchospasm)
PGG2
COX-2 inhibitors
PGH2
COX-1
COX-2
TXA2 (normal platelet function, vasoconstriction)
PGI2 (↓ gastric acid) (↑ gastric mucus) (↑ renal blood flow)
PGE2 PGF2α (inflammation)
ASA NSAIDs

ASA, aspirin; PG, prostaglandin; TX, thromboxane.

QUICK HIT

Administration of aspirin to children with fever increases the risk of Reye syndrome. Acetaminophen, ibuprofen, and other NSAIDs are viable alternatives for pain and fever in children.

A. **Aspirin**, the most common NSAID, blocks prostaglandin synthesis from arachidonic acid in the hypothalamus and in peripheral tissue, which provides its antipyretic, antiplatelet, analgesic, and anti-inflammatory benefits. Unlike other NSAIDs, its inhibitory effect on COX enzymes is irreversible.

B. A major adverse effect of aspirin and NSAIDs (e.g., ibuprofen, indomethacin, naproxen, diclofenac, ketorolac) is increased risk of **GI bleeding**. By blocking prostaglandin synthesis, NSAIDs may result in GI ulcers and hemorrhage. Prostacyclin (PGI2) inhibits gastric acid secretion, whereas prostaglandin (PG) E_2 and $PGF_{2\alpha}$ help synthesize protective mucus in the stomach and small intestine. **COX-2 inhibitors** such as **celecoxib** may be indicated in patients who have a history of GI conditions; these NSAIDs are more specific for the inflammatory mediators (Figure 9-6).

QUICK HIT

Because of the irreversible effect of aspirin on thromboxane production in platelets, it can be used as an anticoagulant. A daily low dose of aspirin has a cardioprotective effect in men.

IV. Opioids

Opioids are useful for severe pain that is uncontrolled by NSAIDs. Opioids exert their effects by interacting with protein receptors in the central nervous system (CNS) and by inhibiting G proteins and adenylyl cyclase in the peripheral nervous system. Each family of opioid receptors—μ, κ, σ, and δ—has its own set of properties and binding potency, which correlates with the amount of analgesia provided. The μ receptors primarily mediate analgesia.

The strong agonists of the various receptor families are **morphine**, **meperidine**, **methadone**, **fentanyl**, and **heroin**. Moderate agonists include codeine and propoxyphene. Some of these agents can produce extreme states of euphoria and become drugs of abuse because of their binding affinity and their intrinsic effects on the CNS. Methadone, which induces less euphoria and has a longer duration of action, is often used to provide controlled withdrawal from addiction to agents such as morphine and heroin.

Opioid overdose can lead to respiratory depression, depression of the cough reflex, pinpoint pupils, constipation, bronchoconstriction, diaphoresis, and urinary retention. Naloxone and naltrexone reverse the adverse effects of opioids. A rapid-acting drug, naloxone, displaces the receptor-bound opioid agents. Its effects are short-lived (approximately 2 hours). However, naltrexone works for up to 48 hours.

QUICK HIT

The miosis seen in opioid overdose is a result of stimulation of the Edinger–Westphal nucleus of the oculomotor nerve, which leads to enhanced parasympathetic stimulation of the eye.

QUICK HIT

Opioids can also be used as effective medications to combat diarrhea and cough.

TABLE 9-12 **Therapeutic Agents for Pain**

Therapeutic Agent (common name, if relevant) [trade name, where appropriate]	Class—Pharmacology and Pharmacokinetics	Indications	Side Effects or Adverse Effects	Contraindications or Precautions to Consider; Notes
Acetaminophen [Tylenol]	Analgesic, antipyretic—reversibly inhibits COX centrally (inactivated peripherally); prostaglandin inhibitor, **not anti-inflammatory**	Pain, fever	Liver toxicity in high doses **(high levels deplete glutathione)**	**Overdose treated with** *N*-acetyl-cysteine (regenerates glutathione); unlike aspirin, **can be used in children, gout, peptic ulcer, and patients with platelet dysfunction**
Acetylsalicylic acid (aspirin)	**Anti-inflammatory, antipyretic, analgesic**—acetylates COX irreversibly	Articular, musculoskeletal pain; chronic pain; **maintenance therapy for preventing clot formation**	GI distress, **GI ulcers, inhibits platelet aggregation**; causes **hypersensitivity reactions (rash)**; reversible hepatic dysfunction	**Contraindicated for children** with the flu or chicken pox (leads to **Reye syndrome), patients with gout**
Ibuprofen [Advil, Motrin]	**NSAID—reversibly inhibits COX** (both COX-1 and COX-2) → decreases prostaglandin synthesis	**Inflammation, pain**	GI distress, **GI ulcers**, coagulation disorders, aplastic anemia, metabolic abnormalities, hypersensitivity, renal damage	

(continued)

TABLE 9-12 Therapeutic Agents for Pain *(Continued)*

Therapeutic Agent (common name, if relevant) [trade name, where appropriate]	Class—Pharmacology and Pharmacokinetics	Indications	Side Effects or Adverse Effects	Contraindications or Precautions to Consider; Notes
Naproxen [Naprosyn, Aleve]	**NSAID—reversibly inhibits COX** (both COX-1 and COX-2) → decreases prostaglandin synthesis	Inflammation, pain	GI distress, **GI ulcers**, coagulation disorders, aplastic anemia, metabolic abnormalities, hypersensitivity, renal damage	
Indomethacin [Indocin]	**NSAID—reversibly inhibits COX** (both COX-1 and COX-2) → decreases prostaglandin synthesis	Acute gout; closes patent ductus arteriosus	GI distress, **GI ulcers**, coagulation disorders, aplastic anemia, metabolic abnormalities, hypersensitivity, renal damage	
Ketorolac [Toradol]	**NSAID—reversibly inhibits COX** (both COX-1 and COX-2) → decreases prostaglandin synthesis; relieves pain and reduces swelling	**Postoperative pain,** severe pain	GI distress, **GI ulcers**, coagulation disorders, aplastic anemia, metabolic abnormalities, hypersensitivity, renal damage	
Celecoxib [Celebrex]	**NSAID—selectively inhibits COX-2**	Rheumatoid arthritis, osteoarthritis; pain, inflammation	**Increased risk of thrombosis; sulfa allergy; less toxic to GI mucosa**	COX-2 selectivity reduces inflammation while minimizing GI adverse effects (ulcers)
Morphine [MS Contin, MSIR, Roxanol]	**Opioid agonist**—converted to more potent morphine-6-glucose	Severe pain; general anesthetic; antitussive; antidiarrheal	Respiratory depression; histamine release; constipation; nausea; miosis	
Meperidine [Demerol]	**Opioid agonist**	**Pain**, acute migraine attacks	**CNS excitation at high doses**; histamine release	**Contraindicated in patients with MAOI** (results in hyperpyrexia)
Fentanyl	**Opioid agonist**	**Pain**; general anesthetic	Prolonged recovery; nausea	
Codeine	**Opioid agonist**	**Pain**; antitussive	**Constipation**	
Oxycodone [Roxicodone]	**Opioid agonist**	Severe pain; general anesthetic	Respiratory depression, constipation, nausea	
Hydromorphone [Dilaudid]	Opioid agonist	**Pain**; antitussive	Respiratory depression, constipation, nausea	
Methadone	**Opioid agonist**—synthetic	Maintenance therapy for **heroin addiction**	Respiratory depression; histamine release; constipation; nausea; miosis	
Tramadol [Ultram]	Analgesic—similar to opioid agonist	Chronic pain of **osteoarthritis**	Nausea, vomiting, constipation, drowsiness	

CNS, central nervous system; COX, cyclooxygenase; GI, gastrointestinal; MAOI, monoamine oxydase inhibitor; MSIR, morphine sulfate instant release; NSAID, nonsteroidal anti-inflammatory drug.

MUSCLE FUNCTION AND DYSFUNCTION *(Figure 9-7)*

FIGURE 9-7 The cross-bridge cycle of skeletal muscle

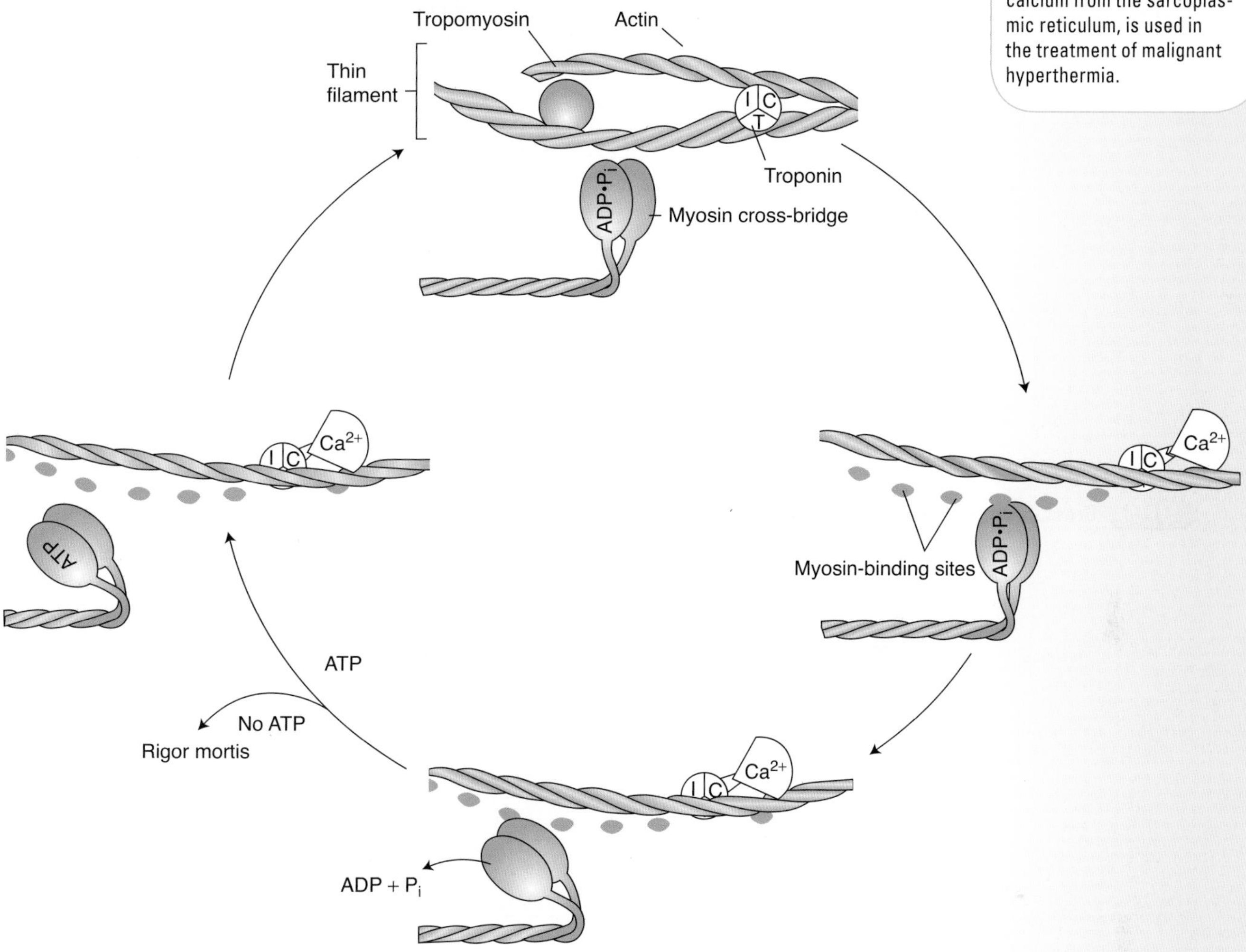
Tropomyosin
Actin
Thin filament
I
C
T
Troponin
ADP•P_i
Myosin cross-bridge
Ca2+
Myosin-binding sites
ATP
No ATP
Rigor mortis
ADP + P_i

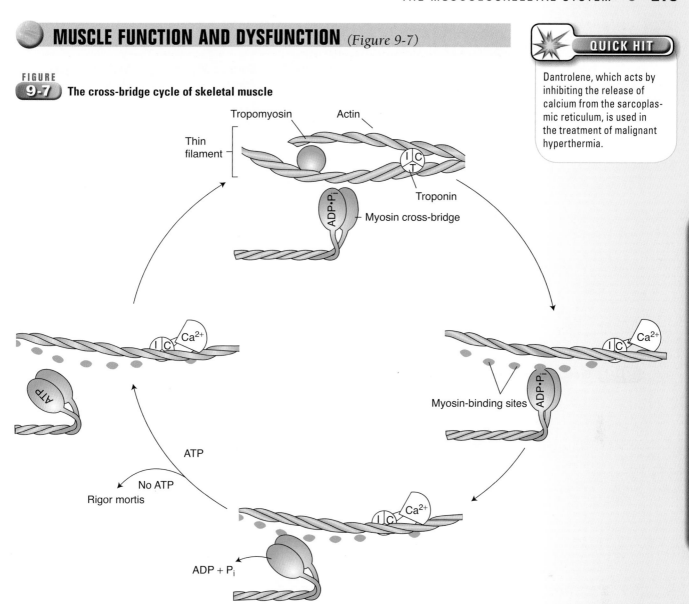

ADP, adenosine diphosphate; ATP, adenosine triphosphate; Ca^{2+}, calcium; P_i, inorganic phospate; T, troponin.

QUICK HIT

Dantrolene, which acts by inhibiting the release of calcium from the sarcoplasmic reticulum, is used in the treatment of malignant hyperthermia.

I. Comparison of muscle fibers *(Table 9-13) (Figure 9-8)*

Muscle can be divided into three subtypes with differing physiologic roles.

A. **Smooth muscle** plays a significant role in the maintenance of the lumens of the respiratory and GI tracts and blood vessels.

B. **Cardiac muscle** contracts the heart and propels blood through the vasculature.

MNEMONIC

Remember the number of nuclei in muscle cells by simply noting **one** heart in the body and **one** nucleus per heart muscle cell; **many** skeletal muscles, so **many** nuclei per skeletal muscle fiber. Also, **location** of nucleus mirrors **location** in human body. The heart is in the center of the body and the nucleus is centrally located. Skeletal muscles predominate in the periphery of the body and the nuclei are at the periphery.

TABLE 9-13 Comparison of Muscle Fibers

Category	Smooth Muscle Fiber	Cardiac Muscle Fiber	Skeletal Muscle Fiber
Nuclei	Centrally located single nucleus	Centrally located single nucleus	Peripherally located multiple nuclei
Banding	No distinct bands	Distinct bands	Distinct bands
Z line (convergence actin filaments)	None; dense bodies present	Present	Present

(continued)

The Musculoskeletal System

TABLE 9-13 **Comparison of Muscle Fibers** *(Continued)*

Category	Smooth Muscle Fiber	Cardiac Muscle Fiber	Skeletal Muscle Fiber
Transverse (T) tubules (membrane invaginations)	None	At Z line; diads	At A–I junction; triads
Junctional communication	Gap junctions	Intercalated disks	None
Neuromuscular junction	None	None	Present
Regeneration	High	None	Some
Calcium source	Sarcoplasmic reticulum; extracellular	Sarcoplasmic reticulum; extracellular	Sarcoplasmic reticulum
Mechanism of calcium release	IP_3 (inositol-1,4,5-triphosphate)	Calcium induced	Depolarization of T tubule
Calcium-binding protein	Calmodulin	Troponin	Troponin

FIGURE 9-8 **Gross, histologic, microscopic anatomy of skeletal muscle**

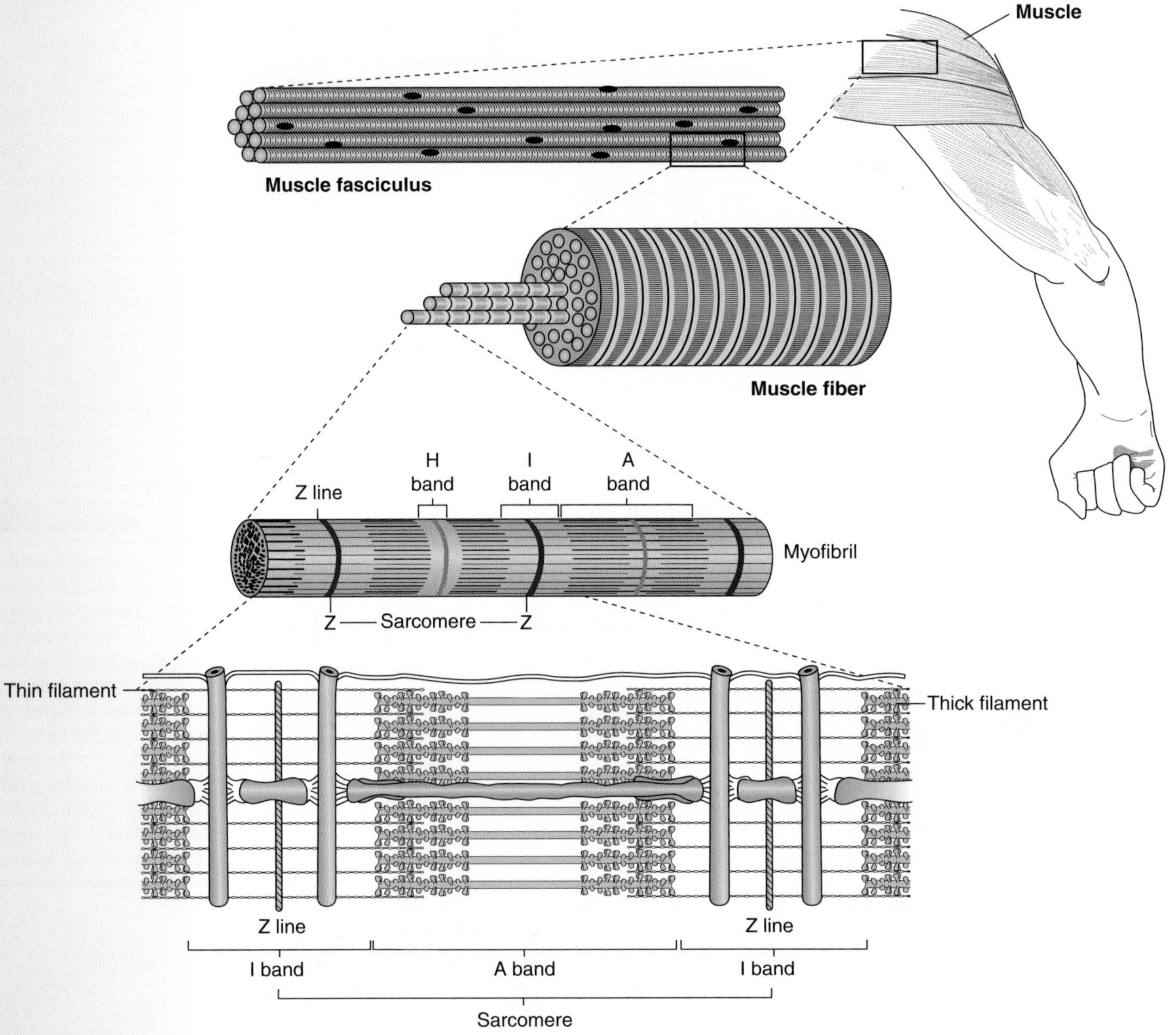
Muscle
Muscle fasciculus
Muscle fiber
H band
I band
A band
Z line
Myofibril
Z — Sarcomere — Z
Thin filament
Thick filament
Z line
Z line
I band
A band
I band
Sarcomere

TABLE 9-14 Types of Skeletal Muscle Fibers

Category	Type 1	Type 2
Action	Sustained force; weight-bearing muscles	Sudden movement; directed action
Lipid stores	Abundant	Few
Glycogen stores	Few	Abundant
Energy utilization	Aerobic; many mitochondria	Anaerobic; few mitochondria; easily fatigued
Twitch	Slow	Fast
Color	Red (owing to blood supply)	White

C. **Skeletal muscle maintains posture and produces movement**. There are two types of skeletal muscle fibers (Table 9-14).

II. Muscle tumors *(Table 9-15)*

Pathology of muscles can take many forms. Metabolic dyscrasias, which can be induced or inherited, are far more common than neoplasms.

QUICK HIT

The embryonal type of rhabdomyosarcoma is related to sarcoma botryoides, resulting in a "bunch of grapes" appearance (see Chapter 8).

TABLE 9-15 Muscle Tumors

	Leiomyoma	Leiomyosarcoma	Rhabdomyosarcoma
Morphology	Benign; elongated nuclei; whorled bundles of smooth muscle cells; no larger than 2 cm	Malignant; "cigar-shaped" nuclei dense bodies	Malignant; embryonal, alveolar, and pleomorphic types; rhabdomyoblast is diagnostic cell
Location	Smooth muscle, **uterus**	Smooth muscle, skin, deep soft tissues	Skeletal muscle, head and neck, genitourinary tract, retroperitoneum
Immunohistochemistry	Antibodies to actin and desmin	Antibodies to vimentin, actin, and desmin	Antibodies to vimentin, actin, desmin, and myoglobin
Prognosis	Indolent course; easily cured	Variable; prognosis worse with increased size	Aggressive; treat with surgery, radiation, chemotherapy
Notes	Afflicts women more often than men; **most common tumor in women**	Uncommon	**Most common soft-tissue sarcoma of childhood** and adolescence

III. Other neuromuscular disorders *(Table 9-16)*

IV. Neuromuscular blocking agents

Neuromuscular blocking agents, which are most often encountered in the operating room, are used to produce the flaccid paralysis that is essential for many procedures, such as abdominal operations and joint replacements. These drugs affect the muscles of the body in a typical order. The small, fast-twitch muscles of the face and eyes are the first to be paralyzed, followed by the muscles of the hand, limbs, and trunk. The intercostal muscles and the diaphragm are the last to be affected. As the effects of neuromuscular blockers wear off, the muscles regain function in the reverse order.

QUICK HIT

Abnormality of the thymus is seen in 65% of patients with myasthenia gravis, 15% being a thymoma, requiring a thymectomy.

QUICK HIT

Pseudohypertrophy is initially caused by muscle hypertrophy. Then as atrophy ensues, an increase in fat and connective tissue deposition occurs.

QUICK HIT

Becker muscular dystrophy is a less common and less severe variant of Duchenne muscular dystrophy that involves the same gene (Xp21) and the dystrophin protein.

TABLE 9-16 **Other Neuromuscular Disorders**

Disorder	Etiology	Clinical Features	Notes
Lactic acidosis	Shock, sepsis, methanol poisoning, metformin toxicity, liver failure, diabetic ketoacidosis	Increased serum lactate; **metabolic acidosis**; increased anion gap	May lead to coma or death
Myasthenia gravis	Acetylcholine receptor **autoantibodies at the neuromuscular junction**; linked to HLA-DR3; associated with thymus disorders	Muscle weakness with use; ptosis; manifests itself in facial, ocular, and limb muscles; proximal muscles affected first	Four times more common in women; diagnosis includes the edrophonium (Tensilon) test; anticholinesterase (e.g., edrophonium) improves condition
Duchenne muscular dystrophy	**X-linked recessive**; deficiency in **dystrophin** leading to lack of actin stabilization	Progressive; proximal muscle weakens, beginning with the pelvic girdle and extending to the shoulder girdle; **pseudohypertrophy** of muscles (e.g., calf); positive Gowers maneuver; leads to death via respiratory or cardiac failure	Increased serum creatine kinase and lactate dehydrogenase; clinical symptoms usually appear by age 5 years with wheelchair dependence by the end of the first decade of life and death in the 20s
Mitochondrial myopathy	Transmitted via mitochondrial DNA (mtDNA); non-Mendelian inheritance	**Ragged red fibers** seen on muscle biopsy; proximal muscle weakness	**Maternal** mode of transmission

HLA, human leukocyte antigen.

QUICK HIT

When succinylcholine is used in combination with halothane, it can cause malignant hyperthermia in certain predisposed individuals. Treatment of this condition, which is characterized by severe, prolonged muscle contractions, involves the use of dantrolene and cooling blankets.

MNEMONIC

Remember MCARDLES syndrome: **M**yoglobinuria; **C**ramping after exercise; **A**ccumulated glycogen; **R**ecessive inheritance; **D**eficiency of muscle glycogen phosphorylase; **L**actate levels fail to rise; **E**levated creatinine kinase; **S**keletal muscle only.

Neuromuscular blocking agents can be categorized in several ways. The most useful system divides them into central-acting and neuromuscular endplate (NMEP) blockers. The NMEP blockers can be further divided into depolarizing and nondepolarizing agents.

Centrally acting neuromuscular blocking drugs include diazepam and baclofen. **Diazepam**, a benzodiazepine, acts at γ-aminobutyric acid (GABA) receptors in the CNS. **Baclofen**, another GABA mimetic, also acts in the CNS to decrease muscle tone. Peripherally acting drugs include curare, succinylcholine, and dantrolene.

Curare acts as a nicotinic antagonist at the motor endplate to produce muscle relaxation. At low doses, this agent binds to and blocks the nicotinic receptor, a competitive blockade that can be overcome by increasing the concentration of acetylcholine. At higher doses, curare and the curare-like agents actually block ion channels at the NMEP (noncompetitive block).

Succinylcholine, the only depolarizing neuromuscular blocking agent, acts by binding to and activating the nicotinic receptor of the NMEP. In phase 1 block, a wave of fasciculations rapidly passes over the patient as the drug is administered. The drug then remains attached to the nicotinic receptor and is not broken down by acetylcholinesterase. In phase 2 block, the membrane of the NMEP repolarizes, the muscles relax, and the succinylcholine continues to block the nicotinic receptor. Plasma cholinesterase quickly breaks down the drug, and its duration of action is only a few minutes. The rapid onset and short duration of action of succinylcholine make it ideal for use during rapid-sequence endotracheal intubation and electroconvulsive therapy.

V. Muscle glycogen storage disorders *(Figure 9-9)*

FIGURE 9-9 Muscle glycogen storage disorders

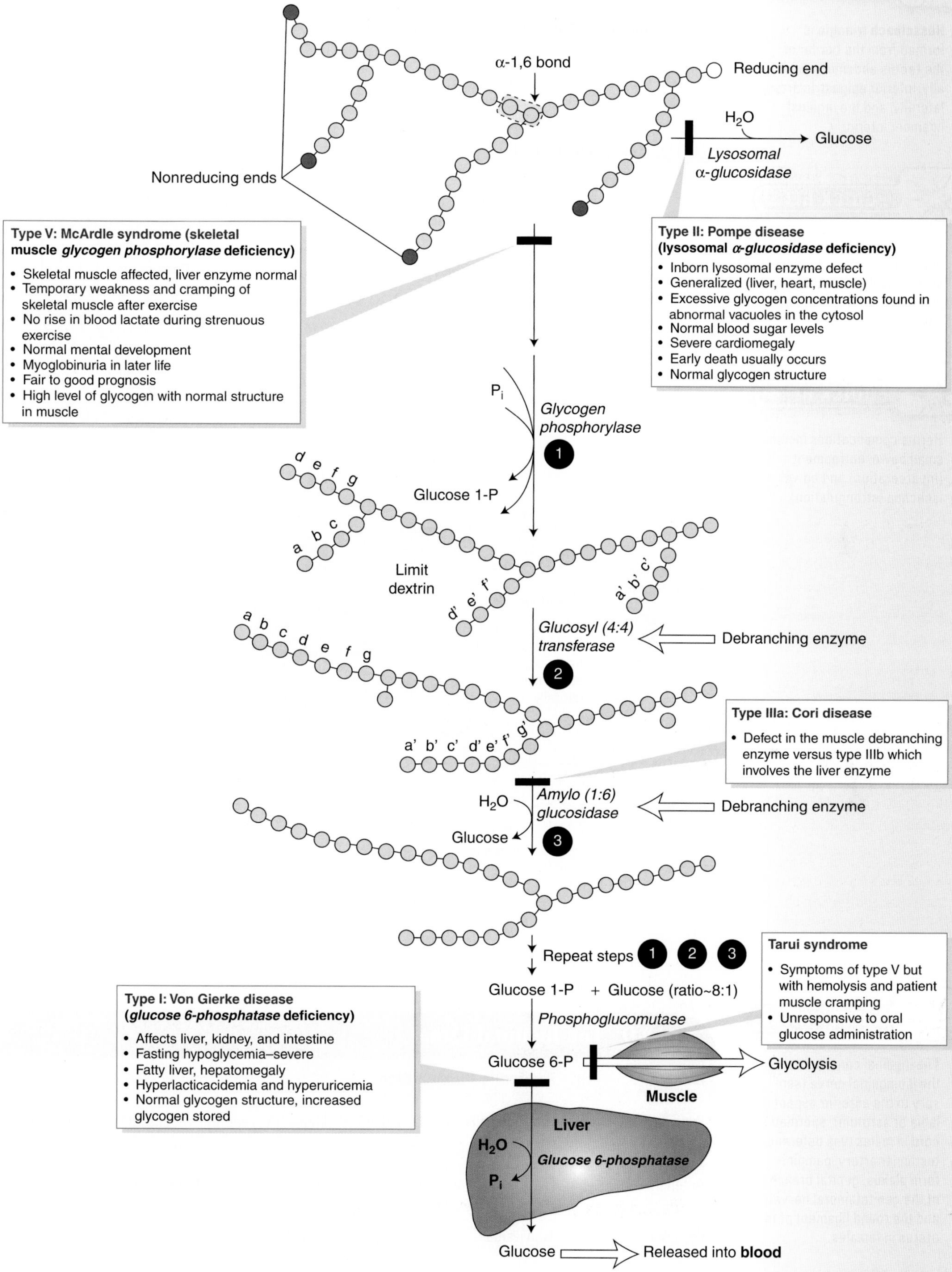
α-1,6 bond
Reducing end
H_2O
Glucose
Lysosomal α-glucosidase
Nonreducing ends
Type V: McArdle syndrome (skeletal muscle *glycogen phosphorylase* deficiency)
• Skeletal muscle affected, liver enzyme normal
• Temporary weakness and cramping of skeletal muscle after exercise
• No rise in blood lactate during strenuous exercise
• Normal mental development
• Myoglobinuria in later life
• Fair to good prognosis
• High level of glycogen with normal structure in muscle
Type II: Pompe disease (lysosomal *α-glucosidase* deficiency)
• Inborn lysosomal enzyme defect
• Generalized (liver, heart, muscle)
• Excessive glycogen concentrations found in abnormal vacuoles in the cytosol
• Normal blood sugar levels
• Severe cardiomegaly
• Early death usually occurs
• Normal glycogen structure
P_i
Glycogen phosphorylase
1
Glucose 1-P
Limit dextrin
Glucosyl (4:4) transferase
2
Debranching enzyme
Type IIIa: Cori disease
• Defect in the muscle debranching enzyme versus type IIIb which involves the liver enzyme
H_2O
Amylo (1:6) glucosidase
Glucose
3
Debranching enzyme
Repeat steps 1 2 3
Glucose 1-P + Glucose (ratio~8:1)
Phosphoglucomutase
Tarui syndrome
• Symptoms of type V but with hemolysis and patient muscle cramping
• Unresponsive to oral glucose administration
Type I: Von Gierke disease (*glucose 6-phosphatase* deficiency)
• Affects liver, kidney, and intestine
• Fasting hypoglycemia–severe
• Fatty liver, hepatomegaly
• Hyperlacticacidemia and hyperuricemia
• Normal glycogen structure, increased glycogen stored
Glucose 6-P
Glycolysis
Muscle
Liver
H_2O
P_i
Glucose 6-phosphatase
Glucose
Released into blood

(Adapted from Champe PC, Harvey RA. *Lippincott's Illustrated Reviews: Biochemistry.* 2nd ed. Philadelphia, PA: Lippincott-Raven; 1994:140. Used by permission of Lippincott Williams & Wilkins.)

The Musculoskeletal System

THE INGUINAL CANAL

I. The inguinal canal *(Figure 9-10) (Table 9-17)*

QUICK HIT

Hesselbach triangle is formed from the border of the rectus abdominis medially, inferior epigastric artery laterally, and the inguinal ligament inferiorly.

QUICK HIT

Hernias may cause small bowel obstruction. However, small bowel obstructions are most commonly caused by adhesions.

QUICK HIT

Hernia complications include small bowel entrapment (incarceration) and bowel ischemia (strangulation).

FIGURE 9-10 The inguinal canal

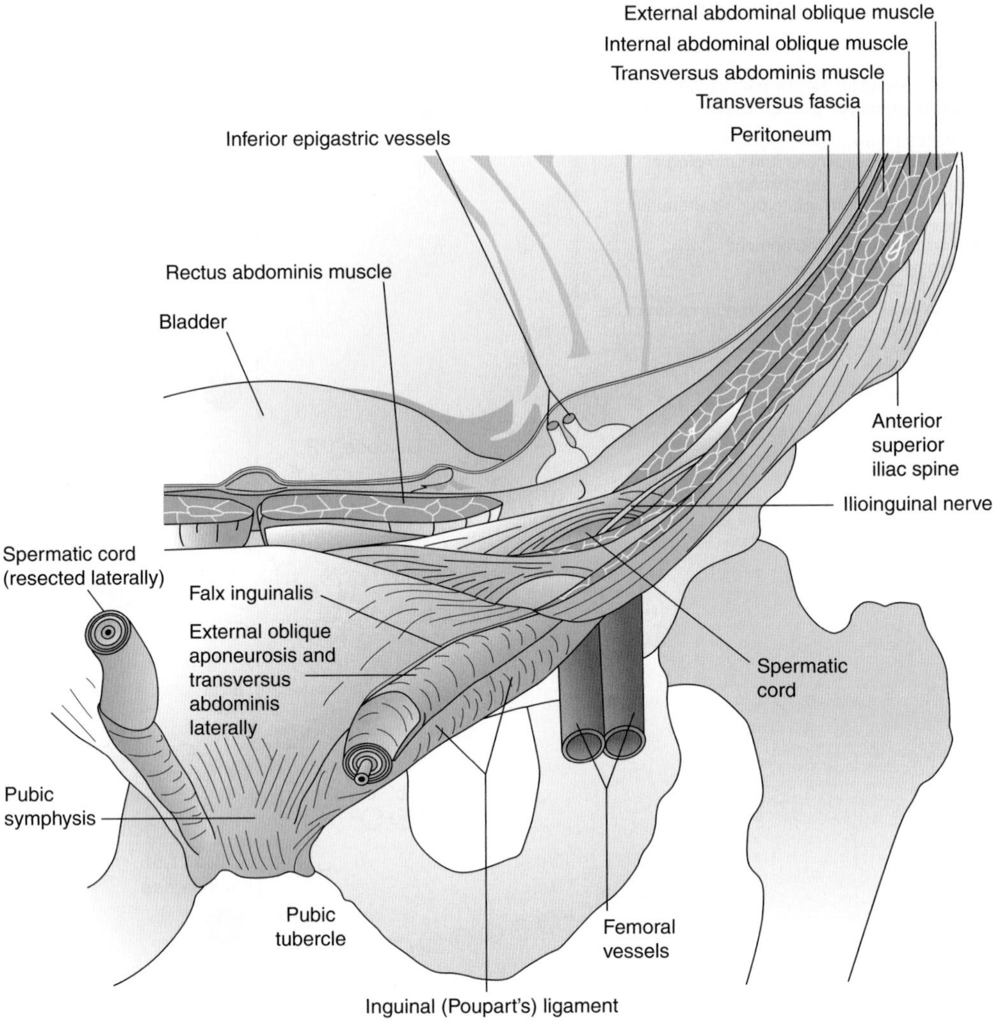

External abdominal oblique muscle
Internal abdominal oblique muscle
Transversus abdominis muscle
Transversus fascia
Peritoneum
Inferior epigastric vessels
Rectus abdominis muscle
Bladder
Anterior superior iliac spine
Ilioinguinal nerve
Spermatic cord (resected laterally)
Falx inguinalis
External oblique aponeurosis and transversus abdominis laterally
Spermatic cord
Pubic symphysis
Pubic tubercle
Femoral vessels
Inguinal (Poupart's) ligament

QUICK HIT

The inguinal canal contains the ilioinguinal nerve (sensory to the anterior aspect of labia or scrotum), spermatic cord in males (vas deferens, testicular artery, pampiniform plexus, genital branch of the genitofemoral nerve), and the round ligament of the uterus in females.

TABLE 9-17 The Inguinal Canal

Border	Anatomic Composition
Superior	Falx inguinalis: internal abdominal oblique (IAO) and transversus abdominis muscles
Inferior	Inguinal ligament
Anterior	External abdominal oblique (EAO) aponeurosis; IAO and transversus abdominis muscles laterally
Posterior	Transversalis fascia; falx inguinalis medially

II. Hernias *(Table 9-18)*

TABLE 9-18 **Hernias**

Hernia	Pathology	Clinical Features	Diagnosis
Direct inguinal hernia	Parietal peritoneum passes directly through the abdominal wall (through the **Hesselbach** triangle)	More common in older males	Medial to inferior epigastric artery; located above pubic tubercle
Indirect inguinal hernia	Parietal peritoneum passes through the internal inguinal ring and follows the inguinal canal; failure of the processus vaginalis to close properly	**Most common** type; occurs in young adult males more frequently than in females	Lateral to inferior epigastric artery; located above and medial to pubic tubercle; hernia sac may enter the scrotum in males
Femoral hernia	Parietal peritoneum passes through the femoral canal	More common in older females	Located below and lateral to pubic tubercle

DERMATOLOGY

I. Skin *(Figure 9-11)*

A. Stratum basale is actively mitotic and gives rise to the other four layers.
B. Epidermis forms from ectoderm and dermis forms from mesoderm.
C. Melanocytes contain melanin pigment and are derived from neural crest.
D. Skin renews every 2 to 3 weeks.
E. Function
   1. Barrier to infection
   2. Thermoregulation
   3. Protection from desiccation
F. Two types of skin
   1. Thick skin (e.g., palms and soles of feet)
      a. Stratum basale (deepest layer)
      b. Stratum spinosum
      c. Stratum granulosum
      d. Stratum lucidum
      e. Stratum corneum (most superficial layer)
   2. Thin skin (e.g., face, genitalia, and back of hands): stratum lucidum is absent in thin skin (although it has all the other layers).

FIGURE 9-11 **Skin histology**

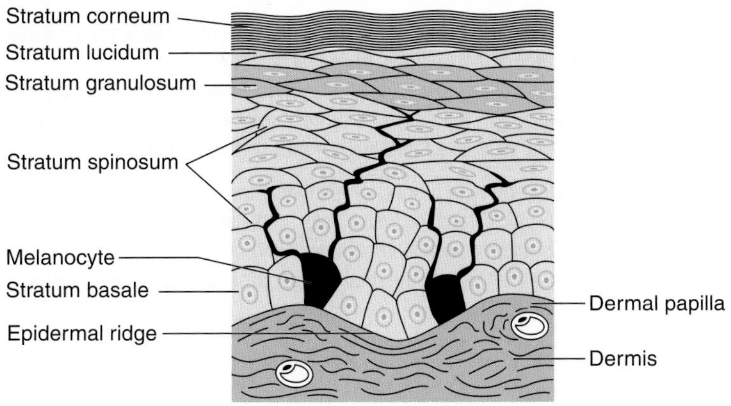
Stratum corneum
Stratum lucidum
Stratum granulosum
Stratum spinosum
Melanocyte
Stratum basale
Epidermal ridge
Dermal papilla
Dermis

QUICK HIT

A lack of pigment, such as in albinism, predisposes one to a variety of skin disorders, including actinic keratosis, basal cell carcinoma, squamous cell carcinoma, and malignant melanoma.

II. Skin disorders *(Table 9-19)*

Skin disorders are often characterized by pruritus, inflammation, and irritability. Skin lesions that are suggestive of malignancy demonstrate asymmetry, irregular borders, variations in color, and increasing size.

- **Skin Cancers** (Table 9-20)

TABLE 9-19 Skin Disorders

Disorder	Description
Keloid scarring	• **Excessive scarring** that occurs after minor trauma • Results in raised, firm lesions on the skin • Occurs more frequently in Blacks • Genetic predisposition is a factor
Xanthomas	• Accumulation of foam-filled histiocytes within the dermis • Often associated with **hyperlipidemia** or lymphoproliferative disorders • Often found on the Achilles tendon, the extensor tendons of the fingers, and the eyelids
Verrucae	• "Warts" • Histology: epidermal hyperplasia, hyperkeratosis, koilocytosis
Seborrheic keratosis	• Common **benign neoplasm** in the elderly • Raised papules and plaques that appear to be "pasted on"; often dark, and can be large
Actinic keratosis	• A series of dysplastic changes that occur before the onset of **squamous cell carcinoma** • A buildup of keratin caused by excessive exposure to sunlight leads to a **"warty"** appearance • Higher incidence in lightly pigmented individuals
Albinism	• **Lack of melanin pigment** production • Ocular type limited to eyes; X linked • Oculocutaneous type involves the skin, eyes, and hair; autosomal recessive; lack of tyrosinase, which converts tyrosine to DOPA (3,4-dihydroxyphenylalanine)
Vitiligo	• Irregular areas of depigmentation, due to **decreased number of melanocytes**
Melasma	• Pregnancy-associated hyperpigmentation
Acanthosis nigricans	• Velvety thickening and **hyperpigmentation** of the axilla, neck, and groin region • Associated with insulin resistance (type 2 diabetes mellitus) and sometimes with occult visceral malignancy
Hemangiomas	• Large-vessel malformation composed of masses of blood-filled channels • **Port-wine stain** birthmarks are the most common manifestation • Cavernous hemangiomas are a subset with large cavernous vascular spaces that can occur in von Hippel–Lindau disease
Psoriasis	• Plaques with **silvery scale**; plaque bleed when scraped (**Auspitz sign**) • Often affects elbows, knees, scalp, hands • Autoimmune etiology; may be associated with psoriatic arthritis • Histology: parakeratotic scaling, increased thickness of the stratum spinosum, decreased thickness of the stratum granulosum
Atopic dermatitis (eczema)	• Dry skin with pruritic inflammatory lesions that become lichenified with chronic scratching, especially in flexural areas • Commonly seen in infants and children • Associated with other atopic diseases (allergic rhinitis, asthma)

TABLE 9-20 **Skin Cancers**

Disorder	Description
Squamous cell carcinoma	• Malignant tumor of the skin associated with excessive exposure to sunlight (UV rays) leading to DNA damage, immunosuppresion, or xeroderma pigmentosum • Rarely metastasizes • Characterized by ulcerated, scaling nodules • Appears microscopically as islands of neoplastic cells with **whorls of keratin** ("pearls") and cells with atypical nuclei at all levels of the epidermis
Basal cell carcinoma	• **Most common skin tumor** • Appears grossly as a pearl-like papule on sun-exposed areas • Appears histologically as a dark cluster with **palisading peripheral cells** • Almost never metastasizes but can cause local invasive tissue destruction

Malignant melanoma	• Aggressive tumor that arises from melanocytes (neural crest origin)
	• Associated with excess exposure to sunlight, immunosuppresion, and xeroderma pigmentosum
	• Associated with the S-100 tumor marker
	• Two growth patterns:
	  • **Benign radial manner** (growth within skin layer)
	  • **Aggressive vertical manner** (growth through deeper layers)

UV, ultraviolet.

MNEMONIC

MElanoma is more likely to **ME**tastasize. Basal and squamous cell carcinoma hardly ever metastasize.

MNEMONIC

Use ABCDE to identify nevi at higher risk for melanoma: **A**symmetry; **B**order irregular; **C**olor irregular; **D**iameter greater than 0.5 cm; **E**levation irregular.

10 The Hematopoietic and Lymphoreticular System

QUICK HIT

Hematopoiesis expands into fetal sites in times of hematologic stress (e.g., sickle cell anemia).

DEVELOPMENT

I. Hematopoiesis timetable

A. **Week 3: Extraembryonic visceral mesoderm** gives rise to **hemangioblasts**, which aggregate and subsequently differentiate into two cell lines:
   1. Endothelial precursor cells, which form capillaries and eventually larger vessels
   2. Primitive hematopoietic stem cells, which form primitive nucleated erythrocytes. These stem cells colonize the developing liver and then the spleen, which become the major sites of fetal hematopoiesis.

B. **Weeks 3 to 9: Yolk sac** produces primitive erythrocytes.

C. Weeks 5 to 6: Intraembryonic visceral mesoderm gives rise to another line of hematopoietic stem cells in the dorsal aorta, near the gonad/mesonephric ridge (the "AGM" region).
   1. These stem cells also migrate and colonize the liver, where they expand in number and become definitive pluripotent hematopoietic stem cells, capable of producing the myeloid and lymphoid cell lines.
   2. These definitive hematopoietic stem cells eventually migrate to the bone marrow.

D. **Weeks 6 to 34: Liver and spleen** produce red blood cells (RBCs).

E. **Week 28 through childhood: Axial** (sternum, pelvis, ribs, cranial bones, vertebrae) and **peripheral** (tibia, femur) **bone marrow** produces RBCs.

F. **Adulthood: Axial skeleton (vertebral bodies, sternum, ribs, and pelvis)** produces RBCs.

II. Hemoglobin structure

A. Normal **hemoglobin** consists of four protein ("globin") subunits and four iron-containing heme prosthetic groups.

B. **Fetal hemoglobin** consists of hemoglobin F, which is composed of two alpha globins and two gamma globins, $\boldsymbol{\alpha_2\gamma_2}$. Compared to adult hemoglobin, fetal hemoglobin has a lower affinity for 2,3-diphosphoglycerate (2,3-DPG) and a higher affinity for oxygen.

C. **Adult hemoglobin** mostly consists of **hemoglobin A**, which is made up of two alpha and two beta globins, $\boldsymbol{\alpha_2\beta_2}$. A small quantity of hemoglobin A_2 may also be found in adult blood, consisting of two alpha and two delta globins, $\alpha_2\delta_2$.

MNEMONIC

To remember the concentrations of the WBCs, think "Never Let Monkeys Eat Bananas."
Neutrophils (65%)
Lymphocytes (25%)
Monocytes (8%)
Eosinophils (3%)
Basophils (<1%)

THE CELLS *(Table 10-1)*

The hematopoietic lymphoreticular system is composed of a multitude of cells. Most of these cells can be found circulating in the bloodstream, although a few are found within peripheral tissues.

TABLE 10-1 **The Cells of the Hematopoietic–Lymphoreticular System**

Cell	Relative Amounts	Life Span	Morphology	Functions	Secretion	Notes
Neutrophils (PMNs)	40%–75% of WBCs; band form 3%–5% of WBCs	Less than 7 days	Multilobed nucleus, azurophilic granules (lysosomes)	Phagocytic; acute inflammatory response	**Myeloperoxidase,** lysozyme, lactoferrin, hydrolytic enzymes	Lysosomes contain lysozyme and myeloperoxidase, which are **bactericidal**
Basophils	<1% of WBCs	Years	Bilobate, basophilic	Allergies	Heparin, histamine, SRS-A	**Bind IgE** antibody to their membrane
Eosinophils	1%–6% of WBCs	Less than 2 weeks in connective tissues	Bilobed, azurophilic granules	Phagocytic for Ag–Ab complexes; **antiparasitic;** inactivated histamine and SRS-A	Histaminase, arylsulfatase	Large numbers found in lamina propria of GI tract
Mast cells	Found in connective tissue	9–18 months	Basophil-like, round nucleus	Bind IgE; mediate **type I hypersensitivity** reaction	ECF, histamine, leukotrienes, heparin, tryptase	**Cromolyn sodium** prevents degranulation by stabilizing membrane
Macrophages	Found **only in tissues,** not in the blood	Extended life in tissues	Ameboid	Phagocytize bacteria, RBCs, and damaged cells; APCs	IL-1, **IL-2,** TNF-α	Activated by LPS and IFN-γ
Monocytes	3%–9% of WBCs	Less than 3 days in the blood	Large, kidney-shaped nucleus	Differentiate into macrophages and osteoclasts	IL-1, IL-6	Chemotactically **attracted to sites of inflammation**
T lymphocytes	15%–18% of WBCs, 75% of lymphocytes	Years	Basophilic, large nucleus, scant cytoplasm	**Cell-mediated immune response**	IL-2, IL-3, IL-4, IL-5, IL-6, IFN-γ, TNF-α, TNF-β	Originate in bone marrow, mature in thymus
B lymphocytes	5%–7% of WBCs, 25% of lymphocytes	Months	Basophilic, large nucleus, scant cytoplasm; plasma cell has clock-faced chromatin distribution	**Humoral immune response**	IFN-α	Differentiate into plasma cells (produce large amounts of Ab specific to an Ag) and long-lived memory cells
Erythrocytes	5×10^6/mL in men, 4.55×10^6/mL in women	120 days	**Anucleate, biconcave disc** (allows for large surface area to volume ratio)	Gas exchange		Anaerobic metabolism exclusively, membrane contains chloride bicarbonate antiport
Platelets	250,000–400,000/mL	7–10 days	Irregularly shaped, membrane bound, anucleate, extremely small	Prevention of bleeding by **clot formation**	Histamine, PDGF, serotonin, TXA_2, clotting factors, thrombospondin (thromboglobulin)	Disorders of number or function can result in bleeding

Ag–Ab, antigen–antibody; APC, antigen-presenting cell; ECF, eosinophilic chemotactic factor; GI, gastrointestinal; IFN, interferon; Ig, immunoglobulin; IL, interleukin; IFN, interferon; LPS, lipopolysaccharide; PDGF, platelet-derived growth factor; PMN, polymorphonuclear neutrophil; RBC, red blood cell; SRS-A, slow-reacting substance of anaphylaxis; TNF, tumor necrosis factor; TXA_2, thromboxane A_2; WBC, white blood cell.

QUICK HIT

All neutrophils are hypersegmented (six to seven segments) in megaloblastic anemia.

QUICK HIT

Slow-reacting substance of anaphylaxis (SRS-A) is composed of leukotriene C_4 and leukotriene D_4, which bronchoconstrict, vasoconstrict, and increase vascular permeability.

MNEMONIC

To remember the causes of eosinophilia, think DNAAACP:

Drugs
Neoplasm
Allergies/**A**sthma
Adrenal insufficiency
Acute interstitial nephritis
Collagen vascular disease
Parasites

> **QUICK HIT**
> Adrenocorticotropin, steroids, estrogens, and androgens cause involution of the thymus.

> **QUICK HIT**
> **Virchow's node** is a left supraclavicular node enlarged by metastasis from gastric carcinoma or other abdominal malignancy.

THE ORGANS OF THE LYMPHORETICULAR SYSTEM

I. Thymus

A. It is derived from the **third pharyngeal pouch**.
B. The cortex contains thymocytes (immature T lymphocytes).
C. The medulla contains mature T lymphocytes and **Hassall corpuscles** (whorl-like bodies that contain keratin). As T lymphocytes mature, they express T cell receptors and cluster of differentiation (CD) receptors. T lymphocytes that recognize "self" undergo apoptosis, whereas those that recognize "nonself" undergo clonal expansion.

II. Lymph nodes *(Figure 10-1)*

A. Derived from **mesenchymal cells**
B. **Outer cortex** contains B lymphocytes.
C. **Inner cortex** (also called the paracortex) contains T lymphocytes and is thymus dependent.
D. **Medulla** contains B lymphocytes, plasma cells, and macrophages.

FIGURE 10-1 The lymph node

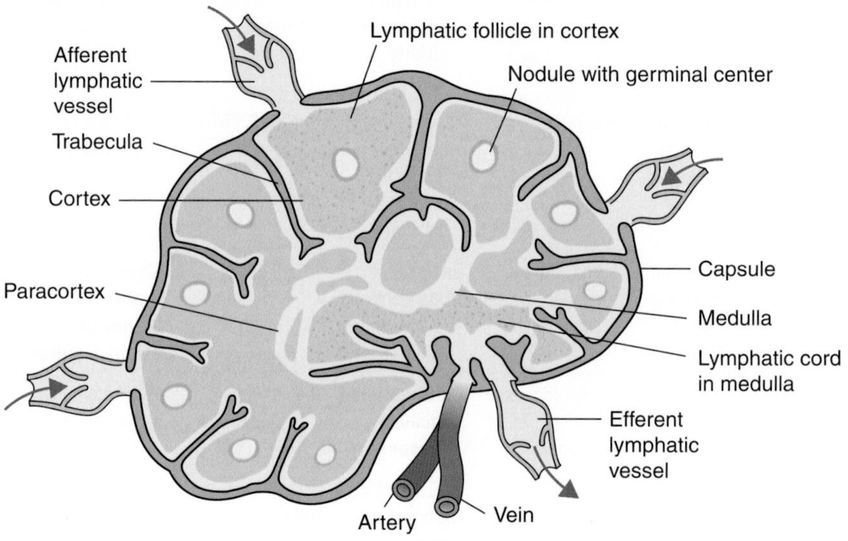

Afferent lymphatic vessel
Lymphatic follicle in cortex
Nodule with germinal center
Trabecula
Cortex
Paracortex
Capsule
Medulla
Lymphatic cord in medulla
Efferent lymphatic vessel
Artery
Vein

III. Lymph

A. It is the fluid that returns lipids, proteins, and water-soluble substances to the circulation via the lymphatic vessels.
B. The **left side of the head, the left thorax, the left upper limb**, and **everything below the diaphragm** drain into the **thoracic duct**. This duct terminates at the junction of the left subclavian and left internal jugular veins.
C. The **right upper quadrant of the body** (right side of the head, right upper limb, and right thorax) empties into the **great vessels of the right side**.

IV. Spleen *(Figure 10-2)*

A. It is derived from **mesenchyme** beginning in the fifth week.
B. **White pulp**: B lymphocytes surround the central artery and T lymphocytes are arranged into periarteriolar lymphatic sheaths (PALS).
C. **Marginal zone**: It is the zone where blood meets spleen parenchyma; antigen-presenting cells (APCs) and macrophages are present.
D. **Red pulp**: It contains splenic (Billroth) cords separated by sinusoids and also has plasma cells, macrophages, lymphocytes, and RBCs.

FIGURE 10-2 The spleen

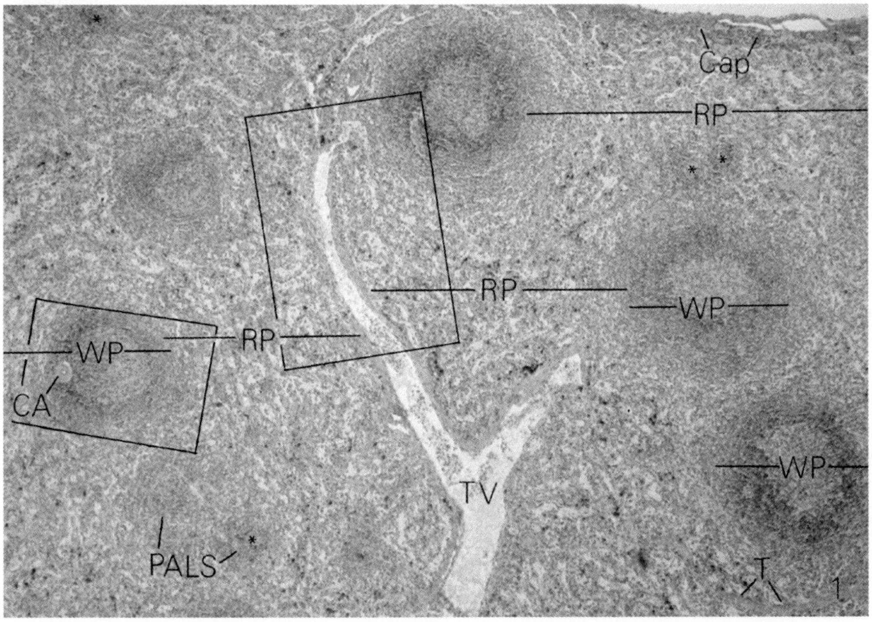
Cap
RP
RP
WP
RP
WP
CA
WP
TV
PALS
T
1

CA, central artery; Cap, capillary; PALS, periarteriolar lymphatic sheaths; RP, red pulp; T, trabeculae; TV, trabecular vein; WP, white pulp. (From Ross MH, Romrell LJ, Kaye GI. *Histology: A Text and Atlas*. 3rd ed. Baltimore, MD: Lippincott Williams & Wilkins; 1995:365. Used by permission of Lippincott Williams & Wilkins.)

V. Liver

A. **Endoderm** of the foregut (**hepatic diverticulum**) grows into the surrounding **mesoderm (septum transversum)**.
B. Hepatic cords from diverticulum, arranged around umbilical and vitelline veins, form **hepatic sinusoids**.
C. It produces **fetal hemoglobin** (HbF) during much of fetal life.
D. It produces **clotting factors** of coagulation cascade.
E. It can function to sequester and break down RBCs if spleen is removed.

VI. Gut-associated lymphatic tissue

A. Found in **tonsils**, **Peyer patches** of the jejunum, **appendix**, and cecum
B. **M cells**: present antigens to lymphocytes and secrete IgA

RED BLOOD CELL PHYSIOLOGY

I. O_2 transport

A. RBCs deliver oxygen from the lungs to the tissues. Deoxyhemoglobin exists in the **tense/taut (T) state**, which has a **low affinity for oxygen**. Binding of the first oxygen molecule requires considerable energy and precipitates a conformational change from the tense state to the **relaxed (R) state**. Binding of further oxygen molecules requires less energy (**positive cooperativity**).
B. Several factors affect hemoglobin affinity for oxygen (Figure 10-3).
C. Hemoglobin binds with carbon monoxide 200 times more readily than with oxygen. The presence of carbon monoxide on one of the four heme sites causes the oxygen to bind with greater affinity. This makes it difficult for the hemoglobin to release the oxygen to the tissues and causes the hemoglobin oxygen dissociation curve to shift to the left. Therefore, increased levels of carbon monoxide can lead to severe hypoxemia while maintaining a normal PO_2.

QUICK HIT

The erythrocyte relies on glucose for energy; 90% is metabolized anaerobically to lactate and 10% by the hexose monophosphate shunt.

QUICK HIT

Carbon monoxide poisoning causes hypoxic injury to the basal ganglia and results in a cherry-red color of the skin and viscera. The treatment is 100% oxygen.

FIGURE 10-3 **Hemoglobin–oxygen dissociation curve**

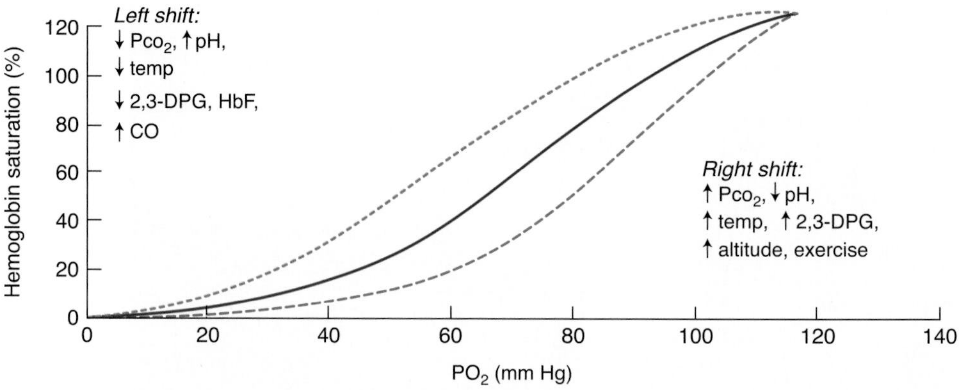
Left shift:
↓ Pco2, ↑ pH,
↓ temp
↓ 2,3-DPG, HbF,
↑ CO
Right shift:
↑ Pco2, ↓ pH,
↑ temp, ↑ 2,3-DPG,
↑ altitude, exercise
Hemoglobin saturation (%)
PO2 (mm Hg)
0
20
40
60
80
100
120
140

2,3-DPG, 2,3-diphosphoglycerate; CO, carbon monoxide; HbF, fetal hemoglobin; PCO_2, partial pressure of carbon dioxide; pH, hydrogen ion concentration; Po_2, partial pressure of oxygen; temp, temperature. Left shift: Hemoglobin (Hgb) molecules have more affinity for oxygen (O_2); Right shift: Hgb molecules have less affinity for O_2.

II. Carbon dioxide transport *(Figure 10-4)*

A. RBCs carry carbon dioxide (CO_2) from the tissues to the lungs. In the tissues, CO_2 diffuses into the RBC, combines with water via **carbonic anhydrase**, and produces carbonic acid. Carbonic acid dissociates into hydrogen ions and bicarbonate. **Bicarbonate leaves** the RBC in exchange for chloride (**chloride shift**). In the lungs, this process is reversed. Thus, **bicarbonate in the plasma** is the **major route** for CO_2 transport to the lungs (90%).

B. Small amounts (5%) of CO_2 are bound to the N-terminus of globin (on hemoglobin) within the RBC. This carbaminohemoglobin favors the taut, oxygen-unloaded state.

C. A small amount (5%) of CO_2 is dissolved in the plasma.

MNEMONIC

To remember which T cells interact with which MHC, think of the "=8" rule: 2 × 4 = 8 and 1 × 8 = 8; thus, MHC **II** goes with CD**4** and MHC **I** goes with CD**8**.

QUICK HIT

The CD4/CD8 ratio is normally 2:1. In AIDS, this ratio is **reversed.**

FIGURE 10-4 **Carbon dioxide transport**

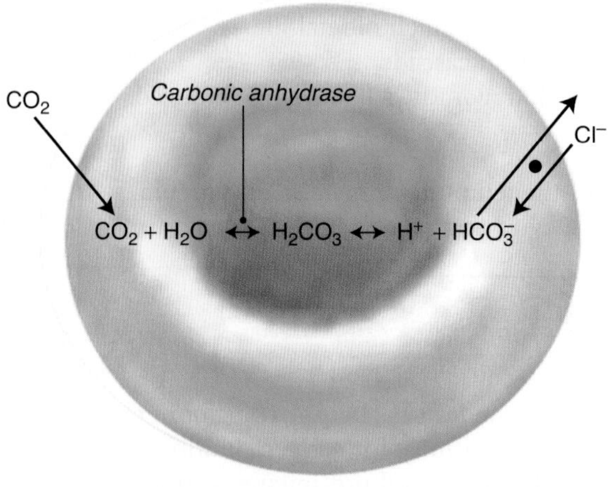
CO2
Carbonic anhydrase
Cl−
CO2 + H2O ↔ H2CO3 ↔ H+ + HCO3−

Cl^-, chloride; CO_2, carbon dioxide; H^+, hydrogen ion; HCO_3^-, bicarbonate; H_2CO_3, carbonic acid; H_2O, water.

LYMPHOCYTE DIFFERENTIATION

T-helper (Th) lymphocytes recognize **major histocompatibility complex (MHC) class II** with **CD4 proteins** on their membranes. They participate in the cellular response to **extracellular** antigens (e.g., bacteria). Cytotoxic T lymphocytes (T-cyt) **recognize MHC class I with CD8 proteins** on their membranes. T-cyt cells are involved in the immune response to **intracellular antigens** (e.g., viruses and obligate intracellular organisms such as Chlamydiae or Rickettsiae). Natural killer (NK) cells are a form of T lymphocytes that do not pass through the thymus for maturation. As one of the body's innate defenses, NK cells kill **tumor cells** and **virus-infected cells** by secreting cytotoxins (perforins). They do not require antibodies to kill, but their potency is increased when antibody is present (i.e., antibody-dependent cellular cytotoxicity [ADCC]).

- **T-cell differentiation** (Figure 10-5)

QUICK HIT

ADCC is one of the mechanisms by which type II hypersensitivity reactions can occur. Other mechanisms are complement-fixing antibodies (e.g., Goodpasture syndrome) and anti–cell surface receptor antibodies (e.g., Graves disease).

FIGURE 10-5 **T-cell differentiation and effect on other immune cells**

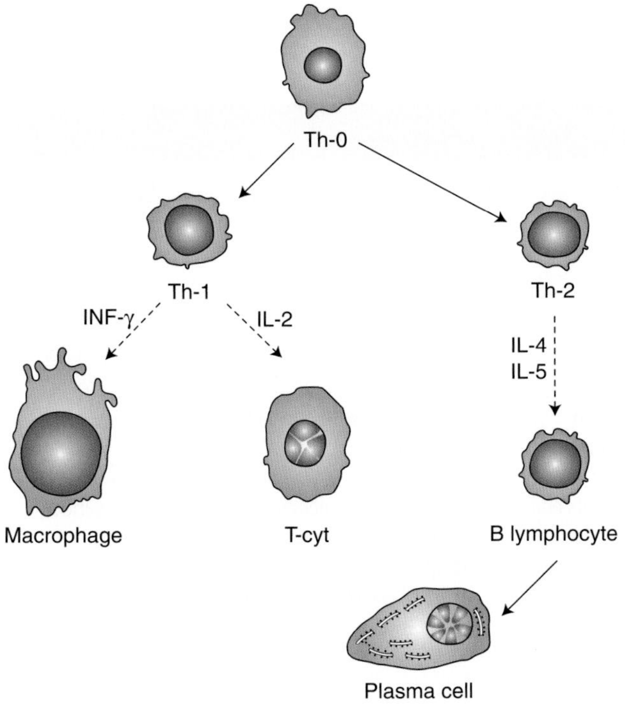
Th-0
Th-1
Th-2
INF-γ
IL-2
IL-4
IL-5
Macrophage
T-cyt
B lymphocyte
Plasma cell

IFN-γ, interferon-γ; IL, interleukin; T-cyt, cytotoxic T lymphocytes; Th, T-helper lymphocytes.

IMMUNOGLOBULINS

I. Characteristics

A. Structure

1. Immunoglobulins are glycoproteins consisting of two identical **heavy (H) chains** and two identical **light (L) chains** linked by **disulfide bonds** in a "Y" shape.
2. **Variable regions** exist on both the L and H chains.
3. The **H chain** is composed of **Fc** and **Fab** fragment. The **L chain** is composed of **Fab** fragment only. The **Fab** is the **antigen-binding fragment**. The **Fc** fragment is **constant** and, in the case of immunoglobulin (Ig) M and IgG, it is **complement binding**. It also contains a **carboxy terminal** and **carbohydrate side chains**.

B. **Antibody diversity** is created by

1. Random recombination of the VJ (L chain) or VDJ (H chain) genes
2. Random combination of H chains with L chains
3. Somatic hypermutation
4. Addition of nucleotides to DNA during recombination by terminal deoxynucleotidyl transferase

C. **Antibody functions**

1. **Opsonization**—in which the antibody promotes phagocytosis
2. **Neutralization**—in which the antibody prevents bacterial adherence to cells and membranes
3. **Complement activation**—in which antibody activates complement, enhancing opsonization and lysis

The Hematopoietic and Lymphoreticular System

MNEMONIC

IgG crosses the placenta during **G**estation.

MNEMONIC

IMmunoGlobulin: IgM is released first, followed by IgG.

D. **Allotype, isotype, and idiotype**
   1. **Allotypes** are Ig epitopes that are different among the members of the same species. It is secondary to polymorphisms in the constant portion of the H chain or L chain. When trying to find appropriate transplant donors, allotypes are matched.
   2. An **isotype** is an Ig epitope that is common to a single class of immunoglobulins. For example, IgG, IgM, and IgA are different isotypes of Ig. It is determined by the constant region of the H chain.
   3. An **idiotype** is an Ig epitope that is specific for a given antigen. It is determined by the antigen-binding site contributed by the variable and hypervariable regions.

II. Types *(Table 10-2)*

TABLE **10-2 Immunoglobulin (Ig) properties**

	IgM	IgG	IgE	IgA	IgD
Percentage of total Ig	9%	75% (most abundant)	0.004% (least abundant)	15%	0.2%
Structure	Monomer or pentamer Pentamer held together by J chain	Monomer	Monomer	Monomer or dimer Dimer held together by J chain (secretory piece)	Monomer
Function	Fixes complement Antigen receptor on B cell surface, **Primary response**	Fixes complement Opsonizes bacteria **Crosses the placenta** Neutralizes bacterial toxins and viruses **Secondary response**	Allergic response **(type I hypersensitivity)** Binds to basophils and mast cells (induces release of mediators) Antihelminthic (by activating eosinophils)	Found in **secretions** (including **breastmilk**) Prevents bacterial and viral attachment to mucous membranes Does not fix complement Picks up secretory - component from epithelial cells before secretion	Unknown May be antigen receptor on B cell surface

COMPLEMENT SYSTEM *(Figure 10-6)*

I. Function of complement
A. Causes **lysis** of target cell
B. Defends against **gram-negative bacteria**

II. Activation of pathways
A. IgG and IgM activate the **classic pathway.**
   1. The activation is initiated by antigen–antibody complexes.
   2. The first step of activation involves formation of the complex by C1, C2, and C4.
B. Antigens activate the **alternative pathway.**
   1. The activation is initiated by microbial surfaces and aggregated IgA.
   2. The first step of activation involves C3.
C. Mannose chains on bacteria activate the **lectin pathway.**
   1. The activation is initiated by mannose-binding lectin (MBL) and associate protease binding to mannose residues.
   2. The first step of activation involves the MBL–mannose complex activating proteases that activate C4 and C2, which then go on to activate the rest of the classical pathway.

III. Properties of complement cascade components
A. **C1**: only component not made in liver (made in gastrointestinal [GI] epithelium)
B. C1–C4: involved in viral neutralization
C. **C3b**: involved in opsonization
D. C3a: produces anaphylatoxin I

MNEMONIC

Remember that **C3a a**ctivates **a**cute inflammation, whereas **C3b b**inds **b**acteria (opsonization).

The Hematopoietic and Lymphoreticular System

E. **C5a**: produces anaphylatoxin II, neutrophil, and macrophage chemotaxis
F. **C5b–C9**: also known as the membrane attack complex (MAC)
G. **C1 inhibitor**: deficiency of this component leads to hereditary angioedema
H. Table 10-3 discusses alterations in the complement cascade (complement deficiencies)

QUICK HIT

The membrane attack complex (MAC) has only one component each of C5b, C6, C7, and C8 but has numerous C9 components.

FIGURE 10-6 Complement pathway

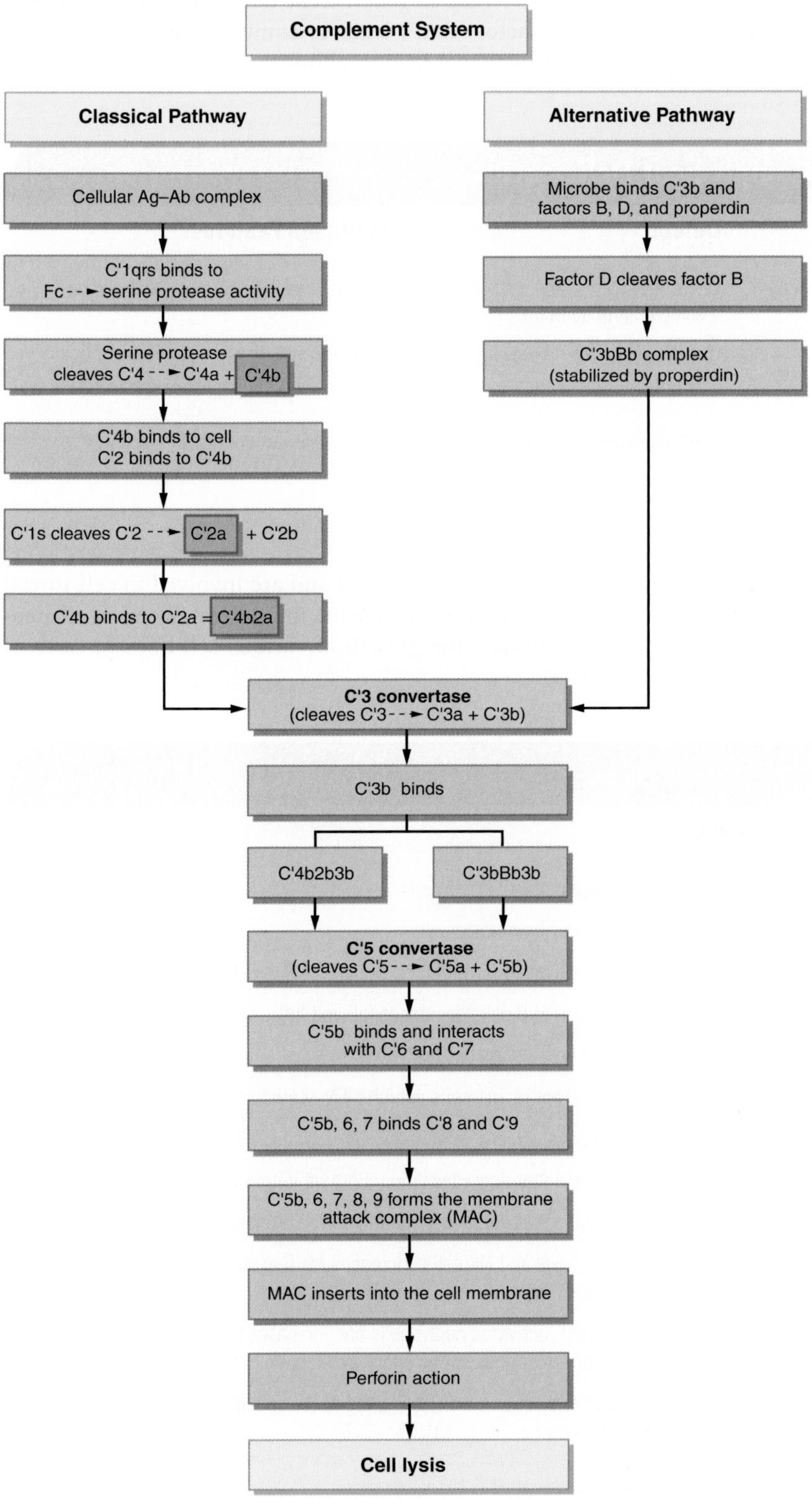
Complement System
Classical Pathway
Alternative Pathway
Cellular Ag–Ab complex
C'1qrs binds to Fc --► serine protease activity
Serine protease cleaves C'4 --► C'4a + C'4b
C'4b binds to cell C'2 binds to C'4b
C'1s cleaves C'2 --► C'2a + C'2b
C'4b binds to C'2a = C'4b2a
Microbe binds C'3b and factors B, D, and properdin
Factor D cleaves factor B
C'3bBb complex (stabilized by properdin)
C'3 convertase (cleaves C'3 --► C'3a + C'3b)
C'3b binds
C'4b2b3b
C'3bBb3b
C'5 convertase (cleaves C'5 --► C'5a + C'5b)
C'5b binds and interacts with C'6 and C'7
C'5b, 6, 7 binds C'8 and C'9
C'5b, 6, 7, 8, 9 forms the membrane attack complex (MAC)
MAC inserts into the cell membrane
Perforin action
Cell lysis

IV. Complement deficiencies

A. Deficiencies of C1, C3, C5, C6, C7, and C8 lead to increased bacterial infections.
B. C1 deficiency results in hereditary angioedema.
C. C2 deficiency is the most common complement deficiency. Manifestations of C2 and C4 deficiencies resemble autoimmune diseases such as systemic lupus erythematosus (SLE).
D. C3 deficiency causes increased susceptibility to *Staphylococcus aureus* and severe, recurrent sinus and respiratory infections.
E. C6, C7, and C8 deficiencies lead to *Neisseria gonorrhoeae* infection and meningitis.
F. Deficiency of decay accelerating factor (DAF) leads to complement-mediated lysis of erythrocytes and paroxysmal nocturnal hemoglobinuria.

MNEMONIC

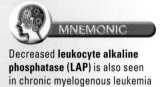

Decreased **leukocyte alkaline phosphatase (LAP)** is also seen in chronic myelogenous leukemia (CML).

TABLE **10-3** Complement Deficiencies

Disease	Defect	Significant Features
Hereditary angioedema	Decreased C1 (first component of complement) inhibitor	Increased capillary permeability; edema
PNH	Deficiency of DAF; increased complement activation	Complement-mediated hemolysis; brown urine in the morning; **decreased LAP**

DAF, decay-accelerating factor; LAP, leukocyte alkaline phosphatase; PNH, paroxysmal nocturnal hemoglobinuria.

V. Cytokines *(Table 10-4)*

Cytokines are hormones that have a low molecular weight and are involved in cell-to-cell communication. Human recombinant cytokines are useful in the management of neoplasms, transplant rejection, and to stimulate the growth of various cell lines in cases of bone marrow suppression (Table 10-5).

TABLE **10-4** Cytokines

Cytokine	Secreted by	Function
IL-1	Macrophages	Endogenous **pyrogen;** stimulates T cells
IL-2	T-helper cells (Th1)	Activates T-helper and T-cytotoxic cells
IL-3	Activated T cells	Stimulates the growth and differentiation of bone marrow stem cells
IL-4	T-helper cells (Th2)	Stimulates the growth of B cells; increases IgE and IgG
IL-5	T-helper cells (Th2)	Differentiation of B cells; increases IgA
IL-10	Monocytes, T-helper cells (Th2)	Inhibits the development of Th1 cells; inhibits IFN-γ production
IL-12	Macrophages	Promotes Th1 cell development; stimulates IFN-γ production
IFN-α	Virus-infected leukocytes	Produces ribonuclease that degrades viral mRNA inhibiting viral protein synthesis
IFN-β	Virus-infected fibroblasts	Produces ribonuclease that degrades viral mRNA inhibiting viral protein synthesis
IFN-γ	T-helper cells (Th1)	Stimulates macrophages and NK cells; increases MHC expression; stimulates phagocytosis and killing
Tumor necrosis factor	Macrophages	At low concentrations, activates neutrophils and increases IL-2 receptor synthesis; at high concentrations, mediates septic shock and results in tumor necrosis
Transforming growth factor	T cells, B cells, and macrophages	Inhibits the growth and activities of T cells; enhances collagen synthesis; dampens the immune response

IFN, interferon; Ig, immunoglobulin; IL, interleukin; MHC, major histocompatibility complex; mRNA, messenger RNA; NK, natural killer.

TABLE 10-5 **Recombinant Cytokines**

Therapeutic Agent (common name, if relevant) [trade name, where appropriate]	Class—Pharmacology and Pharmacokinetics	Indications	Side Effects or Adverse Effects	Contraindications or Precautions to Consider; Notes
Aldesleukin [Proleukin]	Human recombinant **interleukin-2**	**Metastatic renal cell carcinoma, metastatic melanoma, AML**		
Epoetin alfa [Procrit, Epogen]	**Colony-stimulating factor**	**Anemias (especially in renal failure), AIDS**	Hypertension	
Filgrastim [Neupogen]	**Granulocyte-macrophage colony–stimulating factor**	**Recovery of bone marrow (e.g., chemotherapy-induced neutropenia)**		
Sargramostim (Leukine)	**Granulocyte-macrophage colony–stimulating factor**	**Recovery of bone marrow (e.g., bone marrow transplant failure)**	Hypertension	
Interferon α-2a [Roferon A], **α2b** [Intron A], **and α-n3** [Alferon-N]	Antiviral—decreases protein synthesis	**Genital warts, chronic hepatitis B and C, AIDS-related Kaposi sarcoma, laryngeal papillomatosis, hairy cell leukemia, malignant melanoma**	**Flulike symptoms,** headache, malaise, fever, chills, **depression**, **neutropenia,** somnolence, tachycardia	
Interferon β-1a [Avonex, Rebif]	Antiviral—decreases protein synthesis	**Multiple sclerosis**	**Flulike symptoms,** ache, fatigue, fever, pain, chills, depression	
Interferon γ-1b [Actimmune]	Antiviral—decreases protein synthesis	**Chronic granulomatous disease**	Fever, headache, chills, fatigue	
Oprelvekin [Neumega]	**Interleukin-11** stimulates multiple stages of **thrombopoiesis,** increasing the platelet production	**Thrombocytopenia**		
Thrombopoietin	Recombinant human thrombopoietin	**Thrombocytopenia**		

AML, acute myelogenous leukemia.

MNEMONIC

Use **ACID** to help remember immunology of each hypersensitivity reaction:
Anaphylactic: Type I
Cytotoxic: Type II
Immune complex disease: Type III
Delayed hypersensitivity (cell mediated): Type IV

QUICK HIT

An acute allergic reaction is a type I hypersensitivity reaction.

QUICK HIT

Serum sickness is more common than an Arthus reaction.

MNEMONIC

Remember poison **IV**y causes type **IV** hypersensitivity.

QUICK HIT

Graft-versus-host disease (GVHD) is caused by donor lymphocytes attacking recipient cells. It is characterized by elevated bilirubin and liver enzymes and skin lesions. It is seen commonly in bone marrow transplants.

HYPERSENSITIVITY REACTIONS

I. There are four types of hypersensitivity reactions. They vary in onset of symptoms, severity, and mechanism *(Table 10-6)*.

TABLE 10-6 **Hypersensitivity Reactions**

Reaction Type	Description	Example
Type I **(anaphylaxis)**	Mediated by **IgE** antibody bound to mast cells or basophil antigens cross-link antibody Release of **histamine,** SRS-A, eosinophilic chemotactic factor, and platelet-activating factor p-tryptase, leukotrienes	Anaphylaxis Allergic rhinitis (hay fever) Asthma Wheal and flare
Type II (cytotoxic)	Antibody-dependent cellular cytotoxicity Antibody produced to specific cell-surface antigens IgM- and IgG-mediated lysis via complement Immunofluorescence, stains smooth, linear Abs staining in biopsy	Rh incompatibility Goodpasture syndrome Myasthenia gravis Hemolytic anemia Idiopathic thrombocytopenic purpura Rheumatic fever Graves disease Bullous pemphigoid
Type III (immune complex)	**Antigen–antibody complexes** induce inflammatory response Deposition of complexes in tissue	**Arthus reaction** **Serum sickness** Glomerulonephritis Rheumatoid arthritis SLE Polyarteritis nodosa
Type IV (delayed or cell mediated)	**Helper (CD4) Th1 lymphocyte-mediated** Response is delayed (from hours to days) Predominantly mononuclear cell infiltration	Tuberculin (PPD) test GVHD Contact dermatitis Type 1 diabetes mellitus Multiple sclerosis Guillain–Barré syndrome Hashimoto thyroiditis

CD4, cluster of differentiation 4; GVHD, graft-versus-host disease; Ig, immunoglobulin; PPD, purified protein derivative; Rh, rhesus (factor); SLE, systemic lupus erythematosus; SRS-A, slow-reacting substance of anaphylaxis; Th, T-helper.

II. Transplant rejection timeline *(Figure 10-7)*.

FIGURE 10-7 **Transplant rejection timeline**

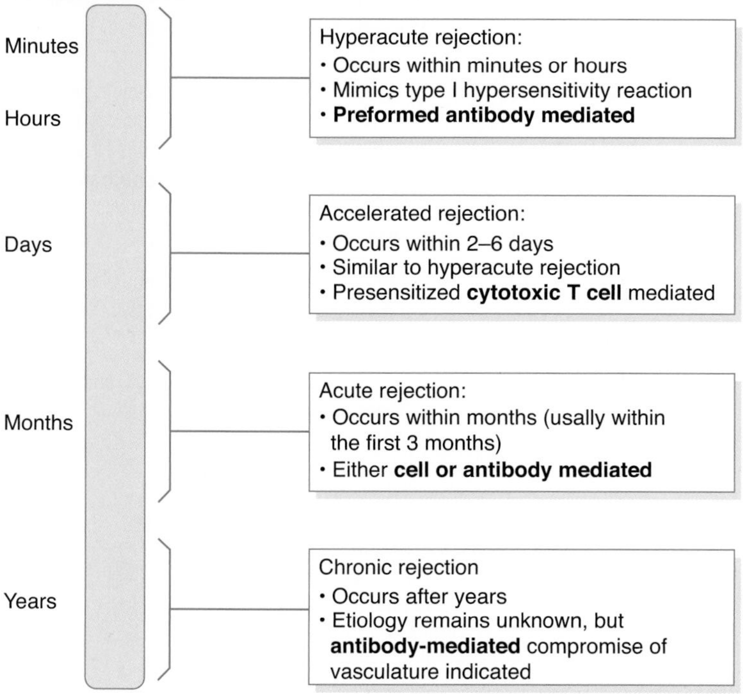
Minutes
Hours
Days
Months
Years
Hyperacute rejection:
• Occurs within minutes or hours
• Mimics type I hypersensitivity reaction
• Preformed antibody mediated
Accelerated rejection:
• Occurs within 2–6 days
• Similar to hyperacute rejection
• Presensitized cytotoxic T cell mediated
Acute rejection:
• Occurs within months (usally within the first 3 months)
• Either cell or antibody mediated
Chronic rejection
• Occurs after years
• Etiology remains unknown, but antibody-mediated compromise of vasculature indicated

IMMUNODEFICIENCIES

I. Diseases affecting the immune system leave the individual prone to infection. The immune system can be affected on any level and at any time—from its development to its most distal signaling mechanisms.

II. Congenital B-cell deficiencies *(Table 10-7)*

TABLE 10-7 **Congenital B-Cell Deficiencies**

Disease	Defect	Significant Features
X-linked agammaglobulinemia (of Bruton)	Lack of maturation of B cells, secondary to defective tyrosine kinase gene	Absence of plasma cells, **low levels of all immunoglobulins**; **recurrent pyogenic infections** beginning after 6 months; lymphoid tissue has **poorly defined germinal centers**
Selective IgA deficiency	Lack of maturation of B cells; failure of gene switching in H chain	**Most common congenital B-cell defect (1 in 600 newborns of European descent);** most appear healthy; **sinus/lung infections**; possible anaphylaxis to blood product transfusions
Common variable immunodeficiency	Failure of terminal B-cell differentiation; defective Ig production	Variable: recurrent infections, autoimmune disorders, chronic lung and/or GI disease, increased risk of lymphoma

GI, gastrointestinal; Ig, immunoglobulin.

MNEMONIC

Remember the features of DiGeorge syndrome by thinking of it as the disease of Ts:
Third and fourth branchial pouch absent
Thymic aplasia
T cells absent
Twenty-**T**wo chromosome deletion
Tetany: Para**T**hyroid (decreased parathyroid hormone results in hypocalcemia).

QUICK HIT

Treat hyper-IgM syndrome with pooled γ-globulin.

QUICK HIT

Measles, a paramyxovirus, results in a T-cell deficiency.

QUICK HIT

Severe combined immunodeficiency (SCID) caused by adenosine deaminase (ADA) deficiency was one of the first diseases successfully treated with gene therapy.

III. Congenital T-cell deficiencies *(Table 10-8)*

TABLE 10-8 Congenital T-Cell Deficiencies

Disease	Defect	Significant Features
Thymic aplasia (DiGeorge syndrome)	Deficiency of development of third and fourth branchial pouches; thymic aplasia leads to T-cell defect; commonly 22q11.2 deletion	Defective development of the thymus, parathyroid glands, ear, mandible, and aortic arch; leads to recurrent infections by **viral and fungal organisms; hypocalcemia** from low parathyroid hormone leads to tetany
Chronic mucocutaneous candidiasis	Lack of T-cell response to *candidiasis*	Recurrent candidal skin and mucous membrane infections; treat infections with fluconazole or ketoconazole
Hyper IgM syndrome	Mutation in $CD4^+$ Th cell interaction with CD40 on B cell prevents class switching; two main types **X linked:** deficiency of CD40 ligand on T cell **AR:** defect in CD40 on B cells	Increased IgM; decreased IgG, IgA, and IgE; normal numbers of T and B cells;
IL-12 receptor deficiency	Deficiency in IL-12 receptor leads to decreased Th1 response	Patients present with disseminated mycobacterial infections

AR, autosomal recessive; CD, cluster of differentiation; Ig, immunoglobulin; IL, interleukin; Th, T-helper.

IV. Congenital combined T- and B-cell deficiencies *(Table 10-9)*

TABLE 10-9 Congenital Combined T- and B-Cell Deficiencies

Disease	Defect	Significant Features
Severe combined immunodeficiency (SCID)	Autosomal recessive (defect in tyrosine kinase zeta-associated protein [ZAP]-70 or adenosine deaminase deficiency); X-linked forms (interleukin [IL]-2 receptor defect)	Triad of severe **recurrent infections** (candidiasis, PCP, fatal or recurrent viral infections [RSV, VZV, HSV, measles, flu, parainfluenza]), **chronic diarrhea, failure to thrive** No thymic shadow on newborn CXR
Wiskott–Aldrich syndrome	X-linked weak IgM response to capsule polysaccharide (e.g., *Streptococcus pneumoniae*)	**Eczema, thrombocytopenia, and recurrent infections;** becomes noticeable in first year of life; low IgM, high IgA
Ataxia–telangiectasia	IgA deficiency and lymphopenia (low T cells)	**Autosomal recessive**; becomes noticeable in first 2 years of life; cerebellar ataxia, poor smooth pursuit of moving target with eyes; telangiectasias of face >5 years; increased cancer risk (lymphoma and acute leukemias); radiation sensitivity (avoid x-rays); average age of death 25 years

CXR, chest x-ray; HSV, herpes simplex virus; Ig, immunoglobulin; PCP, *Pneumocystis carinii* pneumona; RSV, respiratory syncytial virus; VZV, varicella-zoster virus.

V. Plasma cell abnormalities *(Table 10-10)*

TABLE 10-10 **Plasma Cell Abnormalities**

Disease	Etiology	Clinical Features	Notes
Multiple myeloma	Clonal plasma cell tumor	**"Punched-out" lytic bone lesions**, especially in the skull; hypercalcemia; back pain; anemia; hyperglobulinemia; **Bence Jones proteinuria**; renal insufficiency	Rouleaux formation ("stack of coins" appearance) of RBCs on peripheral smear
Waldenström macroglobulinemia	Excessive production of IgM by lymphoid cells	Slowly progressive course; usually in men older than 50 years of age; platelet function abnormal; hyperviscosity syndrome	No bone lesions (which differentiates this from multiple myeloma)
Benign monoclonal gammopathy	Increased production of monoclonal antibodies from an unknown origin	Asymptomatic; occurring in older individuals	Monoclonal spike without Bence Jones proteinuria (versus multiple myeloma)

Ig, immunoglobulin; RBC, red blood cell.

VI. Phagocyte deficiencies *(Table 10-11)*

TABLE 10-11 **Phagocyte Deficiencies**

Disease	Defect	Significant Features
Chronic granulomatous disease (CGD)	Neutrophils **lack NADPH oxidase**; no oxidative burst in macrophages	**X linked** (some AR); susceptible to organisms with catalase (e.g., *Staphylococcus aureus, Escherichia coli, Klebsiella, Aspergillus, Candida*) Diagnosis: **negative nitroblue tetrazolium (NBT) dye** (no yellow to blue-black oxidation) Treatment: prophylactic TMP-SMX, itraconazole, IFN-γ
Chédiak-Higashi syndrome	Defective LYST gene (lysosomal transport); failure of neutrophils to empty lysosomes; giant cytoplasmic granules in neutrophils	Autosomal recessive; presentation triad: **partial albinism; recurrent pyogenic infections** (e.g., *Staphylococcus, Streptococcus*); **neurologic disorders**
Job syndrome	T-helper lymphocytes fail to produce IFN-γ; neutrophils fail to respond to chemotactic stimuli (C5a, LTB4)	High levels of IgE and eosinophils; presentation triad: **eczema; recurrent cold *S. aureus* abscesses; coarse facial features** (broad nose, prominent forehead "frontal bossing," deep-set eyes, doughy skin); commonly have retained primary teeth (2 rows of teeth)
Leukocyte adhesion deficiency	Defect in integrins prevents phagocytes from exiting circulation	Delayed separation of umbilicus; pyogenic infections early in life

IFN-γ, interferon-γ; Ig, immunoglobulin; LTB4, leukotriene B4; NADPH, nicotinamide adenine dinucleotide phosphate; TMP-SMX, trimethoprim-sulfamethoxazole.

QUICK HIT

Interferon-γ (IFN-γ) is used to treat chronic granulomatous disease (CGD).

VII. Acquired immunodeficiencies *(Table 10-12)*

TABLE 10-12 **Acquired Immunodeficiencies**

Disease	Defect	Significant Features
Common variable hypogammaglobulinemia	Acquired or congenital (unknown) B-cell defects	Recurrent pyogenic bacterial infections (e.g., *Streptococcus pneumoniae, Haemophilus influenzae*); decreased IgG production
AIDS	**HIV virus infects CD4 cells and macrophages**	Opportunistic infections (e.g., ***Mycobacterium avium-intracellulare****, Cryptococcus neoformans,* ***Pneumocystis jirovecii****,* and *Candida albicans*); increased tumors (e.g., Kaposi sarcoma)

CD4, cluster of differentiation 4; Ig,immunoglobulin.

IMMUNOSUPPRESSANTS *(Table 10-13)*

TABLE 10-13 **Immunosuppressants**

Therapeutic Agent (common name, if relevant) [trade name, where appropriate]	Class—Pharmacology and Pharmacokinetics	Indications	Side Effects or Adverse Effects	Contraindications or Precautions to Consider; Notes
Cyclosporine [Sandimmune]	Binds **cyclophilins** → complex inhibits **calcineurin** → prevents production of **IL-2, IL-3, and IFN-γ** → inhibits **T-helper cell** activity	**Transplant rejection; selected autoimmune disorder**	**Nephrotoxic,** hepatotoxic; hypertension; **increased incidence of viral infection and lymphoma**	Nephrotoxicity preventable with mannitol diuresis
Tacrolimus (FK506) [Prograf]	Binds to **FK-binding protein** (T-cell transcription factor) → inhibits **calcineurin** → inhibits **IL-2** synthesis and T-cell signal transduction → inhibits **T-cell** activity	**Transplant rejection**	**Nephrotoxic, neurotoxic (peripheral neuropathy); hyperglycemia, hypertension, pleural effusion;** GI disturbances	Potent immunosuppressant

(continued)

TABLE 10-13 **Immunosuppressants**

Therapeutic Agent (common name, if relevant) [trade name, where appropriate]	Class—Pharmacology and Pharmacokinetics	Indications	Side Effects or Adverse Effects	Contraindications or Precautions to Consider; Notes
Azathioprine [Imuran]	**Purine antagonist;** antimetabolite precursor of **6-mercaptopurine →** inhibits nucleic acid synthesis and metabolism → toxic to **proliferating lymphocytes;** blocks both CMI and humoral response	**Transplant (esp. kidney);** acute glomerulonephritis; renal component of lupus; rheumatoid arthritis; hemolytic anemia	**Bone marrow suppression;** rash; fever; nausea; vomiting; hepatotoxicity; malignancy; GI intolerance	Metabolized by xanthine oxidase; **toxic effects may be increased by allopurinol**
Muromonab (OKT3)	**Monoclonal antibody** that binds CD3 on T lymphocytes → blocks cellular interaction with CD3 protein responsible for T-cell signal transduction	Acute rejection of **renal transplants**	**Cytokine release syndrome;** hypersensitivity reaction	
Sirolimus (rapamycin)	Binds to mTOR → inhibits response to **IL-2** → inhibits **T-cell proliferation**	Immunosuppression after **kidney transplantation** (in combination with cyclosporine and corticosteroids)	**Hyperlipidemia, thrombocytopenia, and leukopenia**	
Mycophenolate mofetil [CellCept]	Inhibits de novo **guanine synthesis** → blocks **lymphocyte production**	Prevents rejection after **organ transplantation;** myasthenia gravis	Hypertension, hyperglycemia, hypercholesterolemia, leucopenia, thrombocytopenia	
Daclizumab [Zenapax]	Monoclonal antibody with high affinity for the **IL-2 receptor** on activated T cells → **prevents T-cell activation**	**Prevents rejection after kidney transplantation**		Decreased incidence of opportunistic infections when compared with other immunosuppressants

CD, cluster of differentiation; CMI, cell-mediated immunity; GI, gastrointestinal; IFN, interferon; IL, interleukin; mTOR, mammalian target of rapamycin.

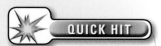

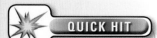

THROMBOSIS AND THE CLOTTING CASCADE *(Figure 10-8)*

Thrombosis is the intravascular coagulation of blood and involves the interaction of platelets, coagulation proteins, and endothelial cells. With intact endothelium, a balance exists between prothrombotic (platelet-derived thromboxane A_2 [TXA_2]) and antithrombotic (endothelium-derived prostaglandin 12 [PGI2]) mediators. With damaged endothelium, exposed collagen causes adhesion of platelets through glycoprotein receptors and **von Willebrand factor (vWF)**. This adhesion triggers platelet release of adenosine diphosphate (ADP), serotonin, histamine, platelet-derived growth factor (PDGF), and TXA_2, resulting in primary plug formation and cessation of bleeding. Stabilization of the primary plug (formation of the secondary plug) is mediated by fibrin and factor XIIIa, a result of activation of the clotting cascade.

Factor XIa in the presence of calcium (Ca^{2+}) activates factor IX. Factor IXa requires Ca^{2+} and a phospholipid to activate factor X. Activated factor X requires Ca^{2+}, phospholipid, and factor Va to activate prothrombin to thrombin. Thrombin and Ca^{2+} activate factor XIII that promotes the cross-linking of fibrin.

- **Key Players in Inhibition of Coagulation**

α1-Antitrypsin	Inhibits factor XIa
α2-Macroglobuli	Inhibits serine proteases
Antithrombin	Inhibits factor Xa and thrombin
Inhibitor of the first component	Inhibits factor XII and kallikrein of complement (C1 INH)
Heparin cofactor II	Inhibits thrombin
Protein C	Inactivates factors Va and VIIIa
Protein S	Is a cofactor for protein C

FIGURE 10-8 Thrombosis and the clotting cascade

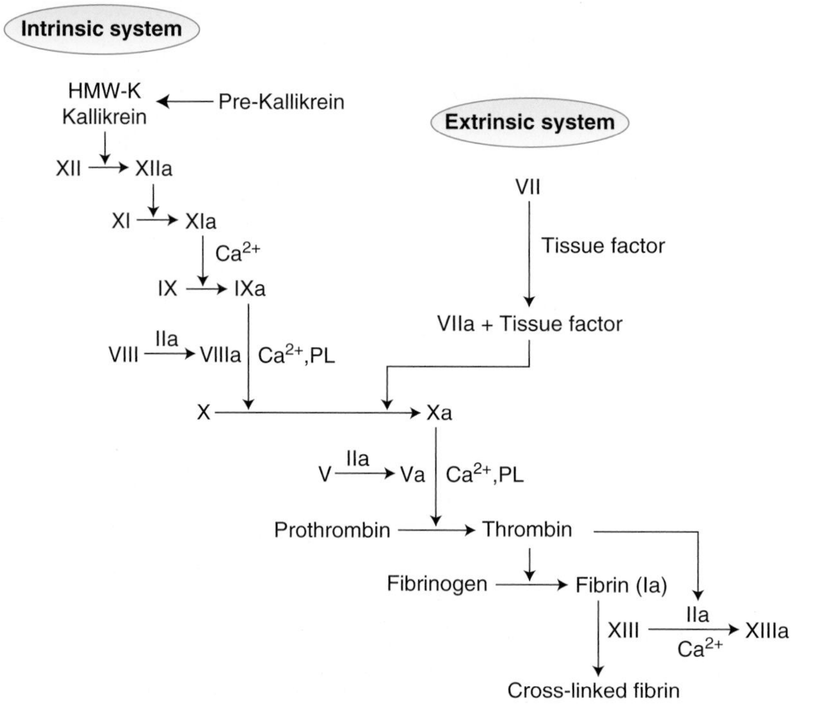
Intrinsic system
HMW-K
Kallikrein
Pre-Kallikrein
Extrinsic system
XII
XIIa
VII
XI
XIa
Ca2+
Tissue factor
IX
IXa
VIIa + Tissue factor
VIII
IIa
VIIIa
Ca2+,PL
X
Xa
V
IIa
Va
Ca2+,PL
Prothrombin
Thrombin
Fibrinogen
Fibrin (Ia)
XIII
IIa
Ca2+
XIIIa
Cross-linked fibrin

Ca^{2+}, calcium; HMW-K, high-molecular-weight kininogen; PL, phospholipid.

QUICK HIT

Aspirin functions as an antithrombotic agent by permanently acetylating cyclooxygenase (COX), thereby inhibiting TXA_2 production. TXA_2 triggers the aggregation of platelets. Aspirin also inhibits prostaglandin formation, but, unlike platelets, endothelium can synthesize new COX.

QUICK HIT

Factors II, VII, IX, and X and **proteins C and S require vitamin K** for their synthesis and are produced in the liver.

QUICK HIT

Vitamin K is administered to newborns in the United States to prevent hemorrhagic diseases.

QUICK HIT

Factor VIII is the only clotting factor increased in liver disease.

QUICK HIT

Partial thromboplastin time (**PTT**) measures the **contact activation pathway.** Therapeutic drug monitoring of heparin is measured using PTT. Heparin overdose is treated with intravenous protamine sulfate.

QUICK HIT

Prothrombin time (**PT**) measures the **tissue factor pathway.** Therapeutic drug monitoring of warfarin is measured using PT. Warfarin overdose is treated with the administration of vitamin K. In acute cases of hemorrhage, fresh frozen plasma may be given to quickly reverse the effects of warfarin.

Clinical Vignette 10-1

CLINICAL PRESENTATION: A 65-year-old man presents to his primary care physician complaining of **bad back pains** for the past several months aggravated by **walking or bending over.** Yesterday, he fell on his right arm while shoveling snow. Patient has no past medical or surgical history, but the patient was recently hospitalized for a **kidney stone.** Physical examination reveals tenderness to palpation over the thoracic and lumbar spine. No splenomegaly or lymphadenopathy. Plain films of the spine show several **lytic lesions in the vertebral bodies at L3–L4 levels.** Plain films of the right upper extremity show lytic lesions in the diaphysis and a **fracture line.**

DIFFERENTIALS: Fibromyalgia, herniated disk (nerve root impingement), osteoarthritis, metastatic bone lesion, and multiple myeloma. The lytic lesions, pathologic fractures, and kidney stones (evidence of hypercalcemia) suggest multiple myeloma.

LABORATORY STUDIES: In addition to the **lytic lesions on the plain film** (Figure 10-9A), **serum and urine electrophoresis** showing M-protein spike would support a diagnosis of multiple myeloma. To confirm a diagnosis of multiple myeloma, a **bone marrow biopsy** showing 10% plasma cells (Figure 10-9B) would need to be performed. A **complete blood count (CBC) showing mild anemia** and **electrolytes showing hypercalcemia and renal insufficiency** are also findings seen in multiple myeloma.

MANAGEMENT: Multiple myeloma has a poor prognosis, with median survival of few months without treatment. Treatment is reserved for patients with advanced disease and includes chemotherapy (alkylating agents), radiation therapy, and transplantation.

QUICK HIT

Osteolytic lesions are secondary to the release of osteoclast-activating factor by the neoplastic plasma cells.

FIGURE **10-9** **Multiple myeloma**

A. Lytic lesions

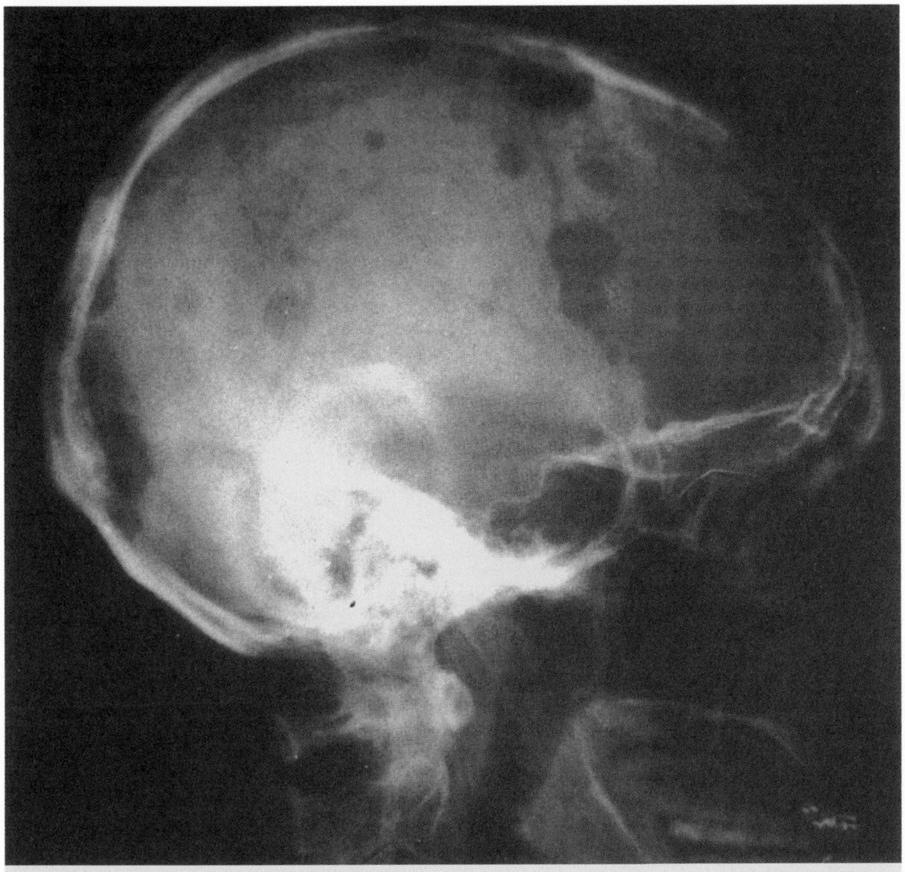

A

(Reproduced with permission from Rubin E, Farber JL. *Pathology.* 3rd ed. Lippincott Williams & Wilkins; 1999.)

FIGURE 10-9 Multiple myeloma *(Continued)*

B. Plasma cells

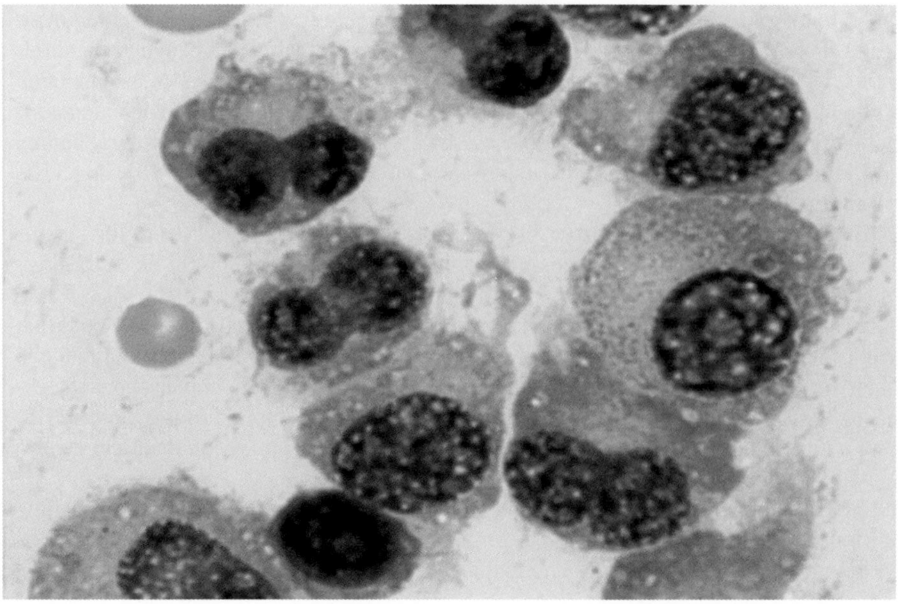

B

(Reproduced with permission from Anderson SC. *Anderson's Atlas of Hematology.* Philadelphia, PA: Wolters Kluwer Health/Lippincott Williams & Wilkins; 2003.)

QUICK HIT

Heparin, sulfonamides, sulfonylureas, valproate, ethanol, gold, antineoplastic agents, chloramphenicol, and benzene result in drug-induced injury to the bone marrow, resulting in a decreased platelet production.

QUICK HIT

Aspirin, ticlopidine, and clopidogrel work globally to reduce the risk of thrombotic occlusion and thromboembolism regardless of the anatomic site.

ANTITHROMBOTIC THERAPEUTIC AGENTS

I. Platelet inhibitors *(Figure 10-10) (Table 10-14)*

Aspirin inhibits thromboxane-mediated platelet aggregation, ticlopidine and clopidogrel block platelet ADP receptors, and argatroban and hirudin inhibit thrombin directly.

A. Aspirin
1. Irreversibly acetylates **platelet cyclooxygenase (COX)**
2. Results in disruption of TXA_2-dependent platelet aggregation
3. Leads to less platelet hemostasis
4. Can be used in acute myocardial infarctions (MIs) or prophylactically to reduce the likelihood of platelet-mediated vascular occlusion

FIGURE 10-10 Inhibition of platelet aggregation pathways

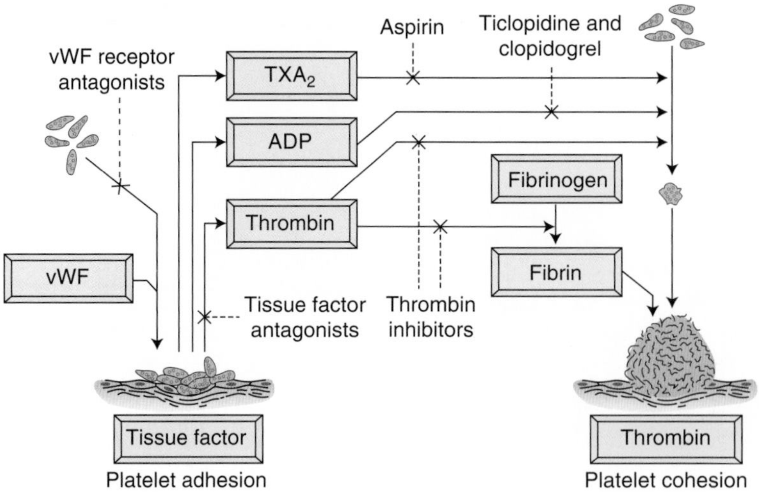
Aspirin
Ticlopidine and clopidogrel
vWF receptor antagonists
TXA2
ADP
Thrombin
Fibrinogen
Fibrin
vWF
Tissue factor antagonists
Thrombin inhibitors
Tissue factor
Platelet adhesion
Thrombin
Platelet cohesion

Aspirin inhibits thromboxane-mediated platelet aggregation, ticlopidine and clopidogrel block platelet ADP receptors, and argatroban and hirudin inhibit thrombin directly. ADP, adenosine diphosphate; TXA_2, thromboxane A_2; vWF, von Willebrand factor.

B. Ticlopidine and clopidogrel
  1. Irreversible **blockage of platelet ADP receptors**
  2. Can be used for the same clinical scenarios in which aspirin has failed
  3. Are at least as safe as aspirin in terms of side effects

QUICK HIT

Low-molecular-weight heparins (LMWHs) such as enoxaparin and dalteparin are much more convenient than standard intravenous heparin therapy because they require no PPT monitoring and are administered subcutaneously. Uses for LMWHs include postsurgical prophylaxis against DVT and the treatment of venous thromboembolism. However, the use of LMWHs is limited in patients with renal failure.

II. Anticoagulants *(Table 10-14)*

A. Heparin
  1. Binds to antithrombin
  2. Greatly **enhances the ability of antithrombin to inhibit coagulation proteases, primarily thrombin**
  3. Is useful in a variety of situations in which anticoagulation is necessary
    a. Deep venous thrombosis (DVT) or pulmonary embolism
    b. Brain attack (thrombotic occlusion)
    c. MI
    d. Others
  4. Leads to **heparin-induced thrombocytopenia** or **thrombosis**, a notable side effect that occurs in 1% to 3% of patients. A heparin-platelet factor 4 antibody is the cause.
  5. Reversal by protamine sulfate

B. Warfarin (Coumadin)
  1. **Impairs vitamin K metabolism**
    a. Low levels of vitamin K prevent y-carboxylation of **clotting factors II, VII, IX, and X.**
    b. Lack of γ-carboxylation leads to **hypofunctional clotting factors II, VII, IX, and X.**
  2. Is used in a variety of clinical scenarios in which oral anticoagulation is required
    a. Atrial fibrillation
    b. Prosthetic valves
    c. DVT or pulmonary embolism
    d. Postoperative anticoagulation
    e. Hypercoagulable states
  3. Use requires care because excessive anticoagulation can lead to hemorrhage.
  4. Reversal by Vitamin K and Factor VIIa

QUICK HIT

The effect of heparin is determined by measuring the activated partial thromboplastin time (aPTT). The effect of warfarin is determined by measuring the PT.

III. Thrombolytics *(Table 10-14)*

A. **Convert plasminogen to plasmin**, which disrupts vascular clot formation
B. Are useful in acute MI, acute ischemic stroke, acute arterial thromboembolic occlusion, severe DVT, and pulmonary embolism
C. Include tissue plasminogen activator (tPA), streptokinase, urokinase, and anistreplase
  1. tPA leads to the most rapid lysis of the clot and results in less systemic fibrinolysis.
  2. However, tPA is also the most expensive.
D. Require careful monitoring because of **increased risk of abnormal bleeding**

IV. Direct thrombin inhibitors *(Table 10-14)*

A. **Do not require antithrombin for activity**
B. Allow for more efficient inhibition of clot-bound fibrin
C. Include hirudin derivatives (lepirudin, bivalirudin, desirudin) and non-hirudin derivatives (argatroban and dabigatran)
D. Various drug-specific indications include prophylaxis of thrombosis in heparin-induced thrombocytopenia or nonvalvular atrial fibrillation, secondary prevention of stroke/transient ischemic attack (TIA), and post-coronary stenting.

TABLE **10-14** **Antithrombotics**

Therapeutic Agent (common name, if relevant) [trade name, where appropriate]	Class—Pharmacology and Pharmacokinetics	Indications	Side Effects or Adverse Effects	Contraindications or Precautions to Consider; Notes
Aspirin	**Platelet inhibitor;** anti-inflammatory, antipyretic, analgesic; **acetylates COX irreversibly** inhibiting the conversion of arachidonic acid to thromboxane A_2	Articular, musculoskeletal pain; chronic pain; acute gout; **maintenance therapy for preventing clot formation**	**Gastric ulcers; bleeding;** causes hypersensitivity reactions (rash); hyperventilation and tinnitus in overdose; **Reye syndrome**	**Contraindicated for children with the flu or chicken pox** (leads to Reye syndrome)
Clopidogrel	**Platelet inhibitor—** irreversibly blocks **ADP receptors,** inhibiting platelet aggregation; prevents **glycoprotein IIb/IIIa** expression which inhibits fibrinogen binding	**Acute coronary syndrome; coronary stenting; prevention of thrombotic stroke**	Bleeding	
Ticlopidine	**Platelet inhibitor—** irreversibly blocks **ADP receptors,** inhibiting platelet aggregation; prevents **glycoprotein IIb/IIIa** expression, which inhibits fibrinogen binding	**Acute coronary syndrome; coronary stenting; prevention of thrombotic stroke**	Bleeding, **neutropenia**	
Abciximab	**Platelet inhibitor— monoclonal antibody** that binds to **glycoprotein receptor IIb/IIIa** on activated platelets → prevents platelet aggregation	**Acute coronary syndrome; PTCA**	Bleeding, thrombocytopenia	
Heparin	**Anticoagulant**—catalyzes the activation of **antithrombin;** decreases thrombin and factor Xa	**Immediate anticoagulation for pulmonary embolism, stroke, angina, myocardial infarction, and deep vein thrombosis**	**Bleeding; osteoporosis; HIT ;** drug–drug interactions; overdose reversed by IV **protamine sulfate**	Fast-acting, short half-life; **laboratory monitoring with PTT; does not cross placenta**
Enoxaparin [Lovenox]	**Anticoagulant—low-molecular-weight heparin;** enhances inhibition of factor Xa and thrombin by increasing **antithrombin** activity **(preferentially increases the inhibition of factor Xa)**	**Prophylaxis of thrombosis**	**Elevated AST/ALT** (reversible); **HIT**	**Caution in recent surgery** or **active bleeding ulcers** or **internal hemorrhages; fewer bleeding complications, increased bioavailability, and longer half-life** compared to unfractionated heparin; no requirement for laboratory monitoring
Fondaparinux [Arixtra]	**Anticoagulant—factor Xa inhibitor**; binds to antithrombin to inactivate Xa	**Prophylaxis or treatment of DVT;** used off-label to treat HIT	Hemorrhage	

(continued)

The Hematopoietic and Lymphoreticular System

TABLE 10-14 **Antithrombotics** *(Continued)*

Therapeutic Agent (common name, if relevant) [trade name, where appropriate]	Class—Pharmacology and Pharmacokinetics	Indications	Side Effects or Adverse Effects	Contraindications or Precautions to Consider; Notes
Warfarin [Coumadin]	**Anticoagulant**—inhibits potassium epoxide regeneration → **interferes with the synthesis of vitamin K–dependent clotting factors II, VII, IX, and X** and **proteins C and S**	**Chronic anticoagulation for thrombotic disorders; atrial fibrillation**	**Bleeding; teratogenic; skin/tissue necrosis; drug–drug interaction**	**Contraindicated in pregnancy and patients with liver, CNS, and hemostatic disease; laboratory monitoring with PT/INR;** 99% exists protein bound; metabolized by and extremely sensitive to **cytochrome P450 system**
Bivalirudin, desirudin	**Anticoagulant—direct thrombin inhibitors**; hirudin derivatives	Bivalirudin: anticoagulation in patients undergoing PTCA at risk for HIT; Desirudin: DVT prophylaxis	**Hemorrhage**	IV administration
Argatroban	**Anticoagulant—direct thrombin inhibitor**	Anticoagulation in patients with **HIT**	**Hemorrhage**	IV administration
Dabigatran [Pradaxa]	**Anticoagulant—direct thrombin inhibitor**	Prevention of thromboembolism in patients with **nonvalvular atrial fibrillation**	**Hemorrhage**	**Reduce dose in patients with moderate renal insufficiency, contraindicated in renal** failure; oral administration
tPA (alteplase)	**Thrombolytic**—binds to **fibrin** in a thrombus → converts entrapped plasminogen to plasmin → fibrinolysis	**Acute myocardial infarction, acute ischemic stroke, and acute pulmonary embolism**	**Hemorrhage;** contraindicated in patients with **active bleeding, history of intracranial bleeding, recent surgery, known bleeding diatheses,** or **severe hypertension**	In cases of acute **ischemic stroke,** should be given **within 3 hours of the onset of symptoms;** treat toxicity with **aminocaproic acid** that inhibits fibrinolysis
Streptokinase [Streptase], **urokinase** [Abbokinase], **anistreplase**	**Thrombolytic—plasminogen-activator converting plasminogen to plasmin → fibrinolysis**	**Lysis of clots**	**Hemorrhage;** contraindicated in patients with **active bleeding, history of intracranial bleeding, recent surgery, known bleeding diatheses,** or **severe hypertension**	**Treat toxicity with aminocaproic acid** that inhibits fibrinolysis

ADP, adenosine diphosphate; ALT, alanine transaminase; AST, aspartate transaminase; CNS, central nervous system; COX, cyclooxygenase; DVT, deep venous thrombosis; HIT, heparin-induced thrombocytopenia; IV, intravenous; PT/INR, prothrombin time/international normalized ratio; PTCA, percutaneous transluminal coronary angioplasty; PTT, partial thromboplastin time; tPA, tissue plasminogen activator.

COAGULATION DISORDERS *(Table 10-15)*

Abnormalities of the coagulation cascade, endothelial cells, or platelets can lead to inappropriate bleeding or clot formation. These coagulopathies can be manifested as symptomatology involving skin, joints, vasculature, or internal organs.

TABLE 10-15 **Coagulation Disorders**

Disease	Etiology	Clinical Features	Notes
Disseminated intravascular coagulation (DIC)	Multifactorial; causes include sepsis, trauma, and neoplasms	**Thrombocytopenia, diffuse hemorrhage,** microthrombus formation, schistocytes	Activation of factors V, VIII, and protein C
Von Willebrand disease (vWD)	**Autosomal dominant** disorder	Impaired platelet adhesion; **decreased factor VIII** (vWF binds factor VIII in the blood); **increased bleeding time**	**Most common hereditary bleeding disorder;** similar deficiency diseases include Bernard–Soulier disease and Glanzmann thrombasthenia
Hemophilia A	**X-linked** factor VIII deficiency	Bleeding into muscle, subcutaneous tissues, and joints	**Most common type of hemophilia;** variable penetrance
Hemophilia B (Christmas disease)	**X-linked** factor IX deficiency	Bleeding into muscle, subcutaneous tissues, and joints	Presentation is identical to hemophilia A
Idiopathic thrombocytopenic purpura (ITP)	**Antiplatelet antibodies**	Thrombocytopenia	Follows upper respiratory tract infection in children and is self-limiting; chronic in adults
Thrombotic thrombocytopenic purpura (TTP)	Idiopathic systemic disease	Hyaline occlusions and microangiopathic hemolytic anemia leading to schistocytes; **classic pentad:** anemia, thrombocytopenia, renal failure, neurologic changes, and fever	May cause neurologic abnormalities

vWF, von Willebrand factor.

MNEMONIC

To remember the classic pentad of TTP, think **FAT RN**:
Fever
Anemia
Thrombocytopenia
Renal failure
Neurologic changes

I. von Willebrand factor deficiency versus hemophilia A *(Table 10-16)*

TABLE 10-16 **von Willebrand Factor (vWF) Deficiency versus Hemophilia A**

	vWF Deficiency	Hemophilia A
Factor VIII: coagulant activity	↓	↓
vWF level	↓	Normal
Ristocetin[a] cofactor activity	↓	Normal
Ristocetin[a] aggregation	↓	Normal
Bleeding time	↑	Normal
Inheritance	**Autosomal dominant**	**X linked**

[a]An antibiotic not used for clinical disease; has platelet aggregation properties.

II. Clotting time algorithm *(Table 10-17)*

TABLE 10-17 **Clotting Time Algorithm**

	PT Normal	PT Prolonged
PTT normal	Factor XIII deficiency	Factor VII deficiency
PTT prolonged	Factors VIII, IX, and XI deficiencies in patients with bleeding; factor XII, prekallikrein, and HMW-K deficiencies in patients without bleeding	Common pathway deficiency: factors V, X, II, and I; severe hepatic diseases; DIC

DIC, disseminated intravascular coagulation; HMW-K, high-molecular-weight kininogen; PT, prothrombin time; PTT, partial thromboplastin time.

Clinical Vignette 10-2

CLINICAL PRESENTATION: A 20-year-old woman presents to her primary care physician with the chief complaint of **frequent and prolonged nosebleeds.** Review of systems is positive for **heavy menstrual flow since menarche** and **easy bruising.** Patient **denies bleeding in joints.** Patient also recently had her wisdom teeth extracted and the oral surgeon had told her she had **bled more than expected.** Physical examination reveals **petechiae in dependent areas** and **multiple ecchymoses** on thigh and upper arms.

DIFFERENTIAL: Coagulation disorder (hemophilia A, hemophilia B, and vitamin K deficiency), platelet disorders (von Willebrand disease, aplastic anemia, Fanconi syndrome, idiopathic thrombocytopenic purpura [ITP], thrombotic thrombocytopenic purpura [TTP], and disseminated intravascular coagulation [DIC]), and increased vascular fragility. In approaching abnormal bleeding, group the differentials according to the pathophysiology (Figure 10-11). Note that this constellation of symptoms is more consistent with a platelet disorder because of the **superficial nature of the bleeding.** On the other hand, **bleeding in joints** suggests hemophilia.

LABORATORY STUDIES: **CBC** should be obtained specifically to measure **platelet counts,** which, if low, define thrombocytopenia. To determine the cause of thrombocytopenia, examination of **peripheral blood smear** and **bone marrow biopsy** might be helpful. A peripheral blood smear may show schistocytes in the case of DIC or TTP (Figure 10-12). **Elevated bleeding time** indicates a *qualitative platelet dysfunction.* **Elevated partial thromboplastin time (PTT)** indicates *defect in contact activation pathway* (factors XII, XI, IX, VIII, X, V, and II). Because hemophilia A and B affect factors VIII and IX, an abnormal PTT is expected in hemophilia. **Elevated prothrombin time (PT)** indicates *defects in the tissue factor pathway* (factors VII, X, V, and II). Production of factors II, VII, IX, and X are vitamin K dependent; because these factors play a role in both contact activation and tissue factor pathways, an elevated PT and PTT is expected in vitamin K deficiency. vWF is a carrier for factor VIII and also contributes to platelet function by binding subendothelium to platelet glycoprotein Ib; thus, abnormalities in bleeding time and PTT are expected. In cases of suspected DIC, **fibrin-split products** (high), **fibrinogen** (low), and **D-dimer** (high) should also be obtained. In this case, the blood studies returned: platelet count = 300 K (normal); bleeding time = 13 seconds (high); PT = 12 seconds (normal); and PTT = 40 seconds (high). Because platelet counts are normal and bleeding time/PTT is elevated, the patient most likely has vWF, which is the most common inherited form of bleeding disorder.

MANAGEMENT: The **underlying cause** should be determined and treated. **Platelet transfusion** depends on cause and severity of thrombocytopenia. Also, **nonsteroidal anti-inflammatory drugs (NSAIDs), anticoagulants, and other antiplatelet agents should be discontinued.**

FIGURE 10-11 Causes of abnormal bleeding

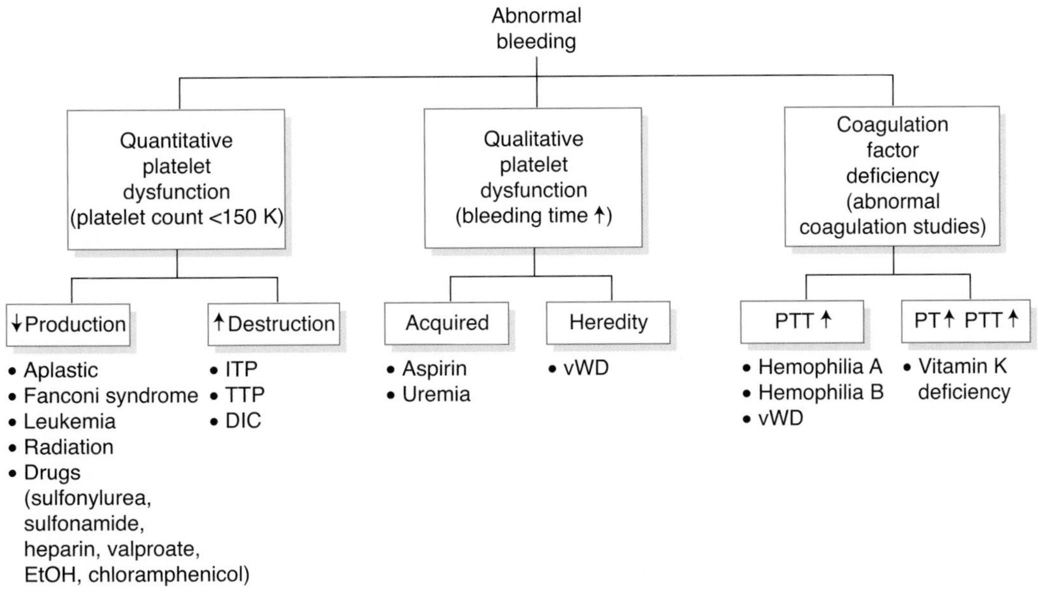
Abnormal bleeding
Quantitative platelet dysfunction (platelet count <150 K)
Qualitative platelet dysfunction (bleeding time ↑)
Coagulation factor deficiency (abnormal coagulation studies)
↓Production
↑Destruction
Acquired
Heredity
PTT ↑
PT↑ PTT↑
• Aplastic
• Fanconi syndrome
• Leukemia
• Radiation
• Drugs (sulfonylurea, sulfonamide, heparin, valproate, EtOH, chloramphenicol)
• ITP
• TTP
• DIC
• Aspirin
• Uremia
• vWD
• Hemophilia A
• Hemophilia B
• vWD
• Vitamin K deficiency

DIC, disseminated intravascular coagulation; EtOH, ethanol; ITP, idiopathic thrombocytopenic purpura; PT, prothrombin time; PTT, partial thromboplastin time; TTP, thrombotic thrombocytopenic purpura; vWD, von Willebrand disease.

FIGURE
10-12 Schistocyte

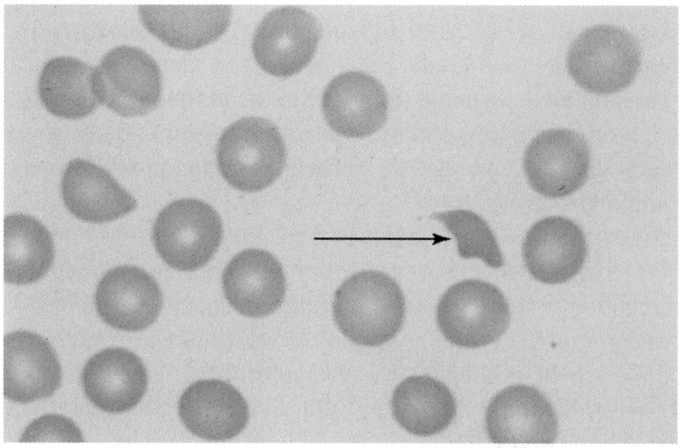

Schistocytes are seen in disseminated intravascular coagulation, thrombotic thrombocytopenic purpura, and hemolytic uremic syndrome. (Reproduced with permission from Anderson SC. *Anderson's Atlas of Hematology.* Philadelphia, PA: Wolters Kluwer Health/Lippincott Williams & Wilkins; 2003.)

QUICK HIT

Staging of lymphoma (Ann Arbor System): (a) one node or organ affected; (b) two nodes or organs on same side of diaphragm affected; (c) both sides of diaphragm, spleen, or other organ affected; and (d) disseminated foci.

LYMPHOMA

Tumors of the lymphoid system present as **enlarged, firm, and fixed painless nodes** and are classified as **Hodgkin** and **non-Hodgkin lymphoma** (Table 10-18).

TABLE 10-18 **Hodgkin versus non-Hodgkin Lymphoma**

Hodgkin Lymphoma	Non-Hodgkin Lymphoma
Number of **Reed–Sternberg cells** (binucleated giant cells) proportional to severity	Malignant neoplasm of lymphocytes (85% B cell, 15% T cell) within lymph nodes (especially periaortic)
Causes **painless cervical lymphadenopathy,** fever, **night sweats**, weight loss, hepatosplenomegaly, and pruritus	Causes painless peripheral lymphadenopathy
Usually affects **young men** (bimodal age distribution)	Usually affects White men younger than 65 years of age
Often curable	Nodular type has better prognosis than diffuse
More reactive lymphocytes signal better prognosis	Small cell type has better prognosis than large cell
Subtypes • Lymphocytic predominance (least common; best prognosis; L/H variant of RS cells; "popcorn" cells) • Mixed cellularity (most frequent, numerous RS cells) • **Nodular sclerosis** (collagen banding, lacunar cells) (most common; women = men; often found in the mediastinum) • Lymphocytic depletion (worst prognosis; rare necrosis and fibrosis of lymphocytic tissue)	**Subtypes** • Small lymphocytic cell (B cell; elderly; indolent course; CLL related) • Follicular cell (cleaved B cells); elderly • Diffuse large cell (**most common non-Hodgkin lymphoma**; elderly and children; usually B cell; **t[14;18];** expression of *bcl-2* oncogene) • Lymphoblastic (T cell; children; **mediastinal mass** progressing to ALL) • Burkitt lymphoma (small, noncleaved B cell, Epstein–Barr virus infection; **"starry-sky"** appearance; **t[8;14];** expression of *c-myc* oncogene) • Cutaneous T cell (mycosis fungoides; Pautrier microabscesses; Sézary syndrome, skin lesions) • Adult T cell (associated with HTLV-1 infection; highly aggressive) • Mantle cell (B cells; poor prognosis) • Marginal cell MALToma (associated with Sjögren syndrome, Hashimoto thyroiditis, and *Helicobacter pylori*) • Intestinal T cell lymphoma (associated with long-term celiac disease; sometimes called "enteropathy-associated T-cell lymphoma")

ALL, acute lymphocytic leukemia; CLL, chronic lymphocytic leukemia; HTLV-1, human T-lymphotropic virus type 1; MALToma, mucosa-associated lymphatic tissue lymphomas; RS, Reed–Sternberg.

LEUKEMIA (*Table 10-19*)

The symptoms of leukemia include fatigue, dyspnea on exertion, bleeding, pallor, and hepatosplenomegaly.

QUICK HIT

Acute lymphocytic leukemia (ALL) is the most common malignancy in children.

TABLE 10-19 Classification of Leukemia

Acute Lymphoblastic	Acute Myeloblastic	Chronic Myeloid	Chronic Lymphocytic
Small lymphoblasts; decreased cytoplasm; predominantly affects **children; PAS (+);** responsive to therapy	Myeloblasts; defect in maturation beyond myeloblast or promyelocyte stage; **Auer rods;** predominantly affects **adults; PAS (−);** poor prognosis	t(9;22) results in **Philadelphia chromosome** (BCR-ABL); leukocytosis; **decreased leukocyte alkaline phosphatase;** splenomegaly; onset at **35–55** years of age; ends in blast crisis	Usually B cells; "smudge cells" in smear; warm AIHA; hypogammaglobulinemia; lymphadenopathy; hepatosplenomegaly; more common in **men >60** years of age

AIHA, autoimmune hemolytic anemia; PAS, periodic acid-Schiff stain.

QUICK HIT

The most common chromosomal translocations tested on the boards are:
t(9;22) (Philadelphia chromosome), associated with chronic myelogenous leukemia (CML) (*BCR-ABL* hybrid)
t(8;14), associated with Burkitt lymphoma (activation of *c-myc*)
t(14;18), associated with follicular lymphoma (activation of *bcl*-2)
t(15;17), associated with M3 type of acute myelogenous leukemia (AML)
t(11;22), associated with Ewing sarcoma
t(11;14), associated with mantle cell lymphoma

ANEMIA (*Table 10-20*)

Anemia, a decrease in circulating RBC mass, is usually defined as hemoglobin <12 g/dL in female patients and <14 g/dL in male patients.

I. Microcytic anemia

A. Iron deficiency
1. **Most common anemia**
2. **Total iron-binding capacity (TIBC) is increased. Serum iron, ferritin**, and **percent transferrin saturation are decreased. Bone marrow iron stores are low.**
3. Occurs in menstruating or pregnant women, infants, and preadolescents
4. Caused by dietary deficiency or bleeding (menorrhagia, GI bleeding, GI cancers, and inflammatory bowel disease)
5. Pale, easy fatigability, and dyspneic; rarely associated with Plummer–Vinson syndrome (characterized by glossitis, esophageal web, and iron-deficiency)

B. Lead poisoning
1. It inhibits heme synthesis (D-ala dehydratase and ferrochelatase).
2. **Basophilic stippling** of RBCs is seen on peripheral smear. Examination of bone marrow may reveal ringed sideroblasts.
3. Finger, wrist, and foot drop occur from neurotoxicity.
4. Renal lesions, GI colic, and gingival lead lines occur.
5. Treatment is chelation with ethylenediaminetetraacetic acid (EDTA), succimer, or dimercaprol.

TABLE 10-20 Classification of Anemia

Microcytic (MCV <80)	Normocytic (MCV 80–100)	Macrocytic (MCV >100)
Iron deficiency	Aplastic anemia	Liver disease
Lead poisoning	Acute blood loss	Vitamin B_{12} deficiency
Sickle cell	Hemolytic anemia	Folate deficiency
Chronic disease	Chronic disease	
Sideroblastic anemia		
Thalassemia		

MCV, mean cell volume.

QUICK HIT

In sickle cell disease, the sixth amino acid of the β-chain of hemoglobin is changed from glutamate to valine. Sickling only occurs when the RBCs are **deoxygenated**. Oxygenated HbS RBCs function normally.

MNEMONIC

Remember the encapsulated bacteria by the phrase "**E**ven **S**ome **P**retty **N**asty **K**illers **H**ave **S**hiny **B**odies"
***E**. coli* (some strains)
***S**trep pneumoniae*
***P**seudomonas aeruginosa*
***N**eisseria meningitidis*
***K**lebsiella pneumoniae*
***H**aemophilus influenzae*
***S**almonella typhi*
Group **B** Strep

C. Sideroblastic anemia
   1. Iron stain of bone marrow reveals ringed sideroblasts.
   2. TIBC is reduced and serum iron is increased.
   3. RBC count is reduced.
D. Sickle cell disease (hemoglobin S [HbS])
   1. It is primarily seen in **Blacks**.
   2. The homozygous form is most severe. Heterozygotes are generally asymptomatic.
   3. Severe hemolytic anemia is seen.
   4. Deoxygenated HbS polymerizes within RBCs, causing the characteristic sickle shape. Sickling leads to painful crises, organ infarction (**autosplenectomy**), and strokes.
   5. Aplastic crises may occur, usually provoked by viral infection (usually parvovirus B19).
   6. Patients are especially susceptible to infection by **encapsulated bacteria** (*Streptococcus pneumoniae* and *Haemophilus influenzae*) and osteomyelitis caused by *Salmonella*.
   7. Sickle cells and Howell–Jolly bodies (due to asplenia) are seen in peripheral blood smear.
   8. Treatment is with **hydroxyurea** to increase HbF.
E. Thalassemia
   1. This is a group of genetic disorders, all in some way deficient in α- or β-globin chain synthesis.
   2. **β-Thalassemia is more common** (especially in people of Mediterranean origin)
      a. The homozygous form, called thalassemia major (also known as Mediterranean or Cooley anemia), causes splenomegaly, bone distortions, hemosiderosis, and increased HbF, and it is fatal in childhood.
      b. The heterozygous form of β-thalassemia (thalassemia minor) causes a minor anemia but has no effect on the life span.
   3. α-Thalassemia is caused by a deletion in one or more of the four α-globin genes; loss of all four genes is incompatible with life. It is seen primarily in patients of Asian or African descent.

II. Normocytic anemias

A. Anemia of chronic disease
   1. Anemia is seen in chronic disease states such as cancer and autoimmune disease due to impaired iron utilization.
   2. It is the second most common anemia.
   3. Usually normocytic, but can be microcytic in longstanding cases
   4. **TIBC is reduced. Ferritin is increased.** Percent transferrin saturation is generally normal.
   5. Low serum iron but high iron stores in the bone marrow are observed.
B. Aplastic anemia
   1. Dysfunctional or deficient multipotent myeloid stem cells lead to pancytopenia.
   2. It is caused by viruses, chemicals, radiation, or renal failure (via decreased erythropoietin), or may be idiopathic.
   3. Drugs causing aplastic anemia include **NSAIDs, benzene,** and **chloramphenicol.**
   4. Symptoms include fatigue, pallor, mucosal bleeding, and petechiae as a result of thrombocytopenia.
   5. Neutropenia occurs, leading to frequent infections.
   6. Marrow is hypocellular, with **fat infiltration**.
C. Anemia caused by acute blood loss
   1. Leads to a **transient normocytic anemia** (however, chronic bleeding can lead to iron deficiency and hence microcytic anemia)
   2. May appear macrocytic because of increased reticulocyte release from bone marrow 7 to 10 days later
D. Hemolytic anemias
   1. Increased RBC destruction leads to an increase in unconjugated bilirubin, hemoglobinemia, hemoglobinuria, and hemosiderosis and decreased serum haptoglobin.

QUICK HIT

Drugs causing hemolytic anemia: penicillin, α-methyldopa, and quinidine. Infectious agents causing hemolytic anemia: *Clostridium* and malarial parasite.

2. Increase in reticulocytes occurs because of additional erythropoiesis.
3. Extracorpuscular (acquired) hemolytic anemias
   a. Warm autoimmune hemolytic immunoglobulin (AIHI) (IgG): associated with lymphoma, spherocytosis, and **positive direct Coombs test**
   b. Cold AIHI (IgM): associated with lymphoid neoplasm, mycoplasma infection, anti-I antibodies, ABO incompatibility, and **Raynaud phenomenon**. It causes hemolysis at low temperatures.
   c. Erythroblastosis fetalis (hemolytic diseases of the newborn): usually caused by Rh blood group incompatibility; can result in kernicterus and death
   d. Infections such as bartonellosis, *Clostridium*, and malaria
4. Intracorpuscular (genetic) hemolytic anemias
   a. Hereditary ovalocytosis (elliptocytosis): **autosomal dominant**
   b. Hereditary spherocytosis: **autosomal dominant; spectrin** deficiency
   c. Paroxysmal nocturnal hemoglobinuria (PNH): deficiency of DAF and decreased leukocyte alkaline phosphatase (LAP)
   d. Glucose-6-phosphate dehydrogenase (G6PD) deficiency: **X linked**; more common in Mediterranean and Blacks; precipitated by oxidative stress (primaquine therapy); **Heinz bodies** are seen.
   e. Pyruvate kinase deficiency: **autosomal recessive**; chronic

III. Macrocytic anemias

A. Liver disease—usually cirrhosis
   1. Excess lipid is added to RBC membrane in diseased liver.
   2. Hypersplenism occurs.
   3. Spur cells are present.

B. Vitamin B_{12} (cobalamin) deficiency
   1. **Megaloblastic anemia** characterized by **hypersegmented neutrophils** (Figure 10-13), macrocytosis, and pancytopenia
   2. Decreased DNA synthesis
   3. Most common form is **pernicious anemia**.
      a. Caused by a deficiency of intrinsic factor secondary to the destruction of parietal cells
      b. Associated with increased incidence of gastric carcinoma and achlorhydria
   4. Other etiologies for vitamin B_{12} deficiency anemia include strict vegetarian diet, distal ileum pathology, bacterial overgrowth, *Diphyllobothrium latum* infection, and type A gastritis
   5. **Neurologic symptoms** caused by demyelination of posterior and lateral columns, ataxia, and paresthesia in distal extremities

FIGURE 10-13 **Hypersegmented neutrophil**

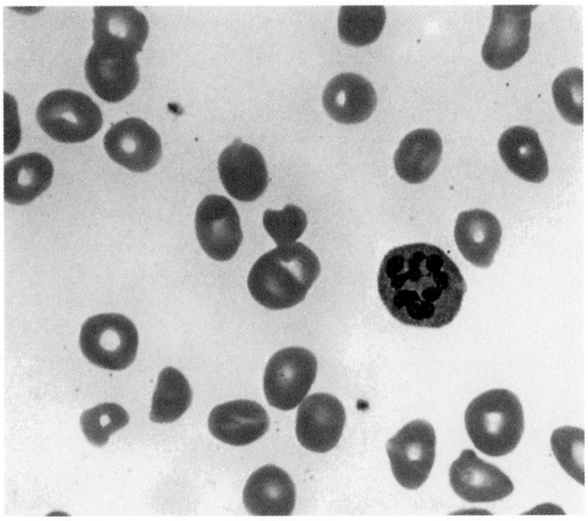

(Reproduced with permission from McClatchey KD. *Clinical Laboratory Medicine.* 2nd ed. Philadelphia, PA: Lippincott Williams & Wilkins; 2002.)

MNEMONIC

Remember the immunoglobulins associated with each type of autoimmune hemolytic anemia: Ig**G** with **warm (Georgia is warm)** and Ig**M** with **cold (Minnesota is cold)**.

QUICK HIT

ABO transfusion reactions are almost always a result of clerical (human) error.

QUICK HIT

Hemolytic disease of the newborn can be prevented with **RhoGAM** (anti-D antibody), which neutralizes the mother's immunogenic response to fetal RBCs that carry the D antigen.

QUICK HIT

Spherocytes are characterized by osmotic fragility in hypotonic solution.

QUICK HIT

The Schilling test is used to diagnose the etiology of pernicious anemia.

MNEMONIC

Remember vitamin **B**$_{12}$, deficiency affects the **B**rain, but folate deficiency is not associated with neurologic symptoms.

C. Folate deficiency
1. It causes megaloblastic anemia; hematologic findings are identical to vitamin B_{12} deficiency.
2. **No neurologic** deficits are present.
3. Folate deficiency can mask vitamin B_{12} deficiency.
4. Etiologies include dietary deficiency, tropical sprue, *Giardia lamblia* infection, oral contraceptives, **antineoplastics** (methotrexate), and pregnancy.

Clinical Vignette 10-3

CLINICAL PRESENTATION: A 28-year-old woman visits her primary care physician for her yearly physical examination. During her review of systems, she tells her physician that she has been feeling **fatigued.** She denies weight loss, diarrhea, and menorrhagia. Physical examination shows **pallor.** Blood studies show: **Hct = 32%, Hg = 11.1 g/dL,** and platelet = 300 K.

DIFFERENTIALS AND LABORATORY STUDIES: This patient is anemic. Figure 10-14 summarizes the approach to anemia. Two laboratory studies critical in working up anemia are (a) **RBC indices** and (b) **peripheral blood smear.** Tables 10-21 and 10-22 summarize the findings expected in each of these studies.

The first step in approaching blood studies for an anemic patient is the **reticulocyte count,** which is used to determine whether the cause of the anemia is from increased destruction of RBCs (high reticulocyte count from compensatory increase in RBC production) or decreased production of RBCs (normal or low reticulocyte count). A high reticulocyte count suggests hemolysis, and the differentials would include causes intrinsic to the RBC such as hereditary spherocytosis, glucose-6-phosphate dehydrogenase (G6PD) deficiency, PNH, and sickle cell anemia. Extrinsic causes of hemolysis include thrombotic thrombocytopenic purpura (TTP), hemolytic uremic syndrome (HUS), artificial heart valve, disseminated intravascular coagulation, warm autoimmune hemolytic anemia (WAIHA), cold autoimmune hemolytic anemia (CAIHA), altered plasma components (high lipids), drugs, and infectious agents; Table 10-23 shows how these hemolytic disorders can be differentiated.

If the reticulocyte count is normal, the next step is to look at the **mean cell volume (MCV)** that categorizes the anemia as hypochromic microcytic (MCV $<$80), normochromic (MCV 80 to 100), and hyperchromic macrocytic (MCV $>$100). If MCV values suggest microcytic anemia, the differentials are iron (Fe) deficiency, anemia of chronic disease, thalassemia, sideroblastic anemia, and lead poisoning. These can be differentiated based on **serum Fe, serum ferritin, and TIBC** (Table 10-24). Also, **lead levels** will be high in lead poisoning. Note that hemolytic anemias can also produce an MCV $<$80. If macrocytic anemia is observed, the differentials include vitamin B_{12} deficiency, folate deficiency, and liver disease. To differentiate, **check B$_{12}$** and **folate levels** and **liver function tests.** If normocytic anemia is observed, the causes could be primary involvement of bone marrow, such as aplastic anemia, or secondary to other underlying disease. **Bone marrow examination** can also be done but is not needed in all patients with anemia.

MANAGEMENT: In acute cases, **transfusion** may be necessary. Otherwise, treat underlying cause of anemia. For iron, vitamin B_{12}, or folate deficiency, **supplement diet** with appropriate nutrient.

FIGURE 10-14 Approach to anemia

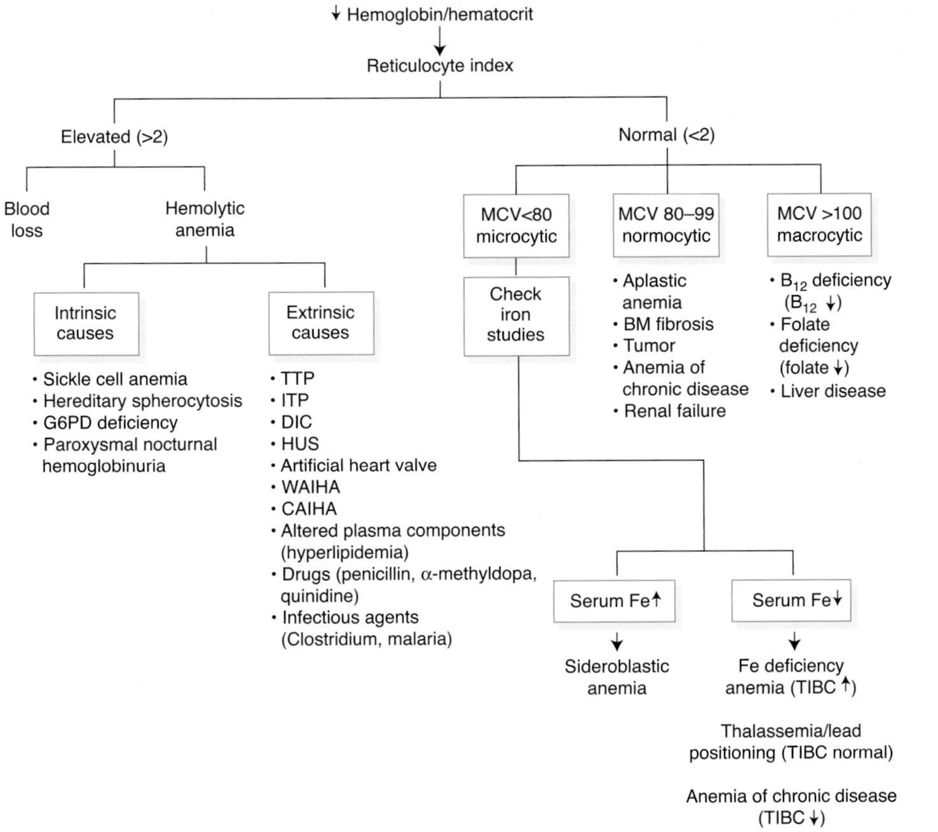

↓ Hemoglobin/hematocrit
Reticulocyte index
Elevated (>2)
Normal (<2)
Blood loss
Hemolytic anemia
Intrinsic causes
Extrinsic causes
• Sickle cell anemia
• Hereditary spherocytosis
• G6PD deficiency
• Paroxysmal nocturnal hemoglobinuria
• TTP
• ITP
• DIC
• HUS
• Artificial heart valve
• WAIHA
• CAIHA
• Altered plasma components (hyperlipidemia)
• Drugs (penicillin, α-methyldopa, quinidine)
• Infectious agents (Clostridium, malaria)
MCV<80 microcytic
MCV 80–99 normocytic
MCV >100 macrocytic
Check iron studies
• Aplastic anemia
• BM fibrosis
• Tumor
• Anemia of chronic disease
• Renal failure
• B12 deficiency (B12 ↓)
• Folate deficiency (folate ↓)
• Liver disease
Serum Fe↑
Serum Fe↓
Sideroblastic anemia
Fe deficiency anemia (TIBC ↑)
Thalassemia/lead positioning (TIBC normal)
Anemia of chronic disease (TIBC ↓)

BM, bone marrow; CAIHA, cold autoimmune hemolytic anemia; DIC, disseminated intravascular coagulation; Fe, iron; G6PD, glucose-6-phosphate dehydrogenase; HUS, hemolytic uremic syndrome; ITP, idiopathic thrombocytopenic purpura; MCV, mean cell volume; TIBC, total iron-binding capacity; TTP, thrombotic thrombocytopenic purpura; WAIHA, warm autoimmune hemolytic anemia.

TABLE 10-21 Approach to Laboratory Blood Studies

Blood Lab Study	Definition	Notes
Hemoglobin (Hgb)	Concentration of Hgb in 100 mL of blood	**Increased:** severe dehydration, erythrocytosis, polycythemia, severe burn, shock, COPD, CHF, high altitudes, drugs (gentamicin, methyldopa) **Decreased:** hyperthyroidism, leukemia, liver disease, hemolytic reaction, overhydration, pregnancy, drugs (acetaminophen, antineoplastic agents, chloramphenicol, hydralazine, MAOI, nitrites, penicillin, tetracycline, sulfonamide)
Hematocrit	Percentage of RBCs in a volume of whole blood; not reliable indicator of anemia immediately after blood loss or blood transfusion	**Increased:** severe dehydration, erythrocytosis, polycythemia, severe burns, shock, high altitudes **Decreased** (defined as anemia): hyperthyroidism, leukemia, liver disease, hemolytic reactions, pregnancy, and causes of macrocytic, normocytic, and microcytic anemia (see below)
MCV	Represents volume of single RBC; indicator of cell size	**Increased** (>100) (defined as macrocytic anemia): vitamin B_{12} deficiency, folate deficiency, liver disease, alcoholism **Decreased** (<80) (defined as microcytic anemia): iron deficiency, thalassemia, lead poisoning, sideroblastic anemia; some hemolytic anemias, possibly anemia of chronic disease
MCHC	Represents average concentration of Hgb in RBC	**Increased:** spherocytosis
MCH	Represents average weight of Hgb in RBCs; confirms accuracy of MCV value	**Increased:** macrocytic anemia (see above) **Decreased:** microcytic anemia (see above)
Reticulocyte count	Reticulocyte is nonnucleated immature RBC formed in bone marrow; increased values indicate accelerated erythropoiesis	**Increased:** hemolytic anemias, sickle cell disease, pregnancy, splenectomy, hemorrhage **Decreased:** aplastic anemia, chronic infection, radiation therapy

CHF, congestive heart failure; COPD, chronic obstructive pulmonary disease; MAOI, monoamine oxidase inhibitor; MCH, mean corpuscular hemoglobin; MCHC, mean corpuscular hemoglobin concentration; MCV, mean cell volume; RBC, red blood cell.

QUICK HIT

Spur cells occur in liver disease and are caused by the reticuloendothelial system "biting" the RBCs.

TABLE 10-22 **Peripheral Blood Smear Findings**

Peripheral Blood Smear	Conditions Associated
Hypersegmented neutrophils (Figure 10-13)	Folate/B_{12} deficiency
Basophilic stippling of RBCs	Lead poisoning
Echinocytes (Burr cells)	Uremia
Spherocytes	Spherocytosis
Microspherocytes	Coombs hemolysis
Schistocytes (fragmented cells, helmet cells) (Figure 10-12)	Disseminated intravascular coagulation, TTP, HUS
Poikilocytes (irregularly shaped cells)	Thalassemia
Target cells	Liver disease, thalassemia
Acanthocytes (spur cells)	Liver disease, abetalipoproteinemia
Sickle cells	Sickle cell anemia
Howell–Jolly bodies	Asplenia
Heinz bodies	Glucose-6-phosphate dehydrogenase deficiency
Teardrop cells	Myeloid metaplasia with myelofibrosis
Sideroblast (ring of small basophilic granules in the periphery of nucleated RBC precursors)	Sideroblastic anemia

HUS, hemolytic uremic syndrome; RBC, red blood cell; TTP, thrombotic thrombocytopenic purpura.

TABLE 10-23 **Differential for Platelet Destruction**

Lab Study	DIC	HUS	TTP	ITP
Blood smear	Schistocytes	Schistocytes	Schistocytes	Normal
PT/PTT	Markedly increased	Normal or mildly increased	Normal or mildly increased	Normal
Fibrin-split products	Increased	Normal	Normal	Normal
Fibrinogen	Decreased	Normal	Normal	Normal
Notes	Platelets trapped in fibrin mesh deposited in blood vessels	***Escherichia coli*** often implicated in pathogenesis; usually occurs in **children**	Idiopathic	Autoimmune: autoantibody-mediated platelet destruction; follows URI in children
	Risk factors: sepsis, trauma, obstetric complications, malignancy, transfusions	Symptoms: anemia, thrombocytopenia, acute renal failure, **bloody diarrhea, abdominal pain, seizures**	**Classic pentad:** anemia, thrombocytopenia, renal failure, **neurologic changes, fever**	

DIC, disseminated intravascular coagulation; HUS, hemolytic uremic syndrome; ITP, idiopathic thrombocytopenic purpura; PT/PTT, prothrombin time/partial thromboplastin time; TTP, thrombotic thrombocytopenic purpura; URI, upper respiratory infection.

TABLE 10-24 **Differential for Microcytic Anemia**

Lab Study	Iron-deficiency Anemia	Beta Thalassemia	Anemia of Chronic Disease	Sideroblastic Anemia
Serum iron	Low	Normal/high	Low	**High**
Serum ferritin	Low	Normal	Normal/high	High
TIBC	High	Normal	Low	Normal/low
% Transferrin saturation	Low (<12%)	Normal/high	Normal (>18%)	High

TIBC, total iron-binding capacity.

MNEMONIC

To remember the findings of TIBC in iron deficiency and chronic disease, use **TIBC**: **T**op = **I**ron, **B**ottom = **C**hronic disease. TIBC levels are high (**top**) in iron-deficiency anemia and low (**bottom**) in chronic disease.

MYELOPROLIFERATIVE DISORDERS

The myeloproliferative disorders include four diseases, all of which have features of hepatosplenomegaly, increased risk of converting into a blastic leukemia, or a spent phase of marrow fibrosis: (1) polycythemia vera, (2) myelofibrosis, (3) essential thrombocythemia, and (4) chronic myelogenous leukemia (CML).

QUICK HIT

Myelodysplastic syndromes also exist: refractory anemia, refractory anemia with ringed sideroblasts, refractory anemia with excess blasts, refractory anemia with excess blasts in transformation, and chronic myelomonocytic leukemia.

I. Polycythemia vera

A. Chronic increase in the number of red cells caused by bone marrow hyperplasia of unknown etiology
B. Clinical manifestations
   1. Presents in middle age
   2. Symptoms include vision disturbances, erythromelalgia (burning pains in the hands/feet, associated with erythema, pallor, or cyanosis), pruritus, facial plethora, hepatosplenomegaly, and thrombosis.
C. Differential diagnosis
   1. Absolute polycythemia vera
      a. Primary polycythemia—**appropriately low erythropoietin levels**
      b. **Secondary polycythemia**—elevated erythropoietin levels
         - Appropriate: response to hypoxia
         - Inappropriate: secondary to inappropriate secretion of erythropoietin (renal cell carcinoma, pheochromocytoma, hepatocellular carcinoma, hemangioblastoma)
   2. Relative polycythemia vera (e.g., dehydration) often caused by a decrease in extracorpuscular volume, thus causing a relative increase in the hematocrit level
D. Diagnosis
   1. Major diagnostic criteria
      a. Increased RBC mass (hematocrit)
      b. Normal arterial oxygen saturation (≥92%)
      c. Splenomegaly
   2. Minor diagnostic criteria
      a. Thrombocytosis
      b. Leukocytosis
      c. Elevated LAP
      d. Elevated serum vitamin B_{12}
   3. Diagnosis requires either all three major criteria *or* increased RBC mass plus normal arterial oxygen saturation plus at least two minor criteria including leukocytosis and thrombocytosis.

II. Myelofibrosis

A. Generalized fibrosis of bone marrow characterized by pancytopenia in the face of increased megakaryocytes in the marrow

B. Clinical manifestations
 1. Presents in patients in their late 50s
 2. **Teardrop deformity** of RBCs occurring along with splenomegaly and extramedullary hematopoiesis
 3. "Dry tap" seen on bone biopsy
C. Differential diagnosis
 1. Primary myelofibrosis
  a. Marrow fibrosis
  b. Extramedullary hematopoiesis
 2. Secondary myelofibrosis
  a. Infections: tuberculosis, osteomyelitis
  b. Metastatic carcinoma
  c. Paget disease

III. Essential thrombocythemia

A. A primary disorder of unknown etiology resulting in increased platelets
B. Clinical manifestations
 1. Thrombocytosis
 2. Megakaryocytic hyperplasia
 3. Splenomegaly
 4. Hemorrhage and thrombosis
 5. Increased bone marrow reticulin and absence of *BCR-ABL* gene

IV. Chronic myelogenous leukemia

A. The t(9,22) translocation of the *ABL* proto-oncogene to *BCR*, creating a *BCR-ABL* fusion gene (Philadelphia chromosome)
B. Clinical manifestations
 1. Hepatosplenomegaly and lymphadenopathy
 2. Normocytic to macrocytic anemia
 3. Platelet derangement (either a thrombocytosis during active phase or thrombocytopenia in spent phase can occur)
 4. Bone marrow hypercellular
 5. Blast crisis in late stages

CHEMOTHERAPEUTICS *(Table 10-25)*

The chemotherapeutics can be classified based on where they act in the cell cycle (mitotic phase, DNA synthesis phase, etc.) and **chemical structure** (e.g., alkylating agent, etoposide, and nitrosoureas).

TABLE 10-25 **Chemotherapeutics**

Therapeutic Agent (common name, if relevant) [trade name, where appropriate]	Class—Pharmacology and Pharmacokinetics	Indications	Side Effects or Adverse Effects	Contraindications or Precautions to Consider; Notes
Methotrexate [Rheumatrex]	**S phase specific antimetabolite—folic acid analog (dihydrofolate reductase inhibitor)** → decreases dTMP → decreases DNA and protein synthesis; **immunosuppressant**	**Acute lymphocytic and myelogenous leukemia, lymphoma,** choriocarcinoma, sarcoma, bone marrow transplant, **abortion, ectopic pregnancy, rheumatoid arthritis, psoriasis**	Oral and GI ulceration, **myelosuppression,** thrombocytopenia, leukopenia, hepatotoxicity, **fibrotic lung disease**, mucositis	**Leucovorin is given as an adjuvant after treatment (reverses myelosuppression)**

(continued)

TABLE 10-25 **Chemotherapeutics** *(Continued)*

Therapeutic Agent (common name, if relevant) [trade name, where appropriate]	Class—Pharmacology and Pharmacokinetics	Indications	Side Effects or Adverse Effects	Contraindications or Precautions to Consider; Notes
5-Fluorouracil	**S phase specific antimetabolite—pyrimidine analog** → bioactivated to 5F-dUMP → binds folic acid → complex inhibits thymidylate synthase → decreases dTMP and DNA synthesis	**Colon cancer, solid tumors, basal cell carcinoma and actinic keratosis (topical)**	**Myelosuppression, photosensitivity**	Acts **synergistically with methotrexate;** myelosuppression is not reversible with leucovorin but with **thymidine**
6-Mercaptopurine [Purinethol]	**S phase specific antimetabolite—purine analog** → inhibits purine synthesis → disrupts DNA and RNA synthesis	**Acute lymphoblastic leukemia;** Crohn disease; ulcerative colitis	**Myelosuppression, liver toxicity** (intrahepatic cholestasis and focal centrilobular necrosis)	Metabolized by **xanthine oxidase,** therefore increased toxicity with **allopurinol**
Cytarabine	**S phase specific antimetabolite—pyrimidine analog**; inhibits DNA polymerase	**AML**	Leukopenia, thrombocytopenia, megaloblastic anemia	
Cyclophosphamide [Cytoxan]	**Cell cycle nonspecific agent—alkylating agent** → cross-links DNA strands → decreases DNA synthesis and prevents cell division → destroys proliferating lymphoid cells; alkylates the resting cells; potent immunosuppressant	**Transplant rejection, rheumatic arthritis, non-Hodgkin lymphoma, breast and ovarian carcinoma**	**GI and bone marrow toxicity, hemorrhagic cystitis** (can be partially prevented by mesna)	Requires bioactivation by liver
Ifosfamide	**Cell cycle nonspecific agent—alkylating agent** → cross-links DNA strands → decreases protein and DNA synthesis → prevents cell division	**Testicular cancer**	**GI and bone marrow toxicity, hemorrhagic cystitis** (can be partially prevented by mesna)	Requires bioactivation by liver
Carmustine, lomustine, semustine, streptozocin	**Cell cycle nonspecific agent (nitrosoureas)—alkylating agent** → cross-links DNA and RNA strands	**Brain tumors** (including **glioblastoma multiforme**)	**CNS toxicity** (dizziness, ataxia)	**Crosses blood–brain barrier to CNS;** requires bioactivation
Cisplatin, carboplatin, oxaliplatin	**Cell cycle nonspecific agent—alkylating agent** → cross-links DNA and RNA strands	**Bladder, testicular, ovarian, and lung carcinomas**	**Nephrotoxicity, acoustic nerve damage**	
Busulfan	**Cell cycle nonspecific agent—alkylating agent** → cross-links DNA and RNA strands	**Chronic myelogenous leukemia**	**Pulmonary fibrosis, hyperpigmentation**	
Doxorubicin [Adriamycin]	**Cell cycle nonspecific agent—generates free radicals; also intercalates into DNA** → breaks DNA; affects plasma membrane	**Hodgkin lymphoma; myeloma;** sarcoma; solid tumors of breast, ovary, and lung	Cardiac changes resulting in cumulative **cardiotoxicity,** myelosuppression, alopecia, and toxic extravasation	Part of the ABVD combination regimen for Hodgkin lymphoma

(continued)

TABLE 10-25 **Chemotherapeutics** *(Continued)*

Therapeutic Agent (common name, if relevant) [trade name, where appropriate]	Class—Pharmacology and Pharmacokinetics	Indications	Side Effects or Adverse Effects	Contraindications or Precautions to Consider; Notes
Daunorubicin [DaunoXome, Cerubidine]	**Cell cycle nonspecific agent—oxidizes free radicals; also intercalates into DNA** → breaks DNA; affects plasma membrane	**Hodgkin lymphoma; myeloma;** sarcoma; solid tumors of breast, ovary, and lung	Cardiac changes resulting in cumulative **cardiotoxicity,** myelosuppression, alopecia, and toxic extravasation	Part of the ABVD combination regimen for Hodgkin lymphoma
Dactinomycin [Cosmegen]	**Cell cycle nonspecific agent—intercalates into DNA**	**Wilms tumor, Ewing sarcoma, rhabdomyosarcoma**	**Skin eruptions, hyperkeratosis, myelosuppression**	
Bleomycin [Blenoxane]	**G2 phase–specific agent—generates free radicals** that bind, intercalate, and cut DNA	**Testicular cancer, Hodgkin disease**	**Pulmonary fibrosis,** fever, **blistering, stomatitis,** hypersensitivity reactions (anaphylaxis)	**Minimal myelosuppression;** part of the A**B**VD regimen for Hodgkin lymphoma
Hydroxyurea [Hydrea]	**S phase–specific agent—binds ribonucleotide reductase** → inhibits formation of DNA	**Melanoma; CML; sickle cell disease**	**Nausea, vomiting, bone marrow suppression**	
Etoposide	**G2 phase specific—inhibits topoisomerase II → increases DNA degradation**	**Small cell lung cancer,** prostate and testicular carcinoma	**Myelosuppression,** nausea, vomiting, **alopecia**	
Prednisone	**Glucocorticoid—inhibits protein synthesis;** reduces lymph node and spleen size; **inhibits cell cycle activity of lymphoid cells; lyses T cells; suppresses antibody, prostaglandin, and leukotriene synthesis; blocks monocyte production of IL-1**	**CLL, Hodgkin lymphoma,** rheumatic arthritis; **autoimmune disorders; allergic reaction; asthma; organ transplantation (esp. during rejection crisis)**	**Osteoporosis, Cushingoid reaction, psychosis, hyperglycemia, immunosuppression, infection, hypertension, cataracts, acne, peptic ulcers**	Part of the MOPP regimen for Hodgkin lymphoma
Tamoxifen [Nolvadex]	**Selective estrogen receptor modulator—competitively binds estrogen receptors; breast (estrogen antagonist):** prevents proliferation of estrogen receptor positive tumor cells; **endometrium (partial agonist);** bone (agonist): decreases bone turnover and increases bone density	**Treats estrogen-dependent breast cancer in postmenopausal women;** reduces contralateral breast cancer; osteoporosis prevention	**May increase the risk of endometrial cancer; hot flashes;** flushing	

(continued)

The Hematopoietic and Lymphoreticular System

TABLE 10-25 **Chemotherapeutics** *(Continued)*

Therapeutic Agent (common name, if relevant) [trade name, where appropriate]	Class—Pharmacology and Pharmacokinetics	Indications	Side Effects or Adverse Effects	Contraindications or Precautions to Consider; Notes
Raloxifene [Evista]	**Selective estrogen receptor modulator—breast (estrogen antagonist); endometrium (estrogen antagonist):** prevents proliferation of endometrium; **bone (estrogen agonist):** decreases bone turnover and increases bone density; **cardiovascular (estrogen agonist):** decreases LDL	**Osteoporosis, breast cancer**	**Hot flashes;** sinusitis; weight gain; muscle pain; leg cramps; **increased risk of blood clots**	Unlike estrogen, raloxifene **does not decrease HDL**
Trastuzumab [Herceptin]	**Monoclonal antibody against HER2;** binds to tumor cells overexpressing HER2 → mediates antibody-dependent cytotoxicity → destruction of tumor cells	**Metastatic breast cancer**	**Cardiotoxicity**	
Imatinib [Gleevec]	**Tyrosine kinase inhibitor—inhibits BCR-ABL tyrosine kinase** (abnormal product of **Philadelphia chromosome** in CML) blocks proliferation → induces apoptosis in BCR-ABL positive cell lines and fresh leukemic cells	**CML,** GI stromal tumors	**Fluid retention**	
Vincristine [Oncovin]	**M phase specific (vinca alkaloid)—blocks polymerization of microtubules** → mitotic spindle cannot form	**Hodgkin lymphoma, Wilms tumor, choriocarcinoma, acute leukemia**	**Peripheral neuritis, areflexia,** paralytic ileus	Part of the MOPP regimen for Hodgkin lymphoma
Vinblastine [Velban]	**M phase specific (vinca alkaloid)—blocks polymerization of microtubules** → mitotic spindle cannot form	**Hodgkin lymphoma, Wilms tumor, choriocarcinoma**	**Myelosuppression**	
Paclitaxel [Taxol]	**M phase specific (Taxol)—stabilizes polymerization of microtubules** → mitotic spindle cannot break down → anaphase cannot occur	**Ovarian and breast cancer**	**Myelosuppression, hypersensitivity**	

ABVD, Adriamycin, bleomycin, vinblastine, and dacarbazine; AML, acute myelogenous leukemia; CLL, chronic lymphoblastic leukemia; CML, chronic myelogenous leukemia; CNS, central nervous system; dTMP, deoxythymidine monophosphate; dUMP, deoxyuridine monophosphate; G1 phase, synthesis of components needed for DNA synthesis; G2 phase, synthesis of components needed for mitosis; GI, gastrointestinal; HDL, high-density lipoprotein; HER2, human epidermal growth factor receptor 2 protein; IL, interleukin; LDL, low-density lipoprotein; MOPP, Mustargen, Oncovin, procarbazine, prednisone; M phase, mitotic phase; S phase, DNA synthesis phase.

Crunch Time Review

The following pages contain high-yield information designed for review in the days just preceding the Step 1 examination.

MOST COMMON

Often on the USMLE exam, the student finds two responses that could potentially answer a question. The National Board of Medical Examiners (NBME) is testing the student to identify the more common of the two responses; for example, the more common cause, site, or type. The following is a high-yield summary of the most common characteristics of the various disorders listed in this text.

Nervous System

Most Common . . .	
Aneurysm of circle of Willis	**Anterior communicating artery, bitemporal hemianopsia**
Blindness	**Diabetic retinopathy**
Blindness—preventable	***Chlamydia trachomatis***
Bacterial meningitis—elderly	***Streptococcus pneumoniae***
Bacterial meningitis—newborns	***Escherichia coli***
Bacterial meningitis—toddlers	***Haemophilus influenzae* type b**
Bacterial meningitis—young adults	***Neisseria meningitidis***
Primary cancer of the brain—child	**Medulloblastoma (cerebellum)**
Primary cancer of the brain—adult	**Astrocytoma (specifically glioblastoma),** meningioma, schwannoma
Dementia	1. **Alzheimer** 2. Multi-infarct dementia
Demyelinating disease	**Multiple sclerosis**
Location of adult brain tumors	**Above tentorium**
Location of childhood brain tumors	**Below tentorium** (Mnemonic: Children are short, they cannot reach above the tentorium.)
Mental retardation	1. **Fetal alcohol syndrome** (most common overall cause) 2. Down syndrome (females) or fragile X (in males) (most common genetic causes)
Motor neuron disease	**Amyotrophic lateral sclerosis (ALS)**
Viral encephalitis	**Herpes simplex virus (HSV)**

Cardiovascular System

Most Common . . .	
Acute mitral insufficiency—children	**Kawasaki disease**
Aneurysm	**Abdominal aorta**
AV fistula	**Penetrating knife wound**
Cancer of the heart—adults	**Metastases**
Cancer of the heart—primary—adults	**Myxoma "ball valve"**
Cancer of the heart—primary—kids	**Rhabdomyoma**
Cardiomyopathy	**Dilated (congestive) cardiomyopathy**
Cause of acute endocarditis	***Staphylococcus aureus***
Cause of subacute endocarditis	**Viridans streptococci**
Congenital cardiac anomaly	**Ventricular septal defect** (membranous > muscular)
Congenital early cyanosis	**Tetralogy of Fallot**
Coronary artery thrombosis	**Left anterior descending**
Death in hypertension	1. **Acute mitral insufficiency** 2. Lenticulostriate stroke 3. Renal failure (benign nephrosclerosis)
Death in the United States	**Ischemic heart disease**
Heart murmur	**Mitral valve prolapse**
Heart valve in bacterial endocarditis	**Mitral**
Heart valve in bacterial endocarditis in IV drug users	**Tricuspid**
Heart valve involved in rheumatic fever	**Mitral** > aortic
Hypertension	1. **Essential (95%)** 2. Renal disease
Hypertension—children	**Renal disease,** cystic disease, Wilms tumor
Hypertension—young women	**Oral contraceptives**
Myocarditis	**Coxsackie B virus**
Right heart failure	**Left heart failure**
Secondary hypertension	**Renal disease**
Sites of atherosclerosis	**Abdominal aorta** > coronary > popliteal > carotid
Vasculitis (of medium and small arteries)	**Temporal arteritis**

AV, atrioventricular; IV, intravenous.

Respiratory System

Most Common . . .	
Cause of pneumonia in debilitated, hospitalized patient	***Klebsiella***
Cause of epiglottitis	***Haemophilus influenzae* type b**
Cause of IV drug user bacteremia/pneumonia	***Staphylococcus aureus***
Cause of opportunistic infection of AIDS	***Pneumocystis jirovecii* is most common overall.**
Death in patients with Alzheimer disease	**Pneumonia**
Fatal genetic defect in Caucasians	**Cystic fibrosis**
Pneumonia—community—atypical	1. ***Mycoplasma*** 2. *Legionella*
Pneumonia—community—typical	1. ***Streptococcus pneumoniae*** 2. *H. influenzae* 3. *Klebsiella*
Pneumonia—hospital acquired	1. ***Klebsiella*** 2. ***Pseudomonas*** 3. ***Escherichia coli***
Pulmonary hypertension	**Chronic obstructive pulmonary disease (COPD)**
Cancer associated with syndrome of inappropriate ADH secretion (SIADH)	**Small cell carcinoma of the lung**
Tracheoesophageal fistula	**Lower esophagus communicates with trachea; upper esophagus ends in blind pouch.**

Gastrointestinal System

Most Common . . .	
Bug in food poisoning	***Staphylococcus aureus***
Bug in gastrointestinal (GI) tract	1. ***Bacteroides*** 2. *Escherichia coli*
Cancer of the appendix	**Carcinoid—rarely metastasizes**
Cancer of the esophagus—malignant	**Adenocarcinoma** > squamous cell carcinoma (in US)
Cancer of the liver	**Metastasis;** lung > GI
Tumor of the liver—primary, benign	**Cavernous hemangioma**
Cancer of the liver—primary	**Hepatocellular carcinoma**
Cancer of the mouth	**Squamous cell carcinoma or mucoepidermoid carcinoma**
Cancer of the mouth—upper lip	**Basal cell carcinoma**
Cancer of the nasal cavities	**Squamous cell carcinoma**
Cancer of the pancreas	**Adenocarcinoma** (usually in the head of pancreas)
Cancer of the salivary glands	**Pleomorphic adenoma**
Cancer of the small bowel	**Carcinoid**—frequent metastasis from ileum
Cancer of the spleen—benign	**Cavernous hemangioma**
Cancer of the stomach	**Gastric adenocarcinoma** (intestinal type or diffuse type)
Cirrhosis	**Alcohol**
Congenital GI anomaly	**Meckel diverticulum**
Diarrhea—children	**Rotavirus**
Dietary deficiency	**Iron**
GI obstruction	1. **Adhesions** 2. Indirect inguinal hernia
Intussusception	**Terminal ileum into cecum**
Liver disease	**Alcoholic liver disease**
Liver infection	**Viral hepatitis (HAV and HBV)**
Lysosomal storage disease	**Gaucher disease**
Portal hypertension	**Cirrhosis**
Protozoal diarrhea	***Giardia***
Site of diverticula	**Sigmoid colon**
Surgical emergency	**Acute appendicitis**
Worm infection in the United States	1. **Pinworm** 2. *Ascaris*

HAV, hepatitis A virus; HBV, hepatitis B virus.

Renal System

Most Common . . .	
Amyloidosis	**Immunologic** (Bence-Jones protein in multiple myeloma is also called the amyloid light chain.)
Death in patients with systemic lupus erythematosus (SLE)	Lupus nephropathy type IV (diffuse proliferative)
End-stage renal disease	**Diabetes**
Glomerulonephritis	**IgA nephropathy (also known as Berger disease)**
Nephrotic syndrome—adults	**Focal segmental glomerulosclerosis**
Nephrotic syndrome—kids	**Minimal change disease**
Renal failure	**Acute tubular necrosis**

Ig, immunoglobulin.

Endocrine System

Most Common . . .	
Addison disease	1. **Autoimmune** 2. Infection
Cancer of the adrenal medulla—adults	**Pheochromocytoma**
Cancer of the adrenal medulla—kids	**Neuroblastoma**
Cancer of the pituitary	1. **Prolactinoma** 2. Somatotropic "acidophilic" adenoma
Cancer of the thyroid	**Papillary carcinoma**
Congenital adrenal hyperplasia	1. **21-Hydroxylase deficiency** 2. 11-Hydroxylase deficiency
Cushing	1. **Exogenous steroid therapy** 2. Primary adrenocorticotropic hormone (ACTH) tumor 3. Adrenal adenoma 4. Ectopic ACTH tumor
Enzyme deficiency	**21-Hydroxylase—95% of congenital adrenal hyperplasia**
Hypercalcemia	**Hyperparathyroidism**
Hyperparathyroidism—primary	1. **Solitary adenomas** 2. Parathyroid hyperplasia 3. Parathyroid carcinoma
Hyperparathyroidism—secondary	**Hypocalcemia due to chronic renal failure**
Hyperthyroidism	**Graves disease**
Hypopituitarism—adults	**Nonfunctioning pituitary adenoma**
Hypopituitarism—kids	**Craniopharyngioma**
Hypothyroidism	**Hashimoto thyroiditis**
Peripheral neuropathy	**Diabetes mellitus**
Thyroid disease	**Goiter**

ACTH, adrenocorticotropic hormone.

Reproductive System

Most Common . . .	
Breast mass (premenopausal)	**Fibrocystic change (premenopausal)**
Breast mass (postmenopausal)	**Breast carcinoma**
Cancer in gynecologic—malignancy	**Endometrial carcinoma**
Cancer in men	**Prostate carcinoma**
Cancer in women	**Uterine leiomyoma (fibroids)**
Cancer in women—malignant	**Breast carcinoma**
Cancer of the breast	**Infiltrating ductal adenocarcinoma**
Cancer of the ovary—benign	**Serous cystadenoma**
Cancer of the ovary—malignant	**Serous cystadenocarcinoma**
Cancer of the placenta—benign	**Cavernous hemangioma**
Cancer of the testicles	**Seminoma**
Cancer that invades the female genitourinary (GU) tract	**Endometrial adenocarcinoma**
Cause of pelvic inflammatory disease (PID)	***Neisseria gonorrhoeae* or *Chlamydia trachomatis***
Chromosomal disorder	**Down syndrome**
Hernia	**Indirect**
Opportunistic infection in AIDS	***Pneumocystis jirovecii***
Sexually transmitted disease	***Chlamydia trachomatis***

Musculoskeletal System

Most Common . . .	
Bacterial arthritis in young adults	***Neisseria gonorrhoeae***
Cancer of the bone	**Metastases from breast and prostate**
Cancer of the bone—primary—adults	**Multiple myeloma**
Cancer of the connective tissue—benign	**Lipoma**
Cancer of the skin	**Basal cell carcinoma**
Carpal bone dislocation	**Lunate**
Carpal bone fracture	**Scaphoid**
Disk herniation	**L4–L5**

The Hematopoietic and Lymphoreticular System

Most Common . . .	
Cancer—leukemia—14-year-old	**Acute lymphoblastic leukemia (ALL)**
Cancer—leukemia—15–39-year-old	**Acute myeloid leukemia (AML)**
Cancer—leukemia—40–60-year-old	**Chronic myelogenous leukemia (CML)**
Cancer—leukemia—>60-year-old	**Chronic lymphocytic leukemia (CLL)**
Cancer in infancy	**Hemangioma**
Cancer in children	1. **Leukemia** 2. Medulloblastoma of cerebellum
Cancer; genetic alteration	**p53**
Cancer; malignant lymphoma in children	**Burkitt lymphoma**
Cancer; site of metastasis	**Regional lymph nodes**
Cancer; site of metastasis (second most common)	**Liver**
Hereditary bleeding disorder	**von Willebrand disease**
Single gene disorder	**Thalassemia**
Type of Hodgkin lymphoma	**Nodular sclerosis Hodgkin lymphoma**
Type of non-Hodgkin lymphoma	**Diffuse large B-cell lymphoma**

QUICK LISTS

The following Quick Lists contain high-yield information organized by basic science subject.

Physiology

Quick List: Important Formulas

	Formula	Notes
Cardiac output	CO = Rate of O_2 consumption / (arterial O_2 content − venous O_2 content) CO = SV × HR	SV = Stroke volume HR = Heart rate
Mean arterial pressure	MAP = CO × TPR MAP = 1/3 SBP + 2/3 DBP	CO = Cardiac output TPR = Total peripheral resistance SBP = Systolic blood pressure DBP = Diastolic blood pressure
Stroke volume	EDV − ESV	EDV = End diastolic volume ESV = End systolic volume
Ejection fraction	SV / EDV × 100	SV = Stroke volume EDV = End diastolic volume
Resistance	$8\eta L / \pi r^4$	η = Viscosity L = Length r = Radius
Net filtration pressure	$(P_C - P_I) - (\pi_C - \pi_I)$	P_C = Hydrostatic capillary pressure P_I = Hydrostatic interstitial pressure π_C = Osmotic capillary pressure π_I = Osmotic interstitial pressure
Glomerular filtration rate	$GFR = K_f (P_{GC} - P_{BS}) - (\pi_{GC} - \pi_{BS})$ $GFR = C_{inulin} = U_{inulin} \times V / P_{inulin}$	K_f = Filtration constant P_{GC} = Hydrostatic pressure in glomerular capillaries P_{BS} = Hydrostatic pressure in Bowman space π_{GC} = Osmotic pressure in glomerular capillaries π_{BS} = Osmotic pressure in Bowman space C_{inulin} = Clearance of para-aminohippuric acid (PAH) U_{inulin} = Urine concentration of PAH V = Urine flow rate P_{inulin} = Plasma concentration of PAH
Effective renal plasma flow	$C_{PAH} = U_{PAH} \times V / P_{PAH}$	C_{PAH} = Clearance of PAH U_{PAH} = Urine concentration of PAH V = Urine flow rate P_{PAH} = Plasma concentration of PAH
Renal blood flow	RPF / (1 − Hct)	RPF = Renal plasma flow Hct = Hematocrit
Filtration fraction	GFR / RPF	GFR = Glomerular filtration rate RPF = Renal plasma flow
Free water clearance	$CH_2O = V - C_{osm}$, where $C_{osm} = U_{osm} V / P_{osm}$	CH_2O = Clearance of water U_{osm} = Urine osmolarity P_{osm} = Plasma osmolarity V = Urine flow rate

Biostatistics

Quick List: Important Formulas

	Formula
Sensitivity	TP / (TP + FN)
Specificity	TN / (TN + FP)
Positive predictive value	TP / (TP + FP)
Negative predictive value	TN / (TN + FN)
Prevalence	TP + FN / (TP + FP +TN + FN) Generally calculated by incidence × duration of disease
Incidence	Generally calculated by number of new cases / susceptible population
Relative risk (RR)	RR = [TP / (TP + FP)] / [FN / (FN + TN)]
Attributable risk (AR)	AR = [TP / (TP + FP)] − [FN / (FN + TN)]

FN, false negative; FP, false positive; TN, true negative; TP, true positive.

Genetics

Quick List: Inherited Diseases

Mode of Inheritance	Diseases
Autosomal dominant diseases	Adult polycystic kidney disease, familial hypercholesterolemia, Marfan syndrome, neurofibromatosis type 1, neurofibromatosis type 2, tuberous sclerosis, von Hippel–Lindau disease, Huntington disease, familial adenomatous polyposis, hereditary spherocytosis, achondroplasia
Autosomal recessive diseases	Cystic fibrosis, albinism, α_1-antitrypsin deficiency, phenylketonuria, thalassemias, sickle cell anemia, glycogen storage disease, mucopolysaccharidoses (except Hunter syndrome), sphingolipidoses (except Fabry disease), infant polycystic kidney disease, hemochromatosis
X-linked dominant diseases	Hypophosphatemic rickets
X-linked recessive diseases	Bruton agammaglobulinemia, Wiskott–Aldrich syndrome, fragile X syndrome, G6PD deficiency, ocular albinism, Lesch–Nyhan syndrome, Duchenne muscular dystrophy, hemophilia A and B, Fabry disease, Hunter syndrome
Mitochondrial diseases	Leber hereditary optic neuropathy, mitochondrial myopathies
Trisomies	Down syndrome (chromosome 21), Edward syndrome (chromosome 18), Patau syndrome (chromosome 13)
Trinucleotide repeat diseases	Huntington disease, myotonic dystrophy, Friedreich ataxia, fragile X syndrome

G6PD, glucose-6-phosphate dehydrogenase.

Pharmacology

Quick List: Important Formulas

	Formula	Notes
Volume of distribution	Total drug in body / plasma concentration	
Clearance	Rate of elimination of drug / plasma concentration	
Half-life	0.7 × volume of distribution / clearance	
Loading dose	Target plasma concentration × volume of distribution / bioavailability	Bioavailability = 1, when medication given IV
Maintenance dose	Target plasma concentration × clearance / bioavailability	Bioavailability = 1, when medication given IV

IV, intravenous.

Quick List: Important Drug Side Effects Based on Organ System *(Figure 1)*

FIGURE 1 **Important drug side effects based on organ system**

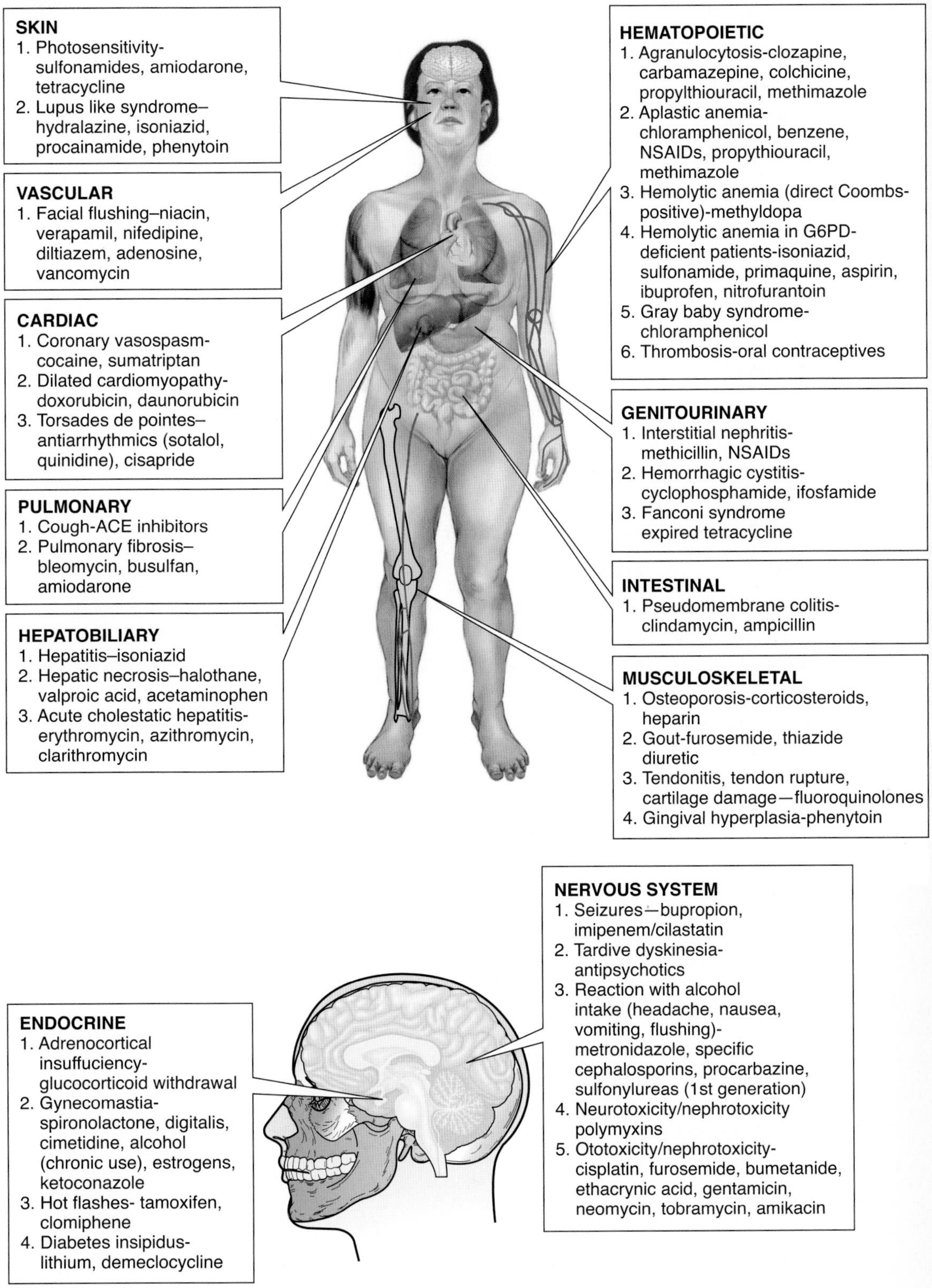
SKIN
1. Photosensitivity-sulfonamides, amiodarone, tetracycline
2. Lupus like syndrome–hydralazine, isoniazid, procainamide, phenytoin
VASCULAR
1. Facial flushing–niacin, verapamil, nifedipine, diltiazem, adenosine, vancomycin
CARDIAC
1. Coronary vasospasm-cocaine, sumatriptan
2. Dilated cardiomyopathy-doxorubicin, daunorubicin
3. Torsades de pointes–antiarrhythmics (sotalol, quinidine), cisapride
PULMONARY
1. Cough-ACE inhibitors
2. Pulmonary fibrosis–bleomycin, busulfan, amiodarone
HEPATOBILIARY
1. Hepatitis–isoniazid
2. Hepatic necrosis–halothane, valproic acid, acetaminophen
3. Acute cholestatic hepatitis-erythromycin, azithromycin, clarithromycin
HEMATOPOIETIC
1. Agranulocytosis-clozapine, carbamazepine, colchicine, propylthiouracil, methimazole
2. Aplastic anemia-chloramphenicol, benzene, NSAIDs, propythiouracil, methimazole
3. Hemolytic anemia (direct Coombs-positive)-methyldopa
4. Hemolytic anemia in G6PD-deficient patients-isoniazid, sulfonamide, primaquine, aspirin, ibuprofen, nitrofurantoin
5. Gray baby syndrome-chloramphenicol
6. Thrombosis-oral contraceptives
GENITOURINARY
1. Interstitial nephritis-methicillin, NSAIDs
2. Hemorrhagic cystitis-cyclophosphamide, ifosfamide
3. Fanconi syndrome expired tetracycline
INTESTINAL
1. Pseudomembrane colitis-clindamycin, ampicillin
MUSCULOSKELETAL
1. Osteoporosis-corticosteroids, heparin
2. Gout-furosemide, thiazide diuretic
3. Tendonitis, tendon rupture, cartilage damage—fluoroquinolones
4. Gingival hyperplasia-phenytoin
NERVOUS SYSTEM
1. Seizures—bupropion, imipenem/cilastatin
2. Tardive dyskinesia-antipsychotics
3. Reaction with alcohol intake (headache, nausea, vomiting, flushing)-metronidazole, specific cephalosporins, procarbazine, sulfonylureas (1st generation)
4. Neurotoxicity/nephrotoxicity polymyxins
5. Ototoxicity/nephrotoxicity-cisplatin, furosemide, bumetanide, ethacrynic acid, gentamicin, neomycin, tobramycin, amikacin
ENDOCRINE
1. Adrenocortical insuffuciency-glucocorticoid withdrawal
2. Gynecomastia-spironolactone, digitalis, cimetidine, alcohol (chronic use), estrogens, ketoconazole
3. Hot flashes- tamoxifen, clomiphene
4. Diabetes insipidus-lithium, demeclocycline

ACE, angiotensin-converting enzyme; G6PD, glucose-6-phosphate dehydrogenase; NSAIDs, nonsteroidal anti-inflammatory drugs.

Quick List: Drugs to Avoid in Pregnancy

Drug	Reason
ACE inhibitors	Fetal renal malformations
Aminoglycosides	Ototoxicity
Atorvastatin	Congenital defects, termination of pregnancy
Chloramphenicol	Gray baby syndrome
Fluoroquinolones	Cartilage damage
Griseofulvin	Teratogenic
Methysergide	Oxytocic effects
Metronidazole	Mutagenesis
Ribavirin	Teratogenic
Sulfonamides	Kernicterus
Tetracyclines	Discolored teeth, inhibition of bone growth
Warfarin	Teratogenic

ACE, angiotensin-converting enzyme.

Quick List: Cytochrome P450 Interactions

Effect	Agent
Inhibitors	Cimetidine, ritonavir (protease inhibitors), amiodarone, ciprofloxacin, ketoconazole, acute alcohol use, macrolides, isoniazid, grapefruit juice, omeprazole, sulfonamides
Inducers	Phenytoin, rifampin, St. John's wort, barbiturates, griseofulvin, carbamazepine

Quick List: Antidotes

Toxic agent	Treatment
Acetaminophen	*N*-acetylcysteine
Amphetamine	Ammonium chloride (acidify urine)
Arsenic	Dimercaprol (BAL), succimer, penicillamine
Aspirin	Activated charcoal, sodium bicarbonate (alkalinize urine), dialysis
Atropine	Physostigmine
Benzodiazepines	Flumazenil
β-Blockers	Atropine, activated charcoal, glucagon, $CaCl_2$
Carbon monoxide	100% oxygen, hyperbaric oxygen
Cocaine	Supportive care, benzodiazepines, calcium channel blockers
Copper	Penicillamine
Cyanide	Sodium thiosulfate; amyl nitrate plus sodium nitrite
Digitalis	Activated charcoal, digoxin immune Fab, potassium (if serum K^+ level is low), possibly atropine
Ethylene glycol (antifreeze)	Fomepizole, ethanol, dialysis
Heparin	Protamine sulfate
Iron	Deferoxamine
Isoniazid	Vitamin B_6
Isopropyl alcohol	Supportive care
Lead	Succimer, EDTA, dimercaprol
Mercury	Dimercaprol
Methanol	Fomepizole, ethanol, dialysis
Methemoglobin	Methylene blue
Opioids	Naloxone, naltrexone
Organophosphates	Atropine, pralidoxime
Streptokinase	Aminocaproic acid
Sulfonylureas	Dextrose, octreotide
tPA	Aminocaproic acid
Tricyclic antidepressants	Gastric lavage, sodium bicarbonate (serum alkalinization), diazepam for seizures
Warfarin	Vitamin K, fresh frozen plasma

BAL, British anti-Lewisite; $CaCl_2$, calcium chloride; EDTA, ethylenediaminetetraacetic acid; tPA, tissue plasminogen activator.

Microbiology

Quick List: Buzzwords for Microbiological Infections

Clinical Characteristics	Organism
Branching rods in oral infections	*Actinomyces israelii*
Burn infections	*Pseudomonas aeruginosa*
Cat bite	*Pasteurella multocida*
Chancroid	*Haemophilus ducreyi*
Clue cells	*Gardnerella vaginalis*
Cold agglutinins	*Mycoplasma pneumoniae*
Currant jelly sputum	*Klebsiella*
Erythema chronicum migrans	Lyme disease
Ghon focus	Primary tuberculosis
Jarisch–Herxheimer reaction	Syphilis—treatment of an asymptomatic patient results in rapid lysis leading to symptoms
Negri bodies	Rabies
Owl's eye	CMV
Pediatric infection (in an unvaccinated patient)	*H. influenzae*
Pneumonia in cystic fibrosis	*Pseudomonas aeruginosa*
Rash on palms or soles	Rocky Mountain spotted fever, secondary syphilis
Reactive arthritis (Reiter syndrome)	Urethritis, conjunctivitis, arthritis
Roth spots in retina	Endocarditis
Slapped cheeks	Parvovirus B19 (erythema infectiosum)
Splinter hemorrhages in fingernails	Endocarditis
Strawberry tongue	Scarlet fever
Suboccipital lymphadenopathy	Rubella
Sulfur granules	*A. israelii*
Tabes dorsalis	Tertiary syphilis
Thumb sign on lateral X-ray	Epiglottis (usually with *H. influenzae*)
Traumatic open wound	*Clostridium perfringens*

CMV, cytomegalovirus.

Quick List: Gram Stain Characteristics of Various Bacteria

Gram Stain Characteristics	Organisms
Gram-positive cocci	*Staphylococcus* (catalase +), *Streptococcus* (catalase −), *Enterococcus* (catalase −)
Gram-positive rods	*Clostridium* (anaerobe), *Corynebacterium, Listeria, Bacillus*
Gram-negative cocci	*Neisseria*
Gram-negative coccoid rods	*Haemophilus influenzae, Pasteurella, Brucella, Bordetella pertussis*
Gram-negative rods	**Lactose fermenters:** *Klebsiella* (fast[a]), *Escherichia coli* (fast), *Enterobacter* (fast), *Citrobacter* (slow), *Serratia* (slow) **Lactose nonfermenters:** *Shigella* (oxidase −), *Salmonella* (oxidase −), *Proteus* (oxidase −), *Pseudomonas* (oxidase +)

[a]Fast fermenter, slow fermenter.

APPENDIX I: **Drug Index**

The therapeutic agents shown in boldface type are those that are often emphasized in the classroom and the clinic. Particular attention should be paid to the information about these agents.

Therapeutic Agent (common name, if relevant) [trade name, where appropriate]	Class—Pharmacology and Pharmacokinetics	Indications	Side Effects or Adverse Effects	Contraindications or Precautions to Consider; Notes
Abacavir (ABC)	**Antiviral, nucleoside reverse transcriptase inhibitor—guanosine analog** → inhibits viral reverse transcriptase → prevents integration of DNA copy of viral genome into host DNA	**AIDS (used in HAART)**	**Neutropenia, anemia, peripheral neuropathy, pancreatitis, lactic acidosis, and hypersensitivity reaction (can be fatal)**	Check HLA-B*5701 test prior to starting ABC to avoid giving to patients at risk for hypersensitivity reactions
Acarbose [Precose]	Hypoglycemic agent; α-glucosidase inhibitor—inhibits intestinal brush border enzyme α-glucosidase → delays sugar hydrolysis and glucose absorption from gut → decreases postprandial hyperglycemia	Oral treatment for type 2 diabetes postprandially	Flatulence, cramps, diarrhea; may reduce absorption of iron	Does not cause reactive hypoglycemia; decreases HbA_{1c}
Acebutolol [Sectral]	Antiarrhythmic (class II)—antihypertensive; β-blocker	Hypertension, PVCs		Cardioselective; intrinsic sympathomimetic activity (useful in treating patients with hypertension who also have bradycardia)
Acetaminophen [Tylenol]	Analgesic, antipyretic—reversibly inhibits COX centrally (inactivated peripherally); prostaglandin inhibitor, **not anti-inflammatory**	Pain, fever	Liver toxicity in high doses **(high levels deplete glutathione)**	**Overdose treated with *N*-acetylcysteine** (regenerates glutathione); **unlike aspirin, can be used in children and patients with gout, peptic ulcer, and platelet dysfunction**
Acetazolamide [Diamox]	**Carbonic anhydrase inhibitor, diuretic—inhibits carbonic anhydrase on PCT and DCT,** which prevents HCO_3^- reabsorption; lose Na^+, HCO_3^-, and K^+ in urine	**Glaucoma; high altitude; metabolic alkalosis; alkalinization of urine; epilepsy**	**Hyperchloremic metabolic acidosis, sulfa drug allergy,** neuropathy, and ammonium toxicity	**Weak diuretic because other sites further downstream along the nephron can compensate for sodium loss;** causes decreased secretion of HCO_3^- in aqueous humor

Acetylcholine	**Muscarinic and nicotinic agonist**	**Eye surgery (miotic)**	**Increased cholinergic stimulation (MNEMONIC: DUMBBELSS—** **D**iarrhea, **U**rination, **M**iosis, **B**ronchoconstriction, **B**radycardia, **E**xcitation of skeletal muscle, **L**acrimation, **S**alivation, **S**weating)	Contraindicated for patients with **peptic ulcer, asthma, hyperthyroidism, or parkinsonism**
Acetylsalicylic acid (aspirin)	**Anti-inflammatory, antipyretic, analgesic**—acetylates COX irreversibly	Articular, musculoskeletal pain; chronic pain; **maintenance therapy for preventing clot formation**	GI distress, **GI ulcers; inhibits platelet aggregation;** causes **hypersensitivity reactions (rash);** reversible hepatic dysfunction	**Contraindicated** for **children** with flu or chicken pox (leads to **Reye syndrome**) and **patients with gout**
ACTH (corticotropin)	Increases production of steroids by the adrenal cortex	Test adrenal function in adrenocortical insufficiency		**Increased cortisol indicates pituitary defect; unchanged cortisol indicates adrenal defect**
Acyclovir [Zovirax]	**Antiviral—guanosine analog;** monophosphorylated by **viral thymidine kinase;** triphosphorylated form **inhibits viral DNA polymerase**	**HSV, VZV, EBV, CMV** (at high doses); **HSV-induced mucocutaneous genital lesions** and **encephalitis**	**Side effects depend on the route of administration: IV—neurotoxicity, renal problems, tremor;** **Oral—diarrhea,** headache; **Topical—local skin irritation**	**Resistant forms lack thymidine kinase**
Adenosine [Adenocard]	**Antiarrhythmic—increases potassium efflux → hyperpolarizes cell**	**Diagnosis and treatment of AV nodal arrhythmias**	**Flushing, hypotension, and chest pain**	Very short acting
Albendazole [Albenza]	Anthelmintic—blocks glucose uptake, resulting in eventual depletion of the parasite's energy stores	*Ascaris* (roundworm), *Ancylostoma* (hookworm), *Trichuris* (whipworm), *Strongyloides;* **cysticercosis, hydatid disease**	**Teratogenic; embryotoxic;** mild nausea, vomiting, and dizziness	Contraindicated in pregnant patients
Albuterol [Proventil, Ventolin]	**Bronchodilation—β_2-agonist, leads to relaxation of smooth muscle**	Asthma, COPD, bronchitis	**Tremor, tachycardia, arrhythmia,** headache, nausea, and vomiting	

(continued)

APPENDIX I: **Drug Index**

Therapeutic Agent (common name, if relevant) [trade name, where appropriate]	Class—Pharmacology and Pharmacokinetics	Indications	Side Effects or Adverse Effects	Contraindications or Precautions to Consider; Notes
Alcohol (EtOH)	Acts at **$GABA_A$ receptor**	Sedative; hypnotic; depressive action on brain; **indicated for methanol and ethylene glycol overdose**	**Intoxication (in order of increasing BAL):** fine motor, coordination, ataxia, lethargy, coma, and respiratory depression **Withdrawal:** nausea, diaphoresis, delirium tremens, and seizures **Fetal alcohol syndrome:** mental retardation, growth deficiencies, microcephaly, and smooth philtrum **Chronic effects of alcoholism:** decreased liver function; Wernicke–Korsakoff syndrome, dilated cardiomyopathy, gynecomastia, and testicular atrophy	Benzodiazepines used for withdrawal symptoms; intoxication treated by thiamine, glucose, folic acid, and multivitamins
Aldesleukin [Proleukin]	Recombinant cytokine—human recombinant IL-2	**Metastatic renal cell carcinoma, metastatic melanoma, AML**		
Alendronate [Fosamax]	Bone stabilizer—bisphosphonate; **pyrophosphate analog;** reduces hydroxyapatite crystal formation, growth, and dissolution, which reduces bone turnover	**Hypercalcemia of malignancy, Paget disease, osteoporosis, hyperparathyroidism**	**Pill-induced esophagitis**	
Allopurinol [Zyloprim]	**Antigout—competitive inhibitor of xanthine oxidase;** converted to oxypurinol by xanthine oxidase, which also produces uric acid → allopurinol and oxypurinol inhibit xanthine oxidase → decreased uric acid production	**Chronic gout therapy;** lymphoma, leukemia (prevents tumor lysis–associated urate nephropathy), and uric acid stones; rheumatic arthritis	Rash; fever; GI problems, hepatotoxicity; inhibition of the metabolism of other drugs; enhances the effect of azathioprine	Should not be used to treat acute gout; inhibition of the metabolism of other drugs; enhances the effect of azathioprine
Alprazolam [Xanax]	Antianxiety—intermediate acting benzodiazepine	**Panic attack; phobia; MNEMONIC:** AL PRAYS when he's in fear	Sedation	Respiratory depression if taken with alcohol
Alprostadil [Vasoprost]	Impotency therapy; **PGE_1 agonist**	**Impotency; maintains patent ductus arteriosus**	Penile pain; prolonged erection; flushing, bradycardia, tachycardia, hypotension, and apnea	

Aluminum hydroxide	**Antacid**—buffers gastric acid by raising the pH; **antidiarrheal—delays gastric emptying**	Peptic ulcer, gastritis, esophageal reflux, and diarrhea	**Constipation,** hypophosphatemia, muscle weakness, **osteodystrophy,** seizures, **and hypokalemia**	Can affect the **absorption, bioavailability,** or **urinary excretion** of drugs by changing **gastric pH, urinary pH,** or **gastric emptying**
Amantadine [Symmetrel]	**Antiviral—antiparkinsonian; inhibits** fusion of lysosomes; inhibits viral penetration and uncoating; increases release of endogenous dopamine	**Influenza A** (prophylaxis and treatment), **Parkinson disease**	**CNS effects** (ataxia, dizziness, slurred speech, nervousness, and seizure); **anticholinergic;** orthostatic hypotension; **livedo reticularis**	Mechanism of viral resistance is mutated M2 protein
Amikacin [Amikin]	**Antibiotic—aminoglycoside,** protein synthesis inhibitor; **irreversibly binds 30S ribosome** subunits; **bacteriostatic** at low concentration; **bactericidal** at high concentration	**Broad spectrum:** gram-negative rods; good for **bone** and **eye** infections; *Proteus, Pseudomonas, Enterobacter, Klebsiella, Escherichia coli*	**Ototoxicity; renal toxicity; neuromuscular blockade;** nausea; vomiting; vertigo; allergic rash	Does not cover anaerobes
Amiloride [Midamor]	Potassium sparing diuretic—binds to intracellular aldosterone steroid receptors in **collecting tubules;** blocks induction of Na^+ channels and Na^+/ATPase synthesis and blocks Na^+ channels directly; lose Na^+ and Cl^- in urine	Hyperaldosteronism, potassium depletion, CHF	**Hyperkalemic metabolic acidosis, gynecomastia** (spironolactone), and antiandrogen effects	Results in decreased secretion of K^+ and H^+, which can lead to **hyperkalemic metabolic acidosis;** often given in combination with a thiazide
Aminocaproic acid [Amicar]	Competitive inhibition of plasminogen activation	Inhibits fibrinolysis; promotes thrombosis		Oral administration
Aminoglutethimide [Cytadren]	Antineoplastic—aromatase inhibitor; cytochrome P450 inhibitor that catalyzes the rate-limiting step of adrenal steroid synthesis	Breast cancer, Cushing syndrome	GI and neurological side effects; transient maculopapular rash	Do not cover anaerobes because oxidative metabolism is required for uptake of these drugs
Aminoglycosides	Antibiotic—**irreversibly binds 30S ribosome** subunits; **bacteriostatic** at low concentration; **bactericidal** at high concentration	**Broad spectrum:** gram-negative rods; good for **bone** and **eye** infections; *Proteus, Pseudomonas, Enterobacter, Klebsiella,* and *Escherichia coli;* also used for tuberculosis	**Ototoxicity, renal toxicity, neuromuscular blockade,** nausea, vomiting, vertigo, allergic rash	Examples include gentamycin, neomycin, and streptomycin
Amiodarone [Cordarone]	**Antiarrhythmic (class III)—K^+ channel blocker**	**Ventricular/supraventricular arrhythmias**	**Hepatotoxicity, thyroid toxicity, pulmonary fibrosis, photodermatitis**	Also functions as class IA, II, and IV antiarrhythmic

(continued)

APPENDIX I: **Drug Index**

Therapeutic Agent (common name, if relevant) [trade name, where appropriate]	**Class—Pharmacology and Pharmacokinetics**	**Indications**	**Side Effects or Adverse Effects**	**Contraindications or Precautions to Consider; Notes**
Amitriptyline [Elavil]	TCAs—inhibit **reuptake** of NE and 5-HT at neuronal synapses	Major depression, panic disorder; sedative; prophylaxis for migraines	Sedation, **α-blocking effects** (orthostatic hypotension), **anticholinergic** (tachycardia, dry mouth, and urinary retention), hallucinations (in elderly), and confusion (in elderly); overdose toxicity results in **convulsions, coma, cardiotoxicity** (arrhythmias), respiratory depression, and hyperpyrexia	
Amlodipine [Norvasc]	**Dihydropyridine Ca^{2+} channel blocker**—block voltage-gated Ca^{2+} channels of **vascular** smooth muscle	**Hypertension, angina pectoris, Prinzmetal angina, Raynaud phenomenon**	Peripheral edema, **flushing, dizziness**, and constipation	
Amobarbital [Amytal sodium]	Sedative-hypnotic; barbiturate; prolongs IPSP duration for GABA receptor	Antiepileptic; cerebral edema; anesthetic	Sedation, respiratory depression	
Amodiaquine	Antimalarial—uncertain mechanism	Suppression and treatment of acute attacks	Headache; GI and visual disturbances; pruritus; prolonged therapy may lead to retinopathy	
Amoxapine	TCAs—inhibit **reuptake** of NE and 5-HT at neuronal synapses	Major depression, panic disorder	Sedation, **α-blocking effects** (orthostatic hypotension), **anticholinergic** (tachycardia, dry mouth, and urinary retention), hallucinations (in elderly), and confusion (in elderly); overdose toxicity results in **convulsions, coma, cardiotoxicity** (arrhythmias), respiratory depression, and hyperpyrexia	
Amoxicillin	**Antibiotic-β-lactam, penicillin derivative,** cell wall inhibitor; same mechanism as penicillin; distinguished by activity against **gram-negative rods;** bactericidal	Gram-positive cocci, gram-positive rods, gram-negative cocci, and **gram-negative rods—extended spectrum:** *Escherichia coli, Proteus, Salmonella, Shigella,* and *Haemophilus influenzae*	**Hypersensitivity reaction; rash when given to mononucleosis patients**	Orally administered; not effective against penicillin-resistant *Staphylococcus*; **can be combined with clavulanic acid** (β-lactamase inhibitor) to enhance spectrum
Amoxicillin/clavulanic acid [Augmentin]	**Antibiotic—clavulanic acid inhibits β-lactamase**			

Amphetamine	**Stimulant—releases NE, dopamine,** and 5-HT	**Narcolepsy; attention-deficit disorder; weight reduction**	**Dilated pupils, psychosis, hallucinations,** increased BP	Contraindicated with MAOI; metabolized by liver
Amphotericin B [Fungizone]	**Antifungal—binds to cell membrane sterols** (especially ergosterol); forms pores in membrane; fungicidal	**Wide spectrum fungal coverage: *Candida, Histoplasma, Cryptococcus, Blastomyces, Aspergillus, Coccidioides, Sporothrix,* and *Mucor***	**Impairment of renal function, hypersensitivity, flushing, fever, shaking chills,** hypotension, thrombophlebitis, anemia, arrhythmias, hypokalemia	**Penetrates CNS poorly;** poor GI absorption, so given IV
Ampicillin	**Antibiotic—β-lactam, penicillin derivative,** cell wall inhibitor; same mechanism as penicillin; distinguished by activity against **gram-negative rods;** bactericidal	Gram-positive cocci, gram-positive rods, gram-negative cocci, and **gram-negatives rods—extended spectrum:** *Escherichia coli, Proteus, Salmonella, Shigella,* and *Haemophilus influenzae*	**Hypersensitivity reaction; rash, when given to mononucleosis patients**	IV administration; not effective against penicillin-resistant *Staphylococcus*; **can be combined with clavulanic acid** (β-lactamase inhibitor) to enhance spectrum
Amprenavir	**Antiviral, protease inhibitor—** protease responsible for final step of viral proliferation; inhibits protease in progeny virions → assembly of nonfunctional viruses	**AIDS (used in HAART)**	**GI irritation (nausea, diarrhea), hyperglycemia, hyperlipidemia, and lipodystrophy**	**All protease inhibitors end in -navir; metabolism occurs by cytochrome P450**
Amrinone [Inocor]	Inotropic agent—**phosphodiesterase inhibitor;** increases contractility via increase in intracellular Ca^{2+}	Acute CHF	**Thrombocytopenia,** arrhythmias, hepatotoxicity, and GI disturbances	Rarely used today because of the side effects
Anastrozole [Arimidex]	Aromatase inhibitor	**Breast cancer** in postmenopausal women; endometriosis	Hot flashes, nausea, and vomiting	Can be used in estrogen receptor–positive or hormone receptor–unknown breast cancer
Anistreplase (APSAC) [Eminase]	**Thrombolytic—plasminogen activator**	Lysis of clots	Hemorrhage	Active compound via deacylation by esterase
Anthraquinone	**Simulant laxative—**reduces absorption of electrolytes and water from gut	Constipation		
α_2-Antiplasmin	Inhibits fibrinolysis			
Aprotinin [Trasylol]	Hemostatic agent—antiplasmin activator	Inhibits fibrinolysis; promotes thrombosis		
Asparaginase [Elspar]	Antineoplastic—deprives cells of asparagines	Cancer	Fever, mental depression, coma, hepatotoxicity	
Aspart [NovoLog]	**Rapid-acting insulin**—*see mechanism for regular insulin*	**Diabetes mellitus** (typically **type 1**), **hyperkalemia, and stress-induced hyperglycemia**	**Hypoglycemia** (diaphoresis, vertigo, and tachycardia); insulin allergy; insulin antibodies; lipodystrophy	

(continued)

APPENDIX I: **Drug Index**

Therapeutic Agent (common name, if relevant) [trade name, where appropriate]	**Class—Pharmacology and Pharmacokinetics**	**Indications**	**Side Effects or Adverse Effects**	**Contraindications or Precautions to Consider; Notes**
Atenolol [Tenormin]	Antihypertensive—**β_1-blocker**	Hypertension, angina	Bradycardia, heart block, fatigue, impotence; **masks signs of hypoglycemia in diabetics**	**Cardioselective**
Atorvastatin [Lipitor]	**Lipid-lowering agent—HMG-CoA reductase inhibitor,** inhibits synthesis of cholesterol precursor mevalonate; **decreases LDL, increases HDL, and decreases TG**	**High LDL, preventative after thrombotic event (e.g., MI or stroke)**	Reversible increase in LFTs; myositis	**Contraindicated in pregnant** or lactating women and children; **increased incidence of rhabdomyolysis when taken with fibric acid, niacin, cyclosporine, and erythromycin**
Atracurium [Tracrium injection]	**Nondepolarizing** neuromuscular blocker			Minimal histamine release
Atropine	**Reversible cholinergic muscarinic blocker**	Dries salivary secretions; Parkinson disease; peptic ulcer; diarrhea; GI spasm; bladder spasm; COPD; asthma; cholinomimetic poisoning; antidiarrheal; antiemetic; high dose: vasodilation as a result of histamine release; mydriasis and cycloplegia (thorough fundus exam, accurate refraction)	Dry mouth, hyperthermia, mydriasis, tachycardia, hot and flushed skin, agitation, delirium; **MNEMONIC: Dry as a bone (dry mouth), hot as a hare (inhibition of sweating), red as a beet (tachycardia, cutaneous vasodilation), blind as a bat (blurring vision), mad as a hatter (hallucinations and delirium)**	Contraindicated in patients with glaucoma and elderly men with BPH
Aurothioglucose [Solganal]	Antirheumatic—gold salt	Rheumatic arthritis	Skin eruption, itching, toxic nephritis, bone marrow suppression	
Aurothiomalate	Antirheumatic—gold salt	Rheumatic arthritis	Skin eruption, itching, toxic nephritis, bone marrow suppression	
Azathioprine [Imuran]	Immunosuppressant—purine **antagonist;** inhibits nucleic acid metabolism; blocks both CMI and humoral response	**Transplant** (especially kidney); **acute glomerulonephritis; renal component of lupus; rheumatoid arthritis**	Bone marrow depression, rash, fever, nausea, vomiting, hepatotoxicity, malignancy, GI intolerance	**Metabolized by xanthine oxidase**
Azithromycin [Zithromax]	**Antibiotic—macrolide,** protein synthesis inhibitor; binds to the 23S RNA of the 50S ribosome subunits → blocks translocation → prevents protein synthesis; bacteriostatic	**First choice for cell wall–deficient bugs: *Mycoplasma, Rickettsia, Chlamydia, Legionella; Corynebacterium diphtheriae;*** gram-positive cocci (*Streptococcus*)	GI discomfort, **acute cholestatic hepatitis, rashes;** increases the concentration of **oral anticoagulants** and theophyllines	Can be used in patients with **streptococcal infections** and **penicillin allergies**

Aztreonam [Azactam]	**Antibiotic—monocyclic β-lactam,** cell wall inhibitor; same mechanism as penicillin (binds to PBP3); bactericidal	**Gram-negative bacteria, especially *Pseudomonas, Klebsiella, Serratia,* and Enterobacteriaceae; no activity against gram-positives or anaerobes**	Rash, GI distress (nausea, vomiting, etc.)	**Does not cross-react with penicillin; synergistic with aminoglycosides;** can be used in patients with **penicillin allergies** and **renal insufficiency who cannot take aminoglycosides**
Bacitracin	Antibiotic—**inhibits cell wall formation; bactericidal**	**Gram-positive** bacteria	**Nephrotoxic**	Topical only
Baclofen [Lioresal]	Skeletal muscle relaxant—**GABA mimetic;** works at the $GABA_B$ receptor	**Muscle spasms,** tetanus contractions, orthopedic manipulation		
BCNU (carmustine)	Antineoplastic—**DNA alkylation**	Cancer	Delayed bone marrow suppression; lung and kidney damage	
Beclomethasone	Corticosteroids—inhibit leukotriene synthesis → reduces inflammation and leads to bronchodilation	Asthma, COPD	**Osteoporosis; cushingoid reaction, psychosis, glucose intolerance, infection, hypertension, cataracts**	
Benserazide	Antiparkinsonian—inhibits decarboxylase (L-DOPA to dopamine) in periphery	Parkinson disease		
Benztropine [Cogentin]	**Antiparkinsonian—muscarinic blocker; H_1 blocker**	Parkinson disease	Sedation, urinary retention, dry mouth, constipation, and mental confusion	Less effective than levodopa in Parkinson disease
Bephenium hydroxynaphthoate	Anthelmintic—cholinergic agonist causing contraction, then relaxation in worm	*Necator* and *Ancylostoma* (hookworms)	Vomiting	
Betamethasone	Glucocorticoid	**Induction of surfactant synthesis in premature infants**		One of two steroids to cross placenta
Bethanechol [Urecholine, Duvoid]	**Muscarinic agonist**	**Atony of bladder; paralytic ileus; MNEMONIC: B**ethanechol stimulates the **b**ladder and **b**owel	**D**iarrhea/**D**ecreased BP, **U**rination, **M**iosis, **B**ronchoconstriction, **E**xcitation of skeletal muscle, **L**acrimation, **S**alivation/**S**weating—**MNEMONIC: DUMBELS**	**Contraindicated in patients with peptic ulcer, asthma, hyperthyroidism, and Parkinson disease**
Bisacodyl [Dulcolax]	**Stimulant laxative;** increases peristalsis	Constipation	Electrolyte imbalances (chronic use); gastric irritation	
Bischloroethylamines (nitrogen mustards) [Mustargen]	Antineoplastic—**DNA alkylation and cross-linking**	Cancer	Nausea, vomiting, bone marrow suppression, alopecia, teratogenicity, carcinogenicity	

(continued)

APPENDIX I: **Drug Index**

Therapeutic Agent (common name, if relevant) [trade name, where appropriate]	Class—Pharmacology and Pharmacokinetics	Indications	Side Effects or Adverse Effects	Contraindications or Precautions to Consider; Notes
Bismuth [Pepto-Bismol]	**Cytoprotectant—binds to ulcer base → protection; allows bicarbonate ion secretion to reestablish pH gradient in the mucous layer**	**Traveler's diarrhea,** peptic ulcer disease		
Black widow spider venom	**Presynaptic neuromuscular junction blocker—overstimulates acetylcholine release**			
Bleomycin [Blenoxane]	**Antineoplastic—generates free radicals that bind, intercalate, and cut DNA**	**Testicular cancer and Hodgkin lymphoma**	**Pulmonary fibrosis,** fever, blistering, stomatitis, hypersensitivity reactions (anaphylaxis)	
Botulinum [Botox, Dysport]	**Neuromuscular blocker—presynaptic neuromuscular junction blocker; prevents acetylcholine release**	Wrinkles, muscle spasm	Paralysis	
Bretylium [Bretylol]	Antiarrhythmic (class III)—K^+ channel blocker; prolongs ventricular action potential, effective refractory period, and blocks NE release	Arrhythmias; refractory ventricular fibrillation and ventricular tachycardia during cardiac arrest	Orthostatic hypotension, nausea, vomiting	
Bromocriptine [Parlodel]	Antiparkinsonian—**agonist at D_2; partial antagonist at D_1**	**Parkinson disease, hyperprolactinemia, acromegaly** (paradoxical effect—releases growth hormone from normal pituitary)	**Inhibits prolactin release;** hallucination, delirium, nausea, vomiting, cardiac arrhythmia, postural hypotension, and erythromelalgia	
Buclizine	Antiemetic	Sedation; parkinsonism		
Budesonide [Rhinocort]	Intranasal glucocorticoids—decrease cytokine synthesis; downregulate inflammatory response in the nasal mucosa	Nasal congestion, allergic rhinitis	Local irritation of nasal mucosa, epistaxis	
Bumetanide [Bumex]	Loop diuretic—inhibits $Na^+/K^+/2Cl^-$ reabsorption in the loop of Henle	CHF, diuresis, pulmonary edema, acute hypercalcemia, acute hyperkalemia, acute renal failure	Ototoxicity, interstitial nephritis, hyperuricemia, acute hypovolemia, hypokalemia, metabolic alkalosis, hyperglycemia, hypocalcemia, hypomagnesemia	
α-Bungarotoxin	Postsynaptic neuromuscular junction blocker; irreversibly binds nicotinic receptor		Paralysis	Component of snake venom

Bupivacaine	Anesthetic—blocks Na^+ channel intracellularly	Local anesthetic	Sleepiness, light-headedness, myocardial depression, hypotension, visual/audio disturbances, restlessness, nystagmus, shivering, tonic–clonic convulsions, death	
Buprenorphine [Buprenex]	Opioid analog—mixed agonist/antagonist action	Treatment of opioid/cocaine dependence	Respiratory depression, sedation, and nausea/vomiting	
Bupropion [Wellbutrin, Zyban]	**Antidepressant—unknown mechanism; thought to be an agonist at D_2, 5-HT**	Major depression, **smoking cessation**	Tachycardia, insomnia, headache, and seizure (especially patients with bulimia)	Does not have sexual side effects such as those occurring with SSRIs
Buspirone [Buspar]	Antidepressant partial agonist at serotonin receptors	Generalized anxiety		**2 weeks for effects to become apparent**
Caffeine [NoDoz]	Stimulant—**adenosine receptor blocker;** stimulates CNS and cardiac muscle; relaxes smooth muscle; produces diuresis; increases cerebrovascular resistance	**Acute migraine attack**	Crosses placenta and into breast milk	**Avoid in patients with peptic ulcer** because it stimulates gastric mucosal secretions
Calcitonin [Calcimar, Miacalcin]	Hypocalcemic agent—anti-osteoporotic agent; **lowers plasma Ca^{2+} and phosphate;** inhibits bone and kidney reabsorption	**Hypercalcemia, Paget disease, osteoporosis**		
Calcium carbonate [TUMS, Caltrate]	**Antacid**—buffers gastric acid by raising pH	Peptic ulcer, gastritis, esophageal reflux, and calcium deficiency	**Hypercalcemia, rebound acid increase, and hypokalemia**	**Can affect the absorption, bioavailability, or urinary excretion of drugs by changing gastric pH, urinary pH, or gastric emptying**
Calcium citrate	Dietary Ca^{2+} supplement	Ca^{2+} deficiency		
Calcium gluconate	Dietary Ca^{2+} supplement	Ca^{2+} deficiency		
Calcium lactate	Dietary Ca^{2+} supplement	Ca^{2+} deficiency		
Captopril [Capoten]	**Antihypertensive—ACE inhibitor** → inhibits conversion of angiotensin I to II → decreases angiotensin II (Ang II) levels → prevents vasoconstriction from Ang II	Hypertension, CHF, post-MI; prevention/treatment of diabetic nephropathy	**Cough, angioedema, hyperkalemia,** renal insufficiency (especially in bilateral renal artery stenosis)	Contraindicated in pregnancy (fetal renal malformation)
Carbachol [Isopto Carbachol]	Antiglaucoma agent—muscarinic cholinergic agonist, works on both muscarinic and nicotinic receptors	Miotic; glaucoma	**DUMBBELSS** (see Acetylcholine)	Contraindicated in patients with peptic ulcer, asthma, hyperthyroidism, and Parkinson disease

(continued)

APPENDIX I: **Drug Index**

Therapeutic Agent (common name, if relevant) [trade name, where appropriate]	**Class—Pharmacology and Pharmacokinetics**	**Indications**	**Side Effects or Adverse Effects**	**Contraindications or Precautions to Consider; Notes**
Carbamazepine [Tegretol]	Antiepileptic—prolongs inactivated state of Na^+ channels; decreases release of glutamate (and other excitatory neurotransmitters)	Epilepsy (partial and **tonic–clonic** [drug of choice]); **trigeminal neuralgia** (drug of choice)	**Agranulocytosis, liver toxicity (check LFTs), and aplastic anemia**	**Induces cytochrome P450**
Carbenicillin	**Antibiotic—β-lactam, penicillin derivative,** cell wall inhibitor; same mechanism as penicillin; distinguished by activity against ***Pseudomonas;*** bactericidal	**Extended spectrum**—*Pseudomonas; Proteus,* and *Enterobacter* species	**Hypersensitivity reactions;** decreased platelet function	Not effective against penicillin-resistant *Staphylococcus*; **can be combined with clavulanic acid** (β-lactamase inhibitor) to enhance spectrum; administered IV
Carbidopa-levodopa [Sinemet]	Antiparkinsonian—inhibits decarboxylase (L-DOPA to dopamine) **in periphery; does not cross BBB**	**Parkinson disease; used with levodopa,** which reduces metabolism of dopamine in periphery and increases its availability in CNS; especially effective for bradykinesia	**Treatment efficacy declines with progression of disease** due to a decrease in healthy dopaminergic neurons required for levodopa's MOA	
Carboplatin [Paraplatin]	Antineoplastic—**cross-links DNA**	Ovarian cancer	Bone marrow suppression and anemia	Contains platinum
Carboprost [Prostin]	Abortive agent—PGF_{2a}	Therapeutic abortion	Nausea, vomiting, diarrhea	
Carvedilol	**Antihypertensive,** antiarrhythmic (class II)—α- and β-blocker	**Hypertension, angina, MI, and antiarrhythmic**	**Impotence, asthma, bradycardia,** AV block, heart failure, sedation, and sleep alterations	
Caspofungin	**Antifungal**—inhibits cell wall synthesis	Invasive aspergillosis or *Candida*	GI irritation, flushing	Administered IV
Castor oil	**Stimulant laxative**—reduces absorption of electrolytes and water from gut; active component is ricinoleic acid	Constipation; labor induction		
Celecoxib [Celebrex]	**NSAID—selectively inhibits COX-2**	Rheumatoid arthritis, osteoarthritis; pain, inflammation	**Increased risk of thrombosis, sulfa allergy, and less toxic to GI mucosa**	COX-2 selectivity reduces inflammation while minimizing GI adverse effects (ulcers)

Cephalosporins	**Antibiotic—β-lactam,** cell wall inhibitor; same mechanism as penicillin, bactericidal, **from first generation to third generation:** **a. Gram-positive** coverage **decreases** **b. Gram-negative** coverage **increases** **c. CNS penetration increases** **d. β-Lactamase resistance increases**	**First generation: Gram + cocci and PEcK** (*Proteus mirabilis, Escherichia coli,* and ***K**lebsiella*); **second generation:** same as first generation + **HENPEcK** (***H.** influenzae **E**nterobacter,* and ***N**eisseria*); **third generation: cephalosporins are used for meningitis, *Klebsiella,* Lyme disease, and gram-negative bacteria**	**Hypersensitivity reaction; pain at injection site; intolerance to alcohol** (cefamandole, cefotetan, moxalactam, and cefoperazone); **hypothrombinemia** (cefamandole, cefoperazone, and moxalactam, due to vitamin K inhibition); **thrombophlebitis; positive Coombs test**	**First generation:** cefazolin, cephalexin; **second generation:** cefaclor, cefoxitin, and cefuroxime; **third generation:** ceftriaxone, cefotaxime, and ceftazidime; **fourth generation:** cefepime; ***Pseudomonas* coverage:** ceftazidime and cefepime; **cross-hypersensitivity with penicillins occurs in 5%–10% of patients**
Chloral hydrate	Anesthetic agent	Sedative (in children), hypnotic	Bitter taste, GI distress	Inexpensive
Chlorambucil [Leukeran]	Antineoplastic—DNA **alkylation and cross-linking**	Cancer	Nausea, vomiting, bone marrow suppression (mild), alopecia, teratogenicity, carcinogenicity, and **pulmonary fibrosis**	
Chloramphenicol [Chloromycetin]	**Antibiotic—protein synthesis inhibitor; inhibits 50S peptidyl transferase activity; bacteriostatic** but bactericidal versus *H. influenzae* and *Neisseria meningitides*	Meningitis (*Haemophilus influenzae Neisseria meningitidis, and Streptococcus pneumoniae*); typhoid fever; *Salmonella; Rickettsia* (Rocky Mountain spotted fever in children); *Bacteroides*	**Fatal aplastic anemia, bone marrow suppression, gray baby syndrome** (cyanosis, vomiting, green stools, and vasomotor collapse due to insufficient glucuronidase in neonatal liver)	Interactions with phenytoin, warfarin, or coumadin; inhibits cytochrome P450; used to treat serious infections after other antibiotics have failed given side effects
Chlordiazepoxide [Librium]	Long-acting benzodiazepine; antianxiety; enhances GABA; increases IPSP amplitude	Sedative, hypnotic, antianxiety, antiepileptic; alcohol withdrawal		
Chlorguanide	Antimalarial—inhibits dihydrofolate reductase	**Prophylaxis for falciparum** malaria; **suppression** of **vivax** malaria	Minor GI upset	
Chloroquine phosphate [Aralen]	Antimalarial—uncertain mechanism	**Suppression of malaria** and treatment of **acute** attack; **amebiasis; clonorchis; rheumatoid arthritis; SLE**	Headache, GI disturbances, visual disturbances, **pruritus;** prolonged therapy may lead to **retinopathy**	
Chloroprocaine	Anesthetic—block Na^+ channel intracellularly	Local anesthetic	Sleepiness, light-headedness, visual/audio disturbances, restlessness, nystagmus, shivering, tonic–clonic convulsions, death	
Chlorpheniramine [Chlor-Trimeton]	Antihistamine—H_1 blocker	Allergies; **motion sickness**	Sedation, CNS depression, atropine-like effects, allergic dermatitis, blood dyscrasias, teratogenicity, acute antihistamine poisoning	

(continued)

APPENDIX I: **Drug Index**

Therapeutic Agent (common name, if relevant) [trade name, where appropriate]	Class—Pharmacology and Pharmacokinetics	Indications	Side Effects or Adverse Effects	Contraindications or Precautions to Consider; Notes
Chlorpromazine [Thorazine]	Antiemetic, antipsychotic—phenothiazines; blocks D_2, α_1, and H_1 receptors	Antipsychotic, antiemetic, hiccups	**Extrapyramidal** (dystonia, akinesia, akathisia, and tardive dyskinesia), **anticholinergic** (dry mouth, constipation), **alpha blockade** (hypotension), **histamine** (sedation); toxicity results in neuroleptic malignant syndrome (rigidity, myoglobinuria, autonomic instability, and hyperpyrexia)	Atropine-like effects fairly common
Chlorpropamide	**Hypoglycemic agent, first-generation sulfonylurea**—closes potassium channel in β-cell membrane → reduces K^+ efflux, increases Ca^{2+} influx → increases secretion of insulin	Oral treatment for type 2 diabetes	**Hypoglycemia,** GI disturbances, muscle weakness, mental confusion	Rarely used due to toxicity
Cholestyramine [Questran]	Lipid-lowering agent—**bile acid resins** act by binding bile acids in the small intestine, forming insoluble complexes that are excreted; decreased bile acids stimulate the liver to increase conversion of cholesterol to bile acids, increasing hepatic LDL receptors, decreasing serum LDL	Reduction of cholesterol	Steatorrhea, constipation, impairment of absorption of drugs/vitamins	**Inhibits warfarin absorption**
Chorionic gonadotropin [Pregnyl]	Infertility therapy—LH-like in action	Treats infertility; induces ovulation; induces masculinization in infertile men; diagnostic for cryptorchidism in young boys		
Cimetidine [Tagamet]	**H_2 blocker—blocks histamine H_2 receptors reversibly → decreases proton secretion by parietal cells**	**Peptic ulcer disease, gastritis, esophageal reflux**	**Gynecomastia, impotence,** decreased libido in males, **confusion, dizziness, and headaches**	**Crosses placenta; decreases renal excretion of creatinine; CYP450 inhibitor**
Ciprofloxacin [Cipro]	**Antibiotic—quinolone, DNA synthesis inhibitor; inhibits DNA gyrase** (topoisomerase II) and **topoisomerase IV** → blocks DNA synthesis; bactericidal	**Gram-negative infections** (especially UTI and bone): *Pseudomonas,* Enterobacteriaceae, and *Neisseria;* **gram-positive infections:** (staphylococci); **intracellular:** ***Legionella***	**GI disturbances, headache, dizziness, phototoxicity, cartilage damage (children, fetus), tendonitis** and **tendon rupture (adults), myalgias (children)**	May elevate theophylline to toxic levels, causing seizure; divalent cations inhibit gut absorption; therefore, quinolones cannot be taken with milk, iron-containing preparations, or antacids.

Cisapride [Propulsid]	**GI stimulant—prokinetic; increases acetylcholine release at myenteric plexus →** increases esophageal tone, gastric/duodenal contractility (improves colon transit time)	Constipation	**Torsades des pointes**	Rarely used; interacts with **erythromycin, ketoconazole, nefazodone, and fluconazole** to produce **Torsades des pointes**
Cisplatin [Platinol]	Antineoplastic—cross-links DNA	Cancer	Bone marrow and renal toxicity, **cystitis, peripheral neuropathy, ototoxicity;** alopecia (severe)	
Citalopram	SSRIs—inhibit **reuptake** of 5-HT at neuronal synapses	Major depression, OCD, anorexia, and bulimia	Inhibits liver enzymes, nausea, agitation, **sexual dysfunction** (anorgasmia), and dystonic reactions	Contraindicated with **MAOIs** secondary to **serotonin syndrome** (hyperthermia, muscle rigidity, and cardiovascular collapse); allows time for antidepressant effect, usually takes 2–3 weeks
Clarithromycin [Biaxin]	**Antibiotic—macrolide,** protein synthesis inhibitor; binds to the 23S RNA of the 50S ribosome subunits → blocks translocation → prevents protein synthesis; bacteriostatic	**First choice for cell wall–deficient bugs: *Mycoplasma, Rickettsia, Chlamydia,* and *Legionella; Corynebacterium diphtheriae;*** gram-positive cocci (*Streptococcus*)	GI discomfort, **acute cholestatic hepatitis,** and **rashes;** increases concentration of **oral anticoagulants** and theophyllines	Can be used in patients with **streptococcal infections** and **penicillin allergies**
Clavulanic acid	β-lactamase inhibitor; synergistic with penicillins			
Clindamycin [Cleocin]	**Antibiotic—protein synthesis inhibitor; binds to 50S subunits →** blocks peptide bond formation; bacteriostatic or bactericidal depending on concentration, site, and organism	**Gram-positive bacteria (*Streptococcus* and *Staphylococcus*); treats anaerobic** infections	Severe diarrhea; **potentially fatal pseudomembranous colitis caused by *Clostridium difficile***	
Clofazimine [Lamprene]	Antibiotic—antileprosy; unknown mechanism	*Mycobacterium leprae*	Turns skin red-brown or black	
Clofibrate [Atromid-S]	Lipid-lowering agent—**up-regulates lipoprotein lipase (periphery) → increases TG clearance; decreases LDL, increases HDL, and decreases TG**	**Increased TG, increased LDL**	Myositis, increased LFTs; increased risk of GI and liver cancer; potentiates anticoagulant drugs; gallstones; mild GI disturbances	
Clomiphene [Clomid]	**Selective estrogen receptor modulator**—binds estrogen receptors in pituitary → prevents normal feedback inhibition, increases LH and FSH release from pituitary → stimulates ovulation	**Stimulates ovulation in infertility, PCOS**	**Hot flashes, ovarian enlargement, multiple gestation pregnancy, and visual disturbances**	

(continued)

Therapeutic Agent (common name, if relevant) [trade name, where appropriate]	Class—Pharmacology and Pharmacokinetics	Indications	Side Effects or Adverse Effects	Contraindications or Precautions to Consider; Notes
Clomipramine	TCAs—inhibit **reuptake** of NE and 5-HT at neuronal synapses	Major depression, OCD, and panic disorder	Sedation, **α-blocking effects** (orthostatic hypotension), **anticholinergic** (tachycardia, dry mouth, and urinary retention), hallucinations (in elderly), and confusion (in elderly); overdose toxicity results in **convulsions, coma, cardiotoxicity** (arrhythmias), respiratory depression, and hyperpyrexia	
Clonazepam [Klonopin]	**Antiepileptic—benzodiazepine**	**Epilepsy (absence of seizures)**		
Clonidine [Catapres]	**Antihypertensive**—centrally acting sympathetic agent (α_2-agonist) → decreases sympathetic outflow from CNS → decreases peripheral resistance	**Hypertension; smoking withdrawal; heroin and cocaine withdrawal**	Drowsiness, **dry mouth; rebound hypertension after abrupt withdrawal**	
Clotrimazole [Lotrimin, Mycelex]	Antifungal—inhibits ergosterol synthesis, preventing cell membrane formation	**Topical use against yeasts, dermatophytes, ringworm, fungi, mold, and oral candidiasis in AIDS**	Burning, itching, and redness when used topically	
Clozapine [Clozaril]	Atypical antipsychotic—blocks D_4, α_1 5-HT, muscarinic receptors	Schizophrenia, useful for positive and negative symptoms	Agranulocytosis, **extrapyramidal** (occurs at a lower rate than typicals), **anticholinergic** (dry mouth, constipation), **alpha blockade** (hypotension), **histamine** (sedation); toxicity results in neuroleptic malignant syndrome (occurs at a lower rate than typicals)	Second-line agent used for refractory schizophrenia; weekly blood counts for patients on this agent due to agranulocytosis
Cocaine	**CNS stimulant—blocks NE, 5-HT, and dopamine reuptake**	**Local anesthetic**	**Vasoconstriction; hypertension; nasal mucus ischemia**	
Codeine	**Opioid agonist**	**Pain;** antitussive	**Constipation**	Converted to morphine 10%
Colchicine	Anti-inflammatory—interrupts **microtubule formation,** thereby interfering with normal mitosis and inhibiting WBC migration and phagocytosis	Acute gout therapy	Diarrhea (common)	Contraindicated in elderly and feeble patients and in patients with GI disturbances, cardiac anomalies, or renal problems

Colestipol [Colestid]	Lipid-lowering agent—**bile acid resin,** impedes fat absorption; **lowers LDL;** binds cholesterol metabolites	Reduction of cholesterol	Steatorrhea, constipation, impaired absorption of drugs and vitamins	
Corticotropin-releasing hormone (CRH)	Increases ACTH production by anterior pituitary	Used in diagnosis of Cushing syndrome		
Cortisol (hydrocortisone) [Hydrocortone, Nutracort]	**Glucocorticoid—induces new protein synthesis; increases gluconeogenesis and lipolysis; reduces peripheral glucose use; catabolic effect on muscle, bone, skin, fat, and lymph tissue; anti-inflammatory; immunosuppressant**	**Adrenal insufficiency; congenital adrenal hyperplasia; diagnosis of pituitary–adrenal disorder; reduces inflammation (especially chronic); leukemia; decreases hypercalcemia**	**Iatrogenic Cushing syndrome, redistribution of fat, acne, insomnia, weight gain, hypokalemia, decrease in skeletal muscle, osteoporosis, hyperglycemia, ulcers, psychosis, cataracts, increased susceptibility to infections, growth suppression in children**	
Cosyntropin [Cortrosyn]	ACTH analog—increases production of steroids by adrenal	Used in diagnosis of adrenocortical insufficiency		
Cromolyn [Nasalcrom, Gastrocom]	**Antiasthmatic—**prevents release of mediators from mast cells → prevents bronchoconstriction and inflammation	Asthma prophylaxis	**Laryngeal edema (rare)**	Not used during acute exacerbation
Cyanocobalamin (Anacobin)	Supplies vitamin B_{12}	B_{12} deficiency		
Cyclobenzaprine [Flexeril]	Centrally acting muscle relaxant	Muscle spasms, tetanus contractions, orthopedic manipulation	Antimuscarinic effects	
Cyclophosphamide [Cytoxan]	Immunosuppressant—**alkylating agent; destroys proliferating lymphoid cells; alkylates resting cells**	**Transplant rejection, rheumatic arthritis**	GI and bone marrow toxicity, **hemorrhagic cystitis**	Coadministration of mesna will prevent hemorrhagic cystitis
Cycloserine [Seromycin]	Antibiotic—analog of o-alanine; interferes with cell wall synthesis	*Mycobacterium*	Psychotic reactions	
Cyclosporine [Sandimmune]	Immunosuppressant—**inhibits T-helper cell activity; inhibits IL-2, IL-3, and IFN-γ formation by T-helper cells**	**Transplant rejection**	**Nephrotoxic, hepatotoxic; hypertension; increased incidence of viral infection and lymphoma**	
Cyproheptadine [Periactin]	Antihistamine—antipruritic; $5\text{-}HT_3$ agonist; histamine blocker	Decreases diarrhea in carcinoid tumors; decreases dumping syndrome	Weight gain	
Cytosine arabinoside [Cytosar-U]	Antineoplastic—inhibits DNA replication and RNA polymerization; competitive inhibitor of dCTP; inhibits chain elongation	Cancer, AML	Severe myelosuppression, stomatitis, alopecia	

(continued)

Therapeutic Agent (common name, if relevant) [trade name, where appropriate]	Class—Pharmacology and Pharmacokinetics	Indications	Side Effects or Adverse Effects	Contraindications or Precautions to Consider; Notes
Dacarbazine (DTIC-Dome)	Antineoplastic—DNA alkylation; strand breakage; inhibits nucleic acid and protein synthesis	Cancer		
Dactinomycin [Cosmegen]	Antineoplastic—intercalates into DNA	Cancer	Skin eruptions, hyperkeratosis	
Danazol [Danocrine]	**Testosterone derivative—weak agonist for androgen, progesterone, and glucocorticoid receptors**	**Endometriosis and fibrocystic disease**	**Masculinization in women, gynecomastia** in men	
Dantrolene [Dantrium]	**Non-centrally acting muscle relaxant—decreases Ca^{2+} from sarcoplasmic reticulum**	**Malignant hyperthermia**	**Hepatotoxic**	
Dapsone [Dapsone]	Antibiotic—related to sulfonamides	*Mycobacterium leprae*	GI disturbances, hemolysis, methemoglobinemia	
Daunorubicin [DaunoXome, Cerubidine]	Antineoplastic—**oxidizes free radicals; intercalates into DNA; breaks DNA;** affects plasma membrane	Cancer	Cardiac changes resulting in cumulative **cardiotoxicity**	
Deferoxamine [Desferal]	**Metal chelator**	**Acute toxicity of iron**	**Hypotensive shock; neurotoxic if long-term use**	
Delavirdine	**Antiviral, nonnucleoside reverse transcriptase inhibitor**—binds viral reverse transcriptase and inhibits movement of protein domains → terminates viral DNA synthesis → prevents integration of viral genome into host DNA	**AIDS (used in HAART)**	**Neutropenia, anemia, peripheral neuropathy, and rash**	
Desflurane [Suprane]	Anesthetic	General anesthetic	Irritating to airway	
Desipramine [Norpramin]	TCAs—inhibit **reuptake** of NE and 5-HT at neuronal synapses	Major depression, panic disorder, and anxiety	Sedation, **α-blocking effects** (orthostatic hypotension), **anticholinergic** (tachycardia, dry mouth, and urinary retention), hallucinations (in elderly), and confusion (in elderly); overdose toxicity results in **convulsions, coma, cardiotoxicity** (arrhythmias), respiratory depression, and hyperpyrexia	Desipramine is the least sedating of the TCA

Desmopressin [DDAVP]	**Antidiuretic—synthetic analog of antidiuretic hormone;** recruits water channels to luminal membrane in collecting duct	Antidiuresis; central (pituitary) diabetes insipidus	Overhydration; allergic reaction; larger doses result in pallor, diarrhea, and hypertension; coronary constriction; chronic rhinopharyngitis	**Synthetic analog to vasopressin; intranasal administration**
Desogestrel	**Progesterone**—binds progesterone receptors	**Endometrial cancer,** amenorrhea, abnormal uterine bleeding, and **prevention of pregnancy**		Also used to prevent endometrial hyperplasia in postmenopausal women taking estrogen
Detemir [Levemir]	**Long-acting insulin**—*see mechanism for regular insulin*	**Diabetes mellitus** (typically **type 1**)	**Hypoglycemia** (diaphoresis, vertigo, tachycardia); insulin allergy; insulin antibodies; lipodystrophy	
Dexamethasone [Decadron, Maxidex]	**Corticosteroid—reduces lymph node and spleen size; inhibits cell cycle activity of lymphoid cells; lyses T cells; suppresses antibody, prostaglandin, and leukotriene synthesis; blocks monocyte production of IL-1**	**Antiemetic; autoimmune disorders; allergic reactions; asthma; organ transplantation (especially during rejection crisis); test for etiology of hypercortisolism**	Insomnia, epigastric disturbances, **cushingoid reaction, psychosis, glucose intolerance, infection, hypertension, cataracts**	
DHEA	Androgen and estrogen precursor	Acne; hair loss; hirsutism; deepening of voice		
Diazepam [Valium]	**Antianxiety, benzodiazepine—enhances GABA; increases IPSP amplitude**	**Sedative, hypnotic, antianxiety, antiepileptic (status epilepticus, grand mal)**	**Sedation**	
Diazepam-binding inhibitor (DBI)	Benzodiazepine receptor antagonist			
Diazoxide	**K^+ channel opener**—hyperpolarizes and relaxes vascular smooth muscle	**Hypertension**	Hypoglycemia (reduces insulin release), hypotension	
Diclofenac [Cataflam, Voltaren]	NSAID—enteric coated			
Dicloxacillin [Dynapen, Pathocil]	**Antibiotic—β-lactam, penicillin derivative,** cell wall inhibitor; same mechanism as penicillin; distinguished by activity against **penicillinase-producing *Staphylococcus*;** bactericidal	**Staphylococcal infections** (except MRSA)	**Hypersensitivity reactions;** interstitial nephritis (methicillin)	Penicillinase resistant; MRSA is resistant to methicillin because of altered penicillin-binding protein target site
Dicyclomine [Bentyl]	Antimuscarinic	Bladder/GI spasm; decreases acid in ulcer		
Didanosine (ddI) [Videx]	**Nucleoside reverse transcriptase inhibitor—guanosine analog →** inhibits viral reverse transcriptase → prevents integration of DNA copy of viral genome into host DNA	**AIDS (used in HAART)**	**Neutropenia, anemia, peripheral neuropathy, pancreatitis, and lactic acidosis**	

(continued)

APPENDIX I: **Drug Index**

Therapeutic Agent (common name, if relevant) [trade name, where appropriate]	**Class—Pharmacology and Pharmacokinetics**	**Indications**	**Side Effects or Adverse Effects**	**Contraindications or Precautions to Consider; Notes**
Diethylcarbamazine [Hetrazan]	Anthelmintic—sensitizes helminths	Filariasis to phagocytosis by macrophages	Headache, malaise, joint pain, anorexia; death of filaria causes swelling and edema of skin, enlarged lymph nodes, hyperpyrexia, and tachycardia	
Digitoxin [Crystodigin]	Inotropic agent—cardiac glycoside; increases cardiac contractility	Severe left ventricular systolic dysfunction; antiarrhythmic	Progressive dysrhythmia, anorexia, nausea, vomiting, headache, fatigue, confusion, blurred vision, altered color perception, halos around dark objects	Contraindicated in patients with right-sided heart failure, diastolic failure; Wolff–Parkinson–White syndrome; ECG changes: increases PR, decreases QT, depresses ST, and inverts T
Digoxin [Lanoxin]	**Inotropic agent—cardiac glycoside; inhibits Na/K/ATPase → indirect inhibition of Na^+/Ca^{2+} exchanger → increases Ca^{2+} → increases cardiac contractility**	**Severe left ventricular systolic dysfunction** (increases contractility), **atrial fibrillation** (decreases conduction at AV node and depresses SA node)	**Progressive dysrhythmia,** anorexia, nausea, vomiting, headache, fatigue, **confusion, blurred vision, altered color perception, halos around dark objects**	Contraindicated in patients with right-sided heart failure, diastolic failure; **ECG changes: increases PR, decreases QT, depresses ST, and inverts T; toxicities of digoxin are increased by renal failure** (decreases excretion), **hypokalemia** (potentiates drug's effects), and **quinidine** (decreases clearance, displaces digoxin)
Diiodohydroxyquin [Yodoxin]	Antiprotozoal—direct action	Amebiasis	Subacute myelo-optic neuropathy	
Diltiazem [Cardizem, Dilacor]	**Non-dihydropyridine Ca^{2+} channel blocker**—block voltage-gated Ca^{2+} channels of **cardiac** smooth muscle	**Hypertension, angina pectoris, arrhythmia**	Cardiac depression, peripheral edema, **flushing, dizzinesss**, and constipation	
Dimenhydrinate [Dramamine]	Antivertigo—antiemetic; H_1 blocker	Emesis, dizziness		
Dimercaprol [British anti-lewisite]	Metal chelator	Arsenic, mercury, or cadmium poisoning	Hypertension, tachycardia, headaches, nausea, vomiting, pain at injection site	
Dinoprostone [Cervidil, Prepidil]	Prostaglandin—PGE_2 analog → cervical dilation, uterine contraction	Induction of labor, termination of pregnancy		
Diphenhydramine [Benadryl]	**Antihistamine—antiemetic; muscarinic blocker; H_1 blocker (first generation)**	**Allergic reactions, asthma, motion sickness, antiemetic, insomnia**	Sedation, CNS depression, **atropine-like effects, allergic dermatitis, blood dyscrasias, teratogenicity,** acute antihistamine poisoning	Rarely used as antiparkinsonian agent

Disopyramide [Norpace]	Antiarrhythmic (class IA)—Na^+ channel blocker	Wolff–Parkinson–White syndrome	Heart failure	Contraindicated in patients with sick sinus syndrome
Disulfiram [Antabuse]	**Antialcoholic agent—inhibits aldehyde dehydrogenase**	**Alcoholism**	**Tachycardia, hyperventilation, nausea**	
Dobutamine [Dobutrex]	**Inotropic agent—β-agonist; positive inotropic effects on the heart and vasodilation**	**Acute** heart failure; **increases cardiac output**		
Docusate	**Stool softener;** by emulsifying stool, makes passage of stool easier	Constipation	Rash	
Doxazosin [Cardura]	Antihypertensive—α_1-blocker	Hypertension, BPH	**Orthostatic hypotension,** dizziness, and headache	First-dose orthostatic hypotension
Doxepin [Sinequan]	TCAs—inhibit **reuptake** of NE and 5-HT at neuronal synapses	Major depression, panic disorder, and potent antihistamine	Sedation, **α-blocking effects** (orthostatic hypotension), **anticholinergic** (tachycardia, dry mouth, and urinary retention), hallucinations (in elderly), and confusion (in elderly); overdose toxicity results in **convulsions, coma, cardiotoxicity** (arrhythmias), respiratory depression, and hyperpyrexia	
Doxorubicin [Adriamycin]	Antineoplastic—oxidizes free radicals; intercalates into DNA; breaks DNA; affects plasma membrane	Cancer	Cardiac changes resulting in cumulative cardiotoxicity	
Doxycycline	**Tetracycline antibiotic—protein synthesis inhibitor; binds 30S ribosome subunits** → prevents attachment of tRNA; bacteriostatic	**Broad spectrum including atypical pathogens: *Chlamydia, Rickettsia, Mycoplasma pneumoniae, Vibrio cholerae, Ureaplasma urealyticum, Francisella tularensis, Helicobacter pylori,* and *Borrelia burgdorferi*** (Lyme disease)	**Liver toxicity, GI distress, depression of bone/teeth development** (less than with tetracycline), **photosensitivity** (less than with tetracycline), **Fanconi syndrome**	**Contraindicated in pregnancy and children; divalent cations inhibit gut absorption, therefore cannot take with milk, antacids, or iron-containing preparations; fecally eliminated**
Dronabinol [Marinol]	Antiemetic—unknown mechanism; binds cannabinoid receptors and inhibits vomiting center in medulla	Antiemetic, appetite stimulant in patients with AIDS	Dry mouth, dizziness, inability to concentrate, disorientation, anxiety, tachycardia, depression, paranoia, psychosis	THC derivative
Echothiophate [Phospholine Iodide]	Antiglaucoma—inhibits cholinesterase; nicotinic receptor stimulator; irreversible	Closed-angle glaucoma	Open-angle glaucoma	
Edetate calcium disodium (calcium EDTA) [Calcium Disodium Versenate]	Metal chelator	Lead toxicity	Nephrotoxic	

(continued)

APPENDIX I: **Drug Index**

Therapeutic Agent (common name, if relevant) [trade name, where appropriate]	Class—Pharmacology and Pharmacokinetics	Indications	Side Effects or Adverse Effects	Contraindications or Precautions to Consider; Notes
Edrophonium [Enlon, Tensilon]	**Cholinesterase inhibitor**	**Diagnosis of myasthenia gravis; emergency anesthetic**		
Efavirenz	Antiviral, nonnucleoside reverse transcriptase inhibitor—**binds viral reverse transcriptase and inhibits movement of protein domains → terminates viral DNA synthesis → prevents integration of viral genome into host DNA**	**AIDS (used in HAART)**	Depression, dizziness, vivid dreams; **teratogenic**	
Emetine	**Antiprotozoal—causes degeneration of nucleus and reticulation of cytoplasm; directly lethal**	**Severe amebic infection**	Diarrhea, nausea, vomiting, abdominal pain; cardiac effects: hypotension, precordial pain, ECG changes	
Emtricitabine (FTC)	**Antiviral, nucleoside reverse transcriptase inhibitor—cytidine analog** → inhibits viral reverse transcriptase → prevents integration of DNA copy of the viral genome into the host DNA	**AIDS (used in HAART)**	**Neutropenia, anemia, peripheral neuropathy, pancreatitis, and lactic acidosis**	
Enalapril [Vasotec]	**Antihypertensive—ACE inhibitor** → inhibits conversion of angiotensin I to II → decreases Ang II levels → prevents vasoconstriction from Ang II	Hypertension, CHF, post-MI; prevention/treatment of diabetic nephropathy	**Cough, angioedema, hyperkalemia,** renal insufficiency (especially in bilateral renal artery stenosis)	Contraindicated in pregnancy (fetal renal malformation)
Encainide	Antiarrhythmia (class IC)—Na^+ channel blocker	Wolff–Parkinson–White syndrome		No antimuscarinic action; no effect on action potential
Enflurane [Ethrane]	Anesthetic agent	General anesthetic	Seizure	Abnormal ECG or seizures
Enfuvirtide	**Antiviral, fusion inhibitor**—binds viral gp41 subunit → inhibits conformation change (required for fusion with CD4 cell) → blocks viral entry and replication	**AIDS (used in patients on antiretroviral therapy with persistent viral replication)**	**Hypersensitivity reactions, reaction at injection site, and bacterial pneumonia**	**Used in combination with other antiretroviral drugs**

Enoxaparin [Lovenox]	Low-molecular-weight heparin; enhances **inhibition of factor Xa and thrombin by increasing antithrombin activity** (preferentially increases the inhibition of factor Xa)	Prophylaxis of thrombosis	**Elevated AST/ALT (reversible); heparin-associated thrombocytopenia**	Caution in recent surgery or active bleeding ulcers or internal hemorrhages; fewer bleeding complications, more bioavailable, and longer half-life than unfractionated heparin; no requirement for monitoring
Ephedrine	Bronchodilation—mixed adrenergic agonist	Stimulates NE release; antitussive; myasthenia gravis	Increases BP	
Epinephrine	Adrenergic agonist	Acute asthma, anaphylactic shock		Activates both α– and β– receptors, but is preferential for β
Eplerenone	**Potassium-sparing diuretic**—binds to intracellular aldosterone steroid receptors in **collecting tubules;** blocks induction of Na^+ channels and Na^+/ATPase synthesis; loss of Na^+, Cl^- in urine	Hyperaldosteronism, potassium depletion, and CHF	**Hyperkalemic metabolic acidosis, gynecomastia** (spironolactone), and antiandrogen effects	Like spironolactone but more selective for mineralocorticoid receptors; results in decreased secretion of K^+ and H^+, which can lead to **hyperkalemic metabolic acidosis;** often given in combination with a thiazide
Epoetin alfa [Procrit, Epogen]	**Colony-stimulating factor**—erythropoietin produced via recombinant DNA technology	**Anemia (especially in renal failure), AIDS**	**Hypertension**	
Epoprostenol [Flolan]	**Prostacyclin—increases cardiac index and stroke volume; decreases pulmonary vascular resistance and mean systemic pressure**	**Pulmonary hypertension**		
Ergotamine [Ergomar]	**Antimigraine—vasoconstriction**	**Acute attack of migraine**	**Gangrene** as a result of vasoconstriction	**Contraindicated in pregnant patients or patients with cardiovascular disease or coronary artery disease**
Erythromycin	**Antibiotic—macrolide,** protein synthesis inhibitor; binds to the 23S RNA of the 50S ribosome subunits → blocks translocation → prevents protein synthesis; bacteriostatic	**First choice for cell wall–deficient bugs: *Mycoplasma, Rickettsia, Chlamydia,* and *Legionella*; *Corynebacterium diphtheriae*;** gram-positive cocci (*Streptococcus*)	GI discomfort, **acute cholestatic hepatitis,** and **rashes;** increases concentration of **oral anticoagulants** and theophyllines	Can be used in patients with **streptococcal infections** and **penicillin allergies**
Esmolol [Brevibloc]	**Antiarrhythmic (class II)—β_1-selective blocker**	**Blocks the effect of catecholamines on heart; decreases the activity of nodal tissue; slows sinus rate; depresses AV conduction**	**Asthma; negative inotropic agent**	Short duration

(continued)

Therapeutic Agent (common name, if relevant) [trade name, where appropriate]	Class—Pharmacology and Pharmacokinetics	Indications	Side Effects or Adverse Effects	Contraindications or Precautions to Consider; Notes
Estrogen [Estratab, Premarin]	**Growth and development of female organs; linear bone growth; epiphyseal closure; endometrial growth; maintains responsiveness of breasts, uterus, and vagina; inhibits bone resorption; increases hepatic production of α_2 globulins, coagulation factors II, VII, IX, and X, and HDL; decreases antithrombin and cholesterol**	**Osteoporosis; contraception; can be used in combination with progesterone**	**Small increased incidence of breast and endometrial cancers; blood clots; may lead to sodium and water retention; nausea; breast tenderness; hyperpigmentation; increased risk of bleeding, gallbladder disease, migraines, hypertension**	
Etanercept	Recombinant form of human TNF receptor → binds TNF → decreases inflammatory response	Rheumatoid arthritis, psoriasis, and ankylosing spondylitis	**Infections**	
Ethacrynic acid [Edecrin]	Phenoxyacetic acid derivative diuretic—prevents cotransport of Na^+, K^+, and Cl^- in **thick ascending limb;** loss of Na^+, Cl^-, Ca^{2+}, and K^+ in urine	**Diuresis in patients with sulfa drug allergy**	**Ototoxicity, hypokalemic metabolic alkalosis,** and dehydration	**Can be given to patients with sulfa drug allergy,** hyperuricemia, and acute gout
Ethambutol [Myambutol]	Antibiotic—unknown mechanism	*Mycobacterium*	**Optic neuropathy (red-green color blindness);** tolerance develops	
Ether	**Anesthetic agent**	**General anesthetic**	Fire/explosion	No longer used
Ethinyl estradiol	**Estrogen**—binds estrogen receptor	In women: **hypogonadism, ovarian failure, contraception,** and menstrual abnormalities; in men: **androgen-dependent prostate cancer**	**Endometrial cancer, bleeding, and thrombosis**	Used in combination with progestin in patients with intact uterus; increased risk of endometrial cancer with unopposed estrogen therapy; females exposed to diethylstilbestrol in utero have an increased risk of **vaginal clear cell adenocarcinoma**
Ethosuximide	Antiepileptic—**decreases Ca^{2+} conduction**	Epilepsy **(absence seizures)**		
Etidocaine [Duranest]	Anesthetic agent—blocks Na^+ intracellularly	Local anesthetic	Sleepiness, light-headedness, visual/audio disturbances, restlessness, nystagmus, shivering, tonic–clonic convulsions, death, greater toxicity than other local anesthetics	

Etidronate [Didronel]	Bone stabilizer—pyrophosphate analog; reduces hydroxyapatite crystal formation, growth, and dissolution, which reduces bone turnover	Hypercalcemia of malignancy, Paget disease, osteoporosis, hyperparathyroidism		
Etomidate [Amidate]	Anesthetic agent	Induces stage 3 anesthesia	Painful injection; myoclonic movements	
Etoposide	**Antineoplastic—G2 phase specific— inhibits topoisomerase II → increases DNA degradation**	**Small cell lung cancer,** prostate and testicular carcinoma	**Myelosuppression,** nausea, vomiting, **alopecia**	
Etretinate	Vitamin A analog	Severe acne, psoriasis		
Exenatide [Byetta]	Hypoglycemic agent, **incretin mimetic—** agonizes GLP-1 receptors → decreases glucagon, increases insulin, delays gastric emptying	Injectable treatment for **type 2 diabetes**	Mild weight loss, nausea, **hypoglycemia,** constipation, slight risk of pancreatitis	Derived from exendin, a hormone found in Gila monster saliva
Ezetimibe [Zetia]	Antihyperlipidemia; **cholesterol absorption blocker—**prevents cholesterol reabsorption at brush border in small intestine; **decreases LDL; no effect on HDL or TG**	**Increased LDL; hypertriglyceridemia;** cardiac event risk reduction	**Increases LFT (rarely); myopathy,** hepatotoxicity, pancreatitis; abdominal symptoms	No proven clinical benefit; may increase plaque thickness
Famotidine [Pepcid]	**H_2 blocker—reversibly blocks histamine H_2 receptors → reduces gastric acid secretion**	**Peptic ulcer disease, gastritis, and esophageal reflux**	**Gynecomastia;** rare: confusion, dizziness, and headaches	**Crosses placenta; milder side effect profile** than cimetidine and ranitidine
Felodipine [Plendil]	**Dihydropyridine Ca^{2+} channel blocker—** block voltage-gated Ca^{2+} channels of **vascular** smooth muscle	**Hypertension, angina pectoris, Prinzmetal angina, Raynaud phenomenon**	Peripheral edema, **flushing, dizziness,** and constipation	
Fenofibrate	**Lipid-lowering agent—up-regulates lipoprotein lipase (periphery) → increases TG clearance; decreases LDL, increases HDL, and decreases TG**	**Increased TG, increased LDL**	Myositis, increased LFTs	Reduces TG more than other agents
Fentanyl	**Opioid agonist**	**Pain;** general anesthetic	Prolonged recovery; nausea	
Fexofenadine hydrochloride [Allegra]	Antihistamine			
Filgrastim [Neupogen]	**Granulocyte-macrophage colony–stimulating factor**	**Recovery of bone marrow (e.g., chemotherapy-induced neutropenia)**		

(continued)

APPENDIX I: **Drug Index**

Therapeutic Agent (common name, if relevant) [trade name, where appropriate]	Class—Pharmacology and Pharmacokinetics	Indications	Side Effects or Adverse Effects	Contraindications or Precautions to Consider; Notes
Finasteride [Proscar]	**Antiandrogen—5α-reductase inhibitor** → decreases the conversion of testosterone to dihydrotestosterone	**BPH,** male pattern baldness	Decreased libido; decreased ejaculate volume	
Flecainide [Tambocor]	**Antiarrhythmic (class IC)—Na^+ channel blocker**			
Fluconazole [Diflucan]	**Antifungal—inhibits ergosterol synthesis,** preventing cell membrane formation	**Cryptococcal meningitis, mucosal candidiasis, coccidioidomycosis**	**Abdominal pain, nausea, hepatotoxicity**	
Flucytosine [Ancobon]	Antifungal—competitive inhibitor of thymidylate synthetase; impairs DNA synthesis	*Candida, Cryptococcus*	Nausea, vomiting, diarrhea, rash, bone marrow and liver toxicity, enterocolitis	Imported in the fungus via permease
Fludrocortisone [Florinef]	Mineralocorticoid—aldosterone analog	Used with cortisol in adrenal insufficiency		
Flumazenil [Romazicon]	Benzodiazepine receptor antagonist	Alcohol abuse; anxiety		IV only
Flunarizine [Sibelium]	Weak Ca^{2+} channel blocker	Prophylaxis for migraine		
Fluoride	Stabilizes hydroxyapatite crystal structure; stimulates new growth of bone (unknown mechanism)		Nausea, vomiting, neurologic symptoms, arthralgias, arthritis	Stains teeth in toxic amounts
5-Fluorouracil (5-FU)	Antineoplastic**—inhibits thymidylate synthetase; inhibits RNA synthesis**	**Colon and breast cancer**	**Delayed toxicity: nausea, oral and GI ulcers, and bone marrow depression**	
Fluoxetine [Prozac]	SSRIs—inhibit **reuptake** of 5-HT at neuronal synapses	Major depression, OCD, anorexia, bulimia, anxiety	Inhibits liver enzymes, nausea, agitation, **sexual dysfunction** (anorgasmia), and dystonic reactions	Contraindicated with **MAOIs** secondary to **serotonin syndrome** (hyperthermia, muscle rigidity, and cardiovascular collapse); allows time for antidepressant effect, usually takes 2–3 weeks
Fluphenazine [Prolixin]	Antipsychotic—phenothiazine; blocks D_2, α_1, and H_1 receptors	Psychosis	**Extrapyramidal** (dystonia, akinesia, akathisia, and tardive dyskinesia), **anticholinergic** (dry mouth, constipation), **alpha blockade** (hypotension), **and histamine** (sedation); toxicity results in neuroleptic malignant syndrome (rigidity, myoglobinuria, autonomic instability, and hyperpyrexia)	**Extrapyramidal** side effects are more common

Flurazepam [Dalmane]	Benzodiazepine—enhances GABA; increases IPSP amplitude	Sedative, hypnotic, antianxiety, antiepileptic		
Flutamide [Eulexin]	**Antiandrogen—**nonsteroidal, competitive androgen receptor blocker	**Metastatic prostate cancer**		
Fluticasone [Flonase]	Intranasal glucocorticoids—decrease cytokine synthesis, downregulate inflammatory response in the nasal mucosa	Nasal congestion, allergic rhinitis	Local irritation of nasal mucosa, epistaxis	
Fluvastatin [Lescol]	Lipid-lowering agent—inhibits HMG-CoA reductase; lowers LDL	Hyperlipidemia (especially type II)	Liver toxicity, myopathy, mild GI disturbances	Contraindicated in pregnant or lactating women and children
Fluvoxamine [Luvox]	Antidepressant—SSRI	Anxiety; OCD		
Folic acid [Folvite]	**Vitamin—one carbon carrier; nucleic acid synthesis**	**Given to pregnant women to prevent neural tube defects in utero**		**Decreased in pregnancy or with the use of phenytoin and isoniazid**
Foscarnet [Foscavir]	**Antiviral—**nonnucleoside inhibitor of DNA polymerase	**CMV retinitis (resistant to ganciclovir), HSV (resistant to acyclovir)**	Hypocalcemia; CNS, cardiac, and **renal toxicity;** anemia	**Does not require activation by viral kinase**
Fosinopril [Monopril]	**Antihypertensive—ACE inhibitor** → inhibits conversion of angiotensin I to II → decreases Ang II levels → prevents vasoconstriction from Ang II	Hypertension, CHF, post-MI; prevention/treatment of diabetic nephropathy	**Cough, angioedema, hyperkalemia,** renal insufficiency (especially in bilateral renal artery stenosis)	Contraindicated in pregnancy (fetal renal malformation)
Furosemide [Lasix]	Loop diuretic—prevents cotransport of Na^+, K^+, and Cl^- in **thick ascending limb;** loss of Na^+, Cl^-, Ca^{2+}, and K^+ in urine	**Hypertension, CHF,** cirrhosis, nephrotic syndrome, **pulmonary edema,** hypercalcemia	**Potassium wasting, metabolic alkalosis,** hypotension, dehydration, ototoxicity, nephritis, and gout	Do not give in patients with **sulfa drug allergy;** rapid onset and short duration of action, which is ideal for relieving acute edema
Gabapentin [Neurontin]	Antiepileptic—blocks Na^+ channels	Add-on drug for epilepsy		
Ganciclovir [Cytovene]	**Antiviral—guanosine analog;** inhibits viral DNA polymerase	**CMV (especially CMV retinitis in AIDS)**	**Bone marrow suppression** (leukopenia, neutropenia, and thrombocytopenia), **renal impairment, seizures**	**Resistance from lack of thymidine kinase or mutation of viral DNA polymerase; more toxic than acyclovir**
Gemfibrozil	**Lipid-lowering agent—up-regulates lipoprotein lipase (periphery) → increases TG clearance; decreases LDL, increases HDL, and decreases TG**	**Increased TG, increased LDL**	Myositis, increased LFTs; potentiates **anticoagulant drugs;** gallstones; mild GI disturbances	Reduces TG more than other agents; contraindicated in patients with impaired renal or hepatic function and pregnant or lactating women
Gentamicin [Garamycin]	**Antibiotic—aminoglycoside,** protein synthesis inhibitor; irreversibly binds **30S ribosome subunits; bacteriostatic** at low concentration; **bactericidal** at high concentration	**Broad spectrum:** gram-negative rods; good for **bone** and **eye** infections; *Proteus, Pseudomonas, Enterobacter, Klebsiella,* and *Escherichia coli*	**Ototoxicity, renal toxicity, neuromuscular blockade,** nausea, vomiting, vertigo, allergic rash	

(continued)

Therapeutic Agent (common name, if relevant) [trade name, where appropriate]	Class—Pharmacology and Pharmacokinetics	Indications	Side Effects or Adverse Effects	Contraindications or Precautions to Consider; Notes
Gestodene	**Progesterone**—binds progesterone receptors	**Endometrial cancer,** amenorrhea, abnormal uterine bleeding, and **prevention of pregnancy**		Also used to prevent endometrial hyperplasia in postmenopausal women taking estrogen
Glargine [Lantus]	**Long-acting insulin**—*see mechanism for regular insulin*	**Diabetes mellitus** (typically **type 1**)	**Hypoglycemia** (diaphoresis, vertigo, and tachycardia); insulin allergy; insulin antibodies; lipodystrophy	
Glimepiride [Amaryl]	**Hypoglycemic agent, second-generation sulfonylurea**—closes potassium channel in pancreatic β-islet cell membrane → reduces K^+ efflux, increases Ca^{2+} influx → increases secretion of insulin	Oral treatment for **type 2 diabetes**	**Hypoglycemia,** GI disturbances, muscle weakness, mental confusion, weight gain	Not useful in type 1 diabetes mellitus because it requires some β-cell function
Glipizide [Glucotrol]	**Hypoglycemic agent, second-generation sulfonylurea**—closes potassium channel in pancreatic β-islet cell membrane → reduces K^+ efflux, increases Ca^{2+} influx → increases secretion of insulin	Oral treatment for **type 2 diabetes**	**Hypoglycemia,** GI disturbances, muscle weakness, mental confusion, weight gain	Not useful in type 1 diabetes mellitus because it requires some β-cell function
Glyburide [DiaBeta, Micronase]	**Hypoglycemic agent, second-generation sulfonylurea**—closes potassium channel in pancreatic β-islet cell membrane → reduces K^+ efflux, increases Ca^{2+} influx → increases secretion of insulin	Oral treatment for **type 2 diabetes**	**Hypoglycemia,** GI disturbances, muscle weakness, mental confusion, weight gain	Not useful in type 1 diabetes mellitus because it requires some β-cell function
Glyceryl guaiacolate [Fenesin]	**Expectorant—increases bronchial secretions**	**Promotes cough**		
Glycopyrrolate [Robinul]	**Antimuscarinic**	**Bladder/GI spasm; decreases acid in ulcer**		Quaternary amine
GnRH	**Controls release of FSH, LH**	**Stimulates pituitary function**		
Gonadorelin [Lutrepulse]	**Analog of GnRH—controls release of FSH, LH**	**Stimulates pituitary function**		

Griseofulvin [Fulvicin, Grifulvin, Grisactin]	**Antifungal—inhibits cell mitosis by disrupting mitotic spindles; binds to tubulin**	**Dermatophytes (especially *Trichophyton rubrum*)**	**Headache, mental confusion, rash, GI irritation, hepatotoxic, photosensitivity, carcinogenic, teratogenic**	Increases **cytochrome P450** and warfarin metabolism
Growth hormone (somatotropin, somatrem)	**Synthetic analog of growth hormone—causes liver to produce insulin-like growth factors (somatomedins)**	Replacement therapy in children with **growth hormone deficiency, Turner syndrome; burn victims**		
Growth hormone–releasing hormone (GHRH)	**Synthetic analog of GHRH—stimulates the release of growth hormone**	Dwarfism	Pain at injection site	
Guaifenesin [Robitussin]	Expectorant—thins mucus and lubricates irritated respiratory tract	Cough associated with common cold and minor upper respiratory tract infections		Does not suppress cough reflex
Guanethidine [Ismelin]	**Antihypertensive**—interferes with NE release	**Severe hypertension**	Orthostatic hypotension, exercise hypotension, impotence, and diarrhea	**Contraindicated in patients taking TCAs**
Haloperidol [Haldol]	**Antipsychotic**—butyrophenone; blocks D and α_1 receptors	**Schizophrenia, psychosis, acute mania, and Tourette syndrome**	**Extrapyramidal** (dystonia, akinesia, akathisia, and tardive dyskinesia), **endocrine** (galactorrhea), **anticholinergic** (dry mouth, constipation), **alpha blockade** (hypotension), and **histamine** (sedation); prolonged QT syndrome; toxicity results in neuroleptic malignant syndrome (rigidity, myoglobinuria, autonomic instability, and hyperpyrexia)	Extrapyramidal side effects are more common; neuroleptic malignant syndrome is treated with dantrolene and dopamine agonists
Haloprogin [Halotex]	**Antifungal—unknown mechanism; fungistatic**	**Topical for tinea pedis**		
Halothane	**Anesthetic agent**	**General anesthetic**	**Hepatotoxic; malignant hyperthermia (with succinylcholine); arrhythmia**	**Contraindicated in adults**
Heparin	**Anticoagulant—increases PTT by accelerating antithrombin**	**Deep vein thrombosis, pulmonary thrombosis, MI**	**Overdose reversed by IV protamine sulfate;** osteoporosis	**Fast acting; does not cross placenta**
Heroin	**Metabolized to morphine**			**More lipid soluble than morphine**
Hexamethonium	Nicotinic ganglionic blocker	Hypertensive emergency	Severe orthostatic hypotension, blurred vision, constipation, and sexual dysfunction	

(continued)

APPENDIX I: **Drug Index**

Therapeutic Agent (common name, if relevant) [trade name, where appropriate]	Class—Pharmacology and Pharmacokinetics	Indications	Side Effects or Adverse Effects	Contraindications or Precautions to Consider; Notes
Hydralazine [Apresoline]	**Antihypertensive**—increases cGMP smooth muscle relaxation → vasodilates arterioles → afterload reduction	**Severe hypertension, CHF**	**Compensatory tachycardia,** fluid retention, **lupus-like syndrome**	**First-line therapy for hypertension in pregnancy,** used with methyldopa; contraindicated in angina/coronary artery disease because of compensatory tachycardia
Hydrochlorothiazide (HCTZ) [HydroDIURIL]	Thiazide diuretic—inhibits transport of Na^+ and Cl^- into the cells of DCT	**Hypertension, CHF,** idiopathic hypercalciuria, and nephrogenic diabetes insipidus	**Hypokalemia, metabolic alkalosis, mild hyperlipidemia, hyperuricemia,** malaise, **hypercalcemia,** hyperglycemia, and hyponatremia	Do not give in patients with sulfa drug allergy
Hydrocodone and acetaminophen [Bancap-HC]	Opioid agonist	Antitussive, analgesic		
Hydromorphone [Dilaudid]	Opioid agonist	Antitussive, analgesic	Respiratory depression, constipation, nausea	
Hydroxychloroquine [Plaquenil]	Antiprotozoal—antirheumatic	Rheumatic arthritis, malaria	Ocular toxicity (blurred vision)	Contraindicated in patients with psoriasis
Hydroxyurea [Hydrea]	**Antineoplastic—binds ribonucleotide reductase; inhibits formation of DNA**	**Melanoma, chronic myelogenous leukemia, sickle cell disease**	Nausea, vomiting, bone marrow suppression	
Ibuprofen [Advil, Motrin]	**NSAID—reversibly inhibits COX** (both COX-1 and COX-2) → decreases prostaglandin synthesis	**Inflammation, pain**	GI distress, **GI ulcers,** coagulation disorders, aplastic anemia, metabolic abnormalities, hypersensitivity, renal damage	
Ibutilide [Corvert]	Antiarrhythmic (class III)—K^+ channel blocker	Terminates atrial fibrillation and flutter	Prolongs QT interval	
Idazoxan	Antihypertensive—α_2-blocker			
Idoxuridine [Herplex Liquifilm]	Antiviral—thymidine analog; inhibits DNA polymerase; inhibits DNA synthesis	Topical for HSV keratitis	Local irritation; allergic contact keratitis	
Ifosfamide [Ifex]	Antineoplastic—DNA alkylation and cross-linking	Cancer	**Hemorrhagic cystitis**; nephrotoxicity; nausea; vomiting; bone marrow suppression; alopecia; teratogenicity; carcinogenicity	Coadministration of mesna will prevent hemorrhagic cystitis

Imipenem and cilastatin [Primaxin]	**Antibiotic—carbapenem,** cell wall inhibitor; same mechanism as penicillin; bactericidal	**Broad spectrum—gram-positive cocci** (MSSA and *Streptococcus*), **gram-negative rods** (*Pseudomonas* and *Enterobacter* spp.), **anaerobes**	Hypersensitivity reaction, **seizure,** confusion state, and superinfection (pseudomembranous colitis)	Significant side effects limit use to when other drugs have failed or in the case of life-threatening infections; always administered with cilastatin (inhibits renal dehydropeptidase) to reduce inactivation in renal tubules
Imipramine [Tofranil]	TCAs—inhibit **reuptake** of NE and 5-HT at neuronal synapses	Major depression, nocturnal enuresis, and panic disorder	Sedation, **α-blocking effects** (orthostatic hypotension), **anticholinergic** (tachycardia, dry mouth, and urinary retention), hallucinations (in elderly), and confusion (in elderly); overdose toxicity results in **convulsions, coma, cardiotoxicity** (arrhythmias), respiratory depression, and hyperpyrexia	
Indecainide	Antiarrhythmic (class IC) Na^+ channel blockers			No antimuscarinic action; no effect on action potential
Indinavir [Crixivan]	**Antiviral, protease inhibitor—** protease responsible for final step of viral proliferation; inhibits protease in progeny virions → assembly of nonfunctional viruses	**AIDS (used in HAART)**	**GI irritation (nausea, diarrhea), hyperglycemia, hyperlipidemia, lipodystrophy, thrombocytopenia**	**All protease inhibitors ending in -navir; metabolism occurs by cytochrome P450**
Indomethacin [Indocin]	**Anti-inflammatory, NSAID—** reversibly inhibits COX **(both COX-1 and COX-2)→ decreases prostaglandin synthesis**	**Acute gout therapy; closes PDA**	**GI distress,** GI ulcers, **coagulation disorders, aplastic anemia, metabolic abnormalities, hypersensitivity, renal damage**	
Infliximab	Anti-inflammatory—**monoclonal antibody that binds TNF → inhibits proinflammatory effects of TNF**	Crohn disease, **rheumatoid arthritis, and** ankylosing spondylitis	**Infections, fever, hypotension, and** reactivation of latent tuberculosis	
Insulin, regular [Humulin R, Novolin R]	**Short-acting insulin—Liver:** promotes glucose storage as glycogen; increases TG synthesis **Muscle:** facilitates protein and glycogen synthesis **Adipose tissue:** improves TG storage by activating plasma lipoprotein lipase; reduces circulating free fatty acids	**Diabetes mellitus** (typically **type 1**), **hyperkalemia, and stress-induced hyperglycemia**	**Hypoglycemia** (diaphoresis, vertigo, and tachycardia); insulin allergy; insulin antibodies; lipodystrophy	

(continued)

Therapeutic Agent (common name, if relevant) [trade name, where appropriate]	Class—Pharmacology and Pharmacokinetics	Indications	Side Effects or Adverse Effects	Contraindications or Precautions to Consider; Notes
Interferon α-2a [Roferon A], **α-2b** [Intron A], **and α-n3** [Alferon-N]	**Antiviral—glycoproteins—block viral RNA, DNA, and protein synthesis**	**Genital warts, chronic hepatitis B and C, AIDS-related Kaposi sarcoma, laryngeal papillomatosis, hairy cell leukemia**	**Flulike symptoms, neutropenia, depression**	
Interferon β-1a [Avonex, Rebif]	**Antiviral—glycoproteins—block viral RNA, DNA, and protein synthesis**	**Multiple sclerosis**	**Flulike symptoms, neutropenia, depression**	
Interferon γ-1b [Actimmune]	**Antiviral—glycoproteins—block viral RNA, DNA, and protein synthesis**	**Chronic granulomatous disease**	**Flulike symptoms, neutropenia**	
Ipecac (syrup) [Quelidrine]	Expectorant—increases bronchial secretions	Promotes cough		
Ipratropium [Atrovent]	Bronchodilator—muscarinic antagonist; competitively blocks muscarinic receptors → prevents bronchoconstriction	Asthma, COPD		
Isocarboxazid [Marplan]	MAOIs—inhibit **degradation** of NE and 5-HT at neuronal synapses	**Atypical depression** (with hypersomnia, anxiety, sensitivity to rejection, and hypochondriasis)	**Hypertensive episodes** with ingestion of tyramine-containing foods or β-agonists, hyperthermia, and convulsions	Contraindicated with **SSRIs** and **meperidine** secondary to **serotonin syndrome** (hyperthermia, muscle rigidity, and cardiovascular collapse)
Isoflurane	Anesthetic	General anesthetic		Best muscle relaxant, most widely used
Isoniazid (INH)	**Antibiotic**—inhibits synthesis of mycolic acids	***Mycobacterium* treatment (*Mycobacterium tuberculosis and Mycobacterium kansasii*); *Mycobacterium tuberculosis prophylaxis***	**Peripheral and CNS effects as a result of pyridoxine deficiency; liver damage; hemolytic anemia in G6PD deficiency; SLE-like syndromes**	Pyridoxine (Vitamin B_6) can prevent neurotoxicity
Isoproterenol [Isuprel]	Bronchodilator—β-agonist (non-selective); relaxes bronchial smooth muscle through β_2-receptor activity	Asthma	Tachycardia (β_1-receptor activity)	
Isosorbide dinitrate [Isordil]	Antianginal—stimulates the synthesis of cGMP, leading to muscle relaxation via NO formation; vasodilator	Angina, CHF	Headache, orthostatic hypotension, syncope	Long acting
Isotretinoin [Accutane]	**Vitamin A analog**	**Severe acne, psoriasis**	**Keratinization; teratogenic**	

Itraconazole [Sporanox]	**Antifungal—inhibits ergosterol synthesis, preventing cell membrane formation**	Oral for dermatophytoses and onychomycosis; **drug of choice for histoplasmosis, blastomycosis, sporotrichosis, paracoccidioidomycosis**	**GI disturbances, hepatotoxicity**	
Ivermectin	**Anthelmintic—**binds to invertebrate chloride channels → hyperpolarizes parasite nerve and muscle cells → parasite paralysis	Onchocerciasis, strongyloidiasis	Mazzotti-like reaction	Contraindicated in pregnancy
Ketamine [Ketalar]	**Anesthetic agent; blocks NMDA-type glutamate receptors**	**General anesthetic**	**Dissociative anesthesia; catatonia; hallucinations**	
Ketoconazole [Nizoral]	**Antifungal—inhibits ergosterol synthesis, preventing cell membrane formation; inhibits adrenal and gonadal steroid synthesis**	**Chronic mucocutaneous candidiasis, blastomycosis, histoplasmosis, coccidioidomycosis, hypercortisolism, prostate carcinoma**	**GI irritation, gynecomastia, thrombocytopenia, hepatotoxic, rash, fever, chills**	**Inhibits cytochrome P450**
Ketorolac [Toradol]	**NSAID—reversibly inhibits COX** (both COX-1 and COX-2) → decreases prostaglandin synthesis; relieves pain and reduces swelling	**Postoperative pain,** severe pain	GI distress, **GI ulcers,** coagulation disorders, aplastic anemia, metabolic abnormalities, hypersensitivity, renal damage	
Labetalol [Normodyne, Trandate]	**Antihypertensive—nonselective β- and α_1-blocker**	**Hypertension**	**Bronchospasm, bradycardia,** AV block, heart failure, sedation, and sleep alterations	
Lactulose	**Osmotic laxative**	Decreases ammonia in hepatic encephalopathy; constipation	Abdominal bloating, flatulence	Lowers colon pH so that ammonia is trapped and then excreted
Lamivudine (3TC) [Epivir]	**Antiviral, nucleoside reverse transcriptase inhibitor—cytidine analog** → inhibits viral reverse transcriptase → prevents integration of DNA copy of viral genome into host DNA	**AIDS (used in HAART)**	**Neutropenia, anemia, peripheral neuropathy, pancreatitis, and lactic acidosis**	
Lamotrigine [Lamictal]	Antiepileptic—blocks Na^+ channels	Add-on drug for epilepsy		
Lansoprazole	**Proton pump inhibitor—irreversibly inhibits H^+/K^+-ATPase in gastric parietal cells → decreases proton secretion by parietal cells**	Peptic ulcer disease, gastritis, esophageal reflux, **Zollinger–Ellison syndrome**		**Inhibits cytochrome P450;** given with **clarithromycin** and **amoxicillin** for ***Helicobacter pylori***
Latanoprost [Xalatan]	$PGF_{2\alpha}$; increases aqueous humor outflow	Glaucoma	Blurred vision, burning, hyperemia, itching, hyperpigmentation of iris, keratitis	

(continued)

Therapeutic Agent (common name, if relevant) [trade name, where appropriate]	**Class—Pharmacology and Pharmacokinetics**	**Indications**	**Side Effects or Adverse Effects**	**Contraindications or Precautions to Consider; Notes**
Leucovorin	Allows stem cells to bypass the inhibition of dihydrofolate reductase caused by methotrexate	Treats acute toxicity of methotrexate		
Leuprolide [Lupron]	**GnRH analog**—agonist (when given pulsatile), antagonist (when given continuously)	**Infertility** (given pulsatile), **prostate cancer** (given continuous), **uterine fibroids,** endometriosis, precocious puberty	Nausea, vomiting, and antiandrogen effects (testicular atrophy); menopausal symptoms	
Levamisole [Ergamisol]	Anthelmintic—immunostimulatory to host; helps rid the host of parasite	*Ascaris* (roundworm); *Ancylostoma* (hookworm); therapy for immunodeficiency	GI disturbances, rashes, neutropenia	
Levodopa	**Antiparkinsonian agent—precursor of dopamine; administered with carbidopa (most often) or benserazide to inhibit carboxylase deactivation of levodopa in periphery**	**Parkinson disease**		**Inhibited by vitamin B_6; do not give with MAOI or pyridoxine**
Levofloxacin [Levaquin]	**Antibiotic—quinolone; inhibits DNA gyrase** (topoisomerase II) and **topoisomerase IV** → blocks DNA synthesis; bactericidal	**Gram-negative infections (especially UTI and bone): *Pseudomonas,* Enterobacteriaceae, and *Neisseria;* gram-positive infections** (*Staphylococcus, Streptococcus*); **intracellular: *Legionella***	**GI disturbances, headache, dizziness, phototoxicity, cartilage damage (children, fetus), tendonitis and tendon rupture (adults), myalgias (children)**	**May elevate theophylline to toxic levels, causing seizure; contraindicated in pregnant women; divalent cations inhibit gut absorption, therefore cannot be taken with milk, antacids, or iron-containing preparations**
Levomethadyl [Orlaam]	Opioid agonist	Long-lasting maintenance therapy for heroin addiction		
Levonorgestrel [Plan B]	**Progesterone**—binds progesterone receptors	**Endometrial cancer,** amenorrhea, abnormal uterine bleeding, and **prevention of pregnancy**		Also used to prevent endometrial hyperplasia in postmenopausal women taking estrogen
Levothyroxine (T_4) [Levothroid, Synthroid]	Synthetic analog of thyroxine (T_4)	**Hypothyroidism**	Tachycardia, heat intolerance, tremors, and arrhythmia	
Lidocaine [Xylocaine]	**Antiarrhythmic (class IB), anesthetic agent—blocks Na^+ channels intracellularly**	**Local anesthetic; ventricular tachycardia**	**Sleepiness, light-headedness, visual/audio disturbances, restlessness, nystagmus, shivering, tonic–clonic convulsion, death**	**Given with epinephrine to maintain locality and increase duration of anesthetic properties via epinephrine-mediated vasoconstriction**

Linagliptin [Tradjenta]	**Hypoglycemic agent, DPP-IV inhibitor**—prevents degradation of incretin hormones → decreased glucagon, increased insulin	Oral treatment for **type 2 diabetes**	Diarrhea, constipation, edema	
Liraglutide [Victoza]	Hypoglycemic agent**, incretin mimetic**—agonizes GLP-1 receptors → decreases glucagon, increases insulin, delays gastric emptying	Injectable treatment for **type 2 diabetes**	Mild weight loss, nausea, vomiting, diarrhea, slight risk of pancreatitis	Increased incidence of medullary thyroid cancer in animal models
Lisinopril [Prinivil, Zestril]	**Antihypertensive—ACE inhibitor** → inhibits conversion of angiotensin I to II → decreases Ang II levels → prevents vasoconstriction from Ang II	Hypertension, CHF, post-MI; prevention/treatment of diabetic nephropathy	**Cough, angioedema, hyperkalemia,** renal insufficiency (especially in bilateral renal artery stenosis)	Contraindicated in pregnancy (fetal renal malformation)
Lispro [Humalog]	**Rapid-acting insulin—***see mechanism for regular insulin*	**Diabetes mellitus** (typically **type 1**), **hyperkalemia, and stress-induced hyperglycemia**	**Hypoglycemia** (diaphoresis, vertigo, and tachycardia); insulin allergy; insulin antibodies; lipodystrophy	
Lithium [Eskalith, Lithobid, Lithotabs, Lithonate]	Antimanic—unclear mechanism; inhibits regeneration of IP_3 and DAG; important for many second-messenger systems	Bipolar disorder, acute manic events	Tremor, hypothyroidism, polyuria, and teratogenesis	Close monitoring of serum levels required due to narrow therapeutic window
Loperamide [Imodium]	**Antidiarrheal—similar to opioid agonist**	**Oral antidiarrheal**		
Loratadine [Claritin]	**Antihistamine**—H_1 blocker (second generation)	**Seasonal allergies**	**Sedating;** rare: headache, dizziness, fatigue, CNS, weak antiandrogenic effect, leukopenia, and reduced sperm count	**Inhibits metabolism or absorption of some drugs;** less sedating than first-generation H_1 blocker due to decreased CNS entry
Lorazepam [Ativan]	Antianxiety—benzodiazepine; enhances GABA, increases IPSP amplitude	Sedative, hypnotic, antianxiety, antiepileptic; panic attack		
Losartan [Cozaar]	**Antihypertensive—**Ang II receptor blockers → prevents vasoconstriction from Ang II	**Hypertension**	Fetal renal toxicity, **hyperkalemia**	
Lovastatin [Mevacor]	**Lipid-lowering agent—HMG-CoA reductase inhibitors**—inhibits synthesis of cholesterol precursor mevalonate; **decreases LDL, increases HDL, and decreases TG**	**High LDL, preventative after thrombotic event (e.g., MI, stroke)**	Reversible increase in LFTs; myositis	**Contraindicated in pregnant or lactating women and children**
α_2-Macroglobulin	Inhibits fibrinolysis			

(continued)

Therapeutic Agent (common name, if relevant) [trade name, where appropriate]	Class—Pharmacology and Pharmacokinetics	Indications	Side Effects or Adverse Effects	Contraindications or Precautions to Consider; Notes
Magnesium hydroxide (milk of magnesia)	**Antacid, osmotic laxative**—buffers gastric acid by raising pH	Peptic ulcer, gastritis, esophageal reflux, and constipation	**Diarrhea, hyporeflexia, hypotension, cardiac arrest, and hypokalemia**	**Can affect the absorption, bioavailability, or urinary excretion of drugs by changing the gastric pH, urinary pH, or gastric emptying**
Magnesium sulfate, magnesium citrate	**Osmotic laxative**		Magnesium toxicity (in renal insufficiency)	
Malathion	Organophosphate—inhibits cholinesterase	Least toxic organophosphate		
Mannitol [Osmitrol]	Osmotic diuretic—prevents isosmotic reabsorption of filtrate in **PCT, loop of Henle,** and **collecting tubule;** loss of Na^+ and all other filtered solutes in urine	Shock, drug overdose, decreased intracranial or intraocular pressure; maintenance of urine flow in rhabdomyolysis	Pulmonary edema, dehydration; contraindicated in anuria and CHF	Results in increased urine volume; readily filtered and not reabsorbed
Maprotiline	Blocks NE uptake	Major depression	Sedation, orthostatic hypotension	
Maraviroc	**Antiviral, CCR5 antagonist**—inhibits viral CCR5 coreceptor → blocks viral entry to host cell	**AIDS; patients on antiretroviral therapy with persistent viral replication**	**Fever, cough, upper respiratory infections, peripheral neuropathy, dizziness**	
Mebendazole [Vermox]	Anthelmintic—irreversible; inhibits glucose uptake	Hookworm, roundworm, threadworm, some cestodes		
Mecamylamine [Inversine]	Antihypertensive—nicotinic ganglionic blocker	Hypertension emergency; smoking cessation	Decreases GI motility, cycloplegia, hypotension, xerostomia	
Mechlorethamine (nitrogen mustard) [Mustargen]	Antineoplastic—DNA alkylation and cross-linking	Cancer	Nausea, vomiting, bone marrow suppression, alopecia, teratogenicity, carcinogenicity	
Meclizine [Antivert, Bonine]	Antiemetic agent—H_1 blocker	Emesis, vertigo	Teratogenic	
Mefloquine [Lariam]	Antimalarial—uncertain mechanism	Treatment of acute attack of chloroquine-resistant organisms	CNS: dizziness, disorientation, hallucinations, seizure, and depression; GI disturbances; nausea; vomiting; abdominal pain	
Melatonin	Promotes sleep	Clock shifting		Pineal hormone

Melphalan [Alkeran]	Antineoplastic—DNA alkylation and cross-linking	Cancer	Nausea, vomiting, bone marrow suppression (serious), alopecia, teratogenicity, carcinogenicity, pulmonary fibrosis, hypersensitivity	
Menotropin [Pergonal]	Mixture of FSH and LH	Secondary hypogonadism with infertility		
Meperidine [Demerol]	**Opioid agonist**	**Pain,** acute migraine attacks	**CNS excitation at high doses;** histamine release; antimuscarinic effects	**Contraindicated in patients with MAOI** (results in hyperpyrexia)
Mephenesin	Centrally acting muscle relaxant	Muscle spasms, tetanus contractions, orthopedic manipulation	Sedation	
Mepivacaine [Isocaine]	Anesthetic agent—blocks Na^+ channels intracellularly	Local anesthetic	Sleepiness, light-headedness, visual/audio disturbances, restlessness, nystagmus, shivering, tonic–clonic convulsion, death	
6-Mercaptopurine [Purinethol]	Antineoplastic—inhibits purine synthesis; disrupts DNA and RNA synthesis	Childhood leukemias	Myelosuppression	
Meropenem [Merrem]	**Carbapenem**—cell wall inhibitor; same mechanism as penicillin; bactericidal	**Broad spectrum—gram-positive cocci** (MSSA and *Streptococcus*), **gram-negative rods** (*Pseudomonas* and *Enterobacter* spp.), **anaerobes**	Reduced risk of seizure compared to imipenem	Stable to dihydropeptidase I, unlike imipenem
Metformin [Glucophage]	**Hypoglycemic agent, biguanide**—decreases hepatic gluconeogenesis, increases glycolysis → decreases serum glucose levels	First-line oral treatment for **type 2 diabetes**	**Lactic acidosis,** GI upset (diarrhea, nausea, and abdominal pain), metallic taste; decreased B_{12} absorption	Stop drug in patients undergoing studies or procedures involving **contrast**; contraindicated in patients with renal dysfunction
Methadone [Dolophine]	**Opioid agonist—synthetic**	**Maintenance therapy for heroin addiction, pain**	Respiratory depression; histamine release; constipation; nausea; miosis	
Methicillin	**Antibiotic—β-lactam, penicillin derivative,** cell wall inhibitor; same mechanism as penicillin; distinguished by activity against **penicillinase-producing *Staphylococcus*;** bactericidal	***Staphylococcal* infections** (except MRSA)	**Hypersensitivity reactions;** interstitial nephritis (methicillin)	Penicillinase resistant; MRSA is resistant to methicillin because of altered penicillin-binding protein target site
Methimazole [Tapazole]	**Antithyroid agent—inhibits peroxidase enzyme in thyroid → decreases synthesis of thyroid hormone**	**Hyperthyroidism**	**Agranulocytosis**	**Crosses the placenta; can cause fetal goiter, hypothyroidism, and aplasia cutis (fetal scalp defect)**

(continued)

Therapeutic Agent (common name, if relevant) [trade name, where appropriate]	**Class—Pharmacology and Pharmacokinetics**	**Indications**	**Side Effects or Adverse Effects**	**Contraindications or Precautions to Consider; Notes**
Methohexital [Brevital]	Anesthetic agent—barbiturate; prolongs IPSP duration	Antiepileptic; cerebral edema; anesthetic (stage 3 anesthetic)		Ultrashort acting
Methotrexate [Rheumatrex]	Antineoplastic—**folic acid analog (dihydrofolate reductase inhibitor); immunosuppressant**	**Rheumatoid arthritis,** bone marrow transplant, acute lymphocytic and myelogenous leukemia, choriocarcinoma, lung cancer, ectopic pregnancy	Oral and GI ulceration, **myelosuppression,** thrombocytopenia; leukopenia, hepatotoxicity, **fibrotic lung disease**	**Leucovorin is given as an adjuvant after treatment**
Methoxyflurane [Penthrane]	Anesthetic agent	General anesthetic	Nephrotoxic	No longer used
Methylcellulose [Citrucel]	**Bulk-forming laxative**—dietary fiber	Constipation	Impaction above strictures, fluid overload, gas, and bloating	
Methyldopa [Aldomet]	**Antihypertensive—**centrally acting sympathetic agent (α-agonist) $\rightarrow$ decreases sympathetic outflow from CNS	**Hypertension**	Sedation; hemolytic anemia	**Positive Coombs test**
Methylphenidate [Ritalin]	CNS stimulant—amphetamine; releases neurotransmitter from synapse	Stimulant; treatment of choice for **attention deficit hyperactivity disorder**		
Methysergide [Sansert]	**Antimigraine—**5-HT antagonist and weak vasoconstrictor	Prophylaxis of migraine	GI distress; inflammatory fibrosis of kidney, lung, and cardiac valves	**Contraindicated in patients with peripheral vascular disease, coronary artery disease, and pregnancy; patient placed on a drug holiday to prevent tachyphylaxis**
Methyltestosterone [Android, Virilon]	**Androgen—**androgen receptor agonist	**In men: hypogonadism, delayed puberty** (promotes secondary sex characteristics), and impotence; **in women: estrogen receptor–positive breast cancer**	**Masculinization (hirsutism), testicular atrophy,** prostate hyperplasia, prostate cancer, impotence, **stunt growth** (premature epiphyseal plate closure), and hyperlipidemia	Decreases testicular testosterone, leading to Leydig cell inhibition and gonadal atrophy
Metoclopramide [Reglan]	**GI stimulant—prokinetic agent; D_2-receptor antagonist; central and peripheral D_2 antagonism at low doses,** weak 5-HT_3 antagonism at high doses; enhances acetylcholine release, increases resting tone, contractility, lower esophageal sphincter tone, and motility (does not affect colon transit time)	**Diabetic** and **postoperative gastroparesis; nausea;** counteracts nausea of **migraine;** increases stomach motility	Sleepiness, fatigue, headache, insomnia, dizziness, nausea, akathisia, **dystonia,** and tardive dyskinesia	Interacts with **digoxin** and **diabetic agents; contraindicated in small bowel obstruction**

Metocurine [Metubine Iodide]	**Nondepolarizing neuromuscular blocker**			
Metolazone [Mykrox, Zaroxolyn]	Diuretic—decreases Na^+ reabsorption in the distal tubule by inhibiting the Na/Cl^- cotransporter; reduced peripheral resistance	Hypertension, CHF	Hypokalemia, hyperuricemia, hypovolemia, hyperglycemia (especially in diabetics), hypercalcemia, hypersensitivity reaction, Na^+ excretion in advanced renal failure	
Metoprolol [Lopressor, Toprol XL]	**Antihypertensive,** antiarrhythmic (class II)—β_1-selective blocker	**Hypertension, angina, MI, and antiarrhythmic**	**Impotence, asthma, bradycardia,** AV block, heart failure, sedation, and sleep alterations	
Metronidazole [Flagyl]	**Antibiotic, antiprotozoal—** penetrates cell membrane and gives off nitro moiety → forms toxic metabolites → reacts and damages DNA; bactericidal	***Bacteroides fragilis*** (especially for endocarditis and CNS); **pseudomembranous colitis** (*Clostridium difficile*); **amebiasis; giardiasis; trichomoniasis, bacterial vaginosis** (*Gardnerella vaginalis*), **peptic ulcer disease** (part of *Helicobacter pylori* triple therapy)	Nausea, vomiting, **disulfiram-like reaction to alcohol,** metallic taste, paresthesia, stomatitis, carcinogenic and mutagenic	**Contraindicated in pregnancy**
Metyrapone [Metopirone]	Inhibits cortisol synthesis	Diagnosis of pituitary dysfunction		
Mevastatin	Lipid-lowering agent—inhibits **HMG-CoA reductase; lowers LDL**	Hyperlipidemia (especially type II)	**Liver toxicity, myopathy,** mild GI disturbances	**Contraindicated in pregnant** or lactating women or in children
Mexiletine [Mexitil]	Antiarrhythmic (class IB)—Na^+ channel blocker			
Midazolam [Versed]	**Benzodiazepine; short acting**	**Preanesthetic medication; produces antegrade amnesia (loss of memory of events after administration) calming down the patient**	Circulatory and respiratory depression	**Flumazenil antagonizes CNS depression caused by benzodiazepines**
Mifepristone (RU-486)	**Antiprogesterone**—synthetic steroid, progesterone receptor blocker → blocks the effects of progesterone → myometrium contraction	**Termination of intrauterine pregnancy** (emergency postcoital contraceptive)	**Heavy bleeding, uterine cramping,** GI effects (nausea, vomiting, and anorexia)	Controversial "morning after" drug
Miglitol	Hypoglycemic agent, α-glucosidase inhibitor—inhibits intestinal brush border enzyme α-glucosidase→ delays sugar hydrolysis and glucose absorption → decreases postprandial hyperglycemia	Oral treatment for type 2 diabetes postprandially	Flatulence, cramps, and diarrhea; may reduce absorption of iron	Does not cause reactive hypoglycemia; decreases HbA_{1c}
Milrinone [Primacor]	Inotropic agent—phosphodiesterase inhibitor; increases contractility via increase in intracellular Ca^{2+}	CHF		

(continued)

APPENDIX I: **Drug Index**

Therapeutic Agent (common name, if relevant) [trade name, where appropriate]	Class—Pharmacology and Pharmacokinetics	Indications	Side Effects or Adverse Effects	Contraindications or Precautions to Consider; Notes
Mineral oil [Fleet Mineral Oil Enema]	**Laxative—hyperosmolar agent;** draws water into gut lumen → gut distension → promotes peristalsis and evacuation of bowel	**Preoperative patients;** short-term treatment of constipation		May interfere with the absorption of fat-soluble vitamins
Minoxidil [Loniten, Rogaine]	Antihypertensive—**K^+ channel opener →** hyperpolarizes and relaxes vascular smooth muscle	**Severe hypertension**	**Hypertrichosis,** pericardial effusion	
Mirtazapine	α_2-Antagonist → increases release of NE and 5-HT	Major depression (especially with insomnia)	**Weight gain,** dry mouth, increased appetite, and sedation	
Misoprostol [Cytotec]	**Cytoprotectant—PGE_1 analog → increased production and secretion of gastric mucosa barrier; decreased acid production;** cervical dilation, uterine contractions	**Prevents NSAID-induced peptic ulcers;** maintains patent ductus arteriosus; **induction of labor,** termination of pregnancy	**Diarrhea**	**Abortion-inducing drug,** contraindicated in women of childbearing age
Molindone [Moban]	Antipsychotic—blocks D_2 receptors	Psychosis	Parkinsonism, tardive dyskinesia	
Montelukast [Singulair]	**Leukotriene inhibitor;** reduces inflammation	**Asthma**		Not for acute attacks
Moricizine [Ethmozine]	Antiarrhythmic (class IC)—Na^+ channel blockers	Ventricular arrhythmia	Dizziness, nausea	
Morphine [Astramorph, Duramorph, Infumorph, Kadian, MS Contin, Oramorph, MSIR, Roxanol]	Opioid agonist—chronic oral dose converted to more potent morphine-6-glucuronide	Severe pain; general anesthetic; antitussive; antidiarrheal	Respiratory depression; histamine release; constipation; nausea; miosis	
Moxifloxacin [Avelox]	**Antibiotic—quinolone; inhibits DNA gyrase** (topoisomerase II) and **topoisomerase IV** → blocks DNA synthesis; bactericidal	**Less activity against gram-negative infections than other fluoroquinolones; gram-positive infections** *(Staphylococcus, Streptococcus)*; **intracellular: *Legionella*; anaerobes**	**GI disturbances, headache, dizziness, phototoxicity, cartilage damage (children, fetus), tendonitis** and **tendon rupture (adults), myalgias (children)**	**May elevate theophylline to toxic levels, causing seizure; contraindicated in pregnant women; divalent cations inhibit gut absorption, therefore cannot be taken with milk, antacids, or iron-containing preparations**
Muromonab (OKT3)	**Immunosuppressant—monoclonal antibody against CD3 on T lymphocytes**	Acute rejection of **renal transplants**		

Muscarine	**Muscarinic agonist**		Abdominal pain, diarrhea, bronchoconstriction	**Contraindicated in patients with peptic ulcer, asthma, hyperthyroidism, and Parkinson disease**
Nabilone [Cesamet]	Antiemetic—unknown mechanism; binds cannabinoid receptors and inhibits vomiting center in medulla	Emesis	Dry mouth, dizziness, inability to concentrate, disorientation, anxiety, tachycardia, depression, paranoia, psychosis	THC derivative
***N*-Acetylcysteine** [Mucomyst]	Breaks disulfide bonds; **mucolytic** (loosens mucus plugs)—**replenishes glutathione**	**Overdose of acetaminophen; liquefies sputum to assist expulsion;** also used to prevent contrast nephropathy	Unpleasant odor during administration	
Nadolol [Corgard]	Antihypertensive—antianginal; blocker	Hypertension, angina, **esophageal varices**		
Nafcillin	**Antibiotic—β-lactam, penicillin derivative,** cell wall inhibitor; same mechanism as penicillin; distinguished by activity against **penicillinase-producing *Staphylococcus;*** bactericidal	***Staphylococcal* infections** (except MRSA)	**Hypersensitivity reactions**	Penicillinase resistant; MRSA is resistant to methicillin and nafcillin because of altered penicillin-binding protein target site
Nalbuphine [Nubain]	Mixed agonist/antagonist of opioids	Similar to pentazocine		
Nalorphine	Mixed agonist/antagonist of opioids	Antagonizes the effects of morphine	Respiratory depression; analgesia	
Naloxone [Narcan]	**Antagonist of all opioids**	**Drug of choice for opioid antagonism**	**Ineffective to use against barbiturate overdose,** but safe	
Naltrexone [ReVia]	Antagonist of all opioids	Longer action than naloxone; can be used orally		
Naproxen [Naprosyn, Aleve]	**NSAID—reversibly inhibits COX** (both COX-1 and COX-2) → decreases prostaglandin synthesis	Inflammation, pain	GI distress, **GI ulcers,** coagulation disorders, aplastic anemia, metabolic abnormalities, hypersensitivity, renal damage	
Natamycin [Natacyn]	Antifungal—binds to cell membrane sterols (especially ergosterol); forms pores in membrane; fungicidal	Topical for fungal keratitis (eye)		
Nedocromil [Tilade]	Antiasthmatic; stabilizes membranes of mast cells and prevents mediator release	Asthma	Unpleasant taste	Not for acute asthmatic attacks
Nefazodone [Serzone]	Antidepressant—postsynaptic $5\text{-}HT_2$ antagonist	Depression		

(continued)

Therapeutic Agent (common name, if relevant) [trade name, where appropriate]	Class—Pharmacology and Pharmacokinetics	Indications	Side Effects or Adverse Effects	Contraindications or Precautions to Consider; Notes
Nelfinavir	**Antiviral, protease inhibitor—** protease responsible for final step of viral proliferation; inhibits protease in progeny virions → assembly of nonfunctional viruses	**AIDS (used in HAART)**	**GI irritation (nausea, diarrhea), hyperglycemia, hyperlipidemia, and lipodystrophy**	**All protease inhibitors end in -navir; metabolism occurs by cytochrome P450**
Neomycin [Mycifradin, Neosporin]	Antibiotic—aminoglycoside; binds 30S ribosome subunits; bacteriostatic at low concentration; bactericidal at high concentration	Reduction of gut flora	Renal damage, deafness	Inhibits absorption of digitalis; topical use
Neostigmine [Prostigmin]	**Inhibits cholinesterase**	**Paralytic ileus, neurogenic bladder, myasthenia gravis**		
Nevirapine	**Antiviral, nonnucleoside reverse transcriptase inhibitor—**binds viral reverse transcriptase and inhibits movement of protein domains → terminates viral DNA synthesis → prevents integration of viral genome into the host DNA	**AIDS (used in HAART)**	**Neutropenia, anemia, peripheral neuropathy, and rash**	
Niclosamide [Niclocide]	Anthelmintic—inhibits anaerobic metabolism	Tapeworms: *Taenia solium, Taenia saginata, Hymenolepis nana*		
Nicotine [Habitrol, NicoDerm, Nicotrol]	**Nicotinic agonist**	**Stops smoking**		
Nifedipine [Adalat, Procardia]	**Dihydropyridine Ca^{2+} channel blocker—**blocks voltage-gated Ca^{2+} channels of **vascular** smooth muscle	**Hypertension, angina pectoris, Prinzmetal angina, Raynaud phenomenon**	Peripheral edema, **flushing, dizziness**, and constipation	
Nitrofurantoin [Macrobid]	Antibiotic—urinary antiseptic; unknown mechanism of action	Gram-positive and gram-negative bacteria		Contraindicated in patients with renal insufficiency
Nitroglycerin	**Antianginal—stimulates synthesis of cGMP, leading to muscle relaxation via NO formation**	**Angina**	**Headache, orthostatic hypotension, syncope**	**Monday disease; short acting**
Nitrosoureas	Antineoplastic—alkylating agent; lipid-soluble	CNS tumors		
Nitrous oxide	Anesthetic agent	General anesthetic	Hypoxia	

Nizatidine [Axid]	**H_2 blocker—reversibly blocks histamine H_2 receptors → reduces gastric acid secretion**	**Peptic ulcer disease, gastritis, and esophageal reflux**	**Gynecomastia;** rare: confusion, dizziness, and headaches	**Crosses placenta; milder side effect profile** than cimetidine and ranitidine
Norethindrone	**Progesterone**—binds progesterone receptors	**Endometrial cancer,** amenorrhea, abnormal uterine bleeding, and **prevention of pregnancy**		Also used to prevent endometrial hyperplasia in postmenopausal women taking estrogen
Norfloxacin	**Antibiotic—quinolone; inhibits DNA gyrase** (topoisomerase II) and **topoisomerase IV** → blocks DNA synthesis; bactericidal	**Gram-negative infections** (especially UTI and bone): *Pseudomonas,* Enterobacteriaceae, and *Neisseria;* **gram-positive infections** (staphylococci)	**GI disturbances, headache, dizziness, phototoxicity, cartilage damage (children, fetus), tendonitis** and **tendon rupture (adults), myalgias (children)**	May elevate theophylline to toxic levels, causing seizure; divalent cations **inhibit gut absorption, therefore cannot be taken with milk, antacids, or iron-containing preparations**
Norgestimate	**Progesterone**—binds progesterone receptors	**Endometrial cancer,** amenorrhea, abnormal uterine bleeding, and **prevention of pregnancy**		Also used to prevent endometrial hyperplasia in postmenopausal women taking estrogen
Nortriptyline [Pamelor]	TCAs—inhibit **reuptake** of NE and 5-HT at neuronal synapses	Major depression, panic disorder, and anxiety	Sedation, **α-blocking effects** (orthostatic hypotension), **anticholinergic** (tachycardia, dry mouth, and urinary retention), hallucinations (in elderly), and confusion (in elderly); overdose toxicity results in **convulsions, coma, cardiotoxicity** (arrhythmias), respiratory depression, and hyperpyrexia	
NPH [Humulin N, Novolin N]	**Intermediate-acting insulin**—*see mechanism for regular insulin*	**Diabetes mellitus** (typically **type 1**)	**Hypoglycemia** (diaphoresis, vertigo, and tachycardia); insulin allergy; insulin antibodies; lipodystrophy	
Nystatin [Mycostatin]	Antifungal—binds to cell membrane sterols (especially ergosterol) → disrupting fungal membranes; fungicidal	**Mucosal candidal** infections (skin, vaginal, and GI)	Few	Used topically or as mouth rinse; too toxic for systemic use
Octreotide [Sandostatin]	**Synthetic analog of somatostatin**—decreases release of growth hormone, gastrin, secretin, VIP, CCK, glucagon, and insulin	**Acromegaly, glucagonoma, insulinoma carcinoid syndrome**	Nausea, cramps, and gallstones	
Ofloxacin [Floxin]	**Antibiotic—quinolone, DNA synthesis inhibitor; inhibits DNA gyrase** (topoisomerase II) and **topoisomerase IV** → blocks DNA synthesis; bactericidal	**Gram-negative infections** (especially UTI and bone): *Pseudomonas,* Enterobacteriaceae, and *Neisseria;* **gram-positive infections** (staphylococci); **intracellular: *Legionella***	**GI disturbances, headache, dizziness, phototoxicity, cartilage damage (children, fetus), tendonitis and tendon rupture (adults), myalgias (children)**	May elevate theophylline to toxic levels, causing seizure; divalent cations **inhibit gut absorption, therefore cannot be taken with milk, antacids, or iron-containing preparations**

(continued)

Therapeutic Agent (common name, if relevant) [trade name, where appropriate]	Class—Pharmacology and Pharmacokinetics	Indications	Side Effects or Adverse Effects	Contraindications or Precautions to Consider; Notes
Olanzapine [Zyprexa]	Atypical antipsychotic—blocks D_4, α_1, 5-HT, and muscarinic receptors	Schizophrenia, OCD, anxiety disorder, depression, mania, and Tourette syndrome	Agranulocytosis, **weight gain, diabetes; extrapyramidal** (occurs at a lower rate than typicals), **anticholinergic** (dry mouth, constipation), **alpha blockade** (hypotension), **histamine** (sedation); toxicity results in neuroleptic malignant syndrome (occurs at a lower rate than typicals)	
Omeprazole [Prilosec]	**Proton pump inhibitors—irreversibly inhibits H^+/K^+-ATPase in gastric parietal cells → decreases proton secretion by parietal cells**	Peptic ulcer disease, gastritis, esophageal reflux, and **Zollinger–Ellison syndrome**		**Inhibits cytochrome P450;** given with **clarithromycin** and **amoxicillin** for ***Helicobacter pylori***
Ondansetron [Zofran]	**Antiemetic—serotonin antagonist, 5-HT_3 blocker**	**Nausea** (caused by **cancer therapy** or **postoperative state**)	Headache, constipation, dizziness	
Oprelvekin [Neumega]	**IL-11** stimulates multiple stages of **thrombopoiesis,** increasing platelet production	**Thrombocytopenia**		
Orlistat [Xenical]	**Inhibits pancreatic lipases →** alters fat metabolism	**Obesity** (long term)	**Steatorrhea,** GI irritation, reduced absorption of fat-soluble vitamins, and headache	**Used in conjunction with modified diet**
Oseltamivir [Tamiflu]	**Antiviral—inhibits neuraminidase →** decreases release of progeny viruses	**Influenza A and B treatment and prophylaxis**		Begin within 2 days of onset of flu symptoms to decrease the duration and intensity of symptoms
Oxacillin [Bactocill]	Antibiotic—β-lactam; penicillinase resistant	*Staphylococcal* infections		
Oxaprozin [Daypro]	NSAID—mildly uricosuric	Acute gout		Contraindicated in patients with kidney stones
Oxazepam [Serax]	Antianxiety—benzodiazepine; enhances GABA; increases IPSP amplitude	Sedative, hypnotic, antiepileptic, anxiolytic		Recommended for use in elderly
Oxybutynin [Ditropan]	Antimuscarinic	Bladder/GI spasm; decreases acid in ulcer		

Oxycodone [Roxicodone]	**Partial opioid agonist** at mu receptor	Severe pain; general anesthetic	Respiratory depression, constipation, nausea	
Oxytocin [Pitocin, Syntocinon]	**Synthetic analog of oxytocin—stimulates uterine contraction and contraction of breast myoepithelial cells; milk letdown reflex**	**Induces labor; controls uterine hemorrhage**		
Paclitaxel [Taxol]	Antineoplastic—stabilizes polymerization of microtubules	Ovarian and breast cancer		
Pamidronate [Aredia]	Bone stabilizer—pyrophosphate analog; reduces hydroxyapatite crystal formation, growth, and dissolution, which reduces bone turnover	Hypercalcemia of malignancy, Paget disease, osteoporosis, hyperparathyroidism		
Pancuronium [Pavulon]	Nondepolarizing neuromuscular blocker			Minimal histamine release
Paroxetine [Paxil]	SSRIs—inhibit **reuptake** of 5-HT at neuronal synapses	Major depression, OCD, anorexia, and bulimia	Inhibits liver enzymes, nausea, agitation, **sexual dysfunction** (anorgasmia), **and** dystonic reactions	Contraindicated with **MAOIs** secondary to **serotonin syndrome** (hyperthermia, muscle rigidity, and cardiovascular collapse); allows time for antidepressant effect, usually takes 2–3 weeks
Penicillamine [Cuprimine, Depen]	Antiarthritis—anti-gold medicine; not specific; unknown mechanism; arthritis relief	**Rheumatic arthritis; copper poisoning; metal chelator**	Decreases vitamin B_6; bone marrow suppression; proteinuria; autoimmune syndrome	
Penicillin	**Antibiotic—β-lactam, cell wall inhibitor; binds penicillin-binding protein → inhibits transpeptidase** cross-linking of cell wall **→ inhibits bacterial cell wall synthesis → activates autolytic enzymes;** bactericidal	**Gram-positive cocci, gram-positive rods, gram-negative cocci, some anaerobes, enterococci,** and **spirochetes**	**Hypersensitivity reactions, neutropenia, thrombocytopenia, anemia, CNS effects, superinfection** (pseudomembranous colitis)	Not penicillinase resistant
Pentazocine [Talwin]	Mixed agonist/antagonist of opioids	Analgesia		Only mixed agonist/antagonist available orally
Pentobarbital [Nembutal Sodium]	Barbiturate—prolongs IPSP duration	Cerebral edema; anesthetic		
Pergolide [Permax]	Antiparkinsonian—dopamine agonist; inhibits prolactin release	Treats breast engorgement; inhibits lactation		
Phenazocine	Opioid agonist			

(continued)

APPENDIX I: **Drug Index**

Therapeutic Agent (common name, if relevant) [trade name, where appropriate]	Class—Pharmacology and Pharmacokinetics	Indications	Side Effects or Adverse Effects	Contraindications or Precautions to Consider; Notes
Phenelzine	**Antidepressant, MAOIs**—inhibits **degradation** of NE and 5-HT at neuronal synapses	**Atypical depression** (with hypersomnia, anxiety, sensitivity to rejection, and hypochondriasis)	**Hypertensive episodes** with ingestion of tyramine-containing foods or β-agonists, hyperthermia, and convulsions	Contraindicated with **SSRIs** and **meperidine** secondary to **serotonin syndrome** (hyperthermia, muscle rigidity, and cardiovascular collapse)
Phenobarbital	**Barbiturate—prolongs** IPSP duration	**Antiepileptic (partial and tonic–clonic); cerebral edema; anesthetic**	Sedation	Many drug interactions
Phenolphthalein [Ex-Lax]	**Stimulant laxative**—reduces absorption of electrolytes and water from gut	Constipation	Tumorigenic	
Phenoxybenzamine [Dibenzyline]	Antihypertensive—α-blocker; long acting; irreversible	Pheochromocytoma	Nasal congestion, miosis, orthostatic hypotension	
Phentolamine [Regitine]	**Antihypertensive—α-blocker**	**Diagnosis of pheochromocytoma;** hypertension (especially tyrosine induced)		
Phenylbutazone [Butazolidin]	**NSAID**	**Rheumatic arthritis, acute gout**	**Agranulocytosis, aplastic anemia**	
Phenylephrine [Neo-Synephrine, Nostril]	Nasal decongestant—α_1-agonist	Nasal decongestant	Hypertension	
Phenylzin	Antidepressant—MAOI; nonselective but isoenzyme A most important; irreversible	Depression		
Phenytoin [Dilantin]	**Antiepileptic—decreases Na^+ flux**	**Epilepsy (partial and tonic–clonic), digitalis-induced arrhythmia**	**Decreases folic acid; gingival hyperplasia; hirsutism; nystagmus**	**Induces cytochrome P450; saturable elimination**
Physostigmine [Eserine]	**Inhibits cholinesterase**	**Intestinal or bladder atony, glaucoma**		
Pilocarpine [Ocusert]	**Antiglaucoma—muscarinic agonist**	**Xerostomia; narrow- and open-angle glaucoma**	**Focusing problems, nausea, abdominal pain, sweating; high dose: bradycardia, hypotension**	**Contraindicated in patients with peptic ulcer, asthma, hyperthyroidism, and Parkinson disease**
Pindolol [Visken]	Antihypertensive, antiarrhythmic (class II)—β-blocker	Hypertension		

Pioglitazone [Actos]	Hypoglycemic agent, thiazolidinedione — binds PPARγ receptors; improves target cell response to insulin	Oral treatment for **type 2 diabetes**	**Weight gain,** edema, hepatotoxicity; increases LDL and TGs	Contraindicated in CHF
Piperacillin [Pipracil] **piperacillin-tazobactam** [Zosyn]	**Antibiotic—β-lactam, penicillin derivative,** cell wall inhibitor; same mechanism as penicillin; distinguished by activity against ***Pseudomonas*;** bactericidal	**Extended spectrum—** *Pseudomonas*; *Proteus*, and *Enterobacter* species	**Hypersensitivity reactions,** decreased platelet function	Not effective against penicillin-resistant *Staphylococcus*; **can be combined with clavulanic acid** (β-lactamase inhibitor) to enhance spectrum; administered IV
Pirenzepine	**Muscarinic antagonist—blocks M_1 receptors on ECL cells → decreases histamine secretion; blocks M_3 receptors on parietal cells → decreases acid secretion**	Peptic ulcer	**Tachycardia, dry mouth, and blurry vision** (difficulty accommodating)	
Piroxicam [Feldene]	NSAID			Long acting; contraindicated in the elderly
Platelet-activating factor (PAF)	Activation of platelets and PMN aggregation; increases vascular permeability			
Plicamycin [Mithracin]	Antineoplastic—inhibits DNA-directed RNA synthesis; decreases protein synthesis needed for bone reabsorption	Paget disease, hypercalcemia		
Polymyxins (colistin)	**Antibiotic—binds to cell membranes** → disrupt osmotic properties; bactericidal	**Gram-negative bacteria: *Pseudomonas* and coliforms; usually topical; can be used IV or nebulized for difficult-to-treat gram-negative infections**	**Neurotoxic, nephrotoxic** (acute renal tubular necrosis)	
Potassium	**Depresses ectopic pacemaker in hypokalemia**	**Digoxin toxicity**		
Potassium iodide [Thyro-Block]	Expectorant—increases bronchial secretions; high doses decrease release of thyroid hormone	Promotes cough; hyperthyroidism		
Pralidoxime (2-PAM) [Protopam]	**Acetylcholinesterase reactivator**	**Overdose of malathion/parathion organophosphates; must be used before aging occurs**		
Pramlintide [Symlin]	**Hypoglycemic agent, analog of amylin—**a pancreatic hormone secreted with insulin that decreases glucagon and delays gastric emptying	Injectable treatment for **type 2 diabetes**	Nausea, vomiting, hypoglycemia	

(continued)

Therapeutic Agent (common name, if relevant) [trade name, where appropriate]	Class—Pharmacology and Pharmacokinetics	Indications	Side Effects or Adverse Effects	Contraindications or Precautions to Consider; Notes
Pravastatin [Pravachol]	**Lipid-lowering agent—HMG-CoA reductase inhibitor**—inhibits synthesis of cholesterol precursor mevalonate; **decreases LDL, increases HDL, and decreases TG**	**High LDL, preventative after thrombotic event (e.g., MI, stroke)**	Reversible increase in LFTs; myositis	Contraindicated in pregnant or lactating women and children
Praziquantel [Biltricide]	Anthelmintic—increases membrane permeability causing loss of Ca^{2+}	Schistosomes, flukes	GI disturbances, headache, fever, urticaria	
Prazosin [Minipress]	**Antihypertensive—α_1-blocker →** vasodilation → decreases total peripheral resistance	**Pheochromocytoma, hypertension, BPH**	**Orthostatic hypotension,** dizziness, headache	First-dose orthostatic hypotension
Prednisone [Deltasone]	**Glucocorticoid—inhibits protein synthesis; reduces lymph node and spleen size; inhibits cell cycle activity of lymphoid cells; lyses T cells; suppresses antibody, prostaglandin, and leukotriene synthesis; blocks monocyte production of IL-1**	**Rheumatic arthritis, autoimmune disorders, allergic reaction, asthma, COPD, organ transplantation (especially during rejection crisis)**	**Osteoporosis; cushingoid reaction, psychosis, glucose intolerance, infection, hypertension, cataracts**	
Prilocaine [Citanest]	Anesthetic agent—blocks Na^+ channels intracellularly	Local anesthetic	Sleepiness, light-headedness, visual/audio disturbances, restlessness, nystagmus, shivering, tonic–clonic convulsions, death	
Primaquine phosphate	**Antimalarial**—unknown mechanism	Prevents relapse of *Plasmodium ovale* and *Plasmodium vivax* malaria; prophylaxis for *Plasmodium falciparum* malaria	GI disturbances, mild anemia; **marked hemolysis in G6PD-deficient individuals; prolongs QT interval**	
Probenecid [Benemid]	Antigout—increased secretion of uric acid (uricosuric)—competes with uric acid for **reabsorption in the kidney**	Chronic gout therapy	**Caution: should not be used in patients with sulfa allergies;** rash; GI disturbances; drowsiness	Should not be used to treat acute gout or patients with uric acid stones
Probucol [Bifenabid, Lesterol]	Lipid-lowering agent—lowers HDL and LDL; mechanism unknown	Hyperlipidemia	Prolongs QT interval; GI disturbances	Contraindicated in patients with heart disease
Procainamide [Pronestyl, Procanbid]	**Antiarrhythmic (class IA)—Na channel blocker**	**Ventricular arrhythmia**	**Lupus-like syndrome**	

Procaine [Novocain]	Anesthetic agent—blocks Na^+ intracellularly	Local anesthetic	Sleepiness, light-headedness, visual/audio disturbances, restlessness, nystagmus, shivering, tonic–clonic convulsions, death	
Procarbazine [Matulane]	Antineoplastic—DNA alkylation and strand breakage; inhibits nucleic acid and protein synthesis	Cancer		
Prochlorperazine [Compazine]	**Antiemetic—dopamine (D_2 receptor) antagonist**	**Nausea;** counteracts nausea of **migraine**	Teratogenic	
Progesterone [Progestasert]	**Hormone—causes secretory changes in endometrium and breast; necessary to maintain pregnancy**	**Endometrial cancer,** amenorrhea, abnormal uterine bleeding, and **prevention of pregnancy**	**Long-lasting suppression of menses, endometriosis, hirsutism, bleeding disorders, nausea, breast tenderness, hyperpigmentation, gallbladder disease, migraines, hypertension**	Also used to prevent endometrial hyperplasia in postmenopausal women taking estrogen
Prolactin	**Hormone—stimulates lactation**			
Promethazine [Phenergan]	**Antihistamine, antiemetic—** D_2-receptor antagonist; H_1 blocker	Counteracts nausea of **migraine;** allergies; **motion sickness**	Sedation, CNS depression, atropine-like effects, allergic dermatitis, blood dyscrasias, **teratogenicity,** acute antihistamine poisoning	
Propafenone [Rythmol]	Antiarrhythmic (class IC)—Na^+ channel blocker			
Propantheline	**Muscarinic antagonist—blocks M_1 receptors on ECL cells → decreases histamine secretion; blocks M_3 receptors on parietal cells → decreases acid secretion**	Peptic ulcer	**Tachycardia, dry mouth, and blurry vision** (difficulty accommodating)	
Propofol [Diprivan]	Anesthetic agent	General anesthetic; fast-acting for ambulatory or outpatients	Seizure	
Propranolol [Inderal]	β-Blocker, antimigraine—decreases cAMP and calcium currents → increases PR interval, suppresses abnormal pacemakers, especially in AV node	**Ventricular tachycardia, supraventricular tachycardia, and** slowing ventricular rate during **atrial fibrillation and atrial flutter**	**Impotence, exacerbation of asthma, bradycardia,** AV block, CHF, sedation, and sleep alteration	

(continued)

Therapeutic Agent (common name, if relevant) [trade name, where appropriate]	Class—Pharmacology and Pharmacokinetics	Indications	Side Effects or Adverse Effects	Contraindications or Precautions to Consider; Notes
Propylthiouracil [Propyl-Thyracil]	Antithyroid agent—inhibits peroxidase enzyme in thyroid → decreases synthesis of thyroid hormone	**Hyperthyroidism**	**Agranulocytosis**	**Crosses the placenta and can cause fetal goiter and hypothyroidism;** preferred to methimazole in treating pregnant women with moderate to severe hyperthyroidism
Pseudoephedrine [Sudafed]	α- and β-Adrenergic agonist; stimulates bronchial relaxation (β), increases heart rate (β), and vasoconstriction (α)	Nasal decongestant; sinusitis, upper respiratory tract infection	Tachycardia, increased BP, hypersensitivity	Sales limited; precursor for illicit methamphetamine synthesis
Protriptyline [Vivactil]	Antidepressant—TCA; blocks NE, 5-HT, muscarinic, α_1, and histamine receptors	Depression, anxiety	Tremors (NE block), anorexia (5-HT block), anticholinergic (muscarinic block), hypotension (α_1 block), drowsiness (histamine block)	
Psyllium [Perdiem Fiber]	**Bulk-forming laxative**—dietary fiber	Constipation	Impaction above strictures, fluid overload, gas, and bloating	
PTH	Increases plasma Ca^{2+} levels by increasing reabsorption in kidney; activates vitamin D, which aids in Ca^{2+} absorption from gut; resorbs Ca^{2+} from bone; decreases phosphate reabsorption by kidney	Used to distinguish between hypoparathyroidism and pseudohypoparathyroidism		
Pyrantel [Antiminth, Reese's Pinworm Medicine]	Anthelmintic—depolarizing neuromuscular blocker causing spastic paralysis in worms	*Ascaris* (roundworm), *Ancylostoma* (hookworm), threadworm		
Pyrazinamide	Antibiotic—postulated mechanism involves inhibition of enzyme pyrazinamidase → inhibition of fatty acid synthesis	*Mycobacterium*	Impairs liver function	
Pyridostigmine [Mestinon]	**Inhibits cholinesterase**	**Myasthenia gravis**		
Pyrimethamine [Daraprim]	Antimalarial—inhibits dihydrofolate reductase	Malaria	Large doses causes megaloblastic anemia	

Quetiapine [Seroquel]	Atypical antipsychotic—blocks D_2, 5-HT, α_1, and H_1 receptors	Schizophrenia, acute mania	Suicide attempt in major depression, arrhythmia, **extrapyramidal** (occurs at a lower rate than typicals), **anticholinergic** (occurs at lower rate than other agents), **alpha blockade** (hypotension), and **histamine** (sedation); toxicity results in neuroleptic malignant syndrome (occurs at a lower rate than typicals)	
Quinapril [Accupril]	**Antihypertensive—ACE inhibitor** → inhibits conversion of angiotensin I to II → decreases Ang II levels → prevents vasoconstriction from Ang II	Hypertension, CHF, post-MI; prevention/treatment of diabetic nephropathy	**Cough, angioedema, hyperkalemia,** renal insufficiency (especially in bilateral renal artery stenosis)	Contraindicated in pregnancy (fetal renal malformation)
Quinidine [Quinaglute]	**Antiarrhythmic (class IA)— Na^+ channel blocker**	**Arrhythmias, acute malarial infection**	**May precipitate arrhythmias at high doses; nausea; vomiting; diarrhea; cinchonism: tinnitus, headache, nausea, disturbed vision; renal damage; hemolytic anemia; purpura; agranulocytosis**	**Torsades des pointes, inhibits cytochrome P450**
Quinine	**Antimalarial—unknown mechanism**	**Suppression and treatment of acute attack of chloroquine-resistant organism; leg cramps**	**Cinchonism: tinnitus, headache, nausea, disturbed vision; renal damage; hemolytic anemia; purpura; agranulocytosis**	
Quinolones	**Antibiotic—blocks DNA synthesis by inhibiting DNA gyrase**	**Gram-negative infections (especially UTI and bone): *Pseudomonas,* Enterobacteriaceae, and *Neisseria*; gram-positive infections; intracellular: *Legionella***	**GI disturbances, headache, dizziness, phototoxicity, cartilage damage**	**May elevate theophylline to toxic levels, causing seizure; divalent cations inhibit gut absorption, therefore cannot be taken with milk antacids, or iron-containing preparations**
Radioiodide (I-131)	**Destroys thyroid gland**	**Hyperthyroidism**	**Hypothyroidism**	
Raloxifene [Evista]	**Selective estrogen receptor modulator—breast (estrogen antagonist); endometrium (estrogen antagonist):** prevents proliferation of endometrium; **bone (estrogen agonist):** decreases bone turnover, increases bone density; **cardiovascular (estrogen agonist):** decreases LDL	**Osteoporosis, breast cancer**	**Hot flashes,** sinusitis, weight gain, muscle pain, leg cramps, **increased risk of blood clots**	Unlike estrogen, raloxifene **does not decrease HDL**

(continued)

Therapeutic Agent (common name, if relevant) [trade name, where appropriate]	Class—Pharmacology and Pharmacokinetics	Indications	Side Effects or Adverse Effects	Contraindications or Precautions to Consider; Notes
Raltegravir	**Antiviral, integrase inhibitor**—inhibits the final step in integration of viral DNA into host DNA	**HAART**	**Neutropenia, pancreatitis, hepatotoxicity, hyperglycemia**	
Ranitidine [Zantac]	**H_2 blocker—blocks histamine H_2 receptors reversibly → decreases proton secretion by parietal cells**	**Peptic ulcer disease, gastritis, and esophageal reflux**	**Gynecomastia, impotence,** decreased libido in males, **confusion, dizziness, and headaches**	**Crosses placenta; decreases renal excretion of creatinine; cytochrome P450 inhibitor**
Repaglinide [Prandin]	Hypoglycemic agent—**meglitinide; acts at pancreatic islet cell** to reduce K^+ efflux, increases Ca^{2+} influx, **increases secretion of insulin**	Oral treatment for **type 2 diabetes**	**Hypoglycemia**	
Reserpine [Rauserfia]	Antihypertensive—prevents storage of monoamines in synaptic vesicle	Hypertension	**Mental depression,** sedation, nasal stuffiness, and diarrhea	
RhoGAM	**Rh immunoglobulin**	**Prevents hemolytic disease of the newborn**		
Ribavirin	**Antiviral—guanosine analog;** inhibits IMP dehydrogenase → decreases synthesis of guanine nucleotides	**Hepatitis C when given with interferon**	**Hemolytic anemia, elevated bilirubin; teratogen**	
Rifampin [Rifadin]	**Antibiotic—inhibits DNA-dependent RNA polymerase**	***Mycobacterium*; reduces resistance to dapsone when used in treatment of leprosy; prophylaxis in close contacts of people with *Neisseria meningitidis* meningitis**	**Turns body fluid orange in color; liver damage**	**Interferes with birth control pills by increasing estrogen metabolism; induces cytochrome P450**
Risedronate [Actonel]	**Bone stabilizer—bisphosphonate; pyrophosphate analog;** reduces hydroxyapatite crystal formation, growth, and dissolution, which reduces bone turnover	**Hypercalcemia of malignancy, Paget disease, osteoporosis, hyperparathyroidism**	**Pill-induced esophagitis**	

Risperidone	Atypical antipsychotic—blocks D_2, 5-HT, α_1, and H_2 receptors	Schizophrenia, useful for positive and negative symptoms	Agranulocytosis, **extrapyramidal** (occurs at a lower rate than typicals), **anticholinergic** (occurs at lower rate than other agents), **alpha blockade** (hypotension), and **histamine** (sedation); toxicity results in neuroleptic malignant syndrome (occurs at a lower rate than typicals)	Second-line agent used for refractory schizophrenia
Ritodrine [Yutopar]	B_2-agonist —> uterine relaxation	Inhibits preterm labor		
Ritonavir [Norvir]	**Antiviral, protease inhibitor—** protease responsible for final step of viral proliferation; inhibits protease in progeny virions → assembly of nonfunctional viruses	**AIDS (used in HAART)**	**GI irritation (nausea, diarrhea), hyperglycemia, hyperlipidemia, and lipodystrophy**	**All protease inhibitors end in -navir; metabolism occurs by cytochrome P450**
Rituximab	Monoclonal antibodies; binds to CD20 receptor on tumor cells, resulting in lysis	Non-Hodgkin lymphoma	Fever, rigor, chills; nausea, hypersensitivity; tumor lysis syndrome; irregular heart rhythms; infection; pancytopenia	
Ropivacaine	Anesthetic agent—blocks Na^+ intracellularly	Local anesthetic	Sleepiness, light-headedness, visual/audio disturbances, restlessness, nystagmus, shivering, tonic–clonic convulsion, death	
Rosiglitazone [Avandia]	Hypoglycemic agent, thiazolidinedione — binds PPARγ receptors, improves target cell response to insulin	Oral treatment for **type 2 diabetes**	**Weight gain,** edema, hepatotoxicity; increases LDL, and TGs; **may increase risk of MI**	Contraindicated in CHF
Salmeterol [Serevent]	**Antiasthmatic—long-acting β_2-agonist, leads to relaxation of smooth muscle**	Asthma prophylaxis	**Hand tremor,** headache, nervousness, dizziness, cough, stuffed nose, runny nose, ear pain, muscle pain/cramps, sore throat	Not in acute asthmatic attack
Saquinavir [Invirase]	**Antiviral, protease inhibitor—** protease responsible for final step of viral proliferation; inhibits protease in progeny virions → assembly of nonfunctional viruses	**AIDS (used in HAART)**	**GI irritation (nausea, diarrhea), hyperglycemia, hyperlipidemia, and lipodystrophy**	**All protease inhibitors end in -navir; metabolism occurs by cytochrome P450**
Sargramostim [Leukine]	**Granulocyte-macrophage colony–stimulating factor**	**Recovery of bone marrow (e.g., bone marrow transplant failure)**	Hypertension	
Sarin/soman	Irreversibly inhibits cholinesterase	Rapidly fatal		"Nerve gas"

(continued)

APPENDIX I: Drug Index

Therapeutic Agent (common name, if relevant) [trade name, where appropriate]	Class—Pharmacology and Pharmacokinetics	Indications	Side Effects or Adverse Effects	Contraindications or Precautions to Consider; Notes
Saxagliptin [Onglyza]	**Hypoglycemic agent, DPP-IV inhibitor**—prevents degradation of incretin hormones → decreased glucagon, increased insulin	Oral treatment for **type 2 diabetes**	Diarrhea, constipation, edema	
Scopolamine	**Anticholinergic**—M_1-muscarinic receptor antagonist	**Motion sickness** prophylaxis	**Dry mouth,** drowsiness, and **vision disturbances**	**Delivered transdermally**
Scorpion toxin	Presynaptic neuromuscular junction blocker; overstimulates acetylcholine release			
Secobarbital [Seconal Sodium]	Antiepileptic—anesthetic agent; barbiturate; prolongs IPSP duration	Epilepsy, cerebral edema		
Selegiline [Eldepryl]	Antiparkinsonian—increases dopamine by inhibiting MAO, irreversibly	Parkinson disease		
Senna [Senokot]	**Stimulant laxative;** increases peristalsis	Constipation	Electrolyte imbalances (chronic use); melanosis coli	
Sertraline [Zoloft]	SSRIs—inhibit **reuptake** of 5-HT at neuronal synapses	Major depression, OCD, anorexia, bulimia, and anxiety	Inhibits liver enzymes, nausea, agitation, **sexual dysfunction** (anorgasmia), and dystonic reactions	Contraindicated with **MAOIs** secondary to **serotonin syndrome** (hyperthermia, muscle rigidity, and cardiovascular collapse); allows time for antidepressant effect, usually takes 2–3 weeks
Sevoflurane [Sevorane, Ultane]	Anesthetic agent	General anesthetic		
Sibutramine [Meridia]	**Sympathomimetic serotonin and NE reuptake inhibitor**	**Obesity** (short term and long term)	Hypertension, tachycardia	
Sildenafil [Viagra]	**Phosphodiesterase type 5 inhibitor (cGMP-specific)—increased cGMP** → smooth muscle relaxation → increased blood flow in the corpus cavernosum → penile erection	**Erectile dysfunction**	**Abnormal vision** (impaired blue-green color vision), **UTIs, cardiovascular events, priapism, dyspepsia,** headache, and flushing	Risk of hypotension (fatal) in patient taking nitrates
Simvastatin [Zocor]	Lipid-lowering agent—HMG-CoA **reductase inhibitors**—inhibit synthesis of cholesterol precursor mevalonate; **decreases LDL, increases HDL, and decreases TG**	**High LDL, preventative after thrombotic event (e.g., MI, stroke)**	Reversible increase in LFTs; myositis	Contraindicated in pregnant and lactating women and children

Sitagliptin [Januvia]	**Hypoglycemic agent, DPP-IV inhibitor**—prevents degradation of incretin hormones → decreased glucagon, increased insulin	Oral treatment for **type 2 diabetes**	Diarrhea, constipation, edema	
Sodium nitroprusside	Antianginal—direct release of NO → increases cGMP → vasodilator (arterial dilation)	**Hypertensive emergency, CHF, and angina**	Cyanide toxicity, hypotension	Short acting, given IV
Somatostatin [Zecnil]	**Hormone—decreases release of growth hormone, gastrin, secretin, VIP, CCK, glucagon, and insulin**	**Acromegaly, glucagonoma, insulinoma**	**Nausea, cramps, gallstones**	
Sotalol [Betapace]	Antiarrhythmic (class III)—K^+ channel blocker	Torsades de pointes		
Spectinomycin [Trobicin]	**Aminoglycoside antibiotic**—protein synthesis inhibitor; **irreversibly binds 30S ribosome** subunits; **bacteriostatic** at low concentration; **bactericidal** at high concentration	**Broad spectrum:** gram-negative rods; good for **bone** and **eye** infections; *Proteus, Pseudomonas, Enterobacter, Klebsiella,* and *Escherichia coli*	**Ototoxicity, renal toxicity, neuromuscular blockade,** nausea, vomiting, vertigo, allergic rash, superinfections	Used to treat gonorrhea in those allergic to penicillin
Spironolactone [Aldactone]	Potassium-sparing diuretic—binds to intracellular aldosterone steroid receptors in **collecting tubules;** blocks induction of Na^+ channels and Na^+/ATPase synthesis or blocks Na channels directly (amiloride, triamterene); loss of Na^+, Cl^- in urine	Hyperaldosteronism, potassium depletion, and CHF	**Hyperkalemic metabolic acidosis, gynecomastia** (spironolactone), and antiandrogen effects	Results in decreased secretion of K^+ and H^+, which can lead to **hyperkalemic metabolic acidosis;** often given in combination with a thiazide
Streptokinase [Streptase]	**Thrombolytic—plasminogen activator**	**Lysis of clots**	**Hemorrhage**	
Streptomycin	**Aminoglycoside antibiotic**—protein synthesis inhibitor; **irreversibly binds 30S ribosome** subunits; **bacteriostatic** at low concentration; **bactericidal** at high concentration	**Broad spectrum:** gram-negative rods; good for **bone** and **eye** infections; *Proteus, Pseudomonas, Enterobacter, Klebsiella,* and *Escherichia coli;* **tuberculosis and other mycobacteria**	**Ototoxicity, renal toxicity, neuromuscular blockade, nausea,** vomiting, vertigo, allergic rash, superinfections	
Strychnine	Acts on the postsynaptic Renshaw cell; binds to glycine receptor (mimics effect of tetanus)	Depression	Fatal seizures	Rat poison
Succinylcholine [Anectine]	**Depolarizing neuromuscular blocker**	**Rapid-sequence intubation**	**Increases intraocular pressure; succinylcholine apnea in genetically defective pseudocholinesterase; malignant hyperthermia if given with halothane**	**Contraindicated in patients with glaucoma and patients taking antibiotics**

(continued)

Therapeutic Agent (common name, if relevant) [trade name, where appropriate]	**Class—Pharmacology and Pharmacokinetics**	**Indications**	**Side Effects or Adverse Effects**	**Contraindications or Precautions to Consider; Notes**
Sucralfate [Carafate]	Antiulcer—protective coating of GI lining	Reduces the effect of gastric acid on mucosa	Constipation	
Sulfamethoxazole, sulfisoxazole, sulfadiazine	**Antibiotic—sulfonamide, DNA synthesis inhibitor; competitive inhibitor of dihydropteroate synthetase (blocks folic acid synthesis);** bacteriostatic	**Broad spectrum: gram-positive UTI; chlamydial infection of genital tract and eye; treatment of nocardiosis**	**Forms crystals in kidney and bladder, causing damage; hypersensitivity reaction; photosensitivity; kernicterus (in infants); hemolysis (in G6PD deficiency)**	Displaces other drugs such as warfarin from albumin
Sulfasalazine	**Anti-inflammatory—sulfapyridine (antibacterial)** and **mesalamine (anti-inflammatory)**	Ulcerative colitis, Crohn disease	Malaise, nausea, **sulfonamide toxicity,** and reversible **oligospermia**	**Activated by colonic bacteria**
Sulfinpyrazone [Anturane]	Antigout—increased secretion of uric acid (uricosuric)—competes with uric acid for **reabsorption in the kidney**	Chronic gout therapy	**Caution: should not be used in patients with sulfa allergies;** GI irritation; hypersensitivity reaction; agranulocytosis	Should not be used to treat acute gout or patients with uric acid stones
Sulindac [Clinoril]	Anti-inflammatory—prodrug sulfide	Chronic inflammation (arthritis)		
Sumatriptan [Imitrex]	**Antimigraine—agonist at 5-HT_{1d} receptors**	**Acute attack of migraine**		
Tacrine [Cognex]	**Alzheimer agent—noncompetitive cholinesterase inhibitor; muscarinic agonist**	**Alzheimer disease**	**Hepatotoxicity**	
Tacrolimus (FK506) [Prograf]	**Immunosuppressant—blocks activation of T-cell transcription factors; involved in IL synthesis**	**Transplant rejection**	**Nephrotoxic; neurotoxic; hyperglycemia; GI disturbances**	
Tamoxifen [Nolvadex]	**Selective estrogen receptor modulator—competitively binds estrogen receptors; breast (estrogen antagonist):** prevents proliferation of estrogen receptor positive tumor cells; **endometrium (partial agonist); bone (agonist):** decreases bone turnover, increases bone density	**Treats estrogen-dependent breast cancer in postmenopausal women;** reduces contralateral breast cancer; osteoporosis prevention	**May increase risk of endometrial cancer;** increased risk of blood clots; **hot flashes;** flushing	

Temazepam [Restoril]	Benzodiazepine—enhances GABA, increases IPSP amplitude	Sedative, hypnotic, antianxiety, antiepileptic		
Tenofovir disoproxil fumarate (TDF)	**Antiviral, nucleoside reverse transcriptase inhibitor—adenosine analog** → inhibits viral reverse transcriptase	**HAART**	**Nausea, vomiting, headache, renal dysfunction**	
Terazosin [Hytrin]	Antihypertensive—α_1-blocker	Pheochromocytoma, hypertension, BPH	Postural hypotension	
Terbinafine [Lamisil]	Antifungal—inhibits squalene-2,3-epoxidase	Orally for onychomycosis, topically for dermatophytes	Hepatotoxicity	
Terbutaline [Brethine, Bricanyl, Brethaire]	**β_2-agonist**—bronchodilator; relaxes uterus	**Bronchodilates to treat asthma; inhibits preterm labor;** treatment of uterine hyperstimulation		
Tetanus toxin	**Acts at the presynaptic Renshaw cell; prevents glycine release**		Seizures	
Tetracaine [Pontocaine]	Anesthetic agent—blocks Na^+ channels intracellularly	Local anesthetic	Sleepiness, light-headedness, visual/audio disturbances, restlessness, nystagmus, shivering, tonic–clonic convulsions, death	
Tetracycline [Achromycin, Sumycin, Topicycline]	**Tetracycline antibiotic—protein synthesis inhibitor; binds 30S ribosome subunits** → prevents attachment of tRNA; bacteriostatic	**Broad-spectrum including atypical pathogens: *Chlamydia, Rickettsia, Mycoplasma pneumoniae, V. cholerae, U. urealyticum, Francisella tularensis, Helicobacter pylori,* and *Borrelia burgdorferi*** (Lyme disease)	**Liver toxicity, GI distress, depression of bone/teeth development, photosensitivity, Fanconi syndrome**	**Contraindicated in pregnancy and children; divalent cations inhibit gut absorption, therefore cannot take with milk, antacids, or iron-containing preparations; renally eliminated**
THC (active ingredient in marijuana)	Unknown mechanism; binds cannabinoid receptors and inhibits vomiting center in medulla	Antiemetic	Dry mouth, dizziness, inability to concentrate, disorientation, anxiety, tachycardia, depression, paranoia, psychosis	
Theobromine	Unknown mechanism; stimulates CNS, cardiac muscle; relaxes smooth muscle; produces diuresis; increases cerebral vascular resistance			

(continued)

Therapeutic Agent (common name, if relevant) [trade name, where appropriate]	Class—Pharmacology and Pharmacokinetics	Indications	Side Effects or Adverse Effects	Contraindications or Precautions to Consider; Notes
Theophylline [Aerolate, Elixophyllin, Respbid, Slo-bid, Slo-Phyllin, Theo-24, Theo-Dur, Theolair, Uniphyl]	Methylxanthines—unknown mechanism; postulated to inhibit phosphodiesterase → decreases cAMP hydrolysis → promotes bronchodilation; stimulates CNS, cardiac muscle; relaxes smooth muscle; produces diuresis; increases cerebral vascular resistance	Asthma	Cardiotoxicity, neurotoxicity	Metabolized by cytochrome P450; narrow therapeutic window; tolerance develops
Thiabendazole [Mintezol]	**Anthelmintic**	***Strongyloides; Ancylostoma*** (hookworm); ***Enterobius*** (pinworm); ***Trichuris*** (whipworm)	Vomiting, diarrhea, dizziness, bradycardia, hypotension, paresthesia, yellow vision, angioneurotic edema, perianal rashes	
6-Thioguanine	Antineoplastic—inhibits purine synthesis; disrupts DNA and RNA synthesis	Adult leukemias	Bone marrow suppression	
Thiopental [Pentothal]	Anesthetic agent—barbiturate; prolongs IPSP duration	Antiepileptic; cerebral edema; anesthetic (stage 3 anesthetic)	Laryngospasm during stage 3 induction	
Thioridazine [Mellaril]	Antipsychotic—phenothiazines; muscarinic, blocks D_2 and α_1 receptors	Psychosis	**Extrapyramidal** (dystonia, akinesia, akathisia, and tardive dyskinesia), **anticholinergic** (dry mouth, constipation), **alpha blockade** (hypotension), and **histamine** (sedation); toxicity results in neuroleptic malignant syndrome (rigidity, myoglobinuria, autonomic instability, and hyperpyrexia)	**Cardiac toxicity (prolongs QT interval); atropine-like effects** are very common; antimuscarinic effects exacerbate tardive dyskinesia; visual impairment has been reported
Thiotepa [Thioplex]	Antineoplastic—unknown mechanism	Cancer		
Thiothixene [Navane]	Antipsychotic—thioxanthene; blocks D_2, α_1, and H_1 receptors	Psychosis	Anticholinergic effects	
Thrombopoietin	Recombinant human thrombopoietin	**Thrombocytopenia**		
Ticarcillin [Ticar], **ticarcillin-clavulanate** [Timentin]	**Antibiotic—β-lactam, penicillin derivative,** cell wall inhibitor; same mechanism as penicillin; distinguished by activity against ***Pseudomonas;*** bactericidal	**Extended spectrum**—*Pseudomonas, Proteus,* and *Enterobacter* spp.	**Hypersensitivity reactions,** decreased platelet function	Not effective against penicillin-resistant *Staphylococcus*; can be **combined with clavulanic acid** (β-lactamase inhibitor) to enhance spectrum; administered IV

Ticlopidine [Ticlid]	**Inhibits ADP-induced platelet aggregation;** acts on ADP receptor	**Transient ischemic attack, stroke**		
Timolol [Betimol, Blocadren, Timoptic]	Antiglaucoma—antihypertensive; β-blocker	Hypertension, MI, glaucoma	Asthma, bradycardia	
Tizanidine [Zanaflex]	Centrally acting muscle relaxant—presynaptic inhibition of motor neurons; acts like clonidine on α_2 receptor	Muscle spasms from spinal cord injury; multiple sclerosis		
Tobramycin [Tobrex]	**Antibiotic—aminoglycoside,** protein synthesis inhibitor; **irreversibly binds 30S ribosome** subunits; **bacteriostatic** at low concentration; **bactericidal** at high concentration	**Broad spectrum:** gram-negative rods; good for **bone** and **eye** infections; *Proteus, Pseudomonas, Enterobacter, Klebsiella,* and *Escherichia coli*	**Ototoxicity, renal toxicity, neuromuscular blockade,** nausea, vomiting, vertigo, allergic rash	
Tocainide [Tonocard]	Antiarrhythmic (class IB)—Na^+ channel blocker			
Tolbutamide [Orinase]	**Hypoglycemic agent, first-generation sulfonylurea**—closes potassium channels located in β-cell membrane → reduces K^+ efflux, increases Ca^{2+} influx → increases secretion of insulin	Oral treatment for **type 2 diabetes**	**Hypoglycemia,** GI disturbances, muscle weakness, mental confusion	Rarely used due to toxicity
Tolnaftate [Tinactin, Desenex]	Antifungal—unknown mechanism; bactericidal	Topical against *Trichophyton rubrum, Trichophyton tonsurans,* and *Trichophyton mentagrophytes*		
Topiramate [Topamax]	Antiepileptic—blocks Na^+ channels	Add-on drug for epilepsy		
Torsemide [Demadex]	Loop diuretic; inhibits $Na^+/K^+/Cl^-$ channels	Diuresis	Ototoxicity, metabolic alkalosis, hypokalemia, hyperglycemia, hyperuricemia	
t-PA (alteplase) [Activase]	**Thrombolytic—plasminogen activator**	**Lysis of clots**	**Hemorrhage**	
Tramadol [Ultram]	Analgesic—similar to opioid agonist	Chronic pain of osteoarthritis	Nausea, vomiting, constipation, and drowsiness	
Tranexamic acid (AMCHA) [Cyklokapron]	Thrombotic agent—competitive inhibitor of plasminogen activation	Inhibits fibrinolysis; promotes thrombosis		

(continued)

Therapeutic Agent (common name, if relevant) [trade name, where appropriate]	Class—Pharmacology and Pharmacokinetics	Indications	Side Effects or Adverse Effects	Contraindications or Precautions to Consider; Notes
Tranylcypromine [Parnate]	Antidepressant—MAOI; inhibits degradation of NE and 5-HT at neuronal synapses; nonselective, but isoenzyme A most important; reversible	**Atypical depression** (with hypersomnia, anxiety, sensitivity to rejection, and hypochondriasis)	**Hypertensive episodes** with ingestion of tyramine-containing foods or β-agonists, hyperthermia, and convulsions	Contraindicated with **SSRIs** and **meperidine** secondary to **serotonin syndrome** (hyperthermia, muscle rigidity, and cardiovascular collapse); only reversible MAOI
Trazodone [Desyrel]	Atypical antidepressant—inhibits reuptake of serotonin	Major depression (especially with insomnia), insomnia	Sedation, nausea, **priapism,** and postural hypotension	
Tretinoin [Retin-A]	Retinoids—inhibits microcomedo formation and existing lesions; makes keratinocytes in sebaceous follicles less adherent and easier to remove	Acne, skin cancer	Photosensitivity	
TRH (protirelin) [Relefact TRH]	Stimulates TSH and prolactin release	Diagnosis of thyroid disease		
Triamcinolone	**Glucocorticoid**—inhibits protein synthesis; reduces lymph node and spleen size; inhibits cell cycle activity of lymphoid cells; lyses T cells; suppresses antibody, prostaglandin, and leukotriene synthesis; blocks monocyte production of IL-1	Addison disease, rheumatic arthritis, autoimmune disorders, allergic reaction, asthma, organ transplantation (especially during rejection crisis)	**Osteoporosis, cushingoid reaction, psychosis, glucose intolerance, infection, hypertension, cataracts, peptic ulcers**	
Triamterene [Dyrenium]	Potassium-sparing diuretic—binds to intracellular aldosterone steroid receptors in **collecting tubules;** blocks induction of Na^+ channels and Na^+/ATPase synthesis and blocks Na channels directly; loss of Na^+, Cl^- in urine	Hyperaldosteronism, potassium depletion, and CHF	**Hyperkalemic metabolic acidosis, gynecomastia** (spironolactone), and antiandrogen effects	Results in decreased secretion of K^+ and H^+, which can lead to **hyperkalemic metabolic acidosis;** often given in combination with a thiazide
Triazolam [Halcion]	Benzodiazepine—enhances GABA; increases IPSP amplitude	Sedative, hypnotic, antianxiety	Paranoia; violent behavior; antiepileptic	
Trientine	Metal chelator	Copper poisoning, Wilson disease		
Trifluridine ophthalmic [Viroptic]	Antiviral—thymidine derivative; inhibits DNA polymerase; inhibits DNA synthesis	DNA viruses		

Trihexyphenidyl [Artane]	Antiparkinsonian—muscarinic blocker	Parkinson disease		
Triiodothyronine (T_3) [Triostat]	Synthetic analog of thyroid hormone T_3	**Hypothyroidism**	Tachycardia, heat intolerance, tremors, and arrhythmia	
Trimethaphan [Arfonad]	Antihypertensive—nondepolarizing nicotinic blocker	Hypertension (short term)		
Trimethoprim [Proloprim, Trimpex]	**Antibiotic—DNA synthesis inhibitor; competitive inhibition of dihydrofolate reductase** (blocks folic acid synthesis); bacteriostatic	**Gram-negative UTI; combined with sulfonamides to treat UTI, otitis media, chronic bronchitis, shigellosis, *Salmonella,* and PCP**	Megaloblastic anemia, leukopenia, and granulocytopenia	Supplementation with folic acid may help pancytopenia
TSH (thyrotropin) [Thyrogen]	**Increases output of thyroid hormone**	**Assesses thyroid function; increases uptake of I-131 in thyroid carcinoma**		
d-Tubocurarine [Tubarine]	**Nondepolarizing neuromuscular blocker**	Topical for dermatophytes (especially tinea pedis)	Paralysis	
Undecylenic acid [Desenex]	Antifungal—unknown mechanism; fungistatic			
Urofollitropin [Metrodin]	FSH analog	Infertility		
Urokinase [Abbokinase]	**Thrombolytic agent—plasminogen activator**	**Lysis of clots**	**Hemorrhage**	
Valacyclovir [Valtrex]	**Antiviral—guanosine analog;** inhibits DNA polymerase	**HSV, VZV, EBV, and CMV at high doses**	**GI disturbances, CNS and renal problems, headache, tremor, rash**	**Longer lasting than acyclovir**
Valproic acid [Depakene]	**Antiepileptic—blocks Na^+ channels and increases GABA**	**Epilepsy: partial, absence, and tonic–clonic**	**Liver toxicity, pancreatitis; potentially fatal**	
Valsartan [Diovan]	**Antihypertensive**—Ang II receptor blockers → prevents vasoconstriction from Ang II	**Hypertension**	Fetal renal toxicity, **hyperkalemia**	
Vancomycin [Vancocin]	**Antibiotic—cell wall inhibitor;** binds to D-alanyl-D-alanine portion of cell wall → inhibits cell wall glycopeptide polymerization → stops bacterial cell wall synthesis; usually bactericidal	**Serious infections by gram-positive bacteria: *Streptococcus, Staphylococcus,* and some anaerobes (especially *Clostridium difficile*)**	**Ototoxicity, nephrotoxicity, thrombophlebitis, and diffuse flushing—"red man syndrome" caused by histamine release**	Can prevent red man syndrome by pretreatment with antihistamines and slow infusion; resistance occurs when bacteria change amino acid in cell wall to D-alanyl-D-lactate

(continued)

Therapeutic Agent (common name, if relevant) [trade name, where appropriate]	Class—Pharmacology and Pharmacokinetics	Indications	Side Effects or Adverse Effects	Contraindications or Precautions to Consider; Notes
Vardenafil	**Phosphodiesterase type 5 inhibitor (cGMP-specific)**—increased cGMP → smooth muscle relaxation → increased blood flow in the corpus cavernosum → penile erection	**Erectile dysfunction**	**Abnormal vision** (impaired blue-green color vision), **UTIs, cardiovascular events, priapism, dyspepsia,** headache, and flushing	Risk of hypotension (fatal) in patient taking nitrates
Vasopressin [Pitressin]	**Antidiuretic—recruits water channels to luminal membrane in collecting duct**	**Antidiuresis; treats central diabetes insipidus**	**Overhydration; allergic reaction; larger doses: pallor, diarrhea, and hypertension; coronary constriction; chronic rhinopharyngitis**	**Also known as antidiuretic hormone**
Vecuronium [Norcuron]	Nondepolarizing neuromuscular blocker			
Venlafaxine [Effexor]	**Antidepressant, anti-anxiolytic—serotonin and NE reuptake inhibitor**	**Depression, generalized anxiety disorder, social phobia**	Sweating, **nausea, constipation,** anorexia, somnolence, dry mouth, dizziness, **insomnia, and hypertension;** nervousness, abnormal dreams, tremor, abnormal vision, impotence, and anorgasmia	
Verapamil [Calan, Isoptin]	**Non-dihydropyridine Ca^{2+} channel blockers**—block voltage-gated Ca^{2+} channels of **cardiac** smooth muscle	**Hypertension, angina pectoris, arrhythmia**	Cardiac depression, peripheral edema, **flushing, dizziness**, and constipation	
Vidarabine [Vira-A]	Antiviral—adenosine analog; inhibits DNA polymerase	Herpes (also topical for HSV keratitis); varicella	GI disturbances; CNS, bone marrow suppression; liver and kidney dysfunction	
Vinblastine [Velban]	**Antineoplastic—blocks polymerization of microtubules**	**Hodgkin disease**	Peripheral neuritis	
Vincristine [Oncovin]	**Antineoplastic—blocks polymerization of microtubules**	**Acute leukemia**	**Peripheral neuritis**	
Vitamin A (retinol) [Aquasol A]	Vitamin	Night blindness, xerophthalmia	Hyperkeratosis	
Vitamin B_1 (thiamine)	**Vitamin**	**Alcoholics (prophylaxis for Wernicke–Korsakoff syndrome)**		**Decrease results in beriberi**
Vitamin B_{12} [Cyanocobalamin]	**Vitamin**	**Megaloblastic anemia**		
Vitamin B_2 (riboflavin)	Vitamin—component of flavin compounds: FMN, FAD			Inhibits chlorpromazine; decreased results in skin, oral, and ocular lesions

Vitamin B_3 (nicotinic acid, niacin)	Vitamin—component of nicotinic compounds: NAD, NADH	Maintains integrity of skin, decreases VLDL and LDL, raises HDL	Flushing, pruritus, myopathy, hepatotoxicity	Decrease results in dermatitis, diarrhea, dementia, and death
Vitamin B_5 (pantothenic acid)	Vitamin—component of CoA			
Vitamin B_6 (pyridoxine)	Vitamin	Protein metabolism; neurotransmitter synthesis	Neuritis, convulsions	Isoniazid decreases amount
Vitamin C (ascorbic acid)	Vitamin	Maintains collagen; oxidation—reduction reactions		Decrease results in scurvy
Vitamin D (calcitriol) [Rocaltrol]	**Vitamin**—binds to receptors in cytoplasm; alters gene expression and protein synthesis; **increases bone resorption of Ca^{2+}; increases renal and intestinal absorption of Ca^{2+} and phosphate**	**Rickets, osteomalacia, hypocalcemia, hypoparathyroidism, osteoporosis**		
Vitamin E	**Vitamin—antioxidant**	**Possible prophylaxis for heart disease**		**Decrease results in abortion, creatinuria, and ceroid pigment**
Vitamin K (phytonadione) [Mephyton]	**Vitamin—enhances clotting factors**	**Bleeding disorders**		**Decreased in children of mothers taking phenytoin or phenobarbital**
Voriconazole [Vfend]	**Antifungal—inhibits ergosterol synthesis,** preventing cell membrane formation	Serious invasive fungal infections (**invasive aspergillosis**, invasive candidiasis)	**Vision disturbances (blurred vision, light sensitivity)**, GI disturbances, hepatotoxicity	
Warfarin [Coumadin]	**Anticoagulant—inhibits potassium epoxide regeneration**	**Thrombosis**	**Bleeding**	**Contraindicated in pregnancy, patients with liver, CNS, and hemostatic disease; 99% exists protein bound; extremely sensitive to cytochrome P450 system**
Yohimbine	Impotence therapy—α_2 antagonist			
Zafirlukast [Accolate], montelukast [Singulair]	**Antiasthma** agent—antileukotriene; **blocks leukotriene receptors (leukotriene D_4 [LTD_4]) →** prevents bronchoconstriction and inflammatory cell infiltrate	Asthma (especially aspirin-induced asthma)		
Zanamivir [Relenza]	**Antiviral—inhibits neuraminidase** → decreases release of progeny viruses	**Influenza A and B treatment and prophylaxis**		Begin within 2 days of onset of flu symptoms to decrease the duration and intensity of symptoms

(continued)

Therapeutic Agent (common name, if relevant) [trade name, where appropriate]	Class—Pharmacology and Pharmacokinetics	Indications	Side Effects or Adverse Effects	Contraindications or Precautions to Consider; Notes
Zidovudine (ZDV; formerly azidothymidine [AZT]) [Retrovir]	**Antiviral, nucleoside reverse transcriptase inhibitor**—inhibits viral reverse transcriptase → prevents integration of DNA copy of viral genome into the host DNA	**AIDS (used in HAART); pregnant women with HIV** to reduce fetal transmission	**Neutropenia, anemia** (megaloblastic anemia), **peripheral neuropathy, pancreatitis, and lactic acidosis**	
Zileuton	**Antiasthma agent-5-lipoxygenase inhibitor** → inhibits conversion of arachidonic acid to leukotriene → prevents bronchoconstriction and inflammatory cell infiltrate	**Improves asthma**		
Zolpidem [Ambien]	Binds to benzodiazepine receptor but is not a benzodiazepine	Insomnia		

5-HT, 5-hydroxytryptamine (serotonin); ACE, angiotensin-converting enzyme; ACTH, adrenocorticotropic hormone; ADP, adenosine diphosphate; AMCHA, 4-(aminomethyl) cyclohexane carboxylic acid; AML, acute myelocytic leukemia; APSAC, anisoylated plasminogen streptokinase activator complex; AST/ALT, aspartate aminotransferase/alanine aminotransferase; ATPase, adenosine triphosphatase; AV, atrioventricular; BAL, blood alcohol level; BBB, blood–brain barrier; BCNU, bischloroethylnitrosourea; BP, blood pressure; BPH, benign prostatic hypertrophy; cAMP, cyclic adenosine monophosphate; CCK, cholecystokinin; CCR5, C-C chemokine receptor 5; cGMP, cyclic guanosine monophosphate; CHF, congestive heart failure; CMI, cell-mediated immunity; CMV, cytomegalovirus; CNS, central nervous system; CoA, coenzyme A; COPD, chronic obstructive pulmonary disease; COX, cyclooxygenase; DAG, diacylglycerol; DCT, distal convoluted tubule; dCTP, deoxycytidine triphosphate; DHEA, dehydroepiandrosterone; DPPV-IV, dipeptidyl peptidase-IV; EBV, Epstein–Barr virus; ECG, electrocardiogram, electrocardiography; ECL, enterochromaffin-like; EtOH, ethanol; FAD, flavin adenine dinucleotide; FMN, flavin mononucleotide; FSH, follicle-stimulating hormone; G6PD, Glucose-6-phosphate dehydrogenase; GABA, γ-aminobutyric acid; GI, gastrointestinal; GLP-1, glucagon-like peptide-1; GnRH, gonadotropin-releasing hormone; HAART, highly active antiretroviral therapy; HDL, high-density lipoprotein; HLA, human leukocyte antigen; HMG-CoA, 3-hydroxy-3-methylglutaryl coenzyme A; HSV, herpes simplex virus; IFN, interferon; IL, interleukin; IMP, inosine 5′ monophosphate; IP_3, inositol triphosphate; IPSP, inhibitory postsynaptic potential; IV, intravenous; LDL, low-density lipoprotein; L-DOPA, levodopa (levo-3, 4-dihydroxyphenylalanine); LFT, liver function test; LH, luteinizing hormone; MAO, monoamine oxidase; MAO_b, monoamine oxidase B; MAOI, monoamine oxidase inhibitor; MI, myocardial infarction; MOA, mechanism of action; MRSA, methicillin-resistant *Staphylococcus aureus*; MSIR, morphine sulfate instant release; MSSA, methicillin-sensitive *Staphylococcus aureus*; NAD, nicotinamide adenine dinucleotide; NADH, reduced nicotinamide adenine dinucleotide; NE, norepinephrine; NMDA, N-methyl-D-aspartate; NO, nitric oxide; NPH, neutral protamine Hagedorn; NSAID, nonsteroidal anti-inflammatory drug; OCD, obsessive compulsive disorder; PCOS, polycystic ovary syndrome; PCP, *Pneumocystis carinii* pneumonia; PCT, proximal convoluted tubule; PDA, patent ductus arteriosus; PGE_1, prostaglandin E_1; PGE_2, prostaglandin E_2; $PGF_{2\alpha}$, prostaglandin $F_{2\alpha}$; PMN, polymorphonuclear; PPAR-γ, peroxisome proliferator-activated receptor-γ; PTH, parathyroid hormone; PTT, partial thromboplastin time; PVC, premature ventricular contraction; Rh, rhesus [factor]; SA, sinoatrial; SLE, systemic lupus erythematosus; SSRI, selective serotonin reuptake inhibitor; TCA, tricyclic antidepressant; TG, triglycerides; THC, tetrahydrocannabinol; TNF, tumor necrosis factor; tPA, tissue plasminogen activator; TRH, thyrotropin-releasing hormone; tRNA, transfer RNA; TSH, thyroid-stimulating hormone; UTI, urinary tract infection; VIP, vasoactive intestinal peptide; VLDL, very low-density lipoprotein; VZV, varicella-zoster virus; WBC, white blood cell.

APPENDIX II: **Bug Index**

BACTERIA

Name	Morphology	Pathogenesis	Description of Disease	Laboratory Findings, Notes	Transmission	Prevention and Therapy
Actinomyces israelii	Gram-positive; filamentous; anaerobic	Unknown	Actinomycosis—oral, thoracic, pelvic, or peritoneal abscesses with draining sinus tracts	Forms filaments; sulfur granules	Dental disease or trauma	Penicillin and drainage
Bacillus anthracis	Gram-positive; rod with square ends; capsule of D-glutamate (only protein capsule); non-motile; spore former; aerobic	Anthrax toxin—edema factor (exotoxin); protective antigen for cell entry; lethal factor (zinc MP increases TNF)	Anthrax—three clinical syndromes: cutaneous (black eschar); inhalational (respiratory symptoms and widened mediastinum); and GI (abdominal pain)	Medusa head colonies; catalase positive	Spores from animals (usually cattle)	Attenuated strain human vaccine; penicillin; ciprofloxacin; doxycycline
Bacillus cereus	Gram-positive; rod; spore former; aerobic	Spores germinate when rice is reheated; enterotoxins—emetic toxin (heat stable), diarrhea toxin (heat labile)	Food poisoning—early vomiting and late diarrhea		Enters through the GI tract via reheated rice	Avoid reheated rice and beans; treatment is symptomatic; cephalosporin
Bacteroides fragilis	Gram-negative; bacilli; anaerobic; capsulated; no exotoxin	Capsule; weak endotoxin	Infections below diaphragm; peritonitis; bacteremia; pelvic inflammatory disease; foul-smelling abscess; sepsis	Mixed infections; pleomorphic	Deep penetrating wounds; wound debridement	Metronidazole, clindamycin
Bordetella pertussis	Gram-negative; coccobacilli; capsule	Noninvasive infection of bronchial epithelium; pertussis toxin (two subunits)—A subunit ADP ribosylates adenylate cyclase, increasing cAMP; whereas B subunit causes attachment; tracheal cytotoxin destroys ciliated epithelial cells, resulting in cough	Whooping cough; three stages of disease: catarrhal, paroxysmal coughing, and convalescent	Culture nasopharynx onto 10%–15% blood agar (Bordet-Gengou agar); slide agglutination test	Droplet nuclei	Acellular pertussis vaccine (at 2, 4, and 6 months) or whole inactive cells; erythromycin (use in catarrhal stage or prophylaxis for sick contacts); treatment in paroxysmal coughing stage is supportive
Borrelia burgdorferi	Spirochete; microaerophilic; flagella	Invasion and replication in the bloodstream; immune response to organism results in pathology	Lyme disease—erythema chronicum migrans with involvement of the heart, joints, and CNS	Common in the northeastern, midwestern, and western United States	Deer ticks; serology	Avoid ticks; wear long pants in wooded areas; doxycycline and penicillin

(continued)

BACTERIA *(Continued)*

Name	Morphology	Pathogenesis	Description of Disease	Laboratory Findings, Notes	Transmission	Prevention and Therapy
Brucella spp.	Gram-negative; coccobacillus; facultative; intracellular	Catalase; LPS; inhibits release of peroxidase in macrophages	Undulant fever—macrophages engulf and then rerelease into the bloodstream; granulomas; drenching night sweats	Serology	Contaminated milk and cheese; droplets; contact with infected animals	Pasteurization of dairy products; tetracycline plus streptomycin
Campylobacter jejuni	Gram-negative; comma-shaped bacilli; motile	Enterotoxin with antigenic diversity stimulates cAMP; incubation 2–6 days	Gastroenteritis—greenish, watery, foul-smelling diarrhea followed by bloody stools with fever	Microaerophilic; Campy plate; diarrhea in college students; oxidase positive	Milk, water, poultry	Symptomatic; self-limiting
Chlamydia trachomatis	Obligate intracellular	Replicates within host lysosomes, using host's cellular machinery	Strains A–C: blindness; strains D–K: nongonococcal urethritis, cervicitis; strains L1–L3: lymphogranuloma venereum	Leading cause of preventable blindness in the world; inactive form extracellular (elementary body) and metabolically active form intracellular (reticulate body)	Sexual contact or via birth canal	Tetracycline, azithromycin
Chlamydophila pneumoniae	Obligate intracellular	Replicates within host lysosomes, using host's cellular machinery	Pneumonia, bronchitis, and pharyngitis; rarely, Guillain-Barré syndrome, arthritis, and meningoencephalitis	Cell culture or other advanced lab testing required to make a definitive diagnosis; treatment is usually empiric	Person-to-person	Macrolides (azithromycin, clarithromycin), doxycycline
Chlamydophila psittaci	Obligate intracellular	Replicates within host lysosomes, using host's cellular machinery	Psittacosis—dry cough with CNS symptoms (photophobia and headache)	Giemsa stain; inactive form extracellular (elementary body) and metabolically active form intracellular (reticulate body)	Aerosol of dried bird feces	Tetracycline, quinolones, azithromycin
Clostridium botulinum	Gram-positive; rod; spore former; anaerobic	Botulinum toxin inhibits release of acetylcholine at neuromuscular junction resulting in flaccid paralysis; exotoxins A, B, and E	Botulism (weakness and respiratory paralysis); food, wound, and infant types; floppy baby syndrome; dysphagia; constipation	Toxin in blood	Spores from contaminated food/canned foods	Trivalent antitoxin; sterilization of canned foods; cook to inactivate toxin; respiratory support
Clostridium difficile	Gram-positive; rod; spore former; anaerobic	Exotoxins A and B—A (cholera-like) causes fluid release and hemorrhagic necrosis; B (diphtheria-like) damages mucosa and causes pseudomembrane formation	Antibiotic-associated pseudomembranous colitis; bloody diarrhea	ELISA detects toxin B in the stool sample	Hospital workers	Withdraw causative antibiotics (classically clindamycin); oral metronidazole, oral vancomycin

Clostridium perfringens	Gram-positive; rod; spore former; anaerobic	α-Toxin (damages cell membranes); γ-toxin (tissue necrosis and hemolysis); cholera-like heat-labile enterotoxin (food poisoning—watery diarrhea); spores establish in GI and produce enterotoxins	Gas gangrene; food poisoning; anaerobic cellulites	Large rods found in food; double zone of hemolysis	Grows in traumatized tissue (muscle); spores in food and soil germinate in reheated foods (stews, soups)	Clean and debride wounds; cook food well
Clostridium tetani	Gram-positive; rod; spore former (tennis racquet shaped); anaerobic	Tetanus toxin (exotoxin)—blocks release of inhibitory neurotransmitters	Tetanus: lockjaw (trismus), spastic paralysis (opisthotonos), and sardonic grin (risus sardonicus)	Usually not recovered by culture	Spore entry via wound (e.g., a rusty nail)	Toxoid vaccine (2, 4, 6, and 18 months); booster every 10 years; tetanus Ig (passive immunity); penicillin
Corynebacterium diphtheriae	Gram-positive; rod; club shaped; arranged in V or L form; not spore former	Exotoxin—A subunit ADP ribosylates EF-2, and B subunit binds toxin to the cell; phage conversion	Diphtheria—pseudomembrane forms in the throat; bull neck; systemic toxemia	Tellurite plate (Loffler's medium) grows black colonies	Airborne droplets	Inactivated toxoid vaccine; antitoxin (neutralizes unbound toxin); penicillin; erythromycin
Coxiella burnetii	Obligate intracellular	Unknown	Q fever	Only rickettsia not transmitted to humans by an arthropod vector; occupational hazard for tanners, sheep shearers, and dairy farmers	Inhalation of aerosols of urine and feces; transplacental	Tetracycline
Enterococcus faecalis	Gram-positive; cocci	Lipoteichoic acid	Urinary, biliary, and cardiovascular infections; endocarditis	Catalase negative; bacitracin resistant; variable hemolysis; grows in 6.5% NaCl/Lancefield group D	Normal flora of gut gaining access to blood	Penicillin or ampicillin and an aminoglycoside
Escherichia coli	Gram-negative; bacilli	Endotoxin—septic shock; heat-labile enterotoxin (LT): increased cAMP leads to diarrhea; heat-stable enterotoxin (ST) stimulates guanylate cyclase to cause diarrhea; pili: adhere to epithelium especially in UTIs; verotoxin (O157:H7): Shigella-like toxin in enterohemorrhagic *E. coli* (EHEC) that inhibits 28S rRNA to cause bloody diarrhea	UTI; sepsis; neonatal meningitis; enteropathogenic *E. coli* (EPEC): traveler's diarrhea; enterotoxigenic *E. coli* (ETEC): watery diarrhea; enteroinvasive *E. coli* (EIEC): dysentery; EHEC: bloody diarrhea, hemolytic uremic syndrome	Oxidase—cysteine agar	Transplacental; fecal–oral route; foodborne	UTIs: trimethoprim-sulfamethoxazole, ciprofloxacin; sepsis: cephalosporins; traveler's diarrhea: rehydration
Francisella tularensis	Gram-negative; rod; intracellular	Capsule; intracellular within macrophages; granuloma formation	Painful lymph nodes; glandular and ocular ulcers	Serology	Zoonotic via rabbits and ticks	Live attenuated vaccine; streptomycin; thorough cooking of meat

(continued)

BACTERIA *(Continued)*

Name	Morphology	Pathogenesis	Description of Disease	Laboratory Findings, Notes	Transmission	Prevention and Therapy
Gardnerella vaginalis	Gram variable; bacillus; anaerobic	Unknown	Vaginosis—watery discharge, fishy odor	Clue cells (epithelial cells coated with bacteria); whiff test	Sexually transmitted	Metronidazole
Haemophilus ducreyi	Gram-negative; bacilli	Virulence via pili	Chancroid with pain and purulent exudate	Lesions similar to those of syphilis; lymphadenopathy	Sexually transmitted	Azithromycin, ceftriaxone
Haemophilus influenzae	Gram-negative; coccobacilli; polysaccharide capsule (polyribitol phosphate)	IgA protease degrades antibody and attaches to respiratory tract; capsule (type B) prevents phagocytosis	Infantile meningitis; epiglottitis; number 2 cause of otitis media and sinusitis	Needs heme (factor X) and NAD (factor V) to grow; chocolate agar; check CSF	Respiratory droplets	Hib vaccine (B-type capsule conjugated to diphtheria toxoid as a carrier protein); ceftriaxone
Helicobacter pylori	Gram-negative; bacilli; motile; flagella	Urease results in ammonia production and subsequent gastric damage	Peptic ulcers (type B gastritis)	Microaerophilic; Campy plate; urea breath test; urease positive; serology ELISA; biopsy	Ingestion	Triple therapy: amoxicillin, omeprazole, and clarithromycin; quadruple therapy: bismuth, tetracycline, metronidazole, and omeprazole
Klebsiella pneumoniae	Gram-negative; bacilli; capsule; positive quellung reaction	Large capsule hinders phagocytosis	Pneumonia, particularly in malnourished alcoholics; UTI; bacteremia	Currant jelly sputum (thick bloody sputum)	Aspiration of respiratory droplets	Cephalosporins
Legionella pneumophila	Gram-negative; bacilli	Endotoxin affects smokers, alcoholics, and those older than 55 years of age	Legionnaire disease (atypical pneumonia)	Dieterle silver stain; cysteine required for culture; urine test for Legionella antigen	Aerosol from environmental water sources and contaminated air conditioning system	Erythromycin, quinolones
Listeria monocytogenes	Gram-positive; rod; arranged in V or L form; tumbling motility; not spore former	Grows intracellularly in macrophages; listeriolysin-O cytotoxic	Meningitis and sepsis in newborns and immunocompromised individuals	Small, gray colonies; β-hemolysis; motility; serology	Transferred to humans by animals or their feces; unpasteurized milk; contaminated vegetables, cheese, and cabbage	Ampicillin and gentamicin; trimethoprim-sulfamethoxazole
Moraxella catarrhalis	Gram-negative; diplococcus		Upper respiratory tract infection; number 3 cause of otitis media and sinusitis		Transmitted by respiratory secretions	Azithromycin; penicillin resistant (100% strains make β-lactamase)
Mycobacterium avium-intracellulare (MAC)	Acid-fast bacilli	Unknown	TB-like disease in immunocompromised individuals		From the soil and water to immunocompromised individuals	Azithromycin plus ethambutol plus rifampin

Mycobacterium leprae	Acid-fast bacilli; obligate intracellular	Tuberculoid: cell-mediated response causes damage; lepromatous: anergy of CD8 cells leads to uncontrolled replication	Leprosy—tuberculoid and lepromatous; lesions in cool parts of body	Cannot be grown in culture but is harvested in the footpads of armadillos; acid-fast stain of infected areas; lepra cells (modified mononuclear epithelioid cells containing acid-fast bacilli)	Prolonged contact, especially with the lepromatous form	Dapsone and rifampin for tuberculoid form (6-month treatment); clofazimine, dapsone, and rifampin for lepromatous form (2-year treatment)
Mycobacterium tuberculosis	Acid-fast bacilli; aerobic; high lipid cell walls (mycotic acids and wax D)	Cord factor; granulomas and caseation	Primary TB (chronic pneumonia), secondary TB (reactivation, hemoptysis), military TB (disseminated), latent TB	Ziehl–Neelsen stain; slow-growing (3–8 weeks) on Lowenstein–Jensen medium; niacin positive; PPD positive if >10 cm after 48 hours	Droplets from coughing	BCG vaccine with live attenuated organisms (rarely used in the United States); isoniazid, rifampin, ethambutol, pyrazinamide initially, then isoniazid plus rifampin to complete 6–9 months of therapy
Mycoplasma pneumoniae	Obligate intracellular; not seen on a Gram stain; smallest free-living organism; only bacteria with cholesterol in membrane (no cell wall)	Hydrogen peroxide and lytic enzymes resulting in damage to the respiratory tract	Walking pneumonia; bullous myringitis (inflamed tympanic membrane); common in young adults (college)	Positive cold agglutinin; highest incidence in 5- to 15-year-olds	Respiratory droplets	Erythromycin
Neisseria gonorrhoeae (gonococcus)	Gram-negative; cocci; coffee bean–shaped pairs; no polysaccharide capsule	Endotoxin (lipid A); pili with variation; proteins I, II, III (porin, adhesin, autoagglutination); IgA protease penicillinase plasmid	Urethral and vaginal infections; discharge; salpingitis and PID; neonatal conjunctivitis; septic arthritis	Thayer-Martin agar; only glucose fermentation; oxidase positive; also check for chlamydia caused by common coinfection	Sexual contact; newborns; symptomatic in men but not usually in women	Condoms; erythromycin or silver nitrate in neonates; ceftriaxone; spectinomycin and tetracycline
Neisseria meningitidis (meningococcus)	Gram-negative; diplococci; coffee bean–shaped pairs; polysaccharide capsule (antiphagocytic)	Endotoxin (LPS) contains lipid A; capsule; IgA protease; pili variation; deficiencies in late-acting complement components; asplenic patients	Meningitis; petechial rash; pharyngitis; Waterhouse–Friderichsen syndrome	Glucose and maltose fermentation; oxidase positive; lumbar puncture with high protein and low glucose; grows on Thayer-Martin agar	Respiratory droplets	Vaccine, rifampin, or ciprofloxacin (prophylaxis for close contacts); penicillin G or ceftriaxone
Nocardia asteroides	Acid-fast; gram-positive branching bacillus; aerobic	Lysosome-phagosome fusion inhibited; immunocompromised individuals at risk	Nocardiosis—lung, heart, kidney, and brain abscesses	Forms filaments	Airborne particles from soil; noncommunicable	Sulfonamides
Pasteurella multocida	Gram-negative; coccobacillus;		Diffuse cellulitis, chronic abscess	Nonhemolytic mucoid colonies on blood agar	Bite/scratch of a dog or cat	

(continued)

BACTERIA *(Continued)*

Name	Morphology	Pathogenesis	Description of Disease	Laboratory Findings, Notes	Transmission	Prevention and Therapy
Proteus vulgaris and *mirabilis*	Gram-negative; bacillus	Pili (adherence to renal pelvis); urease (alkalinization urine, increased precipitation, resulting in increased stone formation)	UTI	Urease positive; swarming motility colonies	GU flora	Ciprofloxacin, TMP–SMP
Pseudomonas aeruginosa	Gram-negative; coccobacilli	Pili; A/B toxin similar to diphtheria; flagella; hemolysin	UTI; septicemia; burn infections	Fruity smell; blue-green pigment	Water; environment; opportunistic: patients with catheters, leukemia, burns, cystic fibrosis, ventilatory assistance, neutropenia, chronic lung disease	May express broad resistance to antibiotics
Rickettsia prowazekii	Obligate intracellular	Invasion of the endothelial lining; possible endotoxin	Epidemic typhus		Louse	Tetracycline
Rickettsia rickettsii	Obligate intracellular	Invasion of endothelial lining	Rocky Mountain spotted fever: vasculitis, rash spreads from periphery inward	Weil-Felix reaction (agglutination when patient's serum mixed with OX strain of *Proteus vulgaris*)	*Dermacentor* ticks	Tetracycline
Rickettsia typhi	Obligate intracellular	Invasion of endothelial lining; possible endotoxin	Endemic typhus—rash spreads from the trunk outward		Spread by fleas	Tetracycline
Salmonella spp.	Gram-negative; rod; multiple flagella	Invades mucosa of GI tract; penetration of layers and systemic infection (typhoid fever); flagellar proteins; endotoxin	Typhoid fever, gastroenteritis, sepsis	Lactose-negative; polysaccharide, somatic O antigens and protein flagellar H antigens; (usually poultry) encapsulated; Widal test	Fecal–oral; contaminated food	Fluoroquinolone, ceftriaxone, azithromycin
Shigella spp.	Gram-negative; rod; nonmotile; not spore former	Invades mucosal M cells; presented to macrophage, which increase TNF and IL-1; produces microabscesses and ulcers; begins in small intestine and invades lower colon; Shiga toxin (A/B toxin): works on 28S ribosome and removes the base; low infective dose; invasion into blood is rare	Bacterial dysentery (shigellosis): ulcerative colitis of large intestine, fever, chills, cramps, tenesmus, bloody stool	Rectal swab; three types: *dysenteriae* (rare, most severe), *sonnei* (most common, day care), *flexneri* (gay men)	Fecal–oral route	Public health measures; significant resistance; fluoroquinolone, ceftriaxone, azithromycin

Staphylococcus aureus	Gram-positive; cocci; capsule; protein A in the cell wall; yellow, creamy, grapelike clusters on culture	Rapid growth; protein A (antiphagocytic); enterotoxin (watery diarrhea); toxic shock syndrome toxin; exfoliation; α-toxin; coagulase	Abscesses; pyogenic infections (endocarditis, osteomyelitis); food poisoning; toxic shock syndrome; scalded skin syndrome	Coagulase positive; catalase positive; β-hemolytic; novobiocin sensitive; ferment mannitol	Via the hands from the skin, nasal mucosa; enterotoxin: ham, chicken salad, cottage cheese, processed food	Hand washing; 80% penicillin resistant (make β-lactamase); vancomycin; first-generation cephalosporin; nafcillin, oxacillin
Staphylococcus epidermidis	Gram-positive; cocci; white, creamy, grapelike clusters on culture	Surface glycocalyx	Endocarditis; infection on catheters and implant sites; sepsis in neonates	Coagulase negative; catalase positive; no hemolysis; novobiocin sensitive	On skin; IV drug users	Vancomycin
Staphylococcus saprophyticus	Gram-positive; cocci; creamy, grapelike clusters	Selectively adheres to transitional epithelium	UTI in young women	Coagulase negative; catalase positive; no hemolysis; novobiocin resistant	Many sexual partners	Quinolones, oral cephalosporin
Streptococcus agalactiae	Gram-positive; cocci; diploid; group B *Streptococcus*	Capsular antigen (contains sialic acid blocks opsonization)	Number 1 cause of neonatal sepsis and meningitis	Catalase negative; bacitracin resistant; β-hemolysis; Lancefield group B; hippurate hydrolysis positive	Genital tract of some women	Ampicillin before delivery; penicillin G
Streptococcus pneumoniae	Gram-positive; cocci; lancet shaped; in pairs; polysaccharide capsule (85 different types)	Capsule prevents phagocytosis; IgA protease; adheres to mucosa	Pneumonia; meningitis; bacteremia; upper respiratory infection; otitis media	Catalase negative; α-hemolysis bile soluble; inhibited by optochin; quellung reaction (capsular swelling)	Inhalation of aerosols, which leads to colonization of oropharynx	Polysaccharide capsular vaccine available for high-risk groups; penicillin and erythromycin
Streptococcus pyogenes	Gram-positive; cocci; chains or pairs; rough or smooth hyaluronic acid capsule	M protein (pili); streptokinase (dissolves fibrin); DNase; hyaluronidase; hemolysins: erythrogenic toxin (scarlet fever rash); streptolysin-O and streptolysin-S; exotoxin A (superantigen causing TSS-like syndrome)	Pharyngitis; cellulitis; rheumatic fever; acute glomerulonephritis; TSS-like syndrome	Catalase negative; bacitracin (A disk) sensitive; (β-hemolytic; antistreptolysin-O for serotyping; Lancefield group A; rapid antigen detection test	May colonize skin, throat	Penicillin G (increasing resistance to erythromycin)
Treponema pallidum	Spirochete	Multiplication followed by blood vessel involvement	Syphilis—primary with painless sores, purulent exudate, and induration; secondary with a rash; tertiary (rare) includes CNS involvement and aortitis	Dark field microscopy; screen with RPR or VDRL test for cardiolipin (non-treponemal tests); confirm with FTA-abs or MHA-tp (treponemal specific test); systemic illness can occur with treatment (Jarisch–Herxheimer reaction)	Sexually transmitted; transplacental	Penicillin

(continued)

BACTERIA *(Continued)*

Name	Morphology	Pathogenesis	Description of Disease	Laboratory Findings, Notes	Transmission	Prevention and Therapy
Tropheryma whippelii	Gram-positive; rod actinomycete	Foamy macrophages found in the lamina propria of the jejunum	Whipple disease—steatorrhea, lymphadenopathy, fever, and cough	Visualization of the organism in a biopsy of the small bowel	Unknown	Trimethoprim-sulfamethoxazole
Vibrio cholerae	Gram-negative; comma-shaped rod; polar flagella ADP ribosylates G protein	Pili adhere to gut mucosa; phage-coded cholera toxin: two A active subunits and five B-binding units (A subunit increasing cAMP and causing movement of ions and water out of the cell)	Rice water stools	Fecal specimens culture; agglutination assays	Fecal–oral route via water and food	Vaccine not available in the United States; rehydration; tetracycline, fluoroquinolones, trimethoprim-sulfamethoxazole
Vibrio parahaemolyticus	Gram-negative; comma-shaped rod	Toxin	Explosive diarrhea, cramps, nausea	High-infective dose required	Shellfish; raw or undercooked seafood	Self-limited
Yersinia pestis	Gram-negative; bacillus; intracellular	V and W antigens (active within macrophages); fibrinolysin; F1 protein inhibits phagocytosis	Bubonic plague (with lymph node swelling and bubo); fever; conjunctivitis	Cultures are hazardous and precautions must be taken	Zoonotic via rat fleas	Vaccine; gentamicin, doxycycline

ADP, adenosine diphosphate; BCG, bacille Calmette–Guerin; cAMP, cyclic adenosine monophosphate; CNS, central nervous system; CSF, cerebrospinal fluid; DNase, deoxyribonuclease; ELISA, enzyme-linked immunosorbent assay; FTA-abs, fluorescent treponemal antibody absorption test; GI, gastrointestinal; GU, genitourinary; Hib, *Haemophilus influenzae* type b; Ig, immunoglobulin; IV, intravenous; LPS, lipopolysaccharide; MHA-tp, microhemagglutination assay test; MP, metalloproteinase; NaCl, sodium chloride; NAD, nicotinamide adenine dinucleotide; PID, pelvic inflammatory disease; PPD, purified protein derivative; RPR, rapid plasma reagin; TB, tuberculosis; TNF, tumor necrosis factor; TSS, toxic shock syndrome; UTI, urinary tract infection; VDRL, Venereal Disease Research Laboratory.

VIRUSES

Name	Morphology	Description of Disease	Pathogenesis	Laboratory Findings, Notes	Transmission	Prevention and Therapy
Adenovirus	Nonenveloped DNA virus; double stranded	Pharyngitis or pneumonia; acute gastroenteritis; conjunctivitis	Infects the epithelium of the eyes, respiratory tract, and GI tract	Complement fixation	Respiratory droplets; hand-to-eye; also fecal-oral	Live vaccine for military populations; no treatments
Coronavirus	Enveloped single-stranded positive RNA virus	Common cold	Infects upper respiratory tract	None	Respiratory secretions	None
Coxsackie B virus	Nonenveloped RNA virus; single stranded; linear; positive polarity	Myocarditis, pericarditis, spastic paralysis	Replicates in the pharynx and GI tract and spreads to other tissues	Isolating virus in cell culture; rise in convalescent antibody	Fecal–oral and respiratory	No therapy or prevention
Cytomegalovirus	Enveloped DNA virus; linear; double stranded	Pneumonia, retinitis, and hepatitis in immunocompromised patients; mononucleosis-like syndrome in immunocompromised patients; cytomegalic inclusion disease of fetus	Infects the oropharynx initially; involves lymphocytes	"Owl's eye" nuclear inclusions	Human body fluids; transplacental, organ transplantation	Ganciclovir
Ebola virus	Enveloped RNA virus; single stranded; linear; negative polarity	African hemorrhagic fever—often rapidly fatal	Viral replication in all organs leads to necrosis	Virus isolation; rise in antibody titer	Contact with blood and body secretions	None
Epstein–Barr virus	Enveloped DNA virus; linear; double stranded	Infectious mononucleosis; causes Burkitt lymphoma	Spreads via the lymph nodes and bloodstream to the liver and spleen from the pharyngeal epithelium	Atypical lymphocytes; positive heterophil antibody (Monospot test); common infection of college students	Saliva	None
Hantavirus	Enveloped RNA virus; single stranded; circular, segmented; negative polarity	Hanta pulmonary syndrome—influenza-like followed by acute respiratory failure	Invasion of the respiratory epithelium	PCR assay of viral RNA from lung tissue	Airborne (inhalation of rodent urine and feces); found in southwestern United States	None
Hepatitis A virus	Nonenveloped RNA virus; single stranded; positive polarity	Hepatitis A; causes acute hepatitis; no chronic infection	Replicates in the GI tract; spreads to the liver; hepatocellular injury via cytotoxic T cell response	Detect IgM antibody	Fecal–oral route	Killed viral vaccine; immune globulin during the incubation period may hinder disease

(continued)

VIRUSES *(Continued)*

Name	Morphology	Description of Disease	Pathogenesis	Laboratory Findings, Notes	Transmission	Prevention and Therapy
Hepatitis B virus (HBV)	Enveloped DNA virus; incomplete circular double stranded; polymerase in virion (virion called the Dane particle); surface antigen (HBsAg); core antigen (HBcAg)	Hepatitis B; arthritis; rash; glomerulonephritis; may result in hepatocellular carcinoma	Immune response (CD8 cells) to the virus results in hepatocellular injury; Ag-Ab complexes form	Serologic tests for HBsAg, HBsAb, HBcAb, and HBeAb	Blood, perinatal, sexual	Vaccine; interferon-α; tenofovir, lamivudine inhibit HBV DNA synthesis
Hepatitis C virus (HCV)	Enveloped RNA virus; single stranded; positive polarity	Hepatitis C; possible predisposition to hepatocellular carcinoma	Cytotoxic T cells result in hepatocellular injury	HCV RNA or anti-HCV Ab; currently the most common cause of transfusion-related hepatitis	Blood, perinatal, sexual	Interferon-α; ribavirin
Hepatitis D virus (delta virus)	Enveloped defective RNA virus; single stranded; negative polarity; no polymerase	Hepatitis D	Cytotoxic T cells result in hepatocellular injury; uses hepatitis B surface antigen as a protein coat and can only replicate in hosts already infected with hepatitis B virus	Serologic testing for delta antigen	Blood, perinatal, sexual	Interferon-α; prevention of hepatitis B
Hepatitis E virus (HEV)	Enveloped; single-stranded RNA virus; positive polarity	Hepatitis E; acute hepatitis no chronic disease		Anti-HEV IgM antibody by ELISA	Fecal–oral route	
Herpes simplex virus type 1	Enveloped DNA virus; linear; double stranded	Herpes labialis (fever blisters and cold sores); keratitis; encephalitis	Lesions on the mouth and face initially; travels retrograde and becomes latent in the trigeminal ganglion; recurrences induced by sunlight, stress, and fever	Multinucleated giant cells on Tzanck smear; immunofluorescence of infected cells; in situ hybridization defects; viral DNA	Saliva; direct contact with the lesion	Acyclovir, trifluorothymidine for keratitis
Herpes simplex virus type 2	Enveloped DNA virus; linear; double stranded	Herpes genitalis; meningitis	Vesicular lesions on the genitalia; retrograde passage through the axon and latency in the sacral ganglion; stress-induced recurrences	Multinucleated giant cells on Tzanck smear; immunofluorescence of infected cells; in situ hybridization defects; viral DNA	Sexual, transplacental	Acyclovir
Human herpes virus 6	Enveloped DNA virus; linear; double stranded	Roseola infantum (exanthem subitum)—common disease of children characterized by high fever and rash	Infects T and B cells	PCR or acute and convalescent antibody titers	Saliva	Symptomatic

HIV	Enveloped RNA virus; diploid; single stranded; positive polarity; reverse transcriptase, retrovirus	AIDS	Infects and kills helper T cells via the CD4 receptors and gp120 protein	Screen with ELISA; Western blot test confirms	Sexual, body fluids, perinatal; blood products	AZT to HIV-infected mothers and newborns; HAART; treat opportunistic infections like pneumonia or Kaposi sarcoma
Influenza virus	Enveloped RNA virus; segmented; single stranded; negative polarity; polymerase in virion	Influenza	Infects the epithelium of the respiratory tract via hemagglutinin and neuraminidase on surface spikes; antigenic shift and drift of surface spikes lead to epidemics	Cell culture; hemagglutination inhibition; complement fixation; H and N protein spikes	Respiratory droplets; vaccine composed of inactivated strains of current virus which causes disease	Zanamivir and oseltamivir for both prevention and treatment; vaccine composed of inactivated strains of current virus which causes disease
Measles virus	Enveloped RNA virus; single stranded; negative polarity; polymerase in virion	Measles, subacute sclerosing panencephalitis (SSPE)	Infection spreads via the bloodstream from the upper respiratory tract to the organs; maculopapular rash caused by an immune response (Koplik spots)	Usually not done	Respiratory droplets	Attenuated vaccine; no treatment
Mumps virus	Enveloped RNA virus; single stranded; negative polarity; polymerase in virion	Mumps; sterility owing to bilateral orchitis	Spreads from the upper respiratory tract to the organs (parotid glands, testes, ovaries, and CNS) via the bloodstream	Cell culture and hemadsorption; rise in antiviral antibody	Respiratory droplets	Attenuated vaccine; no treatment
Norwalk virus	Nonenveloped; RNA virus; single stranded; linear; positive polarity	Gastroenteritis	Binds to cells of intestinal brush border; prevents absorption of water and nutrients; blunted villi in jejunum; infiltration with mononuclear cells	Not performed; serology; ELISA for Ag; stool EM	Fecal–oral	Symptomatic treatment
Papillomavirus	Nonenveloped DNA virus; circular; double stranded	Papillomas (warts); condylomata acuminata; cervical and penile carcinoma	dsDNA incorporates into host DNA; E1 and E2 promote DNA replication; E6 and E7 early viral genes inhibit activity of p53 and Rb tumor suppressor genes, respectively	Koilocytes (squamous cell with perinuclear clearing) in lesions; to define type use in situ DNA hybridization	Sexual via direct contact with genital lesions	Interferon-α; liquid nitrogen for warts; vaccine; annual Pap smear for cervical cancer screening

(continued)

VIRUSES *(Continued)*

Name	Morphology	Description of Disease	Pathogenesis	Laboratory Findings, Notes	Transmission	Prevention and Therapy
Parainfluenza	Enveloped; single stranded–RNA virus	Upper respiratory tract infection, croup (laryngotracheobronchitis), bronchiolitis, pneumonia	Two major surface glycoproteins fusion and HN; replication limited to respiratory epithelial cells		Direct person-to-person contact and large droplet aerosols	Supportive
Parvovirus B19	Nonenveloped; DNA virus; single stranded; linear	Erythema infectiosum (fifth disease)—characterized by "slapped cheek" appearance; may cause aplastic crisis in sickle cell disease	Erythema infectiosum—virus causes immune complex deposition; aplastic anemia: virus infects immature RBCs and kills them	Parvovirus-specific IgG/IgM antibody levels; laboratory analysis for viral DNA	Unknown—may be respiratory or direct contact	Self-limited
Poliovirus	Nonenveloped RNA virus; single stranded; positive polarity	Abortive poliomyelitis, aseptic meningitis (more common), paralytic poliomyelitis, progressive post-poliomyelitis muscle atrophy (very rare)	Replicates in the pharynx and GI tract and spreads to the CNS; death of the anterior horn cells in the spinal cord; neurotropic for motor cortex	Isolation from CSF	Fecal–oral	Salk vaccine: inactivated injection; Sabin vaccine: attenuated oral vaccine, given in childhood immunizations; no treatment; **MNEMONIC:** Saber tooth tiger is alive and eats (Sabin vaccine is live oral vaccine)
Rabies virus	Enveloped RNA virus; bullet shape; single stranded; negative polarity RNA; polymerase in virion	Rabies	ACh receptor of neuron binds virus; the virus follows the retrograde direction to invade the CNS and brain, resulting in encephalitis	Negri bodies (eosinophilic inclusion in nerve cell)	Animal (skunks, bats) bites; domestic dogs in developing countries	Before exposure: vaccine; after exposure: antirabies Ig plus inactivated vaccine from human cell culture; no treatment
Reovirus (*Rotavirus*)	Nonenveloped RNA virus; 11 segments; double stranded; RNA polymerase in virion	Gastroenteritis in children	Resistant to stomach acid, thus infects the small intestine	ELISA detects the virus in stool	Respiratory droplets; fecal–oral route	Rehydration with fluids and electrolytes
Respiratory syncytial virus	Enveloped RNA virus; single stranded; negative polarity; polymerase in virion	Pneumonia or bronchiolitis in children	Immune response to lower respiratory tract infection	Multinucleated giant cells	Direct person-to-person contact	Supportive; ribavirin no longer recommended for children

Rhinovirus	Nonenveloped RNA virus; single stranded; positive polarity; numerous serotypes	Common cold	Upper respiratory tract mucosa and conjunctiva infected; replicates at temperatures $<37°$ C; killed by stomach acid	None	Aerosol droplets with hand-to-nose transmission	None
Rubella virus	Enveloped RNA virus; single stranded; positive polarity	Rubella; congenital: cardiovascular and neurologic malformations, especially if infection occurs during the first trimester	Spreads from the nasopharynx to the skin via the bloodstream; rash caused by replication and immune injury; German measles	Growth in cell culture via interference of Coxsackie virus; recent infection in the mother is detected by IgM, IgA	Respiratory droplets	Attenuated vaccine; no treatment
Varicella-zoster virus	Enveloped DNA virus; linear; double stranded	Chickenpox (varicella) in children; shingles (zoster) in adults	Infects respiratory tract and spreads to the liver and skin via the blood; an acute episode followed by latency in the sensory ganglia; numerous crop of vesicles in different stages at different times	Intranuclear inclusions; shingles is usually unilateral and generally follows the distribution of the dermatomes	Chickenpox: respiratory droplets; shingles: reactivation of the latent virus	Attenuated vaccine; famciclovir valacyclovir
Variola virus	Double stranded; DNA	Smallpox (rare)	Respiratory infection; initially replicates in URT; systemic dissemination by lymphatics; replication in multiple organs; extensive rash to hemorrhage of small blood vessels; single crop of vesicles in one stage all at once			Vaccinia variola

ACh, acetylcholine; Ag-Ab, antigen-antibody; AZT, azidothymidine; CD, cluster of differentation; CNS, central nervous system; CSF, cerebrospinal fluid; dsDNA, double-stranded DNA; ELISA, enzyme-linked immunosorbent assay; EM, electron microscopy; GI, gastrointestinal; HAART, highly active antiretroviral therapy; HBcAb, hepatitis B core antibody; HBeAb, hepatitis B e antibody; HBsAb, hepatitis B surface antibody; HBsAg, hepatitis B surface antigen; HN, hemagglutinin-neuraminidase; Ig, immunoglobulin; PCR, polymerase chain reaction; Rb, retinoblastoma; RBC, red blood cell; URT, upper respiratory tract

FUNGI

Name	Morphology	Pathogenesis	Description of Disease	Laboratory Findings, Notes	Transmission	Prevention and Therapy
Aspergillus fumigatus	Filamentous; septate hyphae and dichotomous branching; mold only	Opportunistic; growth of *Aspergillus* in a preexisting cavitary lesion in the lung	Aspergilloma—hemoptysis; invasive aspergillosis in neutropenic individuals	Septate, branching hyphae; "fungus ball" seen on a radiograph	Airborne spores	Amphotericin B, voriconazole; surgery to remove a "fungus ball"
Blastomyces dermatitidis	Dimorphic fungus—mold in the soil but a yeast in tissue	Invades the respiratory tract and may invade the skin or bone	Blastomycosis—granulomatous and suppurative infection of the respiratory tract	Tissue biopsy showing circular yeast with a broad-based bud	Airborne; endemic to North America	Itraconazole; amphotericin B for serious infections
Candida albicans	Pseudohyphae and hyphae on invasion; yeast in normal flora; germ tubes at 37° C; yeast only	Opportunistic in immunosuppressed patients and those with foreign bodies (e.g., catheters); mucocutaneous lesions in children with a T-cell defect	Thrush, chronic mucocutaneous candidiasis, vaginal candidiasis	Colonies on Sabouraud agar; germ tube formation	Part of the normal flora	Oral form can be prevented by nystatin "swish and swallow"; treatment with nystatin; miconazole; amphotericin B; IV amphotericin B, fluconazole, or caspofungin for bloodborne infection
Coccidioides immitis	Dimorphic—mold in the soil, spherule in tissue; barrel-shaped hyphae	Inhalation; spherules, releasing endospores within the respiratory tract	Coccidioidomycosis—an influenza-like illness with fever and cough	Tissue specimen showing spherules	Airborne; endemic to southwestern United States and Latin America	Amphotericin B, itraconazole, ketoconazole
Cryptococcus neoformans	Encapsulated; not dimorphic; yeast only	Usually immunocompromised patients; spreads via the bloodstream	Cryptococcosis, cryptococcal meningitis	Organism with a capsule seen on an India ink preparation; latex agglutination test	Inhalation of airborne yeast cells	Oral fluconazole as preventative in patients with AIDS; amphotericin B with flucytosine as initial therapy for cryptococcal meningitis

Histoplasma capsulatum	Dimorphic—a mold in the soil, a yeast in tissue; septate hyphae	Inhaled spores are engulfed by macrophages and develop into yeast forms intracellularly	Histoplasmosis—granulomas in the lung tissue	Tissue biopsy showing yeast cells visible in macrophages; radioimmunoassay for *Histoplasma* RNA and DNA	Airborne; endemic to Ohio and Mississippi River valleys; found in bird droppings	Amphotericin B, itraconazole
Mucor spp.	Nonseptate hyphae that branch at near right angles; mold only	Invades the nasal sinuses, lungs, and GI tract	Tissue necrosis	Nonseptate hyphae seen microscopically	Airborne	Amphotericin B; debridement of necrotic tissue
Pneumocystis jirovecii	Respiratory pathogen	Alveolar inflammation	Pneumonia	Silver stain	Inhalation by immunocompromised individual	Trimethoprim-sulfamethoxazole; pentamidine
Sporothrix schenckii	Thermally dimorphic fungus	Inflammation and swelling of the lymph nodes and vessels	Sporotrichosis ("rose gardener's disease")	Cigar-shaped budding cells	Thorn prick	Protection during gardening; potassium iodide; itraconazole

GI, gastrointestinal; IV, intravenous.

APPENDIX II: **Bug Index**

PARASITES AND PROTOZOA

Name	Morphology	Pathogenesis	Description of Disease	Laboratory Findings, Notes	Transmission	Prevention and Therapy
Ascaris lumbricoides	Intestinal parasite	Larvae in the lung and a heavy worm burden in gastrointestinal tract	Ascariasis—intestinal obstruction, abdominal pain, coughing, nausea	Eosinophilia; eggs in feces	Contaminated food or soil	Maintain sanitary conditions; ivermectin or mebendazole
Entamoeba histolytica	Intestinal protozoan, cigar-shaped cysts, four nuclei	Trophozoite form invades the colon	Amebic dysentery, liver abscess, flask-shaped ulcers	Trophozoites or cysts seen in stool	Fecal–oral	Maintain sanitary conditions; metronidazole with iodoquinol or paromomycin; steroids exacerbate
Enterobius vermicularis	Intestinal parasite	Worms migrate to anus at night to lay eggs; results in perianal pruritus	Pinworm infection—anal pruritus, vaginal irritation, and cystitis	Eggs on "Scotch tape" test (tape applied to the anus and then viewed under a microscope)	Reinfection by self; fecal–oral contact; egg ingestion	Mebendazole
Giardia lamblia	Intestinal protozoan; pear shaped; flagella; tumbling motility; two nuclei; four flagella	Interfere with fat and protein absorption	Giardiasis—acute diarrhea, flatulence, bloating	Trophozoites or cysts in stool	Fecal–oral	Do not drink untreated water from streams or rivers; metronidazole
Leishmania donovani	Protozoan	Organs of the reticuloendothelial system are destroyed by macrophages infected with the protozoan	Cutaneous leishmaniasis—ulcerating papules that heal slowly; visceral leishmaniasis ("kala-azar")—hyperpigmentation of the skin, massive splenomegaly, fever, anemia, and malaise	Biopsy of reticuloendothelial tissue shows the infected macrophages	Female Phlebotomus sandfly transmits the disease from the infected host to a human	Protection from sandfly bites; sodium stibogluconate (antimony compound) for cutaneous form; liposomal amphotericin B for visceral form
Plasmodium spp.	Blood and tissue protozoan; signet ring trophozoites in RBCs; banana-shaped gametocytes (*Plasmodium falciparum*)	Sporozoites from bite enter the bloodstream and invade hepatocytes (exoerythrocytic phase); merozoites invade the RBCs (erythrocytic phase)	Malaria—fever, chills, hepatomegaly, splenomegaly; symptoms in cyclical pattern (3 days for *P. malariae;* 2 days for *P. ovale, P. falciparum, P. vivax*); tissue anoxia	Blood smear shows organisms; *P. falciparum* is acute and needs immediate treatment	Female *Anopheles* mosquito	Insecticides or protection from bites; chloroquine, quinine, atovaquone-proguanil, mefloquine, artemether/lumefantrine

Schistosoma spp.	Blood fluke; eggs have spine (*S. mansoni* has large lateral spine, *S. haematobium* has a terminal spine, *S. japonicum* has a small lateral spine); two sexes	Eggs lead to inflammation, fibrosis, and granuloma formation	Schistosomiasis—pipestem fibrosis of liver; *S. haematobium* affects the bladder; *S. mansoni* affects the mesenteric vessels	Eggs in the stool or urine	Penetration of the skin by cercariae	Maintain sanitary conditions; praziquantel
Taenia sp.	Cestode: *T. solium—pork* tapeworm; *T. saginata—*beef; *Diphyllobothrium latum—fish;* four suckers and circle of hooks; 5–10 uterine branches	Encyst in tissue (eyes, brain, muscle) resulting in mass lesions	Taeniasis and cysticercosis	Gravid proglottids in stool	Eating raw or undercooked meat (taeniasis), or fecal–oral (cysticercosis)	Cook meat and maintain sanitary conditions; albendazole or praziquantel
Toxoplasma gondii	Tissue protozoan	Infects macrophages; infects the brain, liver, eyes	Toxoplasmosis	Serologic; high morbidity and mortality	Ingestion of cysts; cat feces; transplacental	Cook meat and avoid cat feces; sulfadiazine positive, pyrimethamine
Trichinella spiralis	Intestinal parasite	Muscle inflammation	Trichinosis—periorbital edema, myositis, fever, and diarrhea	Larvae on muscle biopsy; eosinophilia by 14th day; double-barreled egg	Eating raw or undercooked meat	Cook meat; thiabendazole
Trichomonas vaginalis	Urogenital protozoan; pear shaped; flagella; trophozoites	Attaches to the wall of the vagina	Trichomoniasis—itching and burning with greenish discharge from the vagina (strawberry cervix)	Visible in secretions	Sexual transmission	Treat both partners; metronidazole
Trypanosoma brucei (African)	Blood and tissue protozoan	Infects the brain and leads to encephalitis	Sleeping sickness—fever, enlarged lymph nodes, somnolence, coma, death	Visible in the blood	Tsetse fly (in Africa)	Protection from bites; insecticide; suramin
Trypanosoma cruzi (American)	Blood and tissue protozoan	Amastigotes attack cells, especially cardiac muscle cells	Chagas disease—dilated cardiomyopathy, megaesophagus, megacolon	Visible in the blood	Reduviid bugs (in Latin America) (also known as "kissing bugs")	Protect from bites; insecticide; nifurtimox

RBC, red blood cell.

Index

NOTE: Page numbers followed by *f* indicate figures; *t* indicates tables.

M

N